Pediatric Infectious Diseases

Pediatric Infectious Diseases

Editor: Caroline Francis

AMERICAN
MEDICAL PUBLISHERS
www.americanmedicalpublishers.com

AMERICAN
MEDICAL PUBLISHERS
www.americanmedicalpublishers.com

Cataloging-in-Publication Data

Pediatric infectious diseases / edited by Caroline Francis.
p. cm.
Includes bibliographical references and index.
ISBN 978-1-63927-426-0
1. Communicable diseases in children. 2. Infection in children. 3. Children--Diseases. I. Francis, Caroline.
RJ401 .P43 2022
618.929--dc23

American Medical Publishers,
41 Flatbush Avenue,
1st Floor, New York,
NY 11217, USA

ISBN 978-1-63927-426-0 (Hardback)

Contents

Preface

Pediatrics is a branch of medicine that is concerned with the assessment, diagnosis and treatment of diseases in children. An important specialization in this field is the prevention and control of pediatric infectious diseases. Under the scope of this field is a wide spectrum of complicated, severe or recurrent infections, infections acquired during travel, unexplained fevers, etc. Pediatric infectious diseases comprise of blood infections, tuberculosis, bone and joint infections, respiratory infections, gonococcal infections, eczema, cellulitis, toxic shock syndrome, walking syndrome, etc. Diarrhea is a common disease in children. It may be caused by viral or bacterial infections as well as due to lactose intolerance. The book aims to shed light on some of the unexplored aspects of pediatrics and the recent researches in this domain. The objective of this book is to give a general view of the different pediatric infectious diseases, and their management strategies. It is a vital tool for all researching or studying pediatrics and infectious diseases as it gives incredible insights into emerging trends and concepts.

Various studies have approached the subject by analyzing it with a single perspective, but the present book provides diverse methodologies and techniques to address this field. This book contains theories and applications needed for understanding the subject from different perspectives. The aim is to keep the readers informed about the progresses in the field; therefore, the contributions were carefully examined to compile novel researches by specialists from across the globe.

Indeed, the job of the editor is the most crucial and challenging in compiling all chapters into a single book. In the end, I would extend my sincere thanks to the chapter authors for their profound work. I am also thankful for the support provided by my family and colleagues during the compilation of this book.

Editor

1

Plasma Levels of Inter-α Inhibitor Proteins in Children with Acute Dengue Virus Infection

Penelope Koraka[1], Yow-Pin Lim[2], Michael D. Shin[2], Tatty E. Setiati[3], Albert T. A. Mairuhu[4,5], Eric C. M. van Gorp[1,4], Augustinus Soemantri[3], Albert D. M. E. Osterhaus[1], Byron E. E. Martina[1]*

1 Department of Virology, Erasmus Medical Center, Rotterdam, The Netherlands, **2** ProThera Biologics, Inc., East Providence, Rhode Island, United States of America, **3** Pediatric Department, Dr. Kariadi Hospital, Semarang, Indonesia, **4** Department of Internal Medicine, Slotervaart Hospital, Amsterdam, The Netherlands, **5** Division of Thrombosis and Haemostasis, Beth Israel Deaconess Medical Center, Boston, Massachusetts, United States of America

Abstract

Background: Inter-α inhibitor proteins (IaIp) belong to a family of protease inhibitors that are involved in the haemostatic and the vascular system. Dengue viruses (DENV) infections are characterized by coagulopathy and increased vascular permeability. In this study we measured the concentration of IaIp during DENV infections and evaluated its potential as a biomarker.

Methods and Findings: Concentrations of IaIp were measured in patients with acute DENV infections using a quantitative, competitive enzyme linked immunoassay. Concentrations of IaIp measured in pediatric patients suffering from severe DENV infections were significantly lower than in healthy controls.

Conclusions: This is the first report to demonstrate changes in concentration of IaIp during viral infections. The data also highlight the potential of IaIp as a biological marker for severity of DENV infections.

Editor: Antonio Bertoletti, Singapore Institute for Clinical Sciences, Singapore

Funding: The project was partly funded by the Royal Dutch Academy of Arts and Sciences (KNAW) grant number 99-MED-04, ProThera Biologics and Viroclinics BV. The funders played a role in study design, decision to publish and in data collection and analysis, but no role in preparation of the manuscript.

Competing Interests: None of the authors declare conflict of interest apart from Yow-Pin Lim who holds a significant interest in ProThera Biologics. Albert Osterhaus is a part time employee (CSO) of Viroclinics BV (for details go to www.erasmusmc.nl). The stated competing interests do not alter the authors' adherence to all the PLoS ONE policies on sharing data and materials.

* E-mail: b.martina@erasmusmc.nl

Introduction

Dengue viruses (DENV) are members of the family *Flaviviridae*, genus *Flavivirus*, and are among the most widely distributed arboviruses world wide that are estimated to infect more than 50 million people annually. DENV infection is usually asymptomatic or may lead to uncomplicated "flu-like" disease with fever, myalgia, arthralgia and rash. At the time of defervescence up to 5% of cases may develop dengue hemorrhagic fever and/or dengue shock syndrome (DHF/DSS). Mortality rates are usually around 1%. However, during large outbreaks of DENV infections if supportive intensive care of the patients is not applied promptly these figure can be much higher. Although the epidemiology is changing, DHF/DSS is still mainly a disease of children, being the leading cause of hospitalization and death among children in South East Asia.

Inter-α inhibitor proteins (IaIp) belong to a family of structurally related serine protease inhibitors that are naturally and abundantly found in human plasma. The major forms in human plasma are the inter-α inhibitor, consisting of two heavy chains and a light chain called bikunin, and the pre-α inhibitor, consisting of one heavy chain and a light-bikunin chain [1]. The physiological functions of these proteins have only recently begun to be revealed. Members of the IaIp family have been involved in physiological as well as pathological activities such as tumor invasion, metastasis and inflammation. For instance, bikunin has been shown to inhibit plasmin, thereby exerting anti-inflammatory and anti-fibrinolytic activities [2].

The potential of IaIp as a diagnostic and prognostic biomarker as well as its therapeutic potential has been demonstrated in bacterial sepsis [3,4]. However, the role of IaIp during viral infections has not been investigated. In this report we describe the plasma concentrations of IaIp in children with DENV infections and how these concentrations correlate with disease severity.

Materials and Methods

Ethics Statement

Written informed consent for blood sampling was obtained from all patients (their parents or legal guardians) included in the studies described in this manuscript. The studies have been approved by the ethics committee of the hospitals involved (Dr. Kariadi Hospital, Semarang, Indonesia and Sophia Children's Hospital, Rotterdam, The Netherlands).

Children infected with DENV were selected from a longitudinal cohort study (n = 200) conducted in Dr. Kariadi Hospital, Semarang Indonesia [5]. Plasma samples were collected on day of hospital admission (day 0), as well as 7 and 30 days later. Day 0 (D0) samples were used to confirm DENV infection by a real time RT-PCR assay. Samples from healthy individuals (n = 37) matching demography and age of the DENV patients were used to determine

Table 1. Characteristics of patients included in the study.

Characteristics	DF patients n=7	DHF patients n=15	DSS patients n=11	RSV patients n=12	Healthy controls n=37
Age range (median)	3–14 (12) years	4–13 (10) years	5–12 (6) years	2–6 (4) months	3–6 (4.3) years
Gender, (male n)	4	6	4	7	19
Origin	Indonesia	Indonesia	Indonesia	The Netherlands	Indonesia
Duration of fever range (median)	2–4 (3) days	3–6 (4) days	2–5 (4) days	1–5 (3) days	n.a.
Hematocryte % range (median)*	33–43 (37.8)	33–53 (39.3)	32–51 (41)	n.a.	n.a.
Platelet count cells x $10^3/mm^3$ * (median)	57–186 (106)	14–207 (66)	10–90 (43)	n.a.	n.a.
Albumin g/l range (median) *	2.0–4.2 (3.7)	1.9–4.3 (3.60	1.0–3.8 (3.2)	n.a.	n.a.
AT III % range (median) *	51–110 (85)	75–120 (97)	50–110 (51)	n.a.	n.a.
APTT sec range (median) *	39–76 (48)	38–84 (53)	49–120 (68)	n.a.	n.a.

*on time of admission.
n.a.: not applicable.

baseline values of IaIp. These healthy control samples were collected from healthy children that were enrolled in a prospective cohort study (unpublished data) and resided in the same areas as the DENV patients (Semarang, Indonesia), have the same genetic background (Javanese, Indonesian) and matching age and gender. No DENV-specific antibodies were detected in these samples. Samples from 12 children infected with respiratory syncytial virus (RSV), collected on day of admission to hospital (D0) and 30 days later were used for comparison. The characteristics of these patients have been described elsewhere [6].

Concentrations of IaIp in plasma samples were measured with a quantitative competitive enzyme linked immunoassay with a monoclonal antibody against human IaIp (MAb 69.26) as previously described [4]. All the samples were analyzed in a blinded fashion. The non-parametric Mann-Whitney test (GraphPad version 4) was used for statistical evaluation of the IaIp concentrations in the respective groups of patients. Analyses of correlations were done with the Spearman's rho test using SPSS version 11.0.1.

Results

Patient's characteristics

In order to exclude patients with clinical picture similar to DENV of other aetiology, the criteria for patient selection was confirmation of DENV infection by demonstrating viral RNA in the D0 samples and complete sampling procedure, i.e. availability of plasma samples from D0, D7 and D30. Based on these criteria, 33 patients were selected to measure the levels of IaIp out of the 200 patients included in the cohort study (Table 1). The cohort consisted of 14 males, 19 females and the median age of the patients was 8 years (range 3–14 years). Seven patients were classified with DF, 15 with DHF, and 11 with DSS according to the WHO criteria [7]. Based on the serological profile of the patients (IgM/IgG ratio) 5 patients could be classified as primary DENV infections whereas the remaining 28 patients had a secondary DENV infection. DENV 1 and 3 were the predominant serotypes (n = 14 and n = 13, respectively), while DENV-2 and DENV-4 were only detected in a few patients (n = 4 and n = 2 respectively), suggesting that all four serotypes of DENV were circulating in Semarang at the time of sampling.

Concentration of IaIp in acute viral infections

First, we measured IaIp levels in healthy young children to establish baseline level (median 393 μg/ml, range 236–658 μg/ml) in the study population (Figure 1). Next, we measured the levels of this molecule in plasma from patients with acute systemic (DENV) and non-systemic (RSV) viral infections upon hospital admission. Patients of both groups required hospitalization, indicating that these infections were severe. Both the DENV (median 165, range 56–281 μg/ml) and RSV (median 217, range 145–553 μg/ml) patient groups had significantly lower levels of IaIp on D0 compared to the healthy control group ($P<0.0001$ and $P<0.0001$ respectively).

Concentration of IaIp in DENV infections correlate with disease severity

Several mediators involved in hemostasis have been associated with DENV-associated disease severity. Therefore, we sought to investigate the association of IaIp concentration with development of DHF and/or DSS. Patients experiencing mild DF, had similar levels of IaIp as patients with acute RSV (D0 median 202, range 109–261μg/ml, $P = 0.5867$). It is worth noting that the patient in this group, with the lowest concentration of IaIp was classified with "severe DF" i.e. experienced hemorrhagic manifestations but did not meet all criteria of WHO to be classified as DHF grade I-IV. Patients experiencing hemorrhagic fever (DHF grades I-IV) had

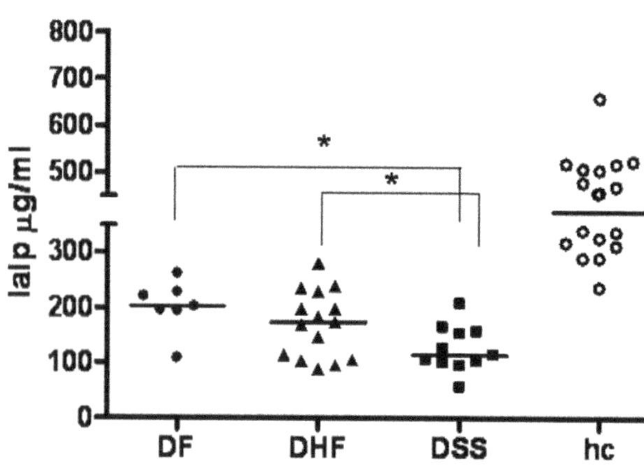

Figure 1. Concentration of IaIp in patients with varying DENV disease severity (day of admission to the hospital) and in healthy controls (hc). *: statistically significant differences with the Mann-Whitney test. Straight lines represent the median.

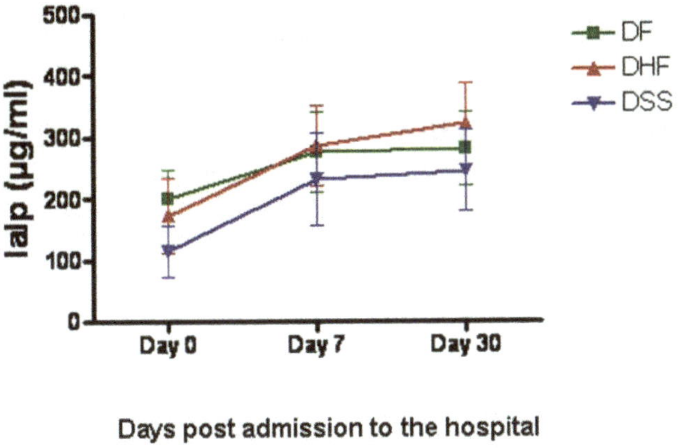

Figure 2. Concentration of IaIp in DENV infected patients with varying disease severity on different time points after infection. Data are depicted as mean ± standard deviation.

significantly lower levels of IaIp on D0, compared to patients with mild DF (median 151, range 56–281 µg/ml, P = 0.0443), whereas patients with DSS had the lowest levels of IaIp (median 112, range 56–208 µg/ml) compared to DF, DHF-I/II, and RSV groups (P = 0.0028, P = 0.0461, P = 0.0006 respectively). As shown in figure 2, clinical recovery of DHF patients (grades I–IV) was associated with a rapid and significant increase of IaIp within seven days post admission (median 261, range 152–434 µg/ml, P<0.0001). By D30 of follow up the levels of IaIp between patients recovering from DF (median 282, range 236–414 µg/ml), and DHF grades I–IV (median 283, range 179–414 µg/ml) were similar (P = 0.6066), but lower than the level of IaIp in patients recovering from RSV (median 333; range 205–462 µg/ml). However, the concentrations did not reach levels measured in the healthy controls (P<0.0001), suggesting different normalization kinetics of this molecule during DENV infections compared to RSV infection.

Clinical records and laboratory findings from the day of admission of the DENV infected patients were used to look for association of IaIp and clinical and laboratory markers of disease severity (Table 2). Circulating concentrations of IaIp correlated inversely with disease severity (P = 0.041), ascites (P = 0.010), and activated partial thromboplastin time (aPTT, P = 0.001). In addition there was a correlation of IaIp with thrombocytopenia (P = 0.002), anti-thrombin III (ATIII, P = 0.024) and albumin levels (P = 0.018).

Discussion

This study is the first one to demonstrate that IaIp is significantly decreased during acute viral infections. Our data showed that both a systemic (DENV) and a localized (RSV) viral infection can affect the concentration of IaIp, with a more pronounced effect measured in patients with DSS. Several studies have shown that mediators and other soluble factors (including antibodies and cytokines) differ significantly between DHF and DSS groups [8–10].

Plasma levels of IaIp have been shown to be reduced in neonatal and adult bacterial-induced sepsis and the levels correlate inversely with mortality in adult patients with sepsis, prompting investigation of its potential as a prognostic or diagnostic marker [3,4] as well as its therapeutic potential for sepsis and anthrax intoxication [11,12]. Fatal outcome of DSS can be significantly reduced when timely supportive treatment and plasma replacement is given to the patients. In this respect, a biomarker with diagnostic/prognostic potential is of paramount importance to assist supportive treatment. In this study we report significant correlations of IaIp and several markers of DENV disease severity, especially thrombocytopenia, a hallmark of severe DENV induced disease (Table 2). These data warrant further studies, designed to elucidate the prognostic potential of IaIp. In this study, we investigated the plasma levels of IaIp in patients that were severely ill and required hospitalization. Studies should be designed in the future to include infected patients prospectively in order to understand the kinetics and prognostic value of IaIp in the early stages of disease (during fever). In light of the therapeutic value of IaIp in sepsis, the potential of this molecule for treatment of DSS should be explored.

The pathogenesis of DENV infections is poorly understood although several studies have concluded that soluble factors and mediators are implicated in the development of DHF/DSS. The significantly decreased concentrations of IaIp in patients with severe disease, in particular in DSS patients, could explain several pathological phenomena seen in DSS. First, the heavy chains of IaIp molecules are known to inhibit activation of both the alternative and classical pathways of the complement system, both *in vitro* and *in vivo* [13]. In this respect, low levels of IaIp could result in the increased levels of C5a often seen in DHF/DSS patients [14]. Second, IaIp inhibit plasmin via its light chain bikunin [2]. Plasmin has a major role in the fibrinolytic system, as an enzyme that degrades fibrin. Impaired fibrinolysis is a hallmark of DSS [10]. In this report, IaIp levels were found to be associated with coagulation (aPTT) and anti-coagulation (ATIII) factors (Table 2), however more studies are needed in order to elucidate the possible role of IaIp in the pathogenesis of DENV infections. Third, IaIp are synthesized and assembled in the liver and low plasma levels of these molecules may reflect liver involvement.

Taken together, this is the first study to highlight the importance of IaIp in acute viral infections and provide an incentive to study the diagnostic and prognostic role of IaIp during acute DENV infections. Our cohort was carefully chosen to include only patients with confirmed DENV infection as demonstrated by the

Table 2. Correlation of IaIp with clinical and laboratory markers of DENV disease severity measured on day of admission.

Spearman's rho IaIp	severity	Pleural effusion	ascites	Platelet count	Hematocryte	ATIII (%)	aPTT (sec)	Albumin (g/l)
Correlation coefficient	−0.357	−0.248	−0.443	0.514	0.03913	0.492	−0.617	0.415
P value	<u>0.041</u>	0.163	<u>0.010</u>	<u>0.002</u>	0.8289	<u>0.024</u>	<u>0.001</u>	<u>0.018</u>
N	33	33	33	33	33	21	25	32

Significant P values are underlined.
ATIII: anti-thrombin III, aPTT: activated partial thromboplastin time.

presence of viral RNA in acute phase plasma of the patients. Since little is known about the epidemiology of other viral infections in that region with similar clinical presentation to dengue, we chose to study only the subjects from which DENV viral RNA could be recovered. As a result, our cohort was rather small and therefore other relevant questions such as correlation of IaIp levels and primary or secondary DENV infections could not be addressed. Determination of IaIp concentrations in larger cohorts of patients with different genetic backgrounds, in combination with measurement of other biological markers, such as liver enzymes, are necessary to better understand the role of IaIp in the pathogenesis of DENV infections. Studies are ongoing to address these issues.

Author Contributions

Conceived and designed the experiments: PK YPL BM. Performed the experiments: PK MDS TES ATAM. Analyzed the data: PK YPL MDS TES ATAM ECMvG AS ADMEO BM. Contributed reagents/materials/analysis tools: YPL. Wrote the paper: PK ADMEO BM.

References

1. Josic D, Brown MK, Huang F, Lim YP, Rucevic M, et al. (2006) Proteomic characterization of inter-alpha inhibitor proteins from human plasma. Proteomics 6: 2874–2885.
2. Wisniewski HG, Hua JC, Poppers DM, Naime D, Vilcek J, et al. (1996) TNF/IL-1-inducible protein TSG-6 potentiates plasmin inhibition by inter-alpha-inhibitor and exerts a strong anti-inflammatory effect in vivo. J Immunol 156: 1609–1615.
3. Chaaban H, Singh K, Huang J, Siryaporn E, Lim YP, et al. (2009) The role of inter-alpha inhibitor proteins in the diagnosis of neonatal sepsis. J Pediatr 154: 620–622 e621.
4. Lim YP, Bendelja K, Opal SM, Siryaporn E, Hixson DC, et al. (2003) Correlation between mortality and the levels of inter-alpha inhibitors in the plasma of patients with severe sepsis. J Infect Dis 188: 919–926.
5. Setiati TE, Mairuhu AT, Koraka P, Supriatna M, Mac Gillavry MR, et al. (2007) Dengue disease severity in Indonesian children: an evaluation of the World Health Organization classification system. BMC Infect Dis 7: 22.
6. Brandenburg AH, Kleinjan A, van Het Land B, Moll HA, Timmerman HH, et al. (2000) Type 1-like immune response is found in children with respiratory syncytial virus infection regardless of clinical severity. J Med Virol 62: 267–277.
7. Anonymus (1997) Dengue haemorrhagic fever: diagnosis, treatment, prevention and control. World Health Organization second edition.
8. Koraka P, Murgue B, Deparis X, Van Gorp EC, Setiati TE, et al. (2004) Elevation of soluble VCAM-1 plasma levels in children with acute dengue virus infection of varying severity. J Med Virol 72: 445–450.
9. Koraka P, Suharti C, Setiati TE, Mairuhu AT, Van Gorp E, et al. (2001) Kinetics of dengue virus-specific serum immunoglobulin classes and subclasses correlate with clinical outcome of infection. J Clin Microbiol 39: 4332–4338.
10. Van Gorp EC, Setiati TE, Mairuhu AT, Suharti C, Cate Ht H, et al. (2002) Impaired fibrinolysis in the pathogenesis of dengue hemorrhagic fever. J Med Virol 67: 549–554.
11. Opal SM, Artenstein AW, Cristofaro PA, Jhung JW, Palardy JE, et al. (2005) Inter-alpha-inhibitor proteins are endogenous furin inhibitors and provide protection against experimental anthrax intoxication. Infect Immun 73: 5101–5105.
12. Wu R, Cui X, Lim YP, Bendelja K, Zhou M, et al. (2004) Delayed administration of human inter-alpha inhibitor proteins reduces mortality in sepsis. Crit Care Med 32: 1747–1752.
13. Garantziotis S, Hollingsworth JW, Ghanayem RB, Timberlake S, Zhuo L, et al. (2007) Inter-alpha-trypsin inhibitor attenuates complement activation and complement-induced lung injury. J Immunol 179: 4187–4192.
14. Navarro-Sanchez E, Despres P, Cedillo-Barron L (2005) Innate immune responses to dengue virus. Arch Med Res 36: 425–435.

2

Benznidazole Therapy Modulates Interferon-γ and M2 Muscarinic Receptor Autoantibody Responses in *Trypanosoma cruzi*-Infected Children

Romina A. Cutrullis[1], Guillermo F. Moscatelli[1], Samanta Moroni[1], Bibiana J. Volta[2], Rita L. Cardoni[2], Jaime M. Altcheh[1], Ricardo S. Corral[1], Héctor L. Freilij[1], Patricia B. Petray[1]*

1 Servicio de Parasitología y Enfermedad de Chagas, Hospital de Niños Ricardo Gutiérrez, Buenos Aires, Argentina, **2** Instituto Nacional de Parasitología Dr. M. Fatala Chabén, Administración Nacional de Laboratorios e Institutos de Salud Dr. C.G. Malbrán, Buenos Aires, Argentina

Abstract

Objective: The presence of autoantibodies with adrenergic and cholinergic activity, capable of triggering neurotransmitter receptor-mediated effects, has been associated with pathogenesis in *T. cruzi*-infected hosts. The goal of this study was to investigate the production of anti-M2 muscarinic receptor autoantibodies (Anti-M2R AAbs) as well as the IFN-γ profile in children at the early stage of Chagas disease, and to examine whether trypanocidal chemotherapy with benznidazole (BZ) could modify both response patterns.

Methods: This study comprised 30 *T. cruzi*-infected children (mean age: 13.8 years) and 19 uninfected controls (mean age: 12.7 years). Infected patients were treated with BZ and followed-up. Blood samples collected at diagnosis-T0, end of treatment-T1, and six months later-T2 were analysed by ELISA for detection of Anti-M2R AAbs and circulating levels of IFN-γ.

Results: At T0, anti-M2R AAbs were demonstrated in 56.7% of *T. cruzi*-infected patients, whereas uninfected controls were 100% negative. The average age of Anti-M2R AAbs$^+$ patients was higher than that from negative population. Infected children also displayed significantly stronger serum IFN-γ responses than controls. Upon BZ treatment, a significant linear decreasing trend in Anti-M2R AAb reactivity was recorded throughout the follow-up, with 29.7–88.1% decrease at T2. IFN-γ circulating levels also declined by T2.

Conclusion: Anti-M2R AAbs and IFN-γ raise early during chagasic infection in children and are downmodulated by BZ therapy. These findings reinforce the usefulness of early BZ treatment not only to eliminate the parasite but also to reduce potentially pathogenic immune responses.

Editor: Guillermo H. Giambartolomei, National Council of Sciences (CONICET), Argentina

Funding: The study was funded by Bunge & Born Foundation (Argentina) and National Research Council (CONICET, Argentina). The funders had no role in study design, data collection and analysis, decision to publish, or preparation of the manuscript.

Competing Interests: The authors have declared that no competing interests exist.

* E-mail: ppetray@conicet.gov.ar

Introduction

Chagas disease, caused by the protozoan parasite *Trypanosoma cruzi*, is one of the worlds leading causes of heart disease [1]. The disease has two successive phases: an initial acute phase lasting between 30 and 60 days and a chronic phase. A majority of the patients that progress to the chronic phase remains clinically asymptomatic for many years, but around 30% of infected individuals progress to disease associated with cardiac and/or digestive disorders [2]. Cardiac manifestations include abnormalities of the intraventricular conduction system, ventricular arrhythmias, sinus node dysfunction, heart failure, aneurysm, and enlargement and dysfunction of the heart [3]. Arrhythmias can be related with cardiomyopathy by itself or with autonomic nervous system alterations [4]. Heart failure and sudden death are the most common causes of decease in patients with Chagas disease [3,5]. Although clinical signs and symptoms appear several years after infection, pathogenic mechanisms can begin since early stages. Several hypotheses have been proposed to account for pathogenesis in chronic *T. cruzi* infections, including parasite persistence in the myocardium [6], autoimmunity events [7] and tissue injury due to exacerbated inflammatory reactions [8]. Among alterations induced by host self response, there are data supporting autoantibody production, able to interact with β1 adrenergic and muscarinic cholinergic M2 receptors in cardiac tissue [9], leading to early autonomic dysfunction [10,11]. It has been suggested that the presence of these antibodies could be due to molecular mimicry between human β1 adrenergic/M2 muscarinic receptors and C terminal regions of ribosomal proteins of *T. cruzi* [12]. Recently, this group also demonstrated direct binding of antibodies developed by chronic chagasic patients to the native human β1 adrenergic receptor [13].

Regarding the inflammatory response, several studies have demonstrated that cytokines participate in the control of infection as well as in the induction of pathogenesis during *T. cruzi* infection [14]. Lymphocytes as well as mononuclear cells infiltrating the heart tissue of patients with chagasic cardiomyopathy produce significantly more inflammatory cytokines, such as interferon (IFN)-γ, than blood cells from infected asymptomatic individuals [15]. Moreover, the secretion of IFN-γ has been correlated with the severe cardiac form of Chagas disease [16]. *In vitro* experiments have shown that IFN-γ may induce profound changes in the cardiomyocyte gene expression program, with potential consequences for myocardial contractility, electric conduction and rhythm [17].

T. cruzi-infected pediatric patients represent the target population for parasiticidal therapy. Benznidazole (BZ) is the main drug available for the treatment of *T. cruzi* infections. In addition to the direct *in vivo* blocking of parasite growth, BZ-treatment appears to affect host immune regulation [18]. However, little research has been carried out to address the prompt consequences of etiological BZ-treatment on the immune response of children at the early stage of chronic Chagas disease. In this context, we aimed to evaluate the M2 muscarinic receptor autoantibodies (Anti-M2R AAb) response as well as the levels of the proinflammatory cytokine IFN-γ in pediatric patients at the early stage of chronic *T. cruzi* infection. In addition, during the follow-up of BZ-treated patients, we examined whether trypanocidal chemotherapy could modify the patterns of both antibody and cytokine responses.

Materials and Methods

Ethics statement

The study protocol was approved by the Research and Teaching Committee and Bioethics Committee of Ricardo Gutiérrez Children's Hospital. Written consent was required from patients' legal representatives, as well as assent from the patient, as appropriate.

Study population

The prospective follow-up study comprised *T. cruzi*-infected patients admitted to the Parasitology and Chagas Service at Ricardo Gutiérrez Children's Hospital, Buenos Aires, Argentina, for their diagnosis and treatment. Patients with any of the following conditions were excluded: (a) concurrent infections other than *T. cruzi* infection; (b) autoimmune disease; (c) acute or chronic inflammatory process; (d) having received previous etiologic treatment. Age- and sex-matched children seronegative for *T. cruzi* were considered as controls. Our study population (infected patients and uninfected controls) comprised children living in Buenos Aires City and surrounding areas, with similar socioeconomic status. This region is free of vector and is not endemic for Chagas disease, therefore the re-infection is not possible.

Diagnosis criteria

Serologic diagnosis of *T. cruzi* infection was carried out by indirect hemagglutination (IHA, Lab. Polychaco, Buenos Aires, Argentina), enzyme-linked immunosorbent assay (ELISA, Wiener, Rosario, Argentina) and passive particle agglutination test (PPA, Bayer, Buenos Aires, Argentina).

IHA and PPA antibody titers ≥16, as well as ELISA positive values higher than 1.2, were considered reactive. Infants with at least two positive tests were diagnosed as infected by *T. cruzi.*

Therapeutic regimen and treatment follow-up

The standard of medical care for *T. cruzi*-infected children is the etiological treatment. Consequently, all infected infants were treated with BZ (RADANIL®, Roche, Buenos Aires, Argentina) at 5–8 mg/kg/day in 2 daily oral doses, for 60 days. Since diagnosis (T0), patients were followed-up by clinical (electrocardiogram-ECG- and echocardiogram-ECHO) and laboratory (IHA and ELISA for *T. cruzi* serology; hemogram, hepatogram, creatinin) evaluations at 30 days, 60 days (end of treatment, T1) and 6 months after completion of chemotherapy (T2). Additionally, parasitological response to treatment was monitored by qualitative polymerase chain reaction (PCR) to detect the presence of *T. cruzi* DNA in blood samples [19]. Ethical considerations precluded the inclusion of an untreated control group in the study taking into account that immediate administration of benznidazole is crucial to achieve therapeutic success.

Determination of anti-autonomic neurotransmitter antibodies

Serum samples obtained at different times (T0, T1 and T2) of follow-up were stored at −20°C until measuring anti-M2R IgG autoantibody levels by a commercial ELISA kit according to manufacturers instructions (Chagacor, Lab. Lemos S.R.L, Buenos Aires, Argentina).

IFN-γ measurements

Individual IFN-γ serum levels were quantified by double sandwich ELISA (OptEIA Kit for IFN-γ, BD PharMingen, San Jose, CA, USA) according to manufacturer's instructions. Supplied standards were used to generate a standard curve. The assay sensitivity was 2 ng/ml.

Statistical analysis

Data are expressed as mean value ± standard error of the mean (SEM) or median value (interquartile range). IHA titers were $\log_2$-transformed before applying the statistical test. ELISA values were expressed as the ratio (R) between optical densities (OD) determined for each specimen and cut-off value. To compare two groups, Student *t* test or Mann-Whitney test were used. One-way analysis of variance (ANOVA) followed by the Tukey test or Friedman test was applied to evaluate changes before and after treatment. Fisher's exact test was used to compare between-group proportions. *P* values of <0.05 were considered significant. Statistical analyses were carried out using the Prisma 4.0 software (GraphPad, San Diego, CA, USA).

Results

Patients' characteristics

A total of 30 *T. cruzi*-infected patients were enrolled in this study. The mean age was 13.8 years (range, 8–17 years) and female/male ratio was 1 (15 female *vs* 15 male). On the admission, all of them presented positive serology for Chagas disease at least by 2 conventional assays. Anti-*T. cruzi* antibody titers measured by ELISA and IHA tests were 8.8±0.5 and 6.5±0.2, respectively. All children were asymptomatic and without cardiac compromise (normal ECG and ECHO). Route of infection was transplacental in 27% of patients, vectorial in 4.5% and undefined in 68.5%. Maternal origin of congenitally infected children was Argentina in 46% of cases, Bolivia in 46% and Paraguay in 8%. The control group included 19 uninfected children whose mean age was 12.7 years (range, 7–17 years) and female/male ratio was 1.4 (11 female *vs* 8 male). There were no significant differences in the age and sex distribution between *T. cruzi*-infected children and uninfected controls.

Pre-treatment Anti-M2R AAb and IFN-γ responses

Children were examined for the presence of serum Anti-M2R AAb and the results are shown in Figure 1A. AntiM2R AAb reactivity was verified in 56.7% of *T. cruzi*-infected patients, whereas uninfected controls were 100% negative ($p = 0.0001$). The R value (mean ± SEM) in *T. cruzi*-infected patients was 2.2±0.4. The average age of Anti-M2R AAb$^+$ patients was significantly higher than that from negative population: 14.6±0.6 years and 12±0.8 years, respectively ($p = 0.0038$). *T. cruzi*-infected children also displayed higher serum IFN-γ levels compared to uninfected controls ($p = 0.015$) (Figure 1B).

Modulation of Anti-M2R AAb and IFN-γ responses after BZ therapy

In the course of BZ treatment, ten children withdrew from the study due to adverse events (n = 2), moving to another city (n = 4) or not returning (n = 4). Among Anti-M2R AAb$^+$ children at T0, we verified a significant ($p = 0.001$) linear decreasing trend in their autoantibody titers throughout the follow-up (Figure 2A). At T2, ELISA values were significantly lower ($p<0.01$) than those detected at T0, representing a decline ranging between 29.7 and 88.1% of the initial level. No correlation between autoantibody response and heart dysfunction could be established in pediatric chagasic patients, as all children presented normal ECG and ECHO examinations.

Serum concentration of IFN-γ was also determined as shown in Table 1 and Figure 2B. The median value of IFNγ at T2 was significantly lower that that observed at T0 (2.5 pg/ml *vs* 7.5 pg/ml, $p<0.05$). Results for these T0 *vs* T2 pairs of sera revealed a drop in IFN-γ levels that ranged between 10 and 100% of the initial value. No significant differences were observed in the comparison of IFN-γ levels at T0 *vs* T1. We were not able to verify any significant correlation between Anti-M2R AAb and IFN-γ levels. The decrease in Anti-M2R AAb and IFN-γ responses in the lapse between T0 and T2 was accompanied by the negativization of PCR for *T. cruzi* in 94% of chagasic children, showing a rapid decrease in parasite load after treatment.

Changes in anti-*T. cruzi* antibody levels after BZ therapy were also evaluated. However, the analysis of the pairs of sera carried out at T0 and T2 did not show a statistically significant difference: ELISA titers were 8.8±0.5 *vs* 7.7±0.7, respectively ($p = 0.08$) and IHA titers were 6.5±0.2 *vs* 6.2±0.3, respectively ($p = 0.28$). Given that the ascertainment of resolution of *T. cruzi* infection is based upon specific serology reverting to negative, this remaining antibody reactivity prevented the confirmation of cure of treated pediatric patients at the end of the 6-month follow-up.

Discussion

Autoantibodies with adrenergic and cholinergic activity, capable of triggering neurotransmitter receptor-mediated effects, have been detected in human [20] and murine [21] chagasic sera. Although further *in vivo* experiments are necessary to reliably establish the contribution of these antibodies to *T. cruzi*-mediated cardiomyopathy [22], they may promote dysautonomia often found in chronic Chagas patients [23]. Indeed, this kind of autoantibodies are observed with higher frequency in adults with chronic Chagas heart disease than in asymptomatic *T. cruzi*-infected individuals, suggesting that self-reactive antibodies could be used as a premature marker of evolution for Chagas cardiomyopathy [24–26]. In a preliminary report, we demonstrated for the first time the induction of Anti-M2R AAb in pediatric patients at early stages of chronic *T. cruzi* infection [27]. In addition, a clearly decreasing trend in Anti-M2R AAb reactivity down to healthy levels, accompanied by negative conversion of *T. cruzi* serology, was verified by 18–36 months after trypanocidal chemotherapy.

In the present work, an extension of our previous study, we observed a significant reduction in Anti-M2R AAb titers as early as 6 months after completing BZ treatment. Noticeably, the mean age of Anti-M2R AAb$^+$ chagasic children was higher than that recorded for the negative population, further emphasizing the need for early trypanocidal therapy in *T. cruzi*-infected young individuals. Taken together, our findings indicate that in pediatric Chagas patients Anti-M2R AAb may be downregulated promptly upon BZ administration.

In some *T. cruzi*-infected children, pretreatment Anti-M2R AAbs levels were similar to those found in uninfected controls. Whether these patients have better prognosis remains to be elucidated. On the other hand, a subgroup of infected children presented high Anti-M2R AAb reactivity with potential pathogenic consequences. The described association between Anti-M2R AAb and cardiomyocyte dysfunction could be coupled to a putative agonistic activity of anti-muscarinic receptor antibodies, capable of inducing a receptor desensitization phenomenon [28]. It has been reported that adult patients at the early stages of Chagas disease have circulating Anti-M2R AAb linked to abnormal modulation of vagal activity [11]. Furthermore, administration of BZ during the advanced phase of experimental *T. cruzi* infection prevented the development of a more severe form of chronic cardiomyopathy, concomitantly with a decrease in the cardiac M2R-specific antibody response [21].

We searched for any correlation between anti-cardiac autoantibodies and heart dysfunction in our pediatric population with *T. cruzi* infection. In contrast with the findings of another research group who found a high frequency of early electrocardiographic alterations in seropositive children from endemic areas [29], we were unable to detect ECG or ECHO abnormalities. This discrepancy might be attributed to the size and characteristics of

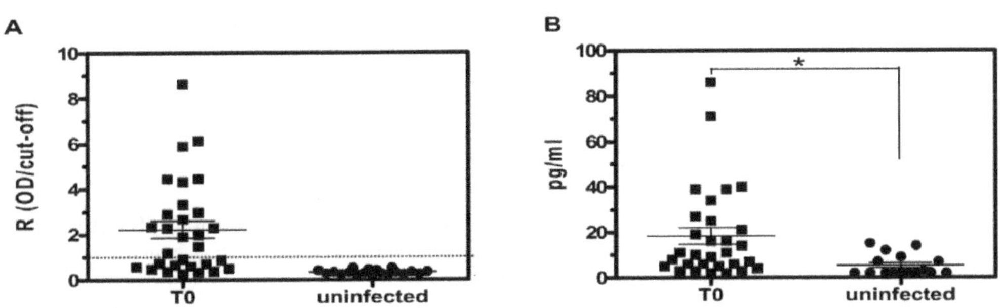

Figure 1. Anti-M2R AAb and IFN-γ profiles in pediatric chagasic patients at T0 and uninfected controls. (A) Distribution of anti-M2R AAb in sera. The group mean and the standard error of the mean are depicted. Dotted line shows cut-off level of the assay. (B) Circulating levels of IFN-γ. The group mean and the standard error of the mean are depicted. * $p = 0.015$ compared to uninfected controls.

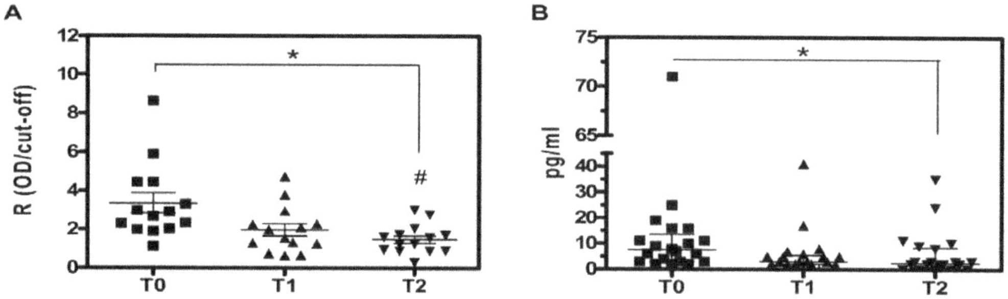

Figure 2. Anti-M2R AAb and IFN-γ profiles in pediatric chagasic patients before and after BZ treatment. (A) Distribution of anti-M2R AAb in sera. Each point represents one patient positive for anti-M2R AAb. The group mean and the standard error of the mean are also depicted. * $p = 0.001$, test for linear trend. # $p < 0.01$, T2 *vs* T0. (B) Circulating levels of IFN-γ. Horizontal lines show median values. * $p < 0.05$, T0 *vs* T2.

the populations evaluated for each study. Unlike our report, de Andrade and co-workers [29] examined a large population of seropositive children from a Chagas-endemic area of central Brazil, where the probability of reinfection, as well as increased pathogenicity of infecting strains of *T. cruzi* prevalent in the zone, could account for the differences observed in ECG profiles. Because antibodies that bind to myocardial cholinergic receptors in patients with Chagas disease have shown to trigger physiological, morphological, enzymatic and molecular alterations [30], it is conceivable that these abnormalities could start from the beginning of *T. cruzi* infection even in asymptomatic individuals with normal ECG and ECHO [26,11].

Clinical and experimental evidences support the involvement of inflammatory cytokines in the pathogenesis of myocardial dysfunction. In this regard, IFN-γ released by infiltrating lymphocytes, both systemically and locally, has been shown to contribute to the impaired cardiac function in the experimental model of autoimmune myocarditis [31]. We herein evaluated the impact of BZ therapy on expression of the inflammatory cytokine IFN-γ in *T. cruzi*-infected children. IFN-γ levels were found to be elevated in *T. cruzi*-infected pediatric patients before initiation of BZ treatment. In agreement with our results, previous studies demonstrated the expression of IFN-γ in young chagasic patients from an endemic region of Paraguay, during the acute and indeterminate stages of infection [32]. In our study population, IFN-γ levels decreased promptly between the time of diagnosis and 6 months after BZ treatment. These findings could well be correlated with the decline in the frequency of peripheral IFN-γ-producing T cells specific for *T. cruzi* observed as early as 12 months after the administration of BZ to chronically infected adults [33]. An exacerbate production of IFN-γ may favour the cytolytic effects of lymphocytes during Chagas disease increasing the chances of myocellular destruction in heart tissue [34]. Consequently, our observations highlight the usefulness of the immunomodulating ability of BZ therapy in *T. cruzi* infection, where a disbalanced inflammatory response becomes detrimental.

Table 1. Distribution of IFN-γ values for *T. cruzi*-infected and uninfected children.

	Median (pg/ml)	P25	P75
Infected			
T0	7.5	3	13.5
T1	3	2	5.5
T2	2.5 *	1	8.5
Uninfected	2	2	8

P25: 25th percentile. P75: 75th percentile. * $p < 0.05$, T2 *vs* T0.

Interestingly, IFN-γ was also associated with a muscarinic receptor-mediated decrease in heart contractility [31]. On the other hand, experimental studies suggested that IFN-γ binding to its specific receptors in the heart may lead to a cholinergic response by interaction of both receptor systems on the surface of atrial cells [35]. Our results indicate that treatment with BZ in the early chronic phase of infection could help prevent the development of immune mechanisms involved in the genesis of severe chronic cardiomyopathy, despite the lack of complete parasite eradication [21]. Although the mechanism by which BZ modulates the production of Anti-M2R AAb and the expression of IFN-γ is unclear, the immunomodulating influence of BZ has been widely documented. Parasiticidal chemotherapy proved capable of modulating phagocyte activation, T-cell profile and the release of immune response mediators, like nitric oxide and cytokines [36]. Accordingly, in pediatric patients acutely infected with *T. cruzi*, elevated circulating levels of CD8 and IL-2 soluble receptors were detected, which decrease after receiving BZ therapy [37]. Whether the impact of BZ treatment on both Anti-M2R AAb and IFN-γ responses is a result of parasite load reduction or a direct effect of the drug on the immune system, is still an open question.

The so far accepted criterion of cure for Chagas disease relies on negative seroconversion of the humoral anti-*T. cruzi* response after etiological treatment. Nevertheless, in pediatric patients initiating therapy at the early chronic stage of infection, negative seroconversion occurs several years after treatment [38], therefore requiring long-term follow-up. Our present findings suggest that the BZ-dependent decline of Anti-M2R AAb and IFN-γ levels might provide a surrogate indicator of early therapeutic success in *T. cruzi*-infected children. Further studies on a larger number of infected individuals are needed to clarify their potential use as novel biomarkers of disease prognosis for those chagasic patients who test positive for Anti-M2R AAb and/or IFN-γ before the onset of treatment.

In conclusion, in pediatric patients the Anti-M2R AAb and the IFN-γ responses are elicited early in the course of *T. cruzi* infection, and decrease after trypanocidal therapy with BZ, even though the negative seroconversion of *T. cruzi*- specific antibodies is not fully accomplished. These findings reinforce the usefulness of BZ treatment and encourage further studies to elucidate the potential use of these immune mediators as biomarkers of disease prognosis.

Author Contributions

Conceived and designed the experiments: PBP RSC RAC HLF. Performed the experiments: RAC BJV GFM SM. Analyzed the data: PBP RSC JMA HLF RAC RLC. Contributed reagents/materials/analysis tools: PBP RSC JMA HLF RLC. Wrote the paper: PBP RAC RSC.

References

1. World Health Organization (2007) Reporte del grupo de trabajo científico sobre la enfermedad de Chagas. Eds.: Guhl F; Lazdins-Helds JK. Available: http://apps.who.int/tdr/publications/tdr-research-publications/reporte-enfermedad-chagas/pdf. Accessed 2011 Sep 2.
2. Bilate AM, Cunha-Neto E (2008) Chagas disease cardiomyopathy: current concepts of an old disease. Rev Inst Med Trop Sao Paulo 50: 67–74.
3. Hagar JM, Rahimtoola SH (1995) Chagas heart disease. Curr Problem Cardiol 20: 825–924.
4. Milei J, Storino R, Jorg M, Chiale P, Schetjman D, et al. (1994) Patogenia. In: Storino R, Milei J, eds. Enfermedad de Chagas. Buenos Aires: Doyma. pp 103–128.
5. Manzullo EC, Chuit R (1999) Risk of death due to chronic chagasic cardiopathy. Mem Inst Oswaldo Cruz 94: 317–320.
6. Tarleton RL (2001) Parasite persistence in the aetiology of Chagas disease. Int J Parasitol 31: 550–554.
7. Leon JS, Godsel LM, Wang K, Engman DM (2001) Cardiac myosin autoimmunity in acute Chagas heart disease. Infect Immun 69: 5643–5649.
8. Rocha MOC, Ribeiro AL, Teixeira MM (2003) Clinical management of chronic Chagasic cardiomyopathy. Frontiers Biosci 8: e44–54.
9. Borda ES, Sterin-Borda L (1996) Antiadrenergic and muscarinic receptor antibodies in Chagas cardiomyopathy. Int J Cardiol 54: 149–156.
10. Ribeiro AL, Moraes RS, Ribeiro JP, Ferlin EL, Tores RM, et al. (2001) Parasympathetic dysautonomia precedes left ventricular systolic dysfunction in Chagas disease. Am Heart J 141: 260–265.
11. Ribeiro ALP, Díaz Giménez LE, Quintero Hernández CC, Campos de Carvalho AC, Teixeira MM, et al. (2007) Early occurrence of anti-muscarinic autoantibodies and abnormal vagal modulation in Chagas disease. Int J Cardiol 117: 59–63.
12. Ferrari I, Levin MJ, Wallukat G, Elies R, Lebesgue D, et al. (1995) Molecular mimicry between the immunodominant ribosomal protein P0 of *Trypanosoma cruzi* and a functional epitope on the human β_1-adrenergic receptor. J Exp Med 182: 59–65.
13. Labovsky V, Smulski CR, Gómez K, Levy G, Levin MJ (2007) Anti-β_1-adrenergic receptor autoantibodies in patients with chronic Chagas heart desease. Clin Exp Immunol 148: 440–449.
14. Gutiérrez FR, Guedes PM, Gazzinelli RT, Silva JS (2009) The role of parasite persistence in pathogenesis of Chagas heart disease. Parasite Immunol 31: 673–685.
15. Gomes JA, Bahia-Oliveira LM, Rocha MO, Martins-Filho OA, Gazzinelli G, et al. (2003) Evidence that development of severe cardiomyopathy in human Chagas' disease is due to a Th1-specific immune response. Infect Immun 71: 1185–1193.
16. Corrêa-Oliveira R, de Assis Silva Gomes J, Moreira Lemos E, Meira Cardoso G, Reis DD, et al. (1999) The role of the immune response on the development of severe clinical forms of human Chagas disease. Mem Inst Oswaldo Cruz 94: 253–255.
17. Cunha-Neto E, Nogueira LG, Teixeira PC, Ramasawmy R, Drigo SA, et al. (2009) Immunological and non-immunological effects of cytokines and chemokines in the pathogenesis of chronic Chagas disease cardiomyopathy. Mem Inst Oswaldo Cruz 104: 252–258.
18. Olivieri BP, Cotta-De-Almeida V, Araujo-Jorge T (2002) Benznidazole treatment following acute *Trypanosoma cruzi* infection triggers CD8+T-cell expansion and promotes resistance to reinfection. Antimicrob Agents Chemother 46: 3790–3796.
19. Villinger F, Hunt D, Mayne A, Vuchetich M, Findley H, et al. (1993) Qualitative and quantitative studies of cytokines synthesized and secreted by non-human primate peripheral blood mononuclear cells. Cytokine 5: 469–479.
20. Goin JC, Borda ES, Auger S, Storino R, Sterin-Borda L (1999) Cardiac M2 muscarinic cholinoreceptor activation by human chagasic autoantibodies: association with bradycardia. Heart 82: 273–278.
21. García S, Ramos CO, Senra JFV, Vilas-Boas F, Rodriguez MM, et al. (2005) Treatment with benznidazole during the chronic phase of experimental Chagasdisease decreases cardiac alterations. Antimicrob Agents Chemother 49: 1521–1528.
22. Benchimol-Barbosa PR (2011) Comments on the article by Ribeiro, et al. 'Enhanced parasympathetic activity in Chagas' disease still stands in need of proof': definitions and biases. Int J Cardiol 146: 88–90.
23. Nussinovitch U, Shoenfeld Y (2011) The diagnostic and clinical significance of anti-muscarinic receptor autoantibodies. Clin Rev Allergy Immunol Jan 5 [Epub ahead of print].
24. Giménez L, Mitelman J, González C, Borda E, Sterin-Borda L (2003) Anticuerpos anti-receptores autonómicos, alteraciones de la variabilidad de la frecuencia cardíaca y arritmias en sujetos con Enfermedad de Chagas. Rev Arg Cardiol 71: 109–113.
25. Talvani A, Rocha MOC, Ribeiro AL, Borda E, Sterin-Borda L, et al. (2006) Levels of anti-M2 and anti-β_1 autoantibodies do not correlate with the degree of heart dysfunction in Chagasheart disease. Microbes Infect 8: 2459–2464.
26. Goin JC, Borda ES, Pérez Leirós C, Storino R, Sterin-Borda L (1994) Identification of antibodies with muscarinic cholinergic activity in human Chagas disease: pathological implications. J Auton Nerv Syst 47: 45–52.
27. Cutrullis RA, Ballering G, Altcheh J, Moscatelli G, Corral R, et al. (2007) Anti-M2 muscarinic receptor autoantibodies in *Trypanosoma cruzi*-infected pediatric patients treated with benznidazole. Rev Patol Trop 36: 141–148.
28. Peraza-Cruces K, Gutiérrez-Guédez L, Castañeda Perozo D, Lankford CR, Rodríguez-Bonfante C, et al. (2008) *Trypanosoma cruzi* infection induces up-regulation of cardiac muscarinic acetylcholine receptors *in vivo* and *in vitro*. Braz J Med Biol Res 41: 796–803.
29. de Andrade AL, Zicker F, Rassi A, Rassi AG, Oliveira RM, et al. (1998) Early electrocardiographic abnormalities in *Trypanosoma cruzi*-seropositive children. Am J Trop Med Hyg 59: 530–534.
30. Marin-Neto JA, Cunha-Neto E, Maciel BC, Simões MV, et al. Pathogenesis of Chronic Chagas Heart Disease. Circulation 115: 1109–1123.
31. Pérez Leirós C, Goren N, Sterin-Borda L, Borda ES (1997) Myocardial dysfunction in an experimental model of autoimmune myocarditis: role of IFN-γ. Neuroimmunomodulation 4: 91–97.
32. Samudio M, Montenegro-James S, Cabral M, Martinez J, Rojas de Arias A (1998) Cytokine responses in *Trypanosoma cruzi*-infected children in Paraguay. Am J Trop Med Hyg 58: 119–121.
33. Laucella SA, Pérez Mazliah D, Bertocchi G, Alvarez MG, Cooley G, et al. (2009) Changes in *Trypanosoma cruzi*-Specific Immune Responses after Treatment: Surrogate Markers of Treatment Efficacy. Clin Infect Dis 49: 1675–1684.
34. Bahia-Oliveira LM, Gomes JA, Rocha MO, Moreira MC, Lemos EM, et al. (1998) IFN-gamma in human Chagas' disease: protection or pathology?. Braz J Med Biol Res 31: 127–131.
35. Borda E, Leirós CP, Sterin-Borda L, de Bracco MM (1991) Cholinergic response of isolated rat atria to recombinant rat interferon-gamma. J Neuroimmunol 32: 53–59.
36. Piaggio E, Roggero E, Pitashny M, Wiertzerbin J, Bottasso OA, et al. (2001) Treatment with benznidazole and its immunomodulating effects on *Trypanosoma cruzi*-infected rats. Parasitol Res 87: 539–547.
37. Moretti E, Basso B, Cervetta L, Brigada A, Barbieri G (2002) Patterns of cytokines and soluble cellular receptors in the sera of children with acute Chagasdisease. Clin Diagn Lab Immunol 9: 1324–1237.
38. Altcheh J, Biancardi M, Lapeña A, Ballering G, Freilij H (2005) Congenital Chagas disease: experience in the Hospital de Niños, Ricardo Gutiérrez, Buenos Aires, Argentina. Rev Soc Bras Med Trop 38: 41–45.

3

IL-12Rβ1 Deficiency in Two of Fifty Children with Severe Tuberculosis from Iran, Morocco, and Turkey

Stéphanie Boisson-Dupuis[1,2,3], Jamila El Baghdadi[4], Nima Parvaneh[5], Aziz Bousfiha[6], Jacinta Bustamante[2,3], Jacqueline Feinberg[2,3], Arina Samarina[2,3], Audrey V. Grant[2,3], Lucile Janniere[2,3], Naima El Hafidi[7], Amal Hassani[8], Daniel Nolan[2,3], Jilali Najib[6], Yildiz Camcioglu[9], Nevin Hatipoglu[10], Cigdem Aydogmus[10], Gonul Tanir[11], Caner Aytekin[11], Melike Keser[12], Ayper Somer[12], Guside Aksu[13], Necil Kutukculer[13], Davood Mansouri[14], Alireza Mahdaviani[15], Setareh Mamishi[5], Alexandre Alcais[1,2,3], Laurent Abel[1,2,3¶], Jean-Laurent Casanova[1,2,3,16*¶]

1 St. Giles Laboratory of Human Genetics of Infectious Diseases, Rockefeller Branch, The Rockefeller University, New York, New York, United States of America, **2** Laboratory of Human Genetics of Infectious Diseases, U980, Institut National de la Santé et de la Recherche Médicale (INSERM), Paris, France, **3** Necker Medical School, University Paris Descartes, Paris, France, **4** Genetics Unit, Military Hospital Mohamed V, Hay Riad Rabat, Morocco, **5** Department of Pediatrics, Infectious Disease Research Center, Teheran University of Medical Sciences, Teheran, Iran, **6** Clinical Immunology Unit, King Hassan II University, Ibn-Rochd Hospital, Casablanca, Morocco, **7** Department of Pediatrics, Rabat Children Hospital, Rabat, Morocco, **8** Department of Pediatrics, Military Hospital Mohamed V, Hay Riad Rabat, Morocco, **9** Infectious Diseases, Clinical Immunology and Allergy Division, Department of Pediatrics, Cerrahpasa Medical School, Istanbul University, Cerrahpasa, Istanbul, Turkey, **10** Department of Pediatric Infectious Diseases and Immunology, Bakirkoy Maternity and Children's State Hospital, Istanbul, Turkey, **11** Dr. Sami Ulus Children's Health and Diseases Training and Research Center, Ankara, Turkey, **12** Department of Pediatric Infectious Diseases and Clinical Immunology, Istanbul University Faculty of Medicine, Istanbul, Turkey, **13** Department of Pediatrics, Ege University Medical School, Izmir, Turkey, **14** Division of Infectious Diseases and Clinical Immunology, National Research Institute of Tuberculosis and Lung Diseases, Shahid Beheshti University of Medical Sciences, Teheran, Iran, **15** Pediatric Respiratory Disease Research Center, NRITLD, Shahid Beheshti University of Medical Sciences, Teheran, Iran, **16** Pediatric Immunology-Hematology Unit, Necker Hospital, Paris, France

Abstract

Background and Objectives: In the last decade, autosomal recessive IL-12Rβ1 deficiency has been diagnosed in four children with severe tuberculosis from three unrelated families from Morocco, Spain, and Turkey, providing proof-of-principle that tuberculosis in otherwise healthy children may result from single-gene inborn errors of immunity. We aimed to estimate the fraction of children developing severe tuberculosis due to IL-12Rβ1 deficiency in areas endemic for tuberculosis and where parental consanguinity is common.

Methods and Principal Findings: We searched for *IL12RB1* mutations in a series of 50 children from Iran, Morocco, and Turkey. All children had established severe pulmonary and/or disseminated tuberculosis requiring hospitalization and were otherwise normally resistant to weakly virulent BCG vaccines and environmental mycobacteria. In one child from Iran and another from Morocco, homozygosity for loss-of-function *IL12RB1* alleles was documented, resulting in complete IL-12Rβ1 deficiency. Despite the small sample studied, our findings suggest that IL-12Rβ1 deficiency is not a very rare cause of pediatric tuberculosis in these countries, where it should be considered in selected children with severe disease.

Significance: This finding may have important medical implications, as recombinant IFN-γ is an effective treatment for mycobacterial infections in IL-12Rβ1-deficient patients. It also provides additional support for the view that severe tuberculosis in childhood may result from a collection of single-gene inborn errors of immunity.

Editor: Pere-Joan Cardona, Fundació Institut Germans Trias i Pujol; Universitat Autònoma de Barcelona CibeRES, Spain

Funding: The Laboratory of Human Genetics of Infectious Diseases is supported in part by grants from the Schlumberger Foundation, the BNP-Paribas Foundation, The Foundation for Medical Research (FRM), the "Institut Universitaire de France," the French National Agency for Research (ANR), the EU-grant HOMITB (HEALTH-F3-2008-200732), the Bill and Melinda Gates Foundation, the St. Giles Foundation, the Jeffrey Modell Foundation and Talecris Biotherapeutics, the Rockefeller University Center for Clinical and Translational Science grant number 5UL1RR024143, the Rockefeller University, and the National Institute of Allergy and Infectious Diseases grant number 1U01AI088685. The funders had no role in study design, data collection and analysis, decision to publish, or preparation of the manuscript. No additional external funding received for this study.

Competing Interests: The authors received funding from Talecris Biotherapeutics. This does not alter the authors' adherence to all the PLoS ONE policies on sharing data and materials.

* E-mail: jean-laurent.casanova@rockefeller.edu

These authors contributed equally to this work.

¶ These authors also contributed equally to this work.

Introduction

"The occurrence of tuberculosis in families led to the view that it was an inherited disease. The demonstration of a characteristic bacterium by Koch in 1882 disposed of this view." Theobald Smith [1]

Tuberculosis (TB) is typically caused by *Mycobacterium tuberculosis* (Mtb) and has probably claimed more lives than any other single infectious disease in human history. It continues to be responsible for almost two million deaths each year [2]. Two main forms of clinical disease have been historically observed in endemic areas, at least until the advent of the first antibiotics, and the further blurring of the overall picture that occurred with the HIV pandemic. The disseminated form in children is acute and results from the hematogenous spread of Mtb during primary infection, whereas the chronic pulmonary form in adults, results from the reactivation of latent Mtb infection [3,4].

A few decades after the discovery of Mtb by Robert Koch in 1882, it became apparent that most people in endemic areas were infected with this bacterium but remained asymptomatic. These findings, obtained at the turn of the twentieth century, were based on both hypersensitivity to subcutaneously [5] and intradermally (Mantoux) administered tuberculin [6] and the growth of Mtb from the lungs of patients dying from other causes [7]. Indeed, only a small fraction of individuals infected with Mtb develop clinical TB in their lifetime. Mtb remains latent in most infected individuals. One century later, the phenomenon of latency, and reactivation thereof, remains largely unexplained, implying that the pathogenesis of adult TB itself is unclear. This is also true for pediatric TB, which occurs in about 5% of infected children during primary infection.

In line with a long tradition of thought, we hypothesize that TB is not only an infectious disease, but also a *bona fide* genetic disorder; more specifically, we hypothesize that TB results from inborn errors of immunity [3,8–12]. The genetic theory of TB, which predates the discovery of Mtb [1,13], was supported from the 1910s onwards by genetic epidemiology surveys, initially based on correlation studies [14,15] and twin studies [16]. Studies in the mouse model conducted from the 1920s onwards also provided strong support for the genetic theory of TB [17]. Finally, over the last decade, adult TB susceptibility chromosomal regions were mapped by candidate gene and genome-wide linkage and association studies [3,8–12,18–20].

The human molecular genetic dissection of pediatric TB was facilitated from 1996 onwards by the dissection of genetic etiologies of the syndrome of Mendelian susceptibility to mycobacterial disease (MSMD), which is characterized by clinical disease caused by weakly virulent mycobacteria, such as BCG vaccines and environmental mycobacteria (EM), in otherwise healthy children who are normally resistant to most other infectious agents [8,21]. In the last 12 years, as many as 15 disorders have been discovered, involving eight genes that control the IL-12-IFN-γ circuit [21–24].

These studies paved the way for the identification of the first children with Mendelian predispositions to *bona fide* TB: autosomal recessive IFN-γR1 deficiency in a child not vaccinated with BCG, autosomal recessive IL-12p40 deficiency in a child who also had disseminated BCG disease (known as BCG-osis), XR-MSMD1 (NEMO) in a child without BCG vaccination [21] and XR-MSMD2 (CYBB) in a child not vaccinated with BCG [23]. More convincingly, in three unrelated families from Morocco, Spain, and Turkey, children bearing two loss-of-function alleles of *IL12RB1* were found to suffer from severe TB in the absence of any signs of MSMD, despite vaccination with BCG and clear exposure to EM [25–27]. The proband in the Moroccan family suffered from BCG-osis [25], leading to the investigation of a sibling with TB, whereas the other two families had no family history of MSMD [26,27]. Indeed, IL-12Rβ1 deficiency has been shown to display incomplete clinical penetrance for the case-definition phenotype of MSMD [28,29].

Based on these studies, the proportion of children with disseminated TB due to monogenic predisposition in endemic areas was proposed, by purely theoretical calculations, to be far from negligible (3% to 30%) [3]. These data and calculations raised two key, general questions: What proportion of children with disseminated TB have a predisposition conferred by single-gene variations? And what are these inborn errors of immunity? As a first approach to tackling this fundamental problem, we attempted to estimate the proportion of children with severe TB due to autosomal recessive IL-12Rβ1 deficiency in three countries endemic for TB, where HIV infection is infrequent, and where consanguineous marriages are common, including Iran, Morocco, and Turkey.

Results

In 48 patients, no rare variations were found. However, we identified two patients carrying homozygous mutations in *IL12RB1*: a mutation in exon 9 in Moroccan P1, leading to the introduction of a stop codon at position 305 (K305X), and a mutation in exon 5 in Iranian P2, leading to the replacement of an arginine residue with a tryptophan residue at position 173 (R173W)(figure 1). These mutations were previously shown not to be polymorphisms by sequencing control samples from various ethnic groups [28,29] and had been further shown to be loss-of-expression and loss-of-function in other patients with MSMD [28,29]. Both mutations lead to complete IL-12Rβ1 deficiency and render the patient's cells completely unresponsive to IL-12. These two patients came from unrelated families, each of which was consanguineous, originating from and living in Morocco (P1) and Iran (P2).

P1 had been vaccinated with BCG at birth, with no adverse reaction. He developed severe pulmonary TB at 13 years of age, leading to his death after three months despite treatment with rifampin, isoniazid, pyrazinamide and streptomycin. The presence of Mtb was confirmed bacteriologically by culture from sputum. The patient was the only member of this family homozygous for the mutant allele of *IL12RB1* (his older brother is heterozygous) (Figure 1).

P2 was diagnosed with severe pulmonary tuberculosis at seven months of age, which was bacteriologically confirmed (from gastric lavage), and treated with isoniazid and rifampin (Figure 1). A paraspinal abcess due to Mtb was diagnosed at six years of age, and was treated by surgical resection and antimycobacterial drugs (isoniazid, rifampin and clarithromycin). P2 also had cutaneous leishmaniasis at the age of five years, successfully treated with Glucantime (meglumine antimoniate) for 20 days. An older brother was found to be homozygous for the mutant allele of *IL12RB1*. This brother had been vaccinated with BCG, with no adverse effect, and developed cutaneous leishmaniasis at the age of seven years and scrofuloderma of the neck at the age of 12 years, which was successfully treated with antimycobacterial drugs (rifampin and isoniazid supplemented with streptomycin for the first two months). Unfortunately, no pathological and microbiological investigations were carried out to ascertain the probable Mtb-linked etiology of scrofuloderma. Another IL-12Rβ1-deficient patient with visceral leishmaniasis has previously been described [30]. All the children of this Iranian family, including

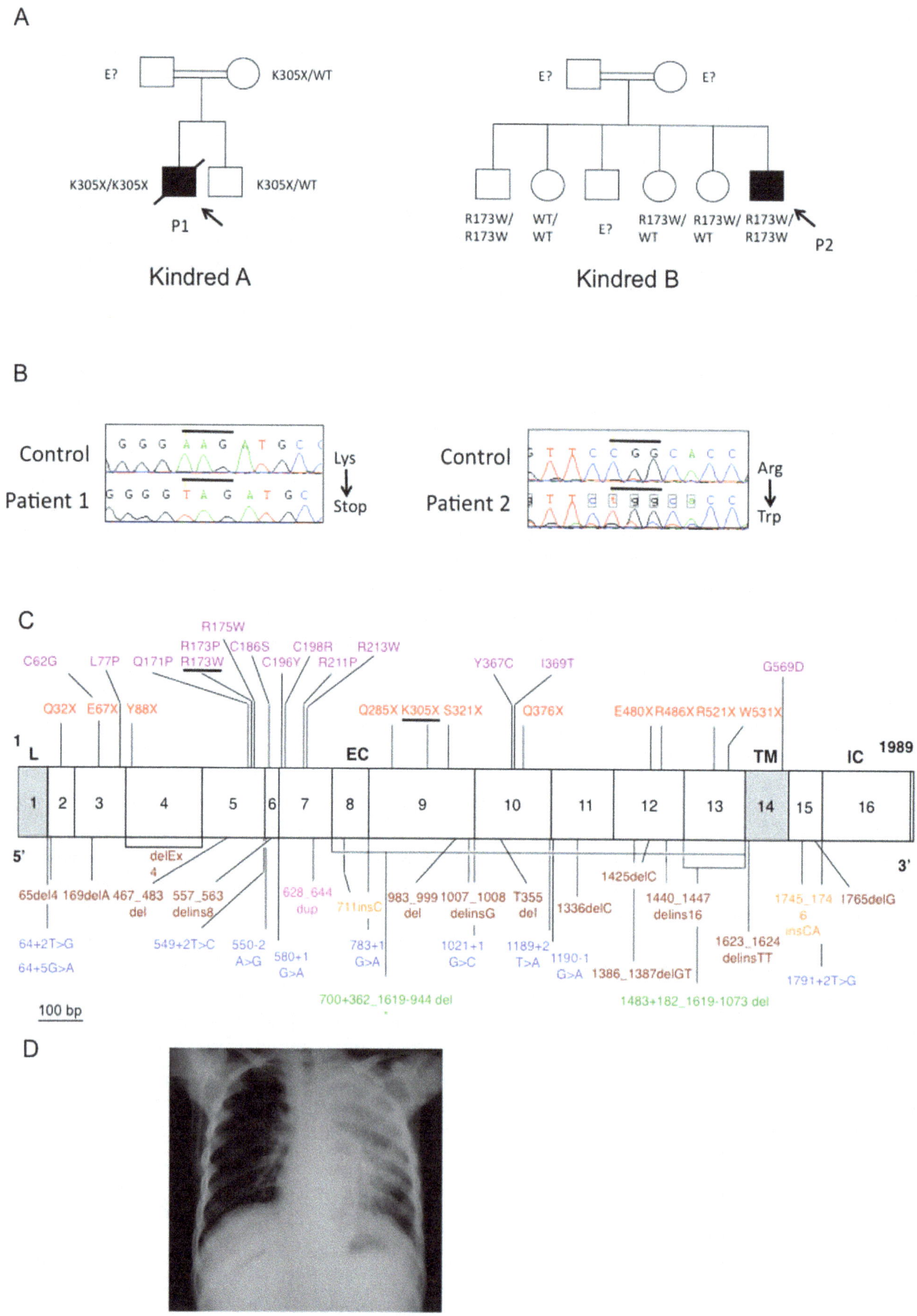
A
E?
K305X/WT
K305X/K305X
K305X/WT
P1
Kindred A
E?
E?
R173W/ R173W
WT/ WT
E?
R173W/ WT
R173W/ WT
R173W/ R173W
P2
Kindred B
B
Control
Patient 1
Lys
Stop
Control
Patient 2
Arg
Trp
C
R175W
R173P
C186S
C198R
R213W
C62G
L77P
Q171P
R173W
C196Y
R211P
Y367C
I369T
G569D
Q32X
E67X
Y88X
Q285X
K305X
S321X
Q376X
E480X
R486X
R521X
W531X
1
L
EC
TM
IC
1989
5'
3'
1 2 3 4 5 6 7 8 9 10 11 12 13 14 15 16
delEx 4
65del4
169delA
467_483 del
557_563 delins8
628_644 dup
711insC
983_999 del
1007_1008 delinsG
T355 del
1336delC
1425delC
1440_1447 delins16
1623_1624 delinsTT
1745_1746 insCA
1765delG
64+2T>G
64+5G>A
549+2T>C
550-2 A>G
580+1 G>A
783+1 G>A
1021+1 G>C
1189+2 T>A
1190-1 G>A
1386_1387delGT
1791+2T>G
700+362_1619-944 del
1483+182_1619-1073 del
100 bp
D

Figure 1. Mendelian mutations in *IL12RB1* leading to severe tuberculosis in two kindreds. A. Pedigree of the two families (A and B) with IL-12Rβ1 deficiency. Each generation is designated by a roman numeral (I–II), and each individual by an Arabic numeral. The double lines connecting the parents indicate consanguinity. The probands are indicated by an arrow, with black indicating *Mycobacterium tuberculosis* disease status. Individuals whose genetic status could not be evaluated are indicated by the symbol "E?". **B.** Electrophoregram showing the genomic sequences of exons 9 and 5 in patients 1 and 2, respectively, compared with a control sequence. **C.** Schematic diagram of the coding region of the IL-12Rβ1 chain containing 17 coding exons and encoding a 662-amino acid protein with a leader sequence (exon1, L), extracellular domain (exons 2 to 13, EC), transmembrane domain (exon 14, TM) and an intracellular cytoplasmic domain (exons 15 to 17, IC). Published and unpublished mutations are indicated as follows: missense mutations are shown in purple, nonsense mutations are shown in red and complex mutations are shown in brown. Splicing mutations are shown in blue, large deletions are shown in green, insertions are shown in orange, and duplication is shown in magenta. * The 700+362_1619-944del mutation is the only mutation resulting in at the expression of a protein at the cell surface. Mutations of P1 (K305X) and P2 (R173W) are underlined. **D.** Chest X ray of patient 1 showing the localization of the disease.

the two IL-12Rβ1-deficient siblings, were vaccinated with BCG at birth, with no adverse reaction (Figure 1). However, none of the children developed clinical disease caused by BCG or environmental mycobacteria. Thus, in summary, P1 and P2 presented a phenotype of severe TB in childhood, without MSMD. The brother of P2 also probably suffered from TB. There was no history of MSMD in either family. All index cases were investigated based on the sole criterion of being children admitted for severe TB to university hospitals in Morocco, Turkey, and Iran.

Discussion

This study shows for the first time, at the population level, that in at least two countries with a high rate of consanguineous marriages (Morocco and Iran) severe TB may result from autosomal recessive IL-12Rβ1 deficiency, in at least some children. We investigated 50 patients, two of whom were found to carry homozygous loss-of-function mutations in *IL12RB1*, giving an overall estimated prevalence of 4%. Given the small size of the sample, this estimate is only a rough one; however, it is quite remarkable that we were able to detect two IL-12Rβ1-deficient patients in a sample of only 50 children. It is difficult to assess the actual prevalence of IL-12Rβ1 deficiency as a genetic etiology of pediatric TB in Morocco (1 in 35 samples); however, P1 is the second child to be diagnosed with TB and IL-12Rβ1 deficiency in this country [25]. P2 is the first IL-12Rβ1-deficient child with TB diagnosed in Iran; however, this is probably not unique, as a young adult patient with TB and IL-12Rβ1 deficiency has also recently been identified in this country [31]. Finally, although we found no IL-12Rβ1-deficient Turkish children with TB in this study, we did identify one such child in a previous study [27]. Overall, IL-12Rβ1 deficiency does not seem to be an exceedingly rare genetic etiology of TB, at least in children from Morocco, Turkey, and Iran. We now need to test more children from these countries, as well as children with severe TB from other regions of the world where parental consanguinity is less common. Our previous identification of two Spanish siblings with TB and IL-12Rβ1 deficiency, born to non-consanguineous parents, suggests that there may be other cases around the world [26]. Overall, our study suggests that IL-12Rβ1 deficiency should be considered in selected children with severe TB, at least in areas with a high prevalence of parental consanguinity. This is important clinically, not only for genetic counseling, but also because recombinant IFN-γ is an effective treatment for mycobacterial disease in patients with IL-12Rβ1 deficiency displaying impaired IFN-γ production [21,32,33].

In this study, we investigated only one gene, *IL12RB1*, because mutations in this gene had previously been found in three unrelated children with TB [25–27]. We focused on its coding region, yet there may be children carrying non-coding and TB-causing mutations in *IL-12RB1*. Moreover, other genes are known to be associated with MSMD and even with childhood TB. Indeed, one child with partial recessive IFN-γR1 deficiency, and others with IL-12p40 deficiency, XR-MSMD1 (NEMO deficiency) and XR-MSMD2 (CYBB deficiency) associated with clinical TB have been identified [21,23]. Mutations in these genes may be responsible for TB in other children, particularly if the morbid alleles concerned display incomplete penetrance for the case-definition phenotype of MSMD, such as *IL12B* and *IL12RB1*. Mutations in other genes possibly but not necessarily related to IFN-γ-mediated immunity, may also be involved. This study adds weight to the hypothesis that severe TB may be attributable to a collection of single-gene mutations, in at least some children. It is not surprising that recessive traits are frequently involved in countries in which the rate of consanguinity is as high as 20% (Morocco and Turkey) or 38% (Iran). However, in our recent large series of 102 families with an IL-12Rβ1-deficient proband with MSMD [29], only 58 families (57%) were clearly consanguineous and 14 probands were compound heterozygous, indicating that complete IL-12Rβ1 deficiency may also occur in non-consanguineous families. Dominant traits may also be involved, consistent with the identification of various dominant MSMD-causing mutations in *IFNGR1*, *IFNGR2*, and *STAT1* [34–37]. We are currently trying to improve our estimate of the percentage of children suffering from genetically determined severe TB by collecting more samples from these three populations (Iran, Morocco and Turkey). We intend to use a genome-wide hypothesis-generating approach, sequencing the 'whole exome' and 'whole genome' of children with TB enrolled in this study [38–40]. The genetic dissection of pediatric TB should have a major impact on our understanding of the pathogenesis of TB and may lead to new therapeutic interventions based on a rational understanding of the pathogenesis.

Methods

We investigated the *IL12RB1* gene in 50 children from three countries in which tuberculosis is endemic: 11 children from Turkey, 4 from Iran, and 35 from Morocco. These countries were selected because they have a high prevalence of consanguineous marriages (around 20% in Morocco and Turkey [41,42] and 38% in Iran [43]), a very low prevalence of HIV (less than 0.1% in Morocco and Turkey and less than 0.15% in Iran) (WHO 2010), a high-quality pediatric care and microbiological diagnosis and a high incidence of TB (25–30 per 100,000 persons/year in Turkey and Iran, and 98 per 100,000 persons/year in Morocco) (WHO 2010). This incidence is slightly higher in urban areas such as 40 per 100,000 persons/year in Istanbul and 122 per 100,000 persons/year in Casablanca. In addition, the Arabs and Berbers in Morocco, the Turks in Turkey, and the Persians in Iran form distinctly different ethnic groups. Our study was conducted in accordance with the Helsinki Declaration, with written informed consent obtained from each patient or the patient's family. The

Table 1. Table indicating the clinical presentations of TB recorded in the fifty patients.

N	Sex	Age	Origin	BCG	Miliary TB	TB Meningitis	Peripheral TB	Mediastinal TB	TB osteitis	Pulmonary TB	Urinary TB
1	F	0.5	Morocco	yes	yes			yes			
2	M	0.25	Morocco	yes	yes						
3	M	1.5	Morocco	yes	yes						
4	F	3	Morocco	yes		yes					
5	F	0.83	Morocco	yes	yes		yes	yes			
6	M	6	Morocco	yes	yes	yes					
7	F	7	Morocco	yes					yes		
8	F	1.16	Morocco	yes	yes	yes					
9	M	9	Morocco	yes			yes	yes			
10	M	11	Morocco	yes				yes			
11	F	3	Morocco	yes			yes			yes	
12	M	10	Morocco	yes				yes			
13	F	3	Morocco	yes	yes		yes				
14	F	12	Morocco	yes				yes			
15	**M**	**13**	**Morocco**	**yes**						yes	
16	M	5	Morocco	yes				yes			
17	F	10	Morocco	yes				yes			
18	F	11	Morocco	yes		yes					
19	M	10	Morocco	yes	yes						
20	F	4	Morocco	yes	yes						
21	M	4	Morocco	yes		yes					
22	M	9	Morocco	yes		yes					
23	F	8	Morocco	yes	yes			yes			
24	F	4	Morocco	yes	yes						
25	F	1.1	Morocco	yes	yes						
26	M	2	Morocco	yes			yes	yes		yes	
27	M	0.5	Morocco	yes	yes						
28	M	10	Morocco	yes			yes	yes		yes	
29	M	3.5	Morocco	yes		yes					
30	F	2	Morocco	yes	yes						
31	M	1.2	Morocco	yes	yes						
32	F	6	Morocco	yes	yes						
33	M	4	Morocco	yes	yes						
34	F	5	Morocco	yes	yes		yes				
35	M	9	Morocco	yes	yes						
36	F	1.8	Turkey	no		yes					
37	F	0.45	Turkey	yes		yes					
38	F	15	Turkey	yes		yes					
39	M	4	Turkey	no				yes			
40	M	3	Turkey	no		yes					
41	F	15	Turkey	yes			yes	yes			
42	M	14	Turkey	no	yes						
43	F	0.75	Turkey	no							yes
44	M	6	Turkey	yes					yes		
45	F	14	Turkey	yes				yes		yes	
46	F	10	Turkey	no	yes	yes				yes	
47	**M**	**0.58**	**Iran**	**yes**			yes			yes	
48	F	12	Iran	yes						yes	
49	F	15	Iran	yes						yes	
50	F	14	Iran	yes						yes	

The two patients presenting with IL-12Rβ1 deficiency are in bold. N means number and age is indicated in years.

IRB was obtained and approved for this study in France (CPP committee C1016) by INSERM and INSERM serves as IRB of record for all institutions/hospitals. The patients herein reported were not described in our recent review of 141 patients with IL-12Rβ1 deficiency, who were selected on the basis of their personal or familial phenotype of MSMD [29]. All the patients studied displayed confirmed severe tuberculosis requiring hospitalisation during childhood, had no classical primary immunodeficiency and were not infected with HIV. All the patients that (i) fulfilled the inclusion criteria, (ii) whose parents agreed to participate and (iii) for whom biological material was recovered, have been analysed. This represents a total of 50 patients. Most (88%) had been vaccinated with BCG, with no adverse effects. The clinical presentations of TB recorded included miliary TB (n = 21), TB meningitis (n = 12), peripheral TB adenitis (n = 9) (i.e. infection of peripheral lymph nodes), mediastinal TB adenitis (n = 14) (i.e. infection of mediastinal lymph nodes), pulmonary TB (n = 10), urinary TB (n = 1) and TB osteitis (n = 2). Most (35) patients presented TB at a single location (Table 1). For all 50 patients, the coding and flanking intron sequences of *IL12RB1* were amplified [44] and sequenced with an ABI 3730x sequencer (Applied Biosystems).

Acknowledgments

We thank Maylis de Suremain, Ron Liebman, Tatiana Kochetkov, Erin Kirk, Yelena Nemirovskaya, Yoann Rose, Martine Courat and Tony Leclerc for technical and secretarial assistance and all members of the Laboratory of Human Genetics of Infectious Diseases for helpful discussions.

Author Contributions

Conceived and designed the experiments: SBD AA LA JLC. Performed the experiments: SBD JF A. Samarina LJ DN. Analyzed the data: SBD LA JLC. Contributed reagents/materials/analysis tools: SBD JEB NP AB JB AG NEH AH JN YC NH C. Aydogmus GT C. Aytekin MK A. Somer GA NK DM AM SM. Wrote the paper: SBD JLC.

References

1. Smith T (1934) Parasitism and disease, Princeton: Princeton University Press 196.
2. WHO (2006) Global tuberculosis control. Surveillance, planning, financing. Geneva: WHO/HTM/TB/ 2006: 362.
3. Alcais A, Fieschi C, Abel L, Casanova JL (2005) Tuberculosis in children and adults: two distinct genetic diseases. J Exp Med 202: 1617–21.
4. Ranke K (1910) Diagnose und Epidemiologie der Lungentuberculose des Kindes. Archiv fuer Kinderheilkunde 54: 279–306.
5. von Pirquet C (1909) Frequency of tuberculosis in childhood. JAMA LII: 675–8.
6. White WC, Graham DA (1909) A quantitative Modification of the von Pirquet tuberculin reaction and its value in diagnosis and prognosis. J Med Res 20: 347–357.
7. Opie EL, Arondon JD (1927) Tubercle bacilli in latent tuberculosis lesions and in lung tissue without tuberculous lesions. Arch Pathol Lab Med 4: 1–21.
8. Casanova JL, Abel L (2002) Genetic dissection of immunity to mycobacteria: the human model. Annu Rev Immunol 20: 581–620.
9. Bellamy R (2005) Genetic susceptibility to tuberculosis. Clin Chest Med 26: 233–46.
10. Schurr E (2007) Is susceptibility to tuberculosis acquired or inherited? J Intern Med 261: 106–11.
11. Alcais A, Quintana-Murci L, Thaler DS, Schurr E, Abel L, et al. (2010) Life-threatening infectious diseases of childhood: single-gene inborn errors of immunity? Ann N Y Acad Sci 1214: 18–33.
12. Casanova JL, Abel L (2007) Primary immunodeficiencies: a fields in its infancy. Science 317: 617–619.
13. Duval CW (1909) Studies in atypical forms of tubercle bacilli isolated directly from the human tissues in cases of primary cervical adenitis: with special reference to the Theobald Smith glycerine bouillon reaction. J Exp Med 11: 403–429.
14. Pearson K (1912) Tuberculosis, heredity and environment. Eugenics Laboratory Lecture Series viii: 694.
15. Pfuffer R (1944) Familial susceptibility to tuberculosis; its importance as a public health problem. Vol5 Cambridge, MA Harvard University Press.
16. Von Verschuer OF (1955) [Tuberculotic twins; follow-up after 20 years.]. Dtsch Med Wochenschr. 80: 1635–7.
17. Fortin A, Abel L, Casanova JL, Gros P (2007) Host genetics of mycobacterial diseases in mice and men: forward genetic studies of BCG-osis and tuberculosis. Annu Rev Genomics Hum Genet 8: 163–92.
18. Baghdadi JE, Orlova M, Alter A, Ranque B, Chentoufi M, et al. (2006) An autosomal dominant major gene confers predisposition to pulmonary tuberculosis in adults. J Exp Med 203: 1679–84.
19. Cobat A, Gallant CJ, Simkin L, Black GF, Stanley K, et al. (2009) Two loci control tuberculin skin test reactivity in an area hyperendemic for tuberculosis. J Exp Med 206: 2583–91.
20. Thye T, Vannberg FO, Wong SH, Owusu-Dabo E, Osei I, et al. (2010) Genome-wide association analyses identifies a susceptibility locus for tuberculosis on chromosome 18q11.2. Nat Genet 42: 739–41.
21. Filipe-Santos O, Bustamante J, Chapgier A, Vogt G, de Beaucoudrey L, et al. (2006) Inborn errors of IL-12/23- and IFN-gamma-mediated immunity: molecular, cellular, and clinical features. Semin Immunol 18: 347–61.
22. Vogt G, Bustamante J, Chapgier A, Feinberg J, Boisson-Dupuis S, et al. (2008) Complementation of a pathogenic IFNGR2 misfolding mutation with modifiers of N-glycosylation. J Exp Med 205: 1729–37.
23. Bustamante J, Arias AA, Vogt G, Picard C, Blancas Galicia L, et al. (2011) Germline but macrophage-tropic CYBB mutations in kindreds with X-linked prédisposition to tuberculous mycobacterial diseases. Nat Immunol 12: 213–21.
24. Hambleton S, Salem S, Bustamante J, Bigley V, Boisson-Dupuis S, et al. Mutations in IRF8 and human dendritic cells immunodeficiency. N Engl J Med, in press.
25. Altare F, Ensser A, Breiman A, Reichenbach J, Baghdadi JE, et al. (2001) Interleukin-12 receptor beta1 deficiency in a patient with abdominal tuberculosis. J Infect Dis 184: 231–6.
26. Caragol I, Raspall M, Fieschi C, Feinberg J, Larrosa MN, et al. (2003) Clinical tuberculosis in 2 of 3 siblings with interleukin-12 receptor beta1 deficiency. Clin Infect Dis 37: 302–6.
27. Ozbek N, Fieschi C, Yilmaz BT, de Beaucoudrey L, Demirhan B, et al. (2005) Interleukin-12 receptor beta 1 chain deficiency in a child with disseminated tuberculosis. Clin Infect Dis 40: e55–8.
28. Fieschi C, Dupuis S, Catherinot E, Feinberg J, Bustamante J, et al. (2003) Low penetrance, broad resistance, and favorable outcome of interleukin 12 receptor beta1 deficiency: medical and immunological implications. J Exp Med 197: 527–35.
29. De Beaucoudrey L, Samarina A, Bustamante J, Cobat A, Boisson-Dupuis S, et al. (2010) Revisiting human IL12RB1 deficiency: a survey of 141 patients from 30 countries. Medicine 89: 381–402.
30. Sanal O, Turkkani G, Gumruk F, Yel L, Secmeer G, et al. (2007) A case of interleukin-12 receptor beta-1 deficiency with recurrent leishmaniasis. Pediatr Infect Dis J 26: 366–8.
31. Tabarsi P, Marjani M, Mansouri N, Farnia P, Boisson-Dupuis S, et al. Lethal tuberculosis in a previously healthy adult with IL-12 receptor deficiency. J Clin Immunol, in press.
32. Holland SM (2000) Treatment of infections in the patient with Mendelian susceptibility to mycobacterial infection. Microbes Infect 2: 1579–90.
33. Alangari AA, Al-Zamil F, Al-Mazrou A, Al-Muhsen S, Boisson-Dupuis S, et al. (2011) Treatment of disseminated mycobacterial infection with high dose IFN-g in a patient with IL-12Rb1 deficiency. Clin Dev Immunol 2011: 691956.
34. Jouanguy E, Lamhamedi-Cherradi S, Lammas D, Dorman SE, Fondanèche MC, et al. (1999) A human IFNGR1 small deletion hotspot associated with dominant susceptibility to mycobacterial infection. Nat Genet 21: 370–8.
35. Rosenzweig SD, Dorman SE, Uzel G, Shaw S, Scurlock A, et al. (2004) A novel mutation in IFN-gamma receptor 2 with dominant negative activity: biological consequences of homozygous and heterozygous states. J Immunol 173: 4000–8.
36. Dupuis S, Dargemont C, Fieschi C, Thomassin N, Rosenzweig S, et al. (2001) Impairment of mycobacterial but not viral immunity by a germline human STAT1 mutation. Science 293: 300–3.
37. Chapgier A, Boisson-Dupuis S, Jouanguy E, Vogt G, Feinberg J, et al. (2006) Novel STAT1 alleles in otherwise healthy patients with mycobacterial disease. PLoS Genet 2: e131.
38. Ng SB, Buckingham KJ, Lee C, Bigham AW, Tabor HK, et al. (2010) Exome sequencing identifies the cause of a Mendelian disorder. Nat Genet 42: 30–5.
39. Bolze A, Byun M, McDonald D, Morgan NV, Abhyankar A, et al. (2010) Whole-exome-sequencing-based discovery of human FADD deficiency. Am J Hum Genet 87: 873–81.
40. Byun M, Abhyankar A, Lelarge V, Plancoulaine S, Palanduz A, et al. (2010) Whole-exome sequencing-based discovery of STIM1 deficiency in a child with fatal classic Kaposi sarcoma. J Exp Med 207: 2307–12.
41. Tadmouri GO, Nair P, Obeid T, Al Ali MT Al Khaja N, et al. (2009) Consanguinity and reproductive health among Arabs. Reproductive Health 6: 17.

4

Post-Pandemic Seroprevalence of Pandemic Influenza A (H1N1) 2009 Infection (Swine Flu) among Children <18 Years in Germany

Rüdiger von Kries[1,9], Susanne Weiss[1,9], Gerhard Falkenhorst[2], Stephan Wirth[3], Petra Kaiser[4], Hans-Iko Huppertz[4], Tobias Tenenbaum[5], Horst Schroten[5], Andrea Streng[6], Johannes Liese[6], Sonu Shai[7], Tim Niehues[7], Hermann Girschick[8], Ellen Kuscher[9], Axel Sauerbrey[9], Jochen Peters[10], Carl Heinz Wirsing von König[11], Simon Rückinger[1], Walter Hampl[12], Detlef Michel[12], Thomas Mertens[1,2]*

1 Institut für Soziale Pädiatrie und Jugendmedizin, Ludwig-Maximilians-Universität, München, Germany, **2** Abteilung für Infektionsepidemiologie, Robert Koch-Institut, Berlin, Germany, **3** Zentrum für Kinder- und Jugendmedizin, Helios Klinikum - Universität Witten/Herdecke, Wuppertal, Germany, **4** Professor-Hess-Kinderklinik, Klinikum Bremen-Mitte, Bremen, Germany, **5** Universitätskinderklinik, Universität Heidelberg, Mannheim, Germany, **6** Universitätskinderklinik, Würzburg, Germany, **7** Helios Klinikum, Krefeld, Germany, **8** Klinik für Kinder- und Jugendmedizin, Vivantes Klinikum im Friedrichshain, Berlin, Germany, **9** Helios Klinikum, Erfurt, Germany, **10** Abteilung für Kinder- und Jugendmedizin, Klinikum Dritter Orden, München-Nymphenburg, Germany, **11** Institut für Hygiene und Laboratoriumsmedizin, Helios Klinikum, Krefeld, Germany, **12** Institut für Virologie, Universitätsklinikum, Ulm, Germany

Abstract

Background: We determined antibodies to the pandemic influenza A (H1N1) 2009 virus in children to assess: the incidence of (H1N1) 2009 infections in the 2009/2010 season in Germany, the proportion of subclinical infections and to compare titers in vaccinated and infected children.

Methodology/Principal Findings: Eight pediatric hospitals distributed over Germany prospectively provided sera from in- or outpatients aged 1 to 17 years from April 1st to July 31st 2010. Vaccination history, recall of infections and sociodemographic factors were ascertained. Antibody titers were measured with a sensitive and specific in-house hemagglutination inhibition test (HIT) and compared to age-matched sera collected during 6 months before the onset of the pandemic in Germany. We analyzed 1420 post-pandemic and 300 pre-pandemic sera. Among unvaccinated children aged 1–4 and 5–17 years the prevalence of HI titers (≥1:10) was 27.1% (95% CI: 23.5–31.3) and 53.5% (95% CI: 50.9–56.2) compared to 1.7% and 5.5%, respectively, for pre-pandemic sera, accounting for a serologically determined incidence of influenza A (H1N1) 2009 during the season 2009/2010 of 25,4% (95% CI : 19.3–30.5) in children aged 1–4 years and 48.0% (95% CI: 42.6–52.0) in 5–17 year old children. Of children with HI titers ≥1:10, 25.5% (95% CI: 22.5–28.8) reported no history of any infectious disease since June 2009. Among vaccinated children, 92% (95%-CI: 87.0–96.6) of the 5–17 year old but only 47.8% (95%-CI: 33.5–66.5) of the 1–4 year old children exhibited HI titers against influenza A virus (H1N1) 2009.

Conclusion: Serologically determined incidence of influenza A (H1N1) 2009 infections in children indicates high infection rates with older children (5–17 years) infected twice as often as younger children. In about a quarter of the children with HI titers after the season 2009/2010 subclinical infections must be assumed. Low HI titers in young children after vaccination with the $AS03_B$-adjuvanted split virion vaccine need further scrutiny.

Editor: Benjamin J. Cowling, University of Hong Kong, Hong Kong

Funding: These authors have no support or funding to report.

Competing Interests: The authors have declared that no competing interests exist.

* E-mail: thomas.mertens@uniklinik-ulm.de

9 These authors contributed equally to this work.

Introduction

In Germany, a total of approximately 223,000 laboratory-confirmed symptomatic cases of pandemic influenza A (H1N1) 2009 infections have been notified from April 1st 2009 until March 31st 2010, accounting for a cumulative incidence of 272 per 100,000. Extrapolation from the 78% of notifications with age information yields an incidence of 468 and 1,110 per 100,000 in age groups 1 to 4 years and 5 to 17 years, respectively. The main wave of the pandemic occurred in weeks 43 to 51 of 2009 (unpublished data, Robert Koch-Institute, Berlin, Germany).

Vaccination with a monovalent $AS03_B$-adjuvanted H1N1-vaccine (Pandemrix®, GSK Pharma GmbH, Munich, Germany) was offered for persons at risk in Germany as of week 44, 2009. For adults and adolescents ≥14 years, ultimate vaccination coverage has been estimated at ~8% on the basis of population-wide telephone surveys [1]. Data on vaccination coverage for <14 year old children are not available.

Seroprevalence studies of antibodies against A (H1N1) 2009 performed after the end of the 2009/2010 influenza season allow for a much better estimation of the cumulative incidence of pandemic A (H1N1) 2009 infections than case surveillance data if corrected for vaccination status [2]. Such data also allow to assess the current proportion of individuals with at least partial protection against A (H1N1) 2009. The proportion of subclinical infections can be estimated if a history of symptomatic infections is documented.

Seroprevalence studies in children are of particular interest since children are supposed to be the driving force of the influenza pandemic [2–5]. Although several seroprevalence studies of A (H1N1) 2009 antibodies have been published [6] there are few studies which include children [2,7,8] and only one also considering vaccination and flu-like disease history as well [7]. No study has compared antibodies against A (H1N1) 2009 after confirmed clinical disease and vaccination with pandemic vaccine in children.

We performed a multi-centre seroprevalence study on children in Germany 1) to assess the incidence of A (H1N1) 2009 infections in the 2009/2010 season, 2) to identify the proportion of subclinical A (H1N1) 2009 infections, and 3) to compare HI antibody titers in vaccinated children and in children after natural infection.

Results

Study population

1555 serum samples and 1511 questionnaires were collected. Fourteen hemolytic sera could not be analyzed and 52 questionnaires were excluded because essential data were missing or children were outside age limits. Merging of the remaining 1541 sera and 1459 questionnaires resulted in 1420 cases, with 373 children (26.3%) 1 to 4 years and 1047 children (73.7%) 5 to 17 years (see table 1). This corresponds to the overall distribution of these age groups in Germany (1–4: 21.2%; 5–17: 78.8%) [9]. The 8 participating hospitals were distributed nationwide.

In the total sample boys and girls were evenly distributed. 84.1% of the children attended school or kindergarten. 70.5% of all children reported a history of one or more infectious disease episodes since June 2009. Influenza A (H1N1) 2009 was suspected by a physician in 97 children (6.8%) and was virologically diagnosed in 25 children (1.8%). Vaccination against seasonal influenza in 2009/2010 or in previous years was reported in 15.7% of all children. Vaccination against influenza A (H1N1) 2009 was reported for 101 of the 1420 children (7.1%).

Hemagglutination inhibition test results - unvaccinated children

Pre-pandemic (control) sera. The pre- and post-pandemic HI titers and the incidence estimates for A (H1N1) 2009 infection based on the difference between post- and pre-pandemic titers are depicted in table 2.

Of the 300 control sera only 2 (1.7%) children <5 years had detectable antibodies in HIT (one child 1:10 and the second child 1:40). In the older age group 10 HIT-positive children were detected (5.5%) including one titer of 1:80 (table 2). To analyze whether these pre-pandemic titers corresponded to high antibody titers against the most recent seasonal influenza A virus (A/Brisbane/59/2007(H1N1)) we tested the sera which were positive for antibodies against the pandemic A (H1N1) 2009 also for

Table 1. Characteristics of the post-pandemic samples.

Variable	Subcategory	Not vaccinated against A(H1N1)2009	Vaccinated against A(H1N1)2009	Unknown vaccination status against A(H1N1)2009	Total
		N = 1307	**N = 101**	**N = 12**	**N = 1420**
		n (column%)	**n (column%)**	**n (column%)**	**n (column%)**
Age	1–4 years	347 (26.6)	23 (22.8)	3 (25.0)	373 (26.3)
	5–17 years	960 (73.4)	78 (77.2)	9 (75.0)	1047 (73.7)
Sex	Male	610 (46.7)	60 (59.4)	3 (25.0)	673 (47.4)
	Female	675 (51.6)	40 (39.6)	9 (75.0)	724 (51.0)
	Missing values	22 (1.7)	1 (1.0)	0 (0.0)	23 (1.6)
(Pre-)school attendance	Yes	1097 (83.9)	89 (88.1)	8 (66.7)	1194 (84.1)
	No	201 (15.4)	11 (10.9)	4 (33.3)	216 (15.2)
	Missing values	9 (0.7)	1 (1.0)	0 (0.0)	10 (0.7)
History of infections	No infection	374 (28.6)	19 (18.8)	3 (25.0)	396 (27.9)
	>=1 infection	914 (69.9)	78 (77.2)	9 (75.0)	1001 (70.5)
	Missing values	19 (1.5)	4 (4.0)	0 (0.0)	23 (1.6)
Diagnosis of A(H1N1) 2009	As suspected by physician	91 (7.0)	6 (5.9)	0 (0.0)	97 (6.8)
	Lab-confirmed	25 (1.9)	0 (0.0)	0 (0.0)	25 (1.8)
	No diagnosis	1030 (78.8)	80 (79.2)	10 (83.3)	1120 (78.9)
	Missing values	161 (12.3)	15 (14.9)	2 (16.7)	178 (12.5)
Seasonal vaccine*	Yes	176 (13.5)	43 (42.6)	4 (33.3)	223 (15.7)
	No	1109 (84.8)	53 (52.5)	3 (25.0)	1165 (82.0)
	Missing values	22 (1.7)	5 (4.9)	5 (41.7)	32 (2.3)

*children having been vaccinated against the seasonal influenza.

Table 2. Pre-and post-pandemic hemagglutination inhibition titers (HIT) ≥1:10 and ≥1:40 for non-vaccinated children aged 1 to 17 years.

HIT	Age-group	Pre-pandemic controls		Post-pandemic samples		Difference: post – pre		
		n/N	(%)	n/N	(%)	(%)	95%CI Lower Limit (%)	95%CI Upper Limit (%)
>=1:10	1–4	2/119	1.7	94/347	27.1	**25.4**	19.3	30.5
	5–17	10/181	5.5	514/960	53.5	**48.0**	42.6	52.0
	all	12/300	4.0	607/1307	46.5	**42.4**	38.5	45.6
>=1:40	1–4	1/119	0.8	80/347	23.1	**22.2**	16.6	27.0
	5–17	4/181	2.2	330/960	34.4	**32.2**	27.7	35.5
	all	5/300	1.7	410/1307	31.4	**29.7**	26.4	32.4

CI = Confidence Interval.

antibodies against this seasonal influenza virus. Four of the 12 children exhibiting antibodies against the pandemic A (H1N1) 2009 were negative for antibodies against the seasonal influenza A virus (geometric mean titer 1:27). By testing additional 96 pre-pandemic sera for antibodies against the seasonal H1N1 virus we found 48.9% positive (geometric mean titer 1:29) and no association between pandemic and seasonal H1N1 titers (Spearman correlation coefficient 0.068, p-value 0.51).

Post-pandemic sera. Of 1307 children not vaccinated with Pandemrix®, HI titers of 1:10 or above were detectable in 607 (46.5%, 95% CI: 44.3–48.8). This percentage was lower for children aged 1 to 4 years (27.1%, 95% CI: 23.5–31.3) and higher for children aged 5 to 17 years (53.5%, 95% CI: 50.9–56.2), p-value<0.0001 (figure 1 and table 2), with no difference between boys and girls.

Logistic regression revealed a higher probability of detectable HI titers by higher age and an influenza A (H1N1) 2009 infection suspected by a physician or diagnosed by virological testing. Except for a lower proportion of children with any detectable HI titers in one center (Berlin) we observed no significant regional variability. School or kindergarten attendance was not associated with HI titers.

More than 40% of the children (13.7%+30.3% = 44.0%; 95%-CI: 39.5–48.9) who had reported no infection since June 2009 had HI titers of ≥1:10. In contrast all 25 children with virologically proven A (H1N1) 2009 infection exhibited a positive HI titer with 80% ≥1:40. Of the children with HI titers ≥1:10 25.5% (95% CI: 22.5–28.8) reported no history of any infectious disease since June 2009 (table 3: (91+41)/(41+95+23+5+91+198+45+20)).

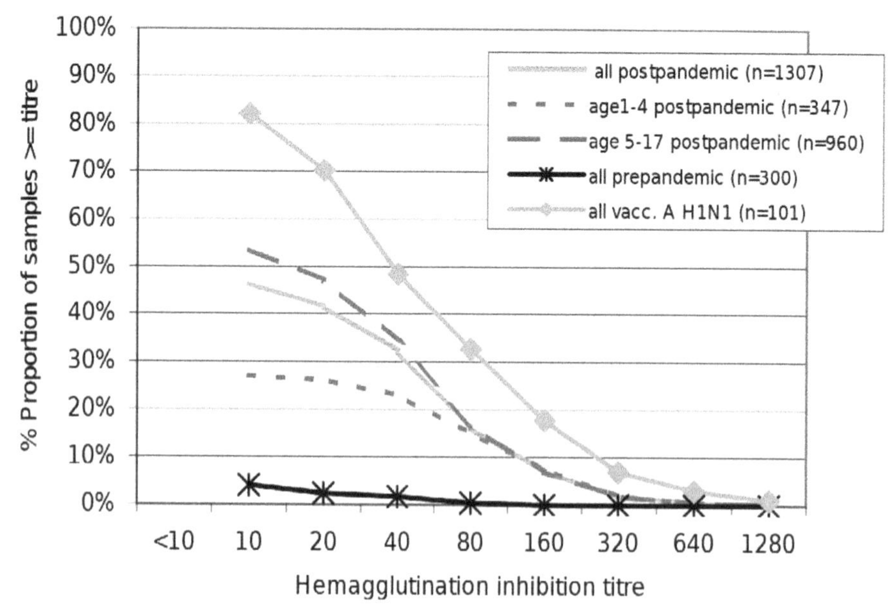

Figure 1. Reverse cumulative distribution curves of hemagglutination inhibition titers for antibodies against influenza A (H1N1) 2009 virus for different strata. Post-pandemic children not vaccinated against influenza A (H1N1) 2009 aged 1–17, thereof 347 aged 1–4 and 960 aged 5–17 were tested and in addition 300 pre-pandemic controls and 101 children vaccinated against influenza A (H1N1) 2009. Children aged 1–4 exhibit lower titers compared to children aged 5–17 and all post-pandemic cases. Titers of pre-pandemic children aged 1–17 are distinctly lower. Children vaccinated against A (H1N1) 2009 exhibit higher titers compared to post-pandemic children having been infected with A (H1N1).

Table 3. History of infections and hemagglutination inhibition titers (HIT) in non-vaccinated children.

HIT		History of infections: No infection reported*	History of infections: One or more infections**	Diagnosis of A(H1N1)2009: Suspected by physician	Diagnosis of A(H1N1)2009: Virologically confirmed	Cumulative missings***	Sum
<1:10	n	168	424	21	0	87	700
	Column% (95%CI)	56.0 (51.4–60.8)	59.1 (56.2–62.2)	23.6 (17.4–32.2)	0.00 (0.2–1.13)	49.4 (43.6–55.9)	
1:10 or 1:20	n	41	95	23	5	33	197
	Column% (95%CI)	13.7 (10.8–17.4)	13.2 (11.3–15.5)	25.8 (19.3–34.6)	20.0 (11.0–37.5)	18.8 (14.6–24.3)	
>=1:40	n	91	198	45	20	56	410
	Column% (95%CI)	30.3 (26.3–35.0)	27.6 (25.0–30.5)	50.6 (42.5–59.7)	80.0 (67.0–91.8)	31.8 (26.6–38.1)	
Total		300	717	89	25	176****	1307

*"Infection" was defined as any infection, since the clinical picture of flu in children may not be confined to typical symptoms of upper or lower respiratory tract infection.
**without suspected or confirmed diagnosis of A (H1N1) 2009.
***Cumulative missing values in "history of infections" or/and "diagnosis of A (H1N1) 2009".
****There were 161 children with missing values for the variable "diagnosis of A (H1N1)" (no such diagnosis; suspected by physician; lab-confirmed) and an additional 19 children with missing values in "history of infections" (no infection; one or more infection) (see table 1). Four children had missing values regarding both variables, therefore the total of missing values was 176 (161+19−4=176).

Hemagglutination inhibition test results – vaccinated children and children after laboratory-confirmed influenza A (H1N1) 2009 infection

All 6 children 1 to 4 years old (100%, 95% CI: 61.0–100) with a history of laboratory-confirmed A (H1N1) 2009 infection exhibited HI titers of 1:80 or above (dashed dark line in figure 2), but only 11 of 23 children in this age group (47.8%, 95% CI: 33.5–66.5) who reported vaccination with Pandemrix® had HI titers ≥1:10, and 21.7% (95% CI: 12.0–40.4) had HI titers ≥1:40 (dark line). The differences between HI titers in children aged 1 to 4 years after natural infection and after vaccination were statistically significant (Kolmogorov-Smirnov test for difference between two curves, p-value: 0.003). For children aged 5 to 17 years no such statistically significant difference (grey dashed line = natural infection; dotted line = vaccinated) was observed (Kolmogorov-Smirnov test, p-value: 0.752).

In addition antibody titers in children vaccinated with Pandemrix® aged 1 to 4 years (dark black line) were significantly lower than in vaccinated children aged 5 to 17 years (grey dotted line) (Kolmogorov-Smirnov test, p-value: 0.0002). In contrast, after natural infection higher titers were observed in the younger children as compared to the older age group. The numbers, however, are small and the difference was not statistically significant (Kolmogorov-Smirnov test, p-value: 0.0941).

There appeared to be an inverse association between the geometric mean HI titers against the A (H1N1) 2009 influenza

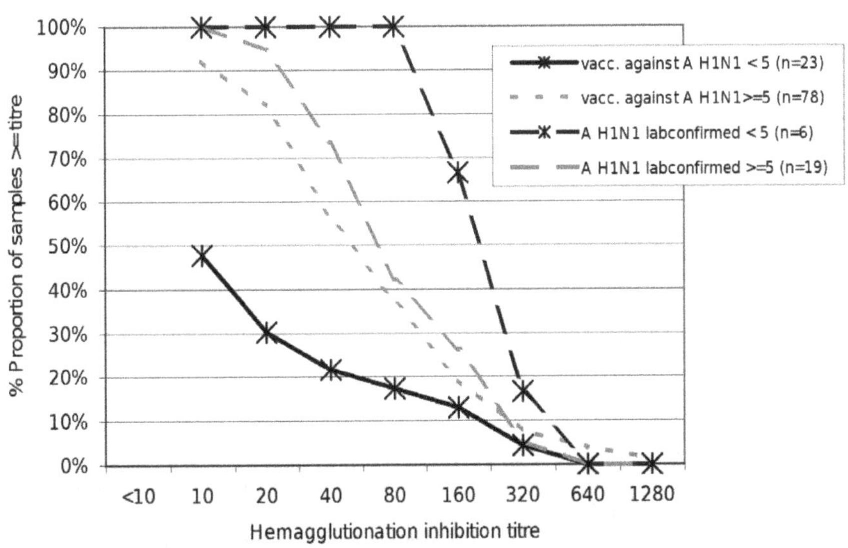

Figure 2. Reverse cumulative distribution curves of children vaccinated against the A (H1N1) 2009 virus <5 years (n = 23), >= 5 years (n = 78) and in children with laboratory-confirmed A (H1N1) 2009 infection <5 years (n = 6), >= 5 years (n = 19). Vaccinated children and children with laboratory-confirmed A (H1N1) infection were mutually exclusive. Children vaccinated against the A (H1N1) 2009 virus exhibit lower titers compared to children with laboratory-confirmed A (H1N1) 2009 infection. This can be observed in both age groups with greater difference in younger children.

virus and previous vaccination with seasonal influenza vaccine. In children vaccinated both with the seasonal and the pandemic vaccine the OR for HI titers ≥1:40 was 0.68; 95% CI 0.46–1.01) compared to children vaccinated with the pandemic vaccine alone.

Discussion

Comparison of seroprevalence against influenza A (H1N1) 2009 in pre- and post-pandemic sera indicates that about a quarter of the unvaccinated preschool (1–4 years) and almost half of the unvaccinated school age children (5–17 years) were infected with influenza A (H1N1) 2009 during the pandemic in Germany. A titer of ≥1:40, usually considered "protective" (i.e. associated with >50% reduction of the risk of contracting influenza) [10], was observed in 23% of preschool and 36% of school age children, taken together vaccinated and unvaccinated (figure 1). A history of pandemic influenza vaccination was reported for ~7% of participating children, a percentage similar to the existing estimate of ~8% for persons >14 years in Germany [11]. HI titers ≥1:40 in as little as 22% of vaccinated children aged 1 to 4 years approximately 4–8 months after vaccination point to a need for further evaluation of the immune response to adjuvanted influenza vaccines in young children although there is a possibility that this is due to chance given that there were only 23 vaccinated children and 6 children with lab-confirmed A (H1N1) 2009 infection <5 years.

The incidence of A (H1N1) 2009 infections in children and adolescents in Germany was similar to those reported from the UK (after first wave) [2] and New Zealand [7], but somewhat lower than after the second wave in UK [8]. As in these studies, we found a considerably higher incidence of infections in school age compared to preschool children, which also corresponds to the reported age-specific incidence of infections from surveillance data in Germany (unpublished data of the Robert Koch-Institute).

Approximately 25% of children with detectable antibodies against A (H1N1) 2009 reported no history of any infectious disease episode during the pandemic influenza season. Disease history in our study is based on parents' or participants' recollection over a period of several months and may therefore not be fully reliable. It is likely that mild events of disease may not have been recalled which would result in an overestimation of subclinical infections. On the other hand, reported infection episodes may have been unrelated to influenza A (H1N1) 2009, which means the proportion of subclinical A (H1N1) 2009 infections could have been even higher. In the study from New Zealand [7], the proportion of subclinical infections was estimated as 45% (for all ages). Smaller studies among contact persons of confirmed cases found proportions of subclinical infections between 9% and 73% [12–14].

In Germany the pandemic vaccine became gradually available starting from the last week of October 2009. While two doses had been recommended initially, the official vaccination recommendation for children (as well as for adults) was changed from a two dose to a single dose regimen as of December 14th 2009 [15]. The vaccine used was an AS03B-adjuvanted split virus vaccine (3.75 μg hemagglutinin) with a half dose recommended for children aged 6 months to 9 years. The lower antibody titers observed in our study in young compared to older children after vaccination are unlikely to be explained by chance. Differential misclassification of the vaccination history against the pandemic influenza virus by the children's age is unlikely. Although we have not ascertained the number of vaccine doses, most children had presumably received one dose only, because by the time the second dose was due (≥3 weeks after the first dose), a second dose was no longer recommended. It remains unclear whether this vaccination regimen is the reason for the lower antibody titers in the young children. Concern regarding a possibly weaker immune response in young children has also been raised for the non-adjuvanted pandemic influenza vaccines [3,16]. Available evidence suggests high seroconversion rates in young children after two doses of AS03B-adjuvanted split virus vaccine (UK) [17] and possibly also after one dose (Spain) [18].

Clinical vaccine effectiveness, however, has been demonstrated for one dose of the vaccine in persons ≥14 years and most recently for children as well [19–21]. In young children, however, vaccine effectiveness appeared to be lower than in adolescents and the 95% CI was wide [21].

For children who had been vaccinated with a seasonal vaccine in previous years, titers after vaccination with the pandemic vaccine were somewhat, but not significantly lower. A similar finding was recently observed in a vaccine effectiveness study of the AS03 adjuvanted influenza A (H1N1) 2009 vaccine for adults [22,23].

This seroprevalence study was performed with an optimized in-house hemagglutination inhibition test which gave clear and highly reproducible results and allowed to determine titers of 1:10 against influenza virus A (H1N1) 2009. We decided not to use a micro neutralization test in addition since the HIT is widely accepted as reference test for detection of subtype-specific influenza antibodies and the inter-assay and inter-laboratory reproducibility and standardization is better for HIT than for micro neutralization ([24,25] and unpublished own data). Furthermore it has been shown in multiple studies that there is a good overall correlation between the results of the two assays for H1N1 [2,8,24].

Instead we optimized the HIT-SOP to reach a high specificity without loosing relevant sensitivity. We found much fewer HIT positive results in the pre-pandemic sera than other studies, where arbitrary cutoffs of 1:32 or 1:40 had to be introduced [2,24, 26,27,28]. We detected only 12 of the 300 control sera repeatedly positive for A (H1N1) 2009 influenza virus antibodies and only 2 in the younger age group of 1 to 4 years, while in the study group all children with virologically proven pandemic A (H1N1) 2009 infection exhibited mainly high antibody titers. Additionally, in a subsample of the control and study sera no correlation between antibodies against seasonal A/Brisbane/59/2007(H1N1) and antibodies against A (H1N1) 2009 influenza was found [28]. Therefore a simple cross reactivity at least between the antibodies against these two H1N1 influenza viruses can be excluded [27]. The prevalence of antibodies against seasonal A H3N2 was very low in sera from the study and control group (data not shown).

The external reference serum pool obtained from the National Institute for Biological Standards and Control (NIBSC), with a defined titer after multi-laboratory testing as 1:180, however, absolutely reproducibly yielded a titer of 1:80 (i.e. practically one twofold dilution lower) in our test. Although the titers determined by our method are slightly lower (one twofold dilution) than determined by other HIT-SOPs, we did not change our method because we had no indication for false negative results and we wanted to minimize false positive results.

In order to allow for a valid estimation of the incidence of A (H1N1) 2009 during the 2009/2010 season we accepted only pre-pandemic sera that were collected within 6 month before onset of the A (H1N1) 2009 pandemic in Germany, thereby assuring that the seasonal influenza virus A experience was as similar as possible in both groups and that the relevance of waning antibody titers was minimized. Within the age groups 1 to 4 and 5 to 17 years the numbers of pre- and post-pandemic sera were collected proportionally by age in order to assure structural homogeneity.

Serum samples from children attending medical care for seroprevalence studies on pandemic influenza, as also used in a recent study from the UK [2], may not be fully representative. A population-based study in children with possibly higher representativity, however, might be fraught with selection bias in case families with a presumed history of influenza A infection were more likely to participate.

In conclusion, serologically determined incidence of influenza A (H1N1) 2009 infections in children indicates overall high infection rates, with older children (5–17 years) infected twice as often as children between 1 and 4 years. In about a quarter of the children with HI titers after the season 2009/2010 subclinical infections must be assumed. Our study provides the first estimate of post-pandemic population partial immunity in this age group in Germany. The observed low HI titers in young children after vaccination with the $AS03_B$-adjuvanted split virion vaccine need further scrutiny.

Methods

Serum and data collection

Eight German pediatric primary care hospitals (Bremen, Berlin, Krefeld, Wuppertal, Erfurt, Würzburg, Mannheim, München) provided sera from April 1st to July 31st 2010 obtained during blood withdrawal for routine laboratory testing from in- or outpatients aged 1 to 17 years. Children with an illness impeding an adequate immune response were excluded, so were children with serious conditions. Eligible children and their parents were informed about the study with age-adapted study descriptions and asked for their written consent. The study was approved by the Ethics Committee of the Bavarian Medical Association.

The following data were collected on a one-page questionnaire filled in by the parents: age and sex of the child, history of infectious disease episodes since June 2009, history of "swine flu" by physician's tentative clinical diagnosis vs. laboratory-confirmed diagnosis, history of pandemic or seasonal influenza vaccination, and kindergarten/school attendance. Questionnaires were sent to the study office in Munich and double-entered into a common data base.

Minimum 400 µl serum samples were sent by cool pack to the virological study laboratory in Ulm for determination of antibody titers. Questionnaires and serum samples were labeled with corresponding anonymous serial numbers. Laboratory staff was not aware of the data collected on the serum donors. Serological results and questionnaire data were linked after the end of the serological testing only.

Pre-pandemic samples

300 control sera for the study were taken from the frozen stored sera bank of the virological institute in Ulm, originally sent for routine virological diagnostic. The sera were selected according to two criteria: 1) the respective blood samples had to be collected between November 2008 and April 2009 and 2) for the age groups 1 to 4 and 5 to 17 years the numbers of pre-pandemic sera were proportionally to the age distribution of sera in the post-pandemic study sample.

Laboratory procedures

For determination of the antibody responses an in-house hemagglutination inhibition test (HIT) was established in Ulm to minimize non-A (H1N1) 2009- specific results [11,24,29]. During establishment of the HIT different buffers, protein additions, and erythrocytes from different species in different concentrations and receptor destroying enzymes (RDE) were evaluated [26].

The study and control sera were tested using the optimized HIT standard operation procedure (SOP). To destroy non-specific inhibitors of influenza virus hemagglutination sera were pretreated with RDE (DENKA Seiken CO Ltd, Tokyo, Japan) [26]. RDE was reconstituted with H_2O and stored frozen in aliquots (100 µl). Before usage RDE stock solution was diluted 1:20 in 0.9% NaCl. 50 µl Serum was mixed with 100 µl RDE and incubated 16–18 h at 37°C. After inactivation 30 min at 56°C, 350 µl hepes saline albumine (HSA, 0.14 M NaCl, 0.025 M hepes, 0.001 M CaCl2+1%BSA (before usage), pH 6.2–6.3) was added (1:10 serum dilution). Two fold serial dilutions (25 µl) of sera were performed using HSA+1% BSA in microtiter plates (round bottom). Influenza-A virus antigens (pandemic A/California/7/2009 (H1N1), seasonal A/Uruguay/716/2007 (H3N2), seasonal A/Brisbane/59/2007 (H1N1), all GlaxoSmithKline, Dresden, Germany) were diluted after HI pre-testing to obtain a solution containing 4 hemagglutinating units (HU). After addition of 25 µl antigen, shaking, and incubation (30 min, room temperature (RT)) 50 µl newborn chicken erythrocytes (Laboratory Dr. Merk&Kollegen, Ochsenhausen, Germany) (0.5% in HSA) were added, plates shaken again, incubated (2 h, RT) and read by 2 independent evaluators using a magnification lens (×10). The titer is defined as the highest serum dilution showing complete inhibition of the agglutination of erythrocytes. A serum control for every serum without addition of antigen and positive (1:80), low positive (1:10) and negative (1:<10) control sera were included for every test. An external reference serum pool was obtained from the Health Protection Agency National Institute for Biological Standards and Control (NIBSC), UK, and used to validate our internal positive control sera. Test results were accepted if the back titration of antigen revealed 4 HU and the control sera yielded correct results. Sera showing non-specific hemagglutination were tested again after absorption (1 h at 4°C) with 50 µl of 40% newborn chicken erythrocyte suspension in HSA. For determination of sensitivity and specificity of our HIT we used the 300 pre-pandemic sera (true negative) and 47 sera available from our diagnostic laboratory at that time including 11 Ulm patients with virologically proven pandemic A (H1N1) 2009 infection and 36 vaccinated co-workers (true positive). Sensitivity was 1.00 and specificity 0.96 for titer ≥1:10. With 14 hemolytic study sera HI titer could not be determined.

Statistical analysis

Reverse cumulative distribution curves were calculated to compare proportions above different threshold hemagglutination inhibition titers for unvaccinated children (by age groups 1–4 years and 5–17 years and for children with laboratory-confirmed A (H1N1) 2009 infection), for children vaccinated against A (H1N1) 2009 and for controls.

Logistic regression models were used to examine differences in HI titers according to age, sex, region, history of infections since June 2009, vaccination against seasonal influenza and kindergarten/school attendance. Chi-square and Kolmogorov-Smirnov tests were used to compare HI titers between different strata of children.

To estimate the incidence of A (H1N1) 2009 infection during the 2009/2010 pandemic in Germany we calculated the difference between the proportion of sera with a HIT titer >1:10 in pre- and post-pandemic samples. Additional evaluations were done using an arbitrary cut-off of ≥1:40 titer, generally assumed to indicate protection. Confidence intervals for the difference in proportion of children achieving titers ≥1:10 and ≥1:40 pre-and post-pandemic were calculated using the Newcombe-Wilson method [30].

All statistical analyses were done with SAS 9.2 and Excel 2003.

Acknowledgments

The excellent assistance of Marlies Just, Claudia Ploil, Thomas Schmid and Ingrid Bennett is highly and most thankfully acknowledged.

Author Contributions

Conceived and designed the experiments: RvK S. Weiss GF S. Wirth PK H-IH TT HS A. Streng JL SS TN HG EK A. Sauerbrey JP CWvK SR WH DM TM. Performed the experiments: TM WH DM. Analyzed the data: RvK S. Weiss SR. Contributed reagents/materials/analysis tools: GF PK H-IH TT HS A. Streng JL SS TN HG EK A. Sauerbrey JP CWvK. Wrote the paper: RvK S. Weiss TM.

References

1. Robert Koch-Institut (2010) Repräsentative telefonische Erhebung zur Impfung gegen die pandemische Influenza (H1N1) 2009. Epidemiol Bull 25: 237–244.
2. Miller E, Hoschler K, Hardelid P, Stanford E, Andrews N, et al. (2010) Incidence of 2009 pandemic influenza A H1N1 infection in England: a cross-sectional serological study. Lancet 375: 1100–1108.
3. Fiore AE, Neuzil KM (2010) 2009 influenza A(H1N1) monovalent vaccines for children. JAMA 303: 73–74.
4. UK Health Protection Agency (2009) Pandemic (H1N1) 2009 in England: an overview of initial epidemiological findings and implications for the second wave. HPA. pp 1–24.
5. Glasser J, Taneri D, Feng Z; Chuang J-H, Tüll P, et al. (2010) Evaluation of targeted influenza vaccination strategies via population modeling. PLoS One 5:pii: e12777.
6. WHO (2010) Seroepidemiological studies of pandemic influenza A (H1N1) 2009 virus. Wkly Epidemiol Rec 24: 229–236.
7. Bandaranayake D, Huang S, Bissielo A, Wood T (2010) Seroprevalence of the 2009 influenza A (H1N1) pandemic in New Zealand. NZ Ministry of Health. pp 1–31.
8. Hardelid P, Andrews NJ, Hoschler K, Stanford E, Baguelin M, et al. (2010) Assessment of baseline age-specific antibody prevalence and incidence of infection to novel influenza AHINI 2009. Health Technol Assess 14: 115–192.
9. Statistisches Bundesamt Deutschland (2008) Bevölkerungsfortschreibung 2008. Fachserie 1 Reihe 1.3: 1–54.
10. Eichelberger M, Golding H, Hess M, Weir J, Subbarao K, et al. (2008) FDA/NIH/WHO public workshop on immune correlates of protection against influenza A viruses in support of pandemic vaccine development, Bethesda, Maryland, US, December 10–11, 2007. Vaccine 26: 4299–4303.
11. Yoon KJ, Janke BH, Swalla RW, Erickson G (2004) Comparison of a commercial H1N1 enzyme-linked immunosorbent assay and hemagglutination inhibition test in detecting serum antibody against swine influenza viruses. J Vet Diagn Invest 16: 197–201.
12. Papenburg J, Baz M, Hamelin ME, Rhéaume C, Carbonneau J, et al. (2008) Household transmission of the 2009 pandemic A/H1N1 influenza virus: elevated laboratory-confirmed secondary attack rates and evidence of asymptomatic infections. Clin Infect Dis 51: 1033–1041.
13. Cowling BJ, Chan KH, Fang VJ, Lau LL, So HC, et al. (2010) Comparative epidemiology of pandemic and seasonal influenza A in households. N Engl J Med 362: 2175–2184.
14. Lee VJ, Yap J, Cook AR, Chen MI, Tay JK, et al. (2010) Effectiveness of public health measures in mitigating pandemic influenza spread: a prospective sero-epidemiological cohort study. J Infect Dis 202: 1319–1326.
15. Robert Koch-Institut, Paul-Ehrlich-Institut (2009) Ergänzende Hinweise des Paul-Ehrlich-Instituts und des Robert Koch-Instituts zur Impfung gegen die Neue Influenza A (H1N1). Epidemiol Bull 50: 519–524.
16. Plennevaux E, Sheldon E, Blatter M, Reeves-Hoche MK, Denis M (2010) Immune response after a single vaccination against 2009 influenza A H1N1 in USA: a preliminary report of two randomised controlled phase 2 trials. Lancet 375: 41–48.
17. Waddington CS, Walker WT, Oeser C, Reiner A, John T, et al. (2010) Safety and immunogenicity of AS03B adjuvanted split virion versus non-adjuvanted whole virion H1N1 influenza vaccine in UK children aged 6 months-12 years: open label, randomised, parallel group, multicentre study. BMJ 340: c2649.
18. Carmona A, Omenaca F, Tejedor JC, Merino JM, Vaman T, et al. (2010) Immunogenicity and safety of AS03-adjuvanted 2009 influenza A H1N1 vaccine in children 6–35 months. Vaccine 28: 5837–5844.
19. Van Buynder PG, Dhaliwal JK, Van Buynder JL, Couturier C, Minville-Leblanc M, et al. (2010) Protective effect of single-dose adjuvanted pandemic influenza vaccine in children. Influenza Other Respi Viruses 4: 171–178.
20. Wichmann O, Stocker P, Poggensee G, Altmann D, Walter D, et al. (2010) Pandemic influenza A(H1N1) 2009 breakthrough infections and estimates of vaccine effectiveness in Germany 2009–2010. Euro Surveill 15:pii: 19561.
21. Andrews N, Waight P, Yung CV, Miller E (2011) Age-specific efffectiveness of an oil-in-water adjuvanted pandemic (H1N1) 2009 vaccine against confirmed infection in high risk groups in England. J Infect Dis 203: 32–9.
22. Janjua NZ, Skowronski DM, Hottes TS, Osei W, Adams E, et al. (2010) Seasonal influenza vaccine and increased risk of pandemic A/H1N1-related illness: first detection of the association in British Columbia, Canada. Clin Infect Dis 51: 1017–1027.
23. Roman F, Vaman T, Kafeja F, Hanon E, Van DP (2010) AS03(A)-Adjuvanted influenza A (H1N1) 2009 vaccine for adults up to 85 years of age. Clin Infect Dis 51: 668–677.
24. Allwinn R, Geiler J, Berger A, Cinatl J, Doerr HW (2010) Determination of serum antibodies against swine-origin influenza A virus H1N1/09 by immunofluorescence, haemagglutination inhibition, and by neutralization tests: how is the prevalence rate of protecting antibodies in humans? Med Microbiol Immunol 199: 117–121.
25. Stephenson I, Heath A, Major D, Newman RW, Hoschler K, et al. (2009) Reproducibility of serologic assays for influenza virus A (H5N1). Emerg Infect Dis 15: 1252–1259.
26. Tandale BV, Pawar SD, Gurav YK, Chadha MS, Koratkar SS, et al. (2010) Seroepidemiology of pandemic influenza A (H1N1) 2009 virus infections in Pune, India. BMC Infect Dis 10: 255.
27. Rizzo C, Rota MC, Bella A, Alfonsi V, Declich S, et al. (2010) Cross-reactive antibody responses to the 2009 A/H1N1v influenza virus in the Italian population in the pre-pandemic period. Vaccine 28: 3558–3562.
28. Zimmer SM, Crevar CJ, Carter DM, Stark JH, Giles BM, et al. (2010) Seroprevalence following the second wave of Pandemic 2009 H1N1 influenza in Pittsburgh, PA, USA. PLoS One 5: e11601.
29. Webster R, Cox N, Stöhr K (2002) WHO Manual on Animal Influenza Diagnosis and Surveillance. CDS/CSR/NCS 2002.5: 1–105.
30. Newcombe RG (1998) Interval estimation for the difference between independent proportions: comparison of eleven methods. Stat Med 17: 873–890.

5

Enhanced Pro-Inflammatory Cytokine Responses following Toll-Like-Receptor Ligation in *Schistosoma haematobium*-Infected Schoolchildren from Rural Gabon

Lynn Meurs[1*⑨], Lucja Labuda[2,3,4⑨], Abena Serwaa Amoah[5¶], Moustapha Mbow[6], Ulysse Ateba Ngoa[3,4], Daniel Adjei Boakye[5], Souleymane Mboup[6], Tandakha Ndiaye Dièye[6], Adrian P. Mountford[7], Joseph D. Turner[7], Peter Gottfried Kremsner[3,4], Katja Polman[1], Maria Yazdanbakhsh[2], Ayola Akim Adegnika[2,3,4]

1 Department of Biomedical Sciences, Institute of Tropical Medicine, Antwerp, Belgium, **2** Department of Parasitology, Leiden University Medical Center, Leiden, The Netherlands, **3** Medical Research Unit, Albert Schweitzer Hospital, Lambaréné, Gabon, **4** Institute of Tropical Medicine, University of Tübingen, Tübingen, Germany, **5** Department of Parasitology, Noguchi Memorial Institute for Medical Research, Accra, Ghana, **6** Laboratory of Immunology, Centre Hospitalier Universitaire Le Dantec, Dakar, Senegal, **7** Department of Biology, University of York, York, United Kingdom

Abstract

Background: *Schistosoma* infection is thought to lead to down-regulation of the host's immune response. This has been shown for adaptive immune responses, but the effect on innate immunity, that initiates and shapes the adaptive response, has not been extensively studied. In a first study to characterize these responses, we investigated the effect of *Schistosoma haematobium* infection on cytokine responses of Gabonese schoolchildren to a number of Toll-like receptor (TLR) ligands.

Methodology: Peripheral blood mononuclear cells (PBMCs) were collected from *S. haematobium*-infected and uninfected schoolchildren from the rural area of Zilé in Gabon. PBMCs were incubated for 24 h and 72 h with various TLR ligands, as well as schistosomal egg antigen (SEA) and adult worm antigen (AWA). Pro-inflammatory TNF-α and anti-inflammatory/regulatory IL-10 cytokine concentrations were determined in culture supernatants.

Principal Findings: Infected children produced higher adaptive IL-10 responses than uninfected children against schistosomal antigens (72 h incubation). On the other hand, infected children had higher TNF-α responses than uninfected children and significantly higher TNF-α to IL-10 ratios in response to FSL-1 and Pam3, ligands of TLR2/6 and TLR2/1 respectively. A similar trend was observed for the TLR4 ligand LPS while Poly(I:C) (Mda5/TLR3 ligand) did not induce substantial cytokine responses (24 h incubation).

Conclusions: This pilot study shows that *Schistosoma*-infected children develop a more pro-inflammatory TLR2-mediated response in the face of a more anti-inflammatory adaptive immune response. This suggests that *S. haematobium* infection does not suppress the host's innate immune system in the context of single TLR ligation.

Editor: Dominik Hartl, Ludwig-Maximilians-Universität München, Germany

Funding: This work was supported by the European Union's sixth framework programme (INCO-CT-2006-032405). Website: http://cordis.europa.eu/fp6/dc/index.cfm?fuseaction=UserSite.FP6HomePage. The funders had no role in study design, data collection and analysis, decision to publish, or preparation of the manuscript.

Competing Interests: The authors have declared that no competing interests exist.

* E-mail: lemurs@itg.be

⑨ These authors contributed equally to this work.

¶ These authors also contributed equally to this work.

Introduction

Schistosomiasis is a parasitic disease of major public health importance and is largely chronic in nature. The WHO estimates that more than 207 million people are infected worldwide [1,2]. Chronic helminth infections are generally assumed to cause down-regulation of immune responses allowing long-term survival of the parasite on the one hand and minimizing immune immunopathology on the other [3] with important consequences to the host's health [4–7]. Effects of schistosomal infection on adaptive immunity are widely studied in this context and it has been shown that chronic schistosomiasis inhibits *in vitro* proliferation of human lymphocytes in response to schistosomal antigens [8,9]. The anti-inflammatory cytokine interleukin (IL)-10 plays an important role in this down-regulation [10–14]. Van den Biggelaar and colleagues have demonstrated that children chronically infected with schistosomes produce more IL-10 together with IL-5 and IL-13 in response to adult worm antigen (AWA), than those free of *Schistosoma* infection [15]. Helminth-induced immunomodulation may also have an impact on other infections and vaccine effectiveness. For example, in filarial infections, IL-10 down-regulates responses to unrelated antigens such as tetanus toxoid

[16,17]. Similar mechanisms might explain the impaired reaction to tetanus toxoid observed in *Schistosoma mansoni*-infected individuals [18]. Another feature of IL-10 is that it might suppress atopy in *Schistosoma haematobium*-infected children [15,19].

Although it is becoming clearer how chronic schistosomiasis impacts on adaptive immune responses in terms of immunoregulation, the effects of schistosomal infection on innate immunity is a less studied area. In general, the innate immune system detects invading pathogens through a set of 'pattern-recognition receptors' (PRRs) which recognize 'pathogen-associated molecular patterns' (PAMPs) [20,21]. Engagement of PRRs, such as Toll-like receptors (TLRs) initiates early immune events prior to the full activation of adaptive immunity. TLRs act as homo- (e.g. TLR3 or TLR4) or heterodimers (e.g. TLR2/1 or TLR2/6), or in combination with other PRRs such as C-type lectins. Most TLRs induce IL-12p70 which in turn promotes differentiation of Th1 cells and inflammatory responses, characterized by production of tumor necrosis factor α (TNF-α) and interferon γ (IFN-γ). On the other hand, C-type lectins can be in part responsible for the induction of anti-inflammatory responses [22]. The interplay between innate receptors is thought to form the signals that will determine the development of adaptive immune responses [21,23].

The present study is part of the SCHISTOINIR project that aims to explore innate immune responses in schistosomiasis (for further information: www.york.ac.uk/res/schistoinir). This pilot study was set out to investigate how chronic schistosomiasis affects the peripheral blood mononuclear cell (PBMC) response to various TLR ligands. Here, we report the results from children living in a *S. haematobium*-endemic rural area near Lambaréné, Gabon.

Methods

Ethics statement

The study was approved by the "Comité d'Ethique Regional Independent de Lambaréné" (CERIL). Written informed consent was obtained from parents or legal guardians of all children participating prior to inclusion into the study.

Study site and population

This pilot study was performed in Zilé, a rural area situated 16 km from Lambaréné, Gabon [24,25]. This area is endemic for *S. haematobium*, but with important focal differences. Within Zilé there are two smaller communities, one with high (PK15) and one with low transmission (PK17), 2 km apart from each other. In June and July 2008, we recruited 17 *S. haematobium*-infected schoolchildren from PK15 and 13 uninfected from PK17, and compared their immune profiles. Study participants had no history of anti-helminthic treatment within the last 3 months prior to this study.

Parasitological examination

S. haematobium infection was determined a maximum of seven days prior to blood collection by examining the residue of 10 ml of urine passed through a filter of 12-μm pore-size (Millipore). Children were classified as *S. haematobium*-infected if at least one *S. haematobium* egg was detected in the urine, or uninfected if three consecutive urine samples were negative. Geometric mean infection intensity was calculated for infected children using the first urine reading. Infections with intestinal helminths *Ascaris lumbricoides* and *Trichuris trichiura* were determined by analyzing one fresh stool sample using the Kato-Katz method 30–45 minutes after preparation [26]. *Necator americanus* larvae were detected in a 7-day coproculture of the same stool sample. To this end the classical charcoal culture procedure was used [27–29]. Infection with *Plasmodium falciparum* and microfilaria was determined by Giemsa-stained thick blood smears [30].

After collection of blood samples, all *S. haematobium*-infected children were treated with a single dose of praziquantel (40 mg/kg), and those with intestinal helminths were given a single dose of albendazole (400 mg). Children with other infections or clinical complaints were provided with appropriate medical care.

Hematology

Hematological parameters were analyzed using the ADVIA® 120 Hematology System (Bayer Health Care) and erythrocyte sedimentation rate was determined manually.

PBMC cultures

PBMCs were isolated from heparinized venous blood by density centrifugation on Ficoll (AZL pharmacy, The Netherlands) and cultured in 200 μl of IMDM supplemented with 5% fetal bovine serum (Greiner Bio-One), 100 U/ml penicillin (Astellas), 10 μg/ml streptomycin, 1 mM pyruvate and 2 mM L-glutamine (Sigma) in 96-well round bottom plates (Nunc). PBMCs were seeded at 1×10^6 cells/well for stimulation with schistosomal egg antigen (SEA) or adult worm antigen (AWA), and at 5×10^5 cells/well for stimulation with specific TLR ligands and phyto-hemagglutinin (PHA; positive control). IMDM medium was used as a negative control. Supernatants were collected after 24 h and 72 h of incubation at 37°C in a 5% CO_2 atmosphere and stored at −80°C until cytokine analysis.

Innate and adaptive stimuli

A panel of four TLR ligands was used:

1. TLR2/1 ligand, Pam3CSK4 (Pam3), a synthetic bacterial triacylated lipopeptide (final concentration of 100 ng/ml; EMC microcollections GmbH),
2. TLR2/6 ligand, FSL-1, a synthetic diacylated lipoprotein mimicking the N-terminal part of LP44 from *Mycoplasma salivarium* (50 ng/ml; InvivoGen),
3. TLR3 ligand polyinosinic-polycytidylic acid (poly(I:C)), a synthetic analogue of viral double-stranded RNA (50 μg/ml; InvivoGen),
4. TLR4 ligand, ultrapure lipopolysaccharide (LPS) derived from *Escherichia coli* (100 ng/ml; InvivoGen).

In addition to the classical innate ligands, we used the schistosomal antigen-containing products SEA and AWA from *S. haematobium* at a final concentration of 10 μg protein/ml. Purified PHA (Remel) was used as a positive control at a final concentration of 2 μg/ml.

Cytokine analysis

Two cytokines were measured in this pilot study; one key pro-inflammatory cytokine, TNF-α [31–33], and the anti-inflammatory/regulatory cytokine IL-10 [12,34–37]. Cytokine concentrations were measured in supernatants from single PBMC cultures by ELISA according to the manufacturer's instructions, using half of the reaction volume (PeliKine Compact™, Human TNF-α and IL-10 ELISA kit, Sanquin).

A pro-inflammatory index was computed as the TNF-α: IL-10 ratio upon stimulation relative to the spontaneously produced TNF-α: IL-10 ratio (i.e. in medium):

$$\frac{[\mathrm{TNF}-\alpha]_{\mathrm{stimulus\ A}}/[\mathrm{IL}-10]_{\mathrm{stimulus\ A}}}{[\mathrm{TNF}-\alpha]_{\mathrm{medium}}/[\mathrm{IL}-10]_{\mathrm{medium}}}$$

Statistical analysis

Differences between schistosome-infected and uninfected groups were determined by the Fisher's exact test for sex and intestinal helminth infections and by the Mann-Whitney U test for helminth infection intensity, body mass index (BMI) and hematological parameters. Age was normally distributed and differences between infection groups were tested using the independent student's T test. As cytokine concentrations were not normally distributed, nonparametric tests were used. Differences in an individual's cytokine response to different stimuli (e.g. medium *versus* stimulus-induced cytokine concentration, or ratio) were tested by the Wilcoxon matched-pair signed-rank test.

Differences between infection groups in cytokine concentrations and pro-inflammatory indices were tested by the Mann-Whitney U test. Cytokine concentrations were corrected for spontaneous cytokine production. This was done by subtracting the spontaneously induced cytokine concentration (i.e. in medium) from the stimulus-induced cytokine concentration. For the pro-inflammatory index, this was done by dividing the stimulus-induced ratio by the spontaneously induced ratio (see formula above). Similarly, Spearman's ρ was calculated to estimate the correlation between cytokine responses and infection intensity.

SPSS 18.0 (SPSS Inc.) and GraphPad Prism 5 (GraphPad Software, Inc.) were used for statistical analysis. Results were considered significant when the *p*-value was <0.05.

Results

Characteristics of the study population

Table 1 shows that the demographic, parasitological and hematological characteristics of the infected and uninfected groups of schoolchildren were comparable. Although *S. haematobium*-infected children tended to be more anemic and to have higher eosinophil levels, there were no significant differences between the groups for any of the parameters. In addition, the prevalence and infection intensity of *A. lumbricoides*, *T. trichiura* or *N. americanus* did not significantly differ between *S. haematobium*-positive and -negative children (data not shown for infection intensity). *S. haematobium* infection intensities were low (<50 epg/10 ml) in 14/17 infected children [38]. Malaria and filariasis are endemic in this area [39]. However, only one study participant was infected with *P. falciparum* and one with microfilariae.

Cytokine responses to TLR-ligands

TLR-induced cytokine production by PBMC cultures from infected and uninfected groups was measured at 24 h (Figure 1A, upper panel). While Pam3, FSL-1 and LPS led to substantial and significant cytokine production in both groups compared to medium control, the TLR3 ligand poly(I:C) did not stimulate significant levels of TNF-α or IL-10. Pam3, FSL-1 and LPS tended to induce the production of greater quantities of the pro-inflammatory cytokine TNF-α in infected compared to uninfected children (Pam3; $p<0.01$), while the production of IL-10 was comparable between the two groups.

There was a stronger pro-inflammatory index for PBMC responses of infected children (Figure 1B, upper panel) upon TLR-stimulation (except poly(I:C)) than those from uninfected children. These differences were significant for both Pam3 and FSL-1 ($p<0.05$) which are ligands for TLR2.

Furthermore, *S. haematobium* infection intensity was positively associated with TLR-2- and TLR-4-mediated TNF-α but not with

Table 1. General characteristics of the study population.

	Uninfected	Infected
N	13	17
Age (mean (range))	10.2 y (7–16)	11.4 y (7–16)
Sex (boys/girls)	8/5	9/8
BMI (median (interquartile range))	15.5 kg/m^2 (2.83)	15.7 kg/m^2 (1.64)
S. haematobium infection intensity (geometric mean (range))	Not applicable	9.8 eggs/10 ml (1–1002)
Intestinal helminth infection (n/total)	5/12	5/11
N. americanus infection(n/total)	1*/12	2/12
A. lumbricoides infection (n/total)	2**/12	2**/11
T. trichiura infection (n/total)	4***/12	2**/11
Malaria (n/total)	1/12	0/17
Microfilariasis (n/total)	0/12	1/17
Erythrocyte sedimentation rate (median (range))	15 mm/h (6–50)	15 mm/h (10–88)
Level of white blood cells (median (range))	8.70•10^3/µl (3.80–10.30)	7.20•10^3/µl (5.00–12.40)
Level of lymphocytes (median (range))	3.22•10^3/µl (1.68–5.00)	3.33•10^3/µl (1.26–4.60)
Level of monocytes (median (range))	0.68•10^3/µl (0.36–1.00)	0.64•10^3/µl (0.49–1.04)
Level of neutrophils (median (range))	2.99•10^3/µl (1.06–6.08)	2.14•10^3/µl (1.05–5.79)
Level of eosinophils (median (range))	0.79•10^3/µl (0.20–1.93)	1.53•10^3/µl (0.50–2.49)
Level of basophils (median (range))	0.09•10^3/µl (0.04–0.27)	0.07•10^3/µl (0.04–0.12)
Level of hemoglobin (median (range))	12.2 g/dl (11.4–13.2)	11.3 g/dl (9.1–13.6)

Thick smears (n = 1) for the diagnosis of blood parasites as well as stool samples (n = 6 for Kato-Katz and n = 5 for coproculture) for the diagnosis of intestinal helminths were missing at random.
* Including one child with a *T. trichiura* - *N. americanus* co-infection.
** Including one child with a *T. trichiura* - *A. lumbricoides* co-infection.
*** Including one child with a *T. trichiura* - *N. americanus* co-infection and another one with a *T. trichiura* - *A. lumbricoides* co-infection.

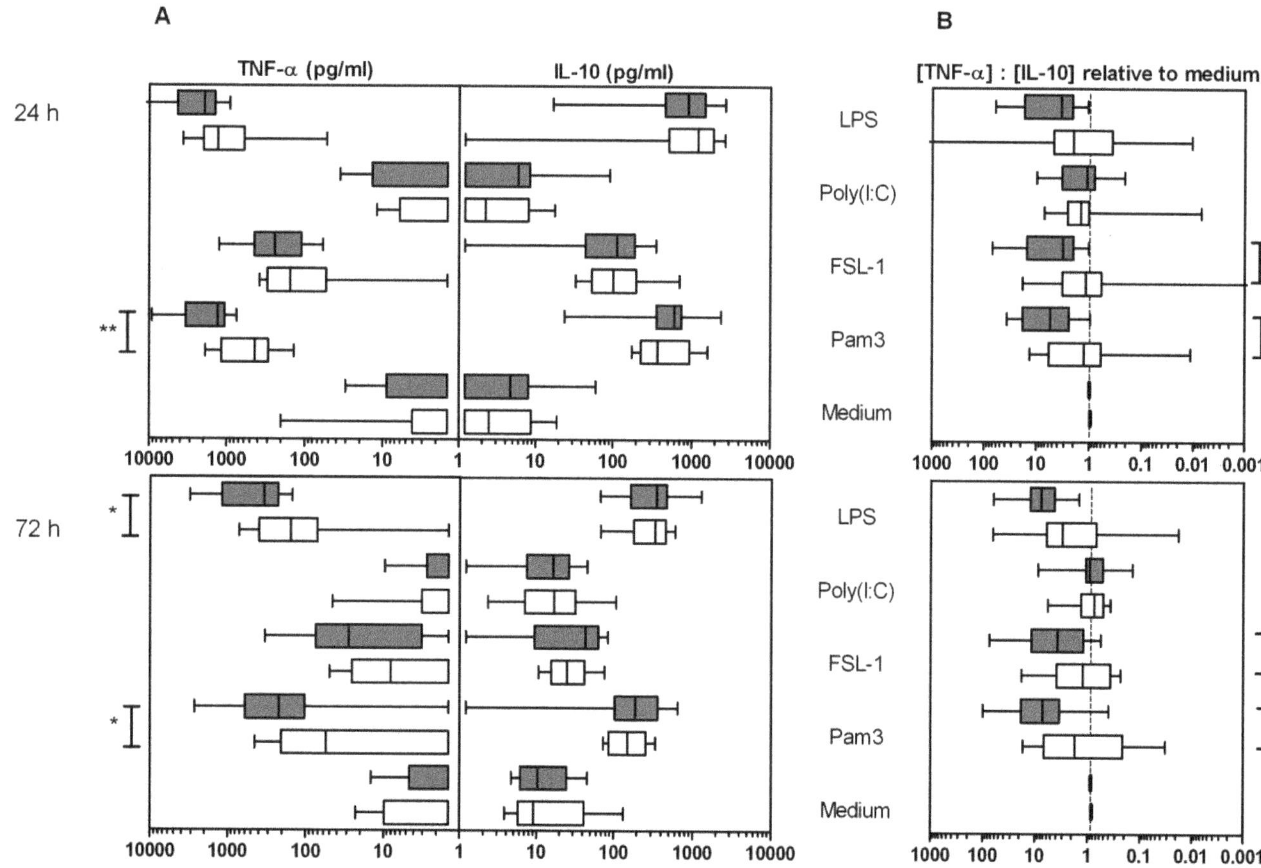

Figure 1. Cytokine production in response to TLR ligands in PBMC cultures. White and grey boxes correspond to *S. haematobium*-free and infected children respectively with the whiskers indicating minimal and maximal concentrations. * $p<0.05$; ** $p<0.01$. **Panel A**: At 24 h, the 'innate' time-point, infected children produced significantly more TNF-α in response to the TLR2/1 ligand Pam3CSK4 (Pam3) compared with uninfected children. TLR-mediated IL-10 production did not significantly deviate between infection groups. When innate cytokine responses faded at 72 h, similar trends were observed. These plots were not adjusted for spontaneous cytokine production. **Panel B**: At both time points, pro-inflammatory indices (i.e. cytokine ratio induced by one of the stimuli relative to the spontaneously produced ratio) induced by the TLR2 ligands, Pam3 and FSL-1, were significantly higher in infected *versus* uninfected children.

IL-10 responses. This was significant for Pam3 ($\rho = 0.80$) and FSL-1 ($\rho = 0.66$). Also, pro-inflammatory indices tended to be positively associated with infection intensity (significant for Pam3 with $\rho = 0.60$).

In order to get an idea of the dynamics of the innate response, TLR responses were also measured after 72 h. Cytokine responses to TLR ligands decreased over time, being less pronounced after 72 h. Nevertheless, the difference between infected and uninfected subjects was similar to that observed in 24 h cultures with a largely pro-inflammatory TLR response in infected subjects (Figure 1, lower panels).

Cytokine responses to schistosomal products

We examined adaptive immune responses by analyzing cytokine production by PBMCs after 72 h of incubation with schistosomal antigens (Figure 2, lower panels). Since these products not only contain antigenic components but also innate ligands [40–47], cytokine production was assessed at both 24 h (innate) and at 72 h (adaptive response).

SEA- and AWA-induced IL-10 was detected in PBMC culture supernatants after 24 h and increased further in 72 h cultures. IL-10 production in infected children was consistently higher than in uninfected children at 24 h but this difference was only significant at 72 h: both SEA- and AWA-induced IL-10 responses were significantly higher in infected children at 72 h (Figure 2A).

After 24 h, AWA-stimulated cultures from infected children secreted significant levels of TNF-α ($p<0.05$ *cf.* medium), while in uninfected children, antigen-induced TNF-α was only detected after 72 h.

After 24 h, the cytokine ratios following stimulation with schistosomal products seemed more anti-inflammatory than pro-inflammatory (i.e. increased IL-10: TNF-α; Figure 2B, upper panel). After 72 h, the pro-inflammatory index tended to increase in uninfected children, and was significantly higher than in infected children upon stimulation with AWA (Figure 2B, lower panel).

Discussion

In this pilot study we investigated the effects of chronic *Schistosoma* infection on TLR-mediated cytokine production. We showed that innate TNF-α responses and TNF-α: IL-10 ratios upon TLR2 stimulation of PBMCs were significantly higher in *S. haematobium*-infected children compared with those without infection, in the face of enhanced regulatory adaptive responses to schistosomal antigens. This suggests that schistosomal infection is associated with elevated pro-inflammatory TLR2 responses.

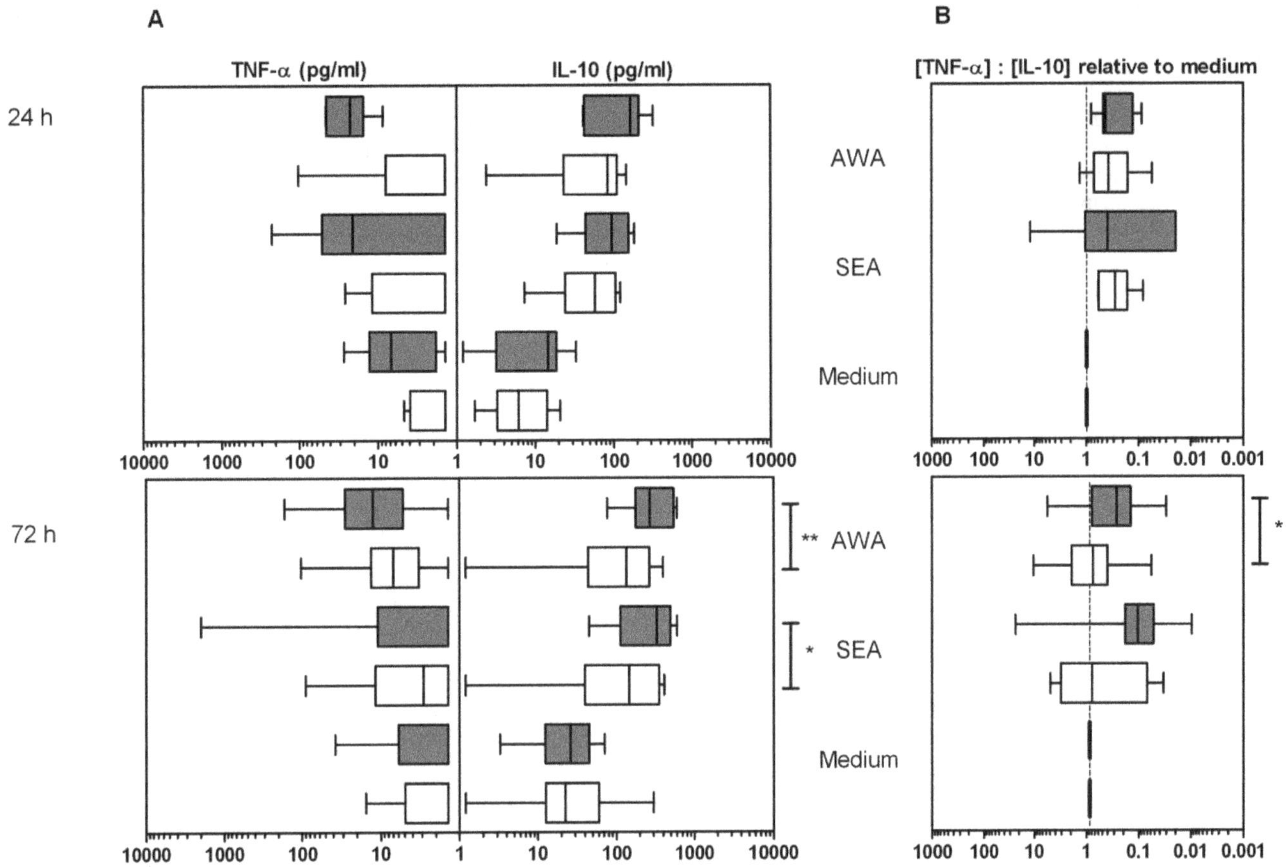

Figure 2. Cytokine production in response to schistosomal products in PBMC cultures. PBMCs were stimulated with schistosomal egg antigen (SEA) or adult worm antigen (AWA). White and grey boxes correspond to *S. haematobium*-free and infected children respectively with the whiskers indicating minimal and maximal concentrations. * $p<0.05$; ** $p<0.01$. **Panel A**: Cytokine production did not differ between groups at 24 h (mainly innate response) but the adaptive IL-10 response after 72 h of incubation to both schistosomal products was significantly higher in infected children than in *S. haematobium*-free children. Furthermore, only infected children produced a significant innate TNF-α response to schistosomal products at 24 h. These plots are not adjusted for spontaneous cytokine production. **Panel B**: After 24 h (predominantly innate), most cytokine ratios induced by schistosomal products were more anti-inflammatory than the ratios induced by medium alone. When the adaptive response had developed after 72 h however, only infected children produced significant anti-inflammatory cytokine balances while pro-inflammatory indices were lower in infected children than in uninfected children (AWA; $p<0.05$).

While cytokine responses upon TLR stimulation tended to decrease over time, the reverse was seen after stimulation with schistosomal products. Although at 24 h, TNF-α levels tended to be more pronounced in infected than in uninfected children, analogous with the observed TLR-mediated cytokine responses, after 72 h of stimulation, PMBCs from *S. haematobium*-infected children produced significantly more IL-10 than uninfected children, as has been described elsewhere [15]. Schistosomal products are more complex than single TLR stimuli. SEA and AWA stimulate the innate immune system through TLRs, C-type lectins and other innate receptors [40–47] but in addition, they contain antigens which can be processed and presented to the T cell receptor forming the basis of acquired immune responses. Schistosomal products are thus able to activate both innate and adaptive pathways. This may explain the observed trend of an initial pro-inflammatory-like immune response. Concurrent with a fading innate cytokine response, a clear anti-inflammatory adaptive response comprising elevated IL-10 was detected in infected children at 72 h.

To our knowledge there are only two other human studies on TLR-mediated cytokine profiles in schistosomiasis. Van der Kleij *et al.* reported reduced TLR responses in Gabonese *S. haematobium*-infected as compared to uninfected children [24]. These results seem to contradict the current findings, but can be explained by differences in the selection of the uninfected control groups. While in the present study both infected and uninfected children were from the same *S. haematobium*-endemic rural area (Zilé), Van der Kleij *et al.* recruited the uninfected control group from a non-endemic neighboring semi-urban area to ensure that the negative subjects were truly negative with no history of exposure. However, when we examined the dataset of the Van der Kleij study to compare the infected (n = 5) and uninfected (n = 10) groups from the same rural area of Zilé, infected children tended to produce higher TNF-α levels as well as higher pro-inflammatory indices in response to LPS than their uninfected counterparts, which is in line with our results.

The second study of TLR-mediated cytokine profiles was carried out in Brazil and also corresponds with our results. Although they did not highlight it, Montenegro *et al.* showed that 48 h whole blood cultures from *S. mansoni*-infected adults produced more TNF-α than those of uninfected adults in response to LPS [48].

In addition, a mouse model of infection pointed towards a similar association between TLR function and schistosomal infection and suggests that schistosomal infection induces elevated pro-inflammatory TLR responses [49].

Few field studies on TLR responses in other helminth infections than schistosomiasis have been published and show varying results. In contrast to *S. haematobium* infection, a negative association has been found between infection with the filarial nematode *Wuchereria bancrofti* and intracellular pro-inflammatory cytokine expression upon TLR stimulation in lymphocytes and monocytes in a population in South India [50,51]. In addition, *W. bancrofti* was associated with reduced pro-inflammatory cytokine responses upon TLR stimulation of PBMCs in a population from the same area with latent tuberculosis [52]. On the other hand, Jackson *et al.* showed infections with intestinal nematodes, i.e. hookworm and *Trichuris trichiura*, to be associated with pro-inflammatory cytokine production, but not with regulatory cytokine production, upon TLR2 and TLR4 stimulation of monocytes from children from Pemba Island [53]. Apparently, the effect of helminth infections on the innate immune responses is species specific; some helminth species may be associated with more pro-inflammatory TLR responses while other helminths are associated with more anti-inflammatory TLR responses. In the present study, *S. haematobium*-infected and uninfected children did not significantly differ with respect to the number and species of other helminth infections. However, information on soil-transmitted helminth infections was not available for some of the participants and we cannot entirely rule out that these infections may have altered the observed innate cytokine responses. In addition, other parasites such as malaria may influence immune balances [54]. The duration as well as the intensity of infection might further influence innate immune responses. It is therefore important to confirm our findings in a larger study population and in varying epidemiological settings.

In conclusion, this pilot study on innate immune responses in schistosomiasis shows a more pro-inflammatory response to single TLR2 ligands in the face of an anti-inflammatory adaptive immune response in *S. haematobium*-infected children. Whilst the precise biological mechanisms for these observations remain to be ascertained, it seems that the commonly accepted view that schistosomal infection suppresses the host's immune system does not hold for ligation of single TLRs. Many receptors – TLRs as well as non-TLRs such as C-type lectins – are involved in innate signaling and their interactions as well as down-stream pathways are at the basis of the immune response to invading pathogens [21,55]. Given the fact that a *Schistosoma* worm is a complex mix of ligands stimulating the innate immune system, further research into this innate cross-talk is necessary.

Acknowledgments

We thank all school children and the Zilé community for their cooperation. Furthermore, we thank Yvonne Kruize for the training she has provided, Sunny Sapthu and Alwin van der Ham for performing most of the ELISAs, Anne Marie Nkoma, Teddy Mabamba, Olivier Kouma and Paule Valerie Mbadinga from the Medical Research Unit of the Albert Schweitzer Hospital in Lambaréné who collected and analyzed stool and urine samples. We would also like to thank Joris Menten from the Institute of Tropical Medicine in Antwerp and Linda May from LUMC for their help on the statistical analysis.

Author Contributions

Conceived and designed the experiments: A.Adegnika LL MY LM KP DB SM TD AM JT PK. Performed the experiments: A.Adegnika A.Amoah LL MM LM UN. Analyzed the data: LM LL A.Amoah MY KP. Contributed reagents/materials/analysis tools: MY. Wrote the paper: LM MY KP.

References

1. Chitsulo L, Engels D, Montresor A, Savioli L (2000) The global status of schistosomiasis and its control. Acta Trop 77: 41–51.
2. WHO website. Available: www.who.int/mediacentre/factsheets/fs115/en/index.html. Accessed 2011 Aug 11.
3. Burke ML, Jones MK, Gobert GN, Li YS, Ellis MK, et al. (2009) Immunopathogenesis of human schistosomiasis. Parasite Immunol 31: 163–176.
4. Diaz A, Allen JE (2007) Mapping immune response profiles: the emerging scenario from helminth immunology. Eur J Immunol 37: 3319–3326.
5. Maizels RM, Yazdanbakhsh M (2003) Immune regulation by helminth parasites: cellular and molecular mechanisms. Nat Rev Immunol 3: 733–744.
6. King CH, Dangerfield-Cha M (2008) The unacknowledged impact of chronic schistosomiasis. Chronic Illn 4: 65–79.
7. Gryseels B, Polman K, Clerinx J, Kestens L (2006) Human schistosomiasis. Lancet 368: 1106–1118.
8. Grogan JL, Kremsner PG, Deelder AM, Yazdanbakhsh M (1998) Antigen-specific proliferation and interferon-gamma and interleukin-5 production are down-regulated during Schistosoma haematobium infection. J Infect Dis 177: 1433–1437.
9. Rocklin RE, Brown AP, Warren KS, Pelley RP, Houba V, et al. (1980) Factors that modify the cellular-immune response in patients infected by Schistosoma mansoni. J Immunol 125: 1916–1923.
10. King CL, Medhat A, Malhotra I, Nafeh M, Helmy A, et al. (1996) Cytokine control of parasite-specific anergy in human urinary schistosomiasis. IL-10 modulates lymphocyte reactivity. J Immunol 156: 4715–4721.
11. Wamachi AN, Mayadev JS, Mungai PL, Magak PL, Ouma JH, et al. (2004) Increased ratio of tumor necrosis factor-alpha to interleukin-10 production is associated with Schistosoma haematobium-induced urinary-tract morbidity. J Infect Dis 190: 2020–2030.
12. Booth M, Mwatha JK, Joseph S, Jones FM, Kadzo H, et al. (2004) Periportal fibrosis in human Schistosoma mansoni infection is associated with low IL-10, low IFN-gamma, high TNF-alpha, or low RANTES, depending on age and gender. J Immunol 172: 1295–1303.
13. Montenegro SM, Miranda P, Mahanty S, Abath FG, Teixeira KM, et al. (1999) Cytokine production in acute versus chronic human Schistosomiasis mansoni: the cross-regulatory role of interferon-gamma and interleukin-10 in the responses of peripheral blood mononuclear cells and splenocytes to parasite antigens. J Infect Dis 179: 1502–1514.
14. Mwatha JK, Kimani G, Kamau T, Mbugua GG, Ouma JH, et al. (1998) High levels of TNF, soluble TNF receptors, soluble ICAM-1, and IFN-gamma, but low levels of IL-5, are associated with hepatosplenic disease in human schistosomiasis mansoni. J Immunol 160: 1992–1999.
15. van den Biggelaar AH, van Ree R, Rodrigues LC, Lell B, Deelder AM, et al. (2000) Decreased atopy in children infected with Schistosoma haematobium: a role for parasite-induced interleukin-10. Lancet 356: 1723–1727.
16. Nookala S, Srinivasan S, Kaliraj P, Narayanan RB, Nutman TB (2004) Impairment of tetanus-specific cellular and humoral responses following tetanus vaccination in human lymphatic filariasis. Infect Immun 72: 2598–2604.
17. Cooper PJ, Espinel I, Paredes W, Guderian RH, Nutman TB (1998) Impaired tetanus-specific cellular and humoral responses following tetanus vaccination in human onchocerciasis: a possible role for interleukin-10. J Infect Dis 178: 1133–1138.
18. Sabin EA, Araujo MI, Carvalho EM, Pearce EJ (1996) Impairment of tetanus toxoid-specific Th1-like immune responses in humans infected with Schistosoma mansoni. J Infect Dis 173: 269–272.
19. Smits HH, Hammad H, van Nimwegen M, Soullie T, Willart MA, et al. (2007) Protective effect of Schistosoma mansoni infection on allergic airway inflammation depends on the intensity and chronicity of infection. J Allergy Clin Immunol 120: 932–940.
20. Iwasaki A, Medzhitov R (2004) Toll-like receptor control of the adaptive immune responses. Nat Immunol 5: 987–995.
21. Lee MS, Kim YJ (2007) Signaling pathways downstream of pattern-recognition receptors and their cross talk. Annu Rev Biochem 76: 447–480.
22. Geijtenbeek TB, Gringhuis SI (2009) Signalling through C-type lectin receptors: shaping immune responses. Nat Rev Immunol 9: 465–479.
23. Chang ZL (2010) Important aspects of Toll-like receptors, ligands and their signaling pathways. Inflamm Res 59: 791–808.
24. van der Kleij D, van den Biggelaar AH, Kruize YC, Retra K, Fillie Y, et al. (2004) Responses to Toll-like receptor ligands in children living in areas where schistosome infections are endemic. J Infect Dis 189: 1044–1051.
25. Retra K, van Riet E, Adegnika AA, Everts B, van Geest S, et al. (2008) Immunologic activity of schistosomal and bacterial TLR2 ligands in Gabonese children. Parasite Immunol 30: 39–46.
26. Katz N, Chaves A, Pellegrino J (1972) A simple device for quantitative stool thick-smear technique in Schistosomiasis mansoni. Rev Inst Med Trop Sao Paulo 14: 397–400.
27. Reiss D, Harrison LM, Bungiro R, Cappello M (2007) Short report: an agar plate method for culturing hookworm larvae: analysis of growth kinetics and infectivity compared with standard coproculture techniques. Am J Trop Med Hyg 77: 1087–1090.

28. Krepel HP, Baeta S, Polderman AM (1992) Human Oesophagostomum infection in northern Togo and Ghana: epidemiological aspects. Ann Trop Med Parasitol 86: 289–300.
29. Polderman AM, Krepel HP, Baeta S, Blotkamp J, Gigase P (1991) Oesophagostomiasis, a common infection of man in northern Togo and Ghana. Am J Trop Med Hyg 44: 336–344.
30. Planche T, Krishna S, Kombila M, Engel K, Faucher JF, et al. (2001) Comparison of methods for the rapid laboratory assessment of children with malaria. Am J Trop Med Hyg 65: 599–602.
31. Abraham E, Anzueto A, Gutierrez G, Tessler S, San Pedro G, et al. (1998) Double-blind randomised controlled trial of monoclonal antibody to human tumour necrosis factor in treatment of septic shock. NORASEPT II Study Group. Lancet 351: 929–933.
32. Martich GD, Boujoukos AJ, Suffredini AF (1993) Response of man to endotoxin. Immunobiology 187: 403–416.
33. Feldmann M, Brennan FM, Maini RN (1996) Role of cytokines in rheumatoid arthritis. Annu Rev Immunol 14: 397–440.
34. Spits H, de Waal MR (1992) Functional characterization of human IL-10. Int Arch Allergy Immunol 99: 8–15.
35. de Vries JE (1995) Immunosuppressive and anti-inflammatory properties of interleukin 10. Ann Med 27: 537–541.
36. Papadakis KA, Targan SR (2000) Role of cytokines in the pathogenesis of inflammatory bowel disease. Annu Rev Med 51: 289–298.
37. Grant AV, Araujo MI, Ponte EV, Oliveira RR, Cruz AA, et al. (2011) Polymorphisms in IL10 are associated with total Immunoglobulin E levels and Schistosoma mansoni infection intensity in a Brazilian population. Genes Immun 12: 46–50.
38. Montresor A, Crompton DWT, Hall A, Bundy DAP, Savioli L (1998) Guidelines for the evaluation of soil-transmitted heminthiasis and schistosomiasis at community level.
39. Wildling E, Winkler S, Kremsner PG, Brandts C, Jenne L, et al. (1995) Malaria epidemiology in the province of Moyen Ogoov, Gabon. Trop Med Parasitol 46: 77–82.
40. Ritter M, Gross O, Kays S, Ruland J, Nimmerjahn F, et al. (2010) Schistosoma mansoni triggers Dectin-2, which activates the Nlrp3 inflammasome and alters adaptive immune responses. Proc Natl Acad Sci U S A 107: 20459–20464.
41. Caldas IR, Campi-Azevedo AC, Oliveira LF, Silveira AM, Oliveira RC, et al. (2008) Human schistosomiasis mansoni: immune responses during acute and chronic phases of the infection. Acta Trop 108: 109–117.
42. Thomas PG (2003) Maturation of dendritic cell 2 phenotype by a helminth glycan uses a Toll-like receptor 4-dependent mechanism. J Immunol 171: 5837–5841.
43. van der Kleij D, Latz E, Brouwers JF, Kruize YC, Schmitz M, et al. (2002) A novel host-parasite lipid cross-talk. Schistosomal lyso-phosphatidylserine activates toll-like receptor 2 and affects immune polarization. J Biol Chem 277: 48122–48129.
44. van Die I (2003) The dendritic cell-specific C-type lectin DC-SIGN is a receptor for Schistosoma mansoni egg antigens and recognizes the glycan antigen Lewis x. Glycobiology 13: 471–478.
45. van Liempt E, van Vliet SJ, Engering A, Garcia Vallejo JJ, Bank CM, et al. (2007) Schistosoma mansoni soluble egg antigens are internalized by human dendritic cells through multiple C-type lectins and suppress TLR-induced dendritic cell activation. Mol Immunol 44: 2605–2615.
46. van Vliet SJ (2005) Carbohydrate profiling reveals a distinctive role for the C-type lectin MGL in the recognition of helminth parasites and tumor antigens by dendritic cells. Int Immunol 17: 661–669.
47. Aksoy E, Zouain CS, Vanhoutte F, Fontaine J, Pavelka N, et al. (2005) Double-stranded RNAs from the helminth parasite Schistosoma activate TLR3 in dendritic cells. J Biol Chem 280: 277–283.
48. Montenegro SM, Abath FG, Domingues AL, Melo WG, Morais CN, et al. (2002) Enhanced interleukin-12 and CD40 ligand activities but reduced Staphylococcus aureus Cowan 1-induced responses suggest a generalized and progressively impaired type 1 cytokine pattern for human schistosomiasis. Infect Immun 70: 5903–5912.
49. Joshi AD, Raymond T, Coelho AL, Kunkel SL, Hogaboam CM (2008) A systemic granulomatous response to Schistosoma mansoni eggs alters responsiveness of bone-marrow-derived macrophages to Toll-like receptor agonists. J Leukoc Biol 83: 314–324.
50. Babu S, Blauvelt CP, Kumaraswami V, Nutman TB (2005) Diminished expression and function of TLR in lymphatic filariasis: a novel mechanism of immune dysregulation. J Immunol 175: 1170–1176.
51. Babu S, Blauvelt CP, Kumaraswami V, Nutman TB (2006) Cutting edge: diminished T cell TLR expression and function modulates the immune response in human filarial infection. J Immunol 176: 3885–3889.
52. Babu S, Bhat SQ, Kumar NP, Anuradha R, Kumaran P, et al. (2009) Attenuation of toll-like receptor expression and function in latent tuberculosis by coexistent filarial infection with restoration following antifilarial chemotherapy. PLoS Negl Trop Dis 3: e489.
53. Jackson JA, Turner JD, Kamal M, Wright V, Bickle Q, et al. (2006) Gastrointestinal nematode infection is associated with variation in innate immune responsiveness. Microbes Infect 8: 487–492.
54. Hartgers FC, Yazdanbakhsh M (2006) Co-infection of helminths and malaria: modulation of the immune responses to malaria. Parasite Immunol 28: 497–506.
55. Carvalho L, Sun J, Kane C, Marshall F, Krawczyk C, et al. (2009) Review series on helminths, immune modulation and the hygiene hypothesis: mechanisms underlying helminth modulation of dendritic cell function. Immunology 126: 28–34.

6

Molecular Analysis of Repeated Methicillin-Resistant *Staphylococcus aureus* Infections in Children

Chih-Jung Chen[1,2,3], Lin-Hui Su[3,4], Tzou-Yien Lin[1,2,3], Yhu-Chering Huang[1,2,3*]

1 Divisions of Pediatric Infectious Diseases, Department of Pediatrics, Chang Gung Children's Hospital and Chang Gung Memorial Hospital, Taoyuan, Taiwan, **2** Pediatric Research Center, Chang Gung Memorial Hospital, Taoyuan, Taiwan, **3** College of Medicine, Chang Gung University, Taoyuan, Taiwan, **4** Department of Laboratory Medicine, Chang Gung Memorial Hospital, Taoyuan, Taiwan

Abstract

Background: Methicillin-resistant *Staphylococcus aureus* (MRSA) is a major pathogen that causes severe morbidity and mortality in hospitalized patients. It is unclear whether repeated MRSA infections in pediatric patients are caused by relapse of previous infecting strains or by acquiring new strains from extrinsic sources. The study aimed to define the genetic relatedness of MRSA isolates from children with repeated infections.

Methodology/Principal Findings: Children with multiple MRSA infections during 2004–2006 were identified in a teaching hospital. Repeated infections were confirmed by chart review and the responsible isolates were genotyped and screened for Panton-Valentine leukocidin (PVL) genes. Two consecutive episodes comprised an infection pair, and strain relatedness was defined for each pair as indistinguishable, highly related, or distinct if the isolates were of the same subtype, the same genotype, or different genotype, respectively. A total of 114 episodes comprising 66 infection pairs were identified in 48 children. The interval of infection pairs ranged from 15 days to 346 days, with a median duration of 57.5 days. Genotypings classified all isolates into 7 genotypes and 31 subtypes. Of 66 pairs, 46 (69.7%), 13 (19.7%) and 7 (10.6%) pairs were caused by indistinguishable, highly related and distinct strains, respectively. Subsequent infections caused by indistinguishable strains were more common for PVL-positive strains (17/18, 94.4%) than for PVL-negative strains (29/48, 60.4%, $P = 0.007$). The strain relatedness was not affected by the durations of interval between infections.

Conclusions/Significance: Most repeated MRSA infections in children are caused by indistinguishable strains even after a long period of interval, suggesting that persistent carriage and relapse of initial infecting strains were responsible for the majority of recurrent MRSA infections.

Editor: Laurent Rénia, BMSI-A*STAR, Singapore

Funding: This study was supported by grants from Chang Gung Memorial Hospital (CMRPG 460111 and CMRPG450123). The funders had no role in study design, data collection and analysis, decision to publish, or preparation of the manuscript.

Competing Interests: The authors have declared that no competing interests exist.

* E-mail: ychuang@adm.cgmh.org.tw

Introduction

Methicillin-resistant *Staphylococcus aureus* (MRSA) is a major pathogen that causes severe morbidity and mortality in hospitalized patients [1,2]. In addition to the increasing methicillin resistance among clinical isolates of *S. aureus*, another growing concern is the emerging community-associated (CA) strains infiltrating hospitals as a major cause of health-care associated (HA) infections [3,4]. The rapid growing CA-MRSA strains harbor a smaller staphylococcal chromosomal cassette *mec* (SCC*mec*) element, produce more exotoxins (e.g., phenol-soluble modulins, Panton-Valentine leukocidin, etc.), and appear more virulent than traditional HA-MRSA strains [5–7]. Evidence further suggests that CA-MRSA as a major nosocomial pathogen may result in increased disease severity and prolonged hospitalization in the infected patients [8,9]. Accordingly, there is a need of more aggressive measures to control the spread of MRSA in hospitals.

The frequently applied strategies in the control of MRSA infections include hand hygiene of healthcare workers, contact isolation of infected patients, and environmental disinfection [10]. Active surveillance of asymptomatic colonized patients, followed by decolonization and/or cohort care, has also been used to prevent MRSA diseases [11]. However, the efficacy of the screening strategy was inconsistent and may be affected by the condition that most MRSA infections were caused by new strains from extrinsic sources or by original colonized strains [12,13].

In this study, we analyzed all clinical MRSA isolates from children with repeated infections in a children's hospital, where MRSA was endemic, during a 3-year period. The aims of the study were to elucidate whether the repeated MRSA infections are relapse of the original strain or re-infection by a new strain, and whether the strain relatedness is affected by the interval of infections or other previously unidentified factors. The findings, we hope, may help to develop a more effective strategy for prevention of MRSA diseases in children at risk of repeated MRSA infections.

Results

During the study period, a total of 82 children with multiple MRSA isolates were identified. Clinical relevance of the isolates

Table 1. Information of infection episodes and infection pairs among children with repeated methicillin-resistant *S. aureus* infections.

Infections in each individual	No. (%) of patients	No. (%) of episodes	No. (%) of infection pairs
2 episodes	36 (71)	72 (63)	36 (55)
3 episodes	9 (19)	27 (24)	18 (27)
4 episodes	1 (2.1)	4 (3.5)	3 (4.5)
5 episodes	1 (2.1)	5 (4.4)	4 (6.1)
6 episodes	1 (2.1)	6 (5.3)	5 (7.6)
Total	48 (100)	114 (100)	66 (100)

was confirmed in 48 children with 2 to 6 discrete episodes of MRSA infection (Table 1). Therefore, a total of 114 episodes (136 isolates) were included for further study. In 16 episodes (13 children), multiple isolates could be found from the respective episode. For the isolates derived from each episode, molecular characterization results indicated that they were indistinguishable from each other. The median duration of intervals between two consecutive episodes was 57.5 days (range, 15 days to 346 days). The duration greater than 6 months was identified in 16 pairs of repeated infection episodes from 15 patients. The longest duration between the recovery of the first and the last isolates from a single patient was 19 months. The common clinical syndromes were wound and lung infections which respectively accounted for 47 (41.2%) and 40 (35.1%) episodes. The detailed characteristics of the repeated infection episodes are displayed in Table 2.

Molecular characterization results indicated that all MRSA isolates belonged to three clonal lineages (ST239, ST59 and ST5) which consisted of 7 genotypes and 31 subtypes (Table 3). PFGE type A were the most predominant type (57.9%), followed by PFGE type D (29.8%) and type C (10.5%). PVL genes were exclusively harbored in isolates of PFGE type D. The distribution of isolation sites differed significantly between major genotypes. Compared to isolates of PFGE types A and F carrying SCC*mec* type III or II (HA genotypes), isolates of PFGE types C, D and AN carrying SCC*mec* type IV or V_T (CA genotypes) were more commonly isolated from wound or pus (10.4% vs. 85.1%, $p<0.001$) but less frequently from sputum (58.2% vs. 2.1%, $P<0.001$) or blood (13.4% vs. 2.1%, $P=0.045$) (Table 3).

The 114 episodes could be further categorized into 66 pairs of repeated MRSA infections (Table 1). Of the 66 infection episode pairs, 46 (69.7%) were caused by indistinguishable strains, 13 (19.7%) were associated with highly related strains, and 7 (10.6%) were caused by distinct strains (Table 4). The detailed PFGE types of MRSA isolates from 12 children with three or more episodes are listed in Table 5. Since these pairs were not independent of each other and the rate of indistinguishable strains can be therefore overestimated, a subsidiary analysis was conducted by including only the first infection pair for each single individual. Among 48 infection pairs in 48 children, 34 (70.8%), 8 (16.7%) and 6 (12.5%) pairs were respectively caused by indistinguishable, related and distinct strains.

The intervals between each paired infection episodes did not differ significantly for infections caused by indistinguishable strains (118.6±98.2 days) compared to those caused by highly related (69.7±96.7 days, $p=0.0985$) or distinct strains (121±126.6 days, $p=0.9593$). The incidence of indistinguishable strains was 74% among 50 infection pairs with interval greater than 30 pairs, which did not differ significantly from that of the 16 infection pairs with interval of 30 days or less (56%, $p=0.217$). Longer intervals of >6 months were found in 16 pairs of infection episodes, and among them, 13 (82%) were caused by indistinguishable strains. Even for the isolates derived from the infection episode pair of longest durations (>11 months), their PFGE types were also indistinguishable. The lack of an association between the length of infection intervals and strain relatedness was further supported by the analysis of episode pairs distributed among 4 arbitrarily categorized durations (<31, 31–90, 91–180 and >180 days, $p=0.404$, Table 4).

The strain relatedness was associated with the genotypes of the preceding isolates. Among the paired infection episodes caused by isolates of the three major genotypes, indistinguishable strains were more common for preceding isolates harboring PVL genes (PFGE type D, 94%) than isolates absent for PVL genes (PFGE type A,

Table 2. Characteristics of repeated methicillin-resistant *Staphylococcus aureus* infections in 48 Taiwanese children.

Characteristic	Total (n = 114)	Infection episode in individuals[1], No. (%)					
		First (n = 48)	Second (n = 48)	Third (n = 12)	Fourth (n = 3)	Fifth (n = 2)	Sixth (n = 1)
Duration from last episode (days)							
Means ± SD	107.7±100.5	-	112.5±101.2	119.6±111.5	60±72.8	29.5±19.1	31
Median	57.5	-	67	61.5	21	29.5	31
Range	15–346	-	15–346	15–306	15–144	16n43	
Clinical syndromes							
Wound infections	47 (41.2)	19 (39.6)	23 (47.9)	4 (33.3)		1 (50)	
Lung infections	40 (35.1)	15 (31.3)	16 (33.3)	4 (16.7)	3 (100)	1 (50)	1 (100)
Primary bacteremia	10 (8.8)	4 (8.3)	4 (8.3)	2 (16.7)			
CVC-associated infections	7 (6.1)	4 (8.3)	2 (4.2)	1 (8.3)			
Ventriculitis	4 (3.5)	2 (4.2)	2 (4.2)				
Others	6 (5.3)	4 (8.3)	1 (2.1)	1 (8.3)			

Abbreviations: CVC, central vascular catheter; SD, standard deviation;
[1]Two and three discrete episodes were identified in 36 and 9 patients, respectively. Four, 5 and 6 episodes were identified in one patient each.

Table 3. Distribution of isolation sites for 7 clones of MRSA responsible for 114 episodes of repeated infections in 48 children.

Lineages	Patterns	No. of PFGE subtypes	Isolation sites, No. (%) of episodes						
			Total	Wound or pus[1]	Sputum[1]	Blood[1]	CVC	CSF	Others
All		31	114	47 (41.2)	40 (35.1)	10 (8.8)	7 (6.1)	4 (3.5)	6 (5.3)
ST239	PFGE A/SCC*mec* III/PVL−	10	42	6 (14.3)	22 (52.4)	4 (9.5)	5 (11.9)	2 (4.8)	3 (7.1)
ST239	PFGE A/SCC*mec* IIIA/PVL−	4	24	1 (4.2)	16 (66.7)	5 (20.8)	0	0	2 (8.3)
ST5	PFGE F/SCC*mec* II/PVL−	1	1	0	1 (100)	0	0	0	0
ST59	PFGE C/SCC*mec* IV/PVL−	8	12	10 (83.3)	1 (8.3)	0	1 (8.3)	0	0
ST59	PFGE D/SCC*mec* V_T/PVL+	6	33	29 (87.9)	0	1 (3.0)	1 (3.0)	1 (3.0)	1 (3.0)
ST59	PFGE D/SCC*mec* IV/PVL+	1	1	1 (100)	0	0	0	0	0
ST59	PFGE AN/SCC*mec* IV/PVL−	1	1	0	0	0	0	1 (100)	0

Abbreviations: CVC, central vascular catheter; HA, hospital-associated genotypes; CA, community-associated genotypes; PFGE, pulsed-field gel electrophoresis; PVL, Panton-Valentine leukocidin; SCC*mec*, staphylococcal cassette chromosome *mec*; ST, multi-locus sequence type.
[1]Comparing to isolates of PFGE C, D and AN, isolates of PFGE type A and F were isolated more commonly from sputum (p<0.001) and blood (p = 0.045) but less frequently from wound/pus (p<0.001).

63% p = 0.012; type C, 67%, p = 0.143, Table 4). Among the highly related strains identified in 13 pairs of repeated infection episodes, all were belonged to subtypes of PFGE type A.

Discussion

Results from this study disclosed that nearly 70% of repeated MRSA infections in children were caused by strains that were genetically indistinguishable from which caused the previous infections. The finding strongly suggested that repeated MRSA infections were frequently caused by relapse of previous infecting strains. The observation was in consistent with two studies addressing the same issue in adult patients [14,15]. Huang et al reported that the same MRSA strain involved in 76% and 72% of repeated infections and infections following colonization, respectively [14]. The close association between colonization and the subsequent clinical infection has also been demonstrated in infants staying in MRSA-endemic neonatal intensive care units [16]. In the present study, since it was a retrospective analysis in nature and we did not survey MRSA colonization at that time, we could not provide the direct evidence of MRSA colonization in these patients and their association with subsequent clinical infection. However, it is reasonable to speculate that, even after effective treatment for clinical infections, colonization of MRSA might still exist in these patients, although direct evidence was not provided in the present study. The acquisition of new strains from other patients, medical care personnel, closed contacts, family members, pets or the environment, though not uncommon, appeared to play a minor role among the repeated MRSA infections observed in this setting. The results also suggest that infection control by standard precaution to break the patient-to-patient or contaminated device-to-patient transmission may at most prevent only 30% of the repeated MRSA infections. Active identification of MRSA colonization, followed by effective decolonization measures, may be required during the health care of children at risk of recurrent MRSA infection.

The genetic diversity of clinical MRSA isolates is usually limited in a defined region within a short period of time [17,18]. Our findings could be a mere coincidence due to the spread of a few endemic clones prevailing in this institute or the neighboring

Table 4. Strain relatedness in 66 pairs of repeated MRSA infection episodes, categorized according to PFGE types of preceding isolates and intervals.

Strain relatedness	No. (%) of patients	No. (%) of episode pairs									
		Total	PFGE types of preceding isolates					Duration of intervals (days)[3]			
			A	C	D	F	AN	15–31	31–90	91–180	>180
Total	48[1]	66	40	6	18	1	1	16	27	7	16
Indistinguishable	34 (71)	46 (70)	25 (63)	4 (67)	17 (94)[2]	0 (0)	0 (0)	9 (56)	18 (67)	6 (86)	13 (81)
Highly related	9 (19)	13 (20)	13 (33)	0 (0)	0 (0)	0 (0)	0 (0)	7 (44)	4 (15)	0 (0)	2 (13)
Distinct	6 (13)	7 (11)	2 (5)	2 (33)	1 (6)	1 (100)	1 (100)	0 (0)	5 (19)	1 (14)	1 (6)

PFGE, pulsed-field gel electrophoresis.
[1]One child had 3 infection pairs caused respectively by indistinguishable strains (2 pairs) and highly related strains (1 pair).
[2]The rate of paired infections caused by indistinguishable strains was higher for PFGE type D (carrying Panton-Valentine leukocidin genes) than for other PFGE types (P = 0.007, Fisher's exact test).
[3]Strain relatedness was not associated with the length of intervals (indistinguishable strains vs. highly related or distinct strains, p = 0.404).

Table 5. Detailed pulsed-field gel electrophoresis patterns of MRSA isolates from 12 children with three or more episodes.

Case No.	Episode					
	First	Second	Third	Fourth	Fifth	Sixth
1	A4	A4	A4			
2	A9	A9	A9			
3	D11	D11	D11			
4	D4	D4	D4			
5	A4	A	A			
6	A10	A10	A38			
7	AN	C38	C38			
8	A4	A12	A			
9	A38	A3	A38			
10	A	A	A23	A23		
11	A38	A38	A38	A38	A38	
12	A3	A10	A10	A10	A10	A10

communities where the pediatric patients came from. Indeed, as noted in the genotyping analysis, there were 3 predominant PFGE clones that belonged to 2 genetic lineages and accounted for the majority (98.2%, Table 3) of repeated MRSA infections in this children's hospital. However, our previous molecular epidemiology studies disclosed that, by PFGE analysis, MRSA in this hospital could be categorized into at least 78 subtypes during the same period of time [19]. In this study, we also identify a total of 31 subtypes among the MRSA isolates studied. The discrimination of the related strains was further increased by the additions of SCC*mec* typing (Table 3). The likelihood of repeatedly getting an identical strain from the exogenous environment should be much less than from a strain which has been persistently carried by the patients. We believe by applying the stringent criteria (same PFGE and SCC*mec* types) of defining the same strain should greatly avoid the bias caused by clonal spread.

It is intriguing that the rate of indistinguishable strains in repeated MRSA infections caused by PVL-positive isolates is significantly higher than that caused by PVL-negative isolates. PFGE type A (ST239) with SCC*mec* III or variants is among one of the six pandemic clones, known as Hungarian clone [20], and has been the most prevalent HA-MRSA clone circulating in major hospitals in Taiwan since early 1990s [21]. PFGE types C and D (ST59 lineage) are both emerging CA-MRSA clones in Taiwan and the PFGE type D/SCC*mec* V_T/PVL-positive clone has become the most predominant cause of *S. aureus* infection in previously healthy Taiwanese children [22,23]. It is unclear why with repeated infections the strain relatedness was correlated with genotypes of preceding isolates. It has been suggested that PVL-positive *S. aureus* strains expressed more abundant cell wall-anchored proteins (e.g., staphylococcal protein A, serine-aspartate repeat proteins C and D) and exhibited a greater affinity to extracellular matrix than did PVL-negative strains [7,24]. Whether PVL-positive MRSA strains possess a greater potential to persistent colonization and facilitate the subsequent relapse infection needs further studies.

The cut-off period of defining distinct infection episodes may have impact in strain relatedness in repeated infections. For instance, a subsequent infection occurred closed to the cessation of antibiotic treatment of prior infection may suggest relapse due to inadequate treatment and increase the incidence of finding the same strains in two episodes. However, the indistinguishable strains in the current study accounted for 56% of subsequent infections occurring between 14 and 31 days. The rate was not greater than those with longer durations of interval (67%, 86% and 81% for interval of 31–90, 91–180 and >180 days, respectively). We also noted that the strain relatedness was not affected by the durations of infection intervals. The data indicated that different cut-off period of defining a new episode did not substantially affect the results or change our conclusion. The finding was compatible with another study addressing this issue in adult populations [14]. For the 46 pairs of repeated infections caused by indistinguishable strains in the present study, 28.3% had intervals greater than 180 days with a maximal duration of 340 days. The long-term carriage of MRSA was also evident in a recent study investigating the duration of MRSA colonization in an adult population [25]. Nearly 50% of the MRSA-carried patients remained colonized in the first year. Since every episode of MRSA infection in our study had been managed with a complete course of antibiotic treatment, the observation might indicate that systemic antibiotic treatment was not sufficient in eradicating MRSA colonization and the immunity against MRSA was incapable of protecting the individual from repeated infection by the same MRSA strains.

There were limitations in this study. Although the indistinguishable strains in infection-infection pair strongly suggested persistent carriage of the same strain to be responsible for MRSA repeated infections, direct evidence by exploring the strain relatedness in colonization-infection pairs was not available in this study with a retrospective-based design. A prospective study incorporating multiple centers and larger patient cohorts will be needed to directly address this issue.

In conclusion, we demonstrated that the majority of repeated MRSA infections in children were caused by the same strains that caused the previous infections even after a long period of intervals. The observation provides new insights into the prevention of MRSA infection. Interruption of transmission may not be sufficient in preventing most of the repeated MRSA infections. Strategies to identify MRSA colonization followed by successful decolonization may be required in children with high risks of MRSA infections.

Materials and Methods

Ethics statement

The study was approved by the institute review boards from Chang Gung Memorial Hospital, which allowed retrieve of the patients list from the electronic microbiology database, review of the medical information and characterizations of the responsible isolates. A waiver of consent was granted given the retrospective nature of the project and anonymous analysis of the data.

Case enrollments

Between January 1, 2004 and December 31, 2006, all clinical isolates of MRSA were collected from the clinical microbiology laboratory of Chang Gung Children's Hospital and stored at −80°C in the research laboratory until use. Information regarding the name and chart number of each patient and the specimen date and source of the respective MRSA isolate was recorded in the hospital's central computer system. In this study, a list of children that were younger than 18 years old and had at least two positive cultures of MRSA was retrieved from the database. If the isolates were not recovered from sterile sites, clinical validation would be performed by reviewing the medical records, aiming to differentiate between MRSA colonization and clinical infection. To define the lung infections, the age-specific clinical criteria for diagnosis of pneumonia was adopted from CDC/NHSN [26], which included a positive chest radiology (e.g. new or progressive and persistent infiltrate, consolidation, cavitation or pneumatoceles in infant) and definitive clinical signs or symptoms (e.g. fever, leucopenia or leukocytosis, new onset or change character of sputum, new onset or worsening cough, dyspnea, rales or bronchial sounds, worsening gas exchange). The diagnosis of wound infections also followed the CDC/NHSN criteria for either surgical sites infection or skin and soft tissue infection where appropriate [26].

Definitions of infection "episodes" and infection "pairs"

For those being determined as true infections, if the associated isolates were derived consecutively with an interval greater than 14 days and a full course of appropriate antimicrobial agents as judged by the in-vitro susceptibility testing were administered, the infections would be considered as distinct infection episodes. Multiple isolates can be identified from different specimens in single episode. Patients with at least 2 separate infection episodes were enrolled for further analysis. Two consecutive episodes comprised a pair of repeated infection. Children with 2 episodes were considered to have one pair of repeated infection. Those with 3 episodes were considered to have 2 pairs of repeated infection (one pair for the first and the second episodes and the other pair for the second and the third episodes) and so on.

Molecular characterizations

All MRSA isolates recovered from the enrolled patients were subjected to molecular characterization. Pulsed-field gel electrophoresis (PFGE) of *SmaI*-digested macro fragments of the respective chromosomal DNA was used to fingerprint the isolates according to methods described previously [19]. The DNA fingerprints generated by PFGE were manually analyzed according to the criteria proposed by Tenover et al [27]. Isolates with PFGE patterns differed by 4 or more than 4 bands were considered distinct and designated as different genotypes. Isolates with identical PFGE patterns or differed by less than 4 bands were considered indistinguishable or highly related and defined as the same genotype or a subtype of an existing genotype, respectively. Genotypes were designated consecutively in an alphabetical order and subtypes of a genotype were labeled with Arabic number suffixes. For consistency, genotypes described in the present study followed those described in our previous reports [19,28]. Only those newly identified PFGE patterns would be assigned with a new genotype name.

The SCC*mec* types I–IV were determined by a multiplex PCR system, whereas type V or V_T was determined by the detection of *ccrC* complex as described previously [29,30]. Control strains for the SCC*mec* typing were kindly provided by Dr. K. Hiramatsu and listed as follows: type I, NCTC10442; type II, N315; type III, 85/2082; type IVa, JCSC4744 and type V, WIS. The control strain for SCC*mec* type V_T was provided by Dr. Chih-Chien Wang at Tri-Service General Hospital, Taipei, Taiwan.

Multilocus sequence typing (MLST) was performed among representative strains of major PFGE types according to the instruction provided in the MLST website (http://www.mlst.net). Briefly, each allele was assigned a number by comparing the respective sequence with those of the known alleles in the *S. aureus* MLST database. The allele numbers at each of the seven loci defined the allelic profile of each isolate. An allelic profile was defined as a sequence type (ST).

Panton-Valentine leukocidin (PVL) has been considered an epidemiological marker for CA-MRSA strains. All isolates were investigated for the presence of the *lukS-PV* and *lukF-PV* genes encoding PVL using a single PCR method as previously described [22].

Determination of genetic relatedness among isolates derived from consecutive infections

Strain relatedness was investigated in isolates accounting for each pair of infection episodes. Isolates derived from a pair of repeated infection were interpreted as indistinguishable if they had the same PFGE patterns as well as the same SCC*mec* elements. Highly related strains were defined if their PFGE patterns were subtypes of the same genotype and they carried the same SCC*mec* elements. Distinct strains were defined if they had different PFGE patterns or carried different SCC*mec* elements.

Statistical analysis

The descriptive statistics were analyzed with SAS 9.1 software (SAS Institute Inc. Cary, NC) for Windows. Categorical variables were compared by chi-square or Fisher's exact test, when appropriate. Differences in means were assessed by the Student *t*-test. Statistical significance was deemed to be $p<0.05$.

Acknowledgments

We thank Dr. K. Hiramatsu and Dr. Chih-Chie Wang for providing the control strains for SCC*mec* typing.

Author Contributions

Conceived and designed the experiments: TYL YCH. Performed the experiments: CJC LHS. Analyzed the data: CJC YCH. Contributed reagents/materials/analysis tools: CJC LHS. Wrote the paper: CJC LHS.

References

1. National Nosocomial Infections Surveillance (NNIS) System Report, data summary from January 1992 through June 2004 (2004) Am J Infect Control 32: 470–485.
2. Klevens RM, Morrison MA, Nadle J, Petit S, Gershman K, et al. (2007) Invasive methicillin-resistant *Staphylococcus aureus* infections in the United States. JAMA 298: 1763–1771.
3. Klevens RM, Edwards JR, Tenover FC, McDonald LC, Horan T, et al. (2006) Changes in the epidemiology of methicillin-resistant *Staphylococcus aureus* in intensive care units in US hospitals, 1992–2003. Clin Infect Dis 42: 389–391.
4. Gonzalez BE, Rueda AM, Shelburne SA, 3rd, Musher DM, Hamill RJ, et al. (2006) Community-associated strains of methicillin-resistant *Staphylococccus aureus* as the cause of healthcare-associated infection. Infect Control Hosp Epidemiol 27: 1051–1056.
5. Wang R, Braughton KR, Kretschmer D, Bach TH, Queck SY, et al. (2007) Identification of novel cytolytic peptides as key virulence determinants for community-associated MRSA. Nat Med 13: 1510–1514.
6. Diep BA, Gill SR, Chang RF, Phan TH, Chen JH, et al. (2006) Complete genome sequence of USA300, an epidemic clone of community-acquired meticillin-resistant *Staphylococcus aureus*. Lancet 367: 731–739.
7. Labandeira-Rey M, Couzon F, Boisset S, Brown EL, Bes M, et al. (2007) *Staphylococcus aureus* Panton-Valentine leukocidin causes necrotizing pneumonia. Science 315: 1130–1133.
8. D'Agata EM, Webb GF, Horn MA, Moellering RC, Jr., Ruan S (2009) Modeling the invasion of community-acquired methicillin-resistant *Staphylococcus aureus* into hospitals. Clin Infect Dis 48: 274–284.
9. Popovich KJ, Weinstein RA, Hota B (2008) Are community-associated methicillin-resistant *Staphylococcus aureus* (MRSA) strains replacing traditional nosocomial MRSA strains? Clin Infect Dis 46: 787–794.
10. Muto CA, Jernigan JA, Ostrowsky BE, Richet HM, Jarvis WR, et al. (2003) SHEA guideline for preventing nosocomial transmission of multidrug-resistant strains of *Staphylococcus aureus* and enterococcus. Infect Control Hosp Epidemiol 24: 362–386.
11. Kotilainen P, Routamaa M, Peltonen R, Evesti P, Eerola E, et al. (2001) Eradication of methicillin-resistant *Staphylococcus aureus* from a health center ward and associated nursing home. Arch Intern Med 161: 859–863.
12. Harbarth S, Fankhauser C, Schrenzel J, Christenson J, Gervaz P, et al. (2008) Universal screening for methicillin-resistant *Staphylococcus aureus* at hospital admission and nosocomial infection in surgical patients. JAMA 299: 1149–1157.

13. Robicsek A, Beaumont JL, Paule SM, Hacek DM, Thomson RB, Jr., et al. (2008) Universal surveillance for methicillin-resistant *Staphylococcus aureus* in 3 affiliated hospitals. Ann Intern Med 148: 409–418.
14. Huang SS, Diekema DJ, Warren DK, Zuccotti G, Winokur PL, et al. (2008) Strain-relatedness of methicillin-resistant *Staphylococcus aureus* isolates recovered from patients with repeated infection. Clin Infect Dis 46: 1241–1247.
15. Liao CH, Lai CC, Chen YH, Huang YT, Hsueh PR (2010) Strain relatedness of methicillin-resistant *Staphylococcus aureus* isolates recovered from patients with repeated bacteremia. Clin Microbiol Infect 16: 463–469.
16. Huang YC, Chou YH, Su LH, Lien RI, Lin TY (2006) Methicillin-resistant *Staphylococcus aureus* colonization and its association with infection among infants hospitalized in neonatal intensive care units. Pediatrics 118: 469–474.
17. Enright MC, Robinson DA, Randle G, Feil EJ, Grundmann H, et al. (2002) The evolutionary history of methicillin-resistant *Staphylococcus aureus* (MRSA). Proc Natl Acad Sci USA 99: 7687–7692.
18. Aires de Sousa M, Crisostomo MI, Sanches IS, Wu JS, Fuzhong J, et al. (2003) Frequent recovery of a single clonal type of multidrug-resistant *Staphylococcus aureus* from patients in two hospitals in Taiwan and China. J Clin Microbiol 41: 159–163.
19. Huang YC, Su LH, Wu TL, Liu CE, Young TG, et al. (2004) Molecular epidemiology of clinical isolates of methicillin-resistant *Staphylococcus aureus* in Taiwan. J Clin Microbiol 42: 307–310.
20. Aires de Sousa M, de Lencastre H (2004) Bridges from hospitals to the laboratory: genetic portraits of methicillin-resistant *Staphylococcus aureus* clones. FEMS Immunol Med Microbiol 40: 101–111.
21. Wang JT, Fang CT, Chen YC, Wu CL, Chen ML, et al. (2007) Staphylococcal cassette chromosome mec in MRSA, Taiwan. Emerg Infect Dis 13: 494–497.
22. Huang YC, Ho CF, Chen CJ, Su LH, Lin TY (2008) Comparative molecular analysis of community-associated and healthcare-associated methicillin-resistant *Staphylococcus aureus* isolates from children in northern Taiwan. Clin Microbiol Infect 14: 1167–1172.
23. Chen CJ, Huang YC (2005) Community-acquired methicillin-resistant *Staphylococcus aureus* in Taiwan. J Microbiol Immunol Infect 38: 376–382.
24. de Bentzmann S, Tristan A, Etienne J, Brousse N, Vandenesch F, et al. (2004) *Staphylococcus aureus* isolates associated with necrotizing pneumonia bind to basement membrane type I and IV collagens and laminin. J Infect Dis 190: 1506–1515.
25. Robicsek A, Beaumont JL, Peterson LR (2009) Duration of colonization with methicillin-resistant *Staphylococcus aureus*. Clin Infect Dis 48: 910–913.
26. Horan TC, Andrus M, Dudeck MA (2008) CDC/NHSN surveillance definition of health care-associated infection and criteria for specfic types of infections in the acute care setting. AM J Infect Control 36: 309–332.
27. Tenover FC, Arbeit RD, Goering RV, Mickelsen PA, Murray BE, et al. (1995) Interpreting chromosomal DNA restriction patterns produced by pulsed-field gel electrophoresis: criteria for bacterial strain typing. J Clin Microbiol 33: 2233–2239.
28. Chen CJ, Su LH, Chiu CH, Lin TY, Wong KS, et al. (2007) Clinical features and molecular characteristics of invasive community-acquired methicillin-resistant *Staphylococcus aureus* infections in Taiwanese children. Diagn Microbiol Infect Dis 59: 287–293.
29. Oliveira DC, de Lencastre H (2002) Multiplex PCR strategy for rapid identification of structural types and variants of the mec element in methicillin-resistant *Staphylococcus aureus*. Antimicrob Agents Chemother 46: 2155–2161.
30. Boyle-Vavra S, Ereshefsky B, Wang CC, Daum RS (2005) Successful multiresistant community-associated methicillin-resistant *Staphylococcus aureus* lineage from Taipei, Taiwan, that carries either the novel Staphylococcal chromosome cassette *mec* (SCC*mec*) type V_T or SCC*mec* type IV. J Clin Microbiol 43: 4719–4730.

7

Association of Differentiation State of CD4+ T Cells and Disease Progression in HIV-1 Perinatally Infected Children

Elizabeth R. Sharp[1], Christian B. Willberg[1], Peter J. Kuebler[1], Jacob Abadi[2], Glenn J. Fennelly[2], Joanna Dobroszycki[2], Andrew A. Wiznia[2], Michael G. Rosenberg[2], Douglas F. Nixon[1]*

1 Division of Experimental Medicine, Department of Medicine, University of California San Francisco, San Francisco, California, United States of America, 2 Jacobi Medical Center, Bronx, New York, United States of America

Abstract

Background: In the USA, most HIV-1 infected children are on antiretroviral drug regimens, with many individuals surviving through adolescence and into adulthood. The course of HIV-1 infection in these children is variable, and understudied.

Methodology/Principal Findings: We determined whether qualitative differences in immune cell subsets could explain a slower disease course in long term survivors with no evidence of immune suppression (LTS-NS; CD4%≥25%) compared to those with severe immune suppression (LTS-SS; CD4%≤15%). Subjects in the LTS-NS group had significantly higher frequencies of naïve (CCR7+CD45RA+) and central memory (CCR7+CD45RA−) CD4+ T cells compared to LTS-SS subjects ($p = 0.0005$ and <0.0001, respectively). Subjects in the rapid progressing group had significantly higher levels of CD4+ T_{EMRA} (CCR7−CD45RA+) cells compared to slow progressing subjects ($p<0.0001$).

Conclusions/Significance: Rapid disease progression in vertical infection is associated with significantly higher levels of CD4+ T_{EMRA} (CCR7−CD45RA+) cells.

Editor: Landon Myer, University of Cape Town, South Africa

Funding: Funding was provided by a grant from the National Institutes of Health AI060379. The funders had no role in study design, data collection and analysis, decision to publish, or preparation of the manuscript.

Competing Interests: The authors have declared that no competing interests exist.

* E-mail: douglas.nixon@ucsf.edu

Introduction

Various studies have sought to determine an association between the control of HIV-1 viremia and magnitude of the HIV-1 specific immune response [1,2,3,4,5]. The results have been inconsistent. The qualitative characteristics of the HIV-1-specific T cell response have become the focus of intense study and it has been suggested that the inability of these responses to control viremia is due to a failure of these cells to fully differentiate [6].

In contrast to other chronic viral infections such as CMV, HIV-1 infection appears to result in a maturational block in the generation of the HIV-1-specific T cell responses with skewing toward an effector memory, T_{EM}, phenotype [6]. This seems to result in an overall decrease in the frequency of fully differentiated effector memory, T_{EMRA}, cells [6,7]. We have previously shown that the frequency and absolute numbers of CD8+ HIV-specific T_{EMRA} cells in early HIV-1 infection negatively correlate with the future viral load set point [8]. As CD4+ T cells are also known to be important in the control of HIV-1 viremia[9,10,11,12,13,14,15,16,17,18], we sought to determine whether alterations in CD4+ T cell subpopulations were associated with disease progression. We chose to study a population of vertically infected children, and categorized them into two progression groups based on CD4% values using revised guidelines published by the CDC in 1994 [19], subjects with no immune suppression (LTS-NS; CD4%≥25%), and subjects with severe immune suppression (LTS-SS; CD4%≥15%). Surprisingly, we found striking differences in the differentiation phenotype of CD4+ T cells between the two groups.

Results

Subject Cohort Characteristics

We analyzed peripheral blood samples from 58 children and adolescents with vertically acquired HIV-1. As described in Materials and Methods, these subjects were divided into two groups of immunological progression based on CDC guidelines. The characteristics of both groups are described in Table 1.

As the children were categorized according to percentage CD4+ T cell count, it was not surprising to find a statistically significant difference in the viral loads between the two groups. Of particular note, all of the patients had some level of ongoing viral replication, as none of them maintained consistently undetectable viral loads. The LTS-NS group contained more African-Americans than the LTS-SS group, but this did not reach significance. The LTS-SS group was slightly older than the LTS-NS group, but again this did not reach significance. There were no significant differences in treatment regimen or adherence levels between the two clinical groups.

Table 1. Patient cohort characteristics.

Immunological Category	N	CD4%	LVL[a]	Age (y)	Sex	Race[b]
No immune suppression - LTS-NS (CD4% ≥25)	30	29.8% (27.1; 34.8)	3.65 (2.85; 4.14)	13.8 (10.9; 16.6)	M = 15 F = 15	H = 9 AA = 20
No immune suppression - LTS-NS (CD4%<15)	28	8.25% (5.5; 11.5)	4.79 (4.37; 5.11)	15.6 (12.5; 18.1)	M = 11 F = 17	H = 13 AA = 13
TOTAL	58	24.5% (8.25; 31.0)	4.28 (3.61; 4.81)	14.3 (11.6; 17.52)	M = 26 F = 32	H = 22 AA = 33

[a]Log viral load.
[b]H = Hispanic; AA = African American.

Comparison of Differentiation Profiles of Bulk and HIV-1-specific CD8+ T cells Between Progression Groups

We first characterized the HIV-1-specific CD8+ T cell population in the two groups. We hypothesized that there would be more fully differentiated CD8+ T_{EMRA} cells in the LTS-NS subjects compared to LTS-SS subjects, both in the total CD8+ T cell population and in Gag-specific CD8+ T cells, as has been observed from studies from adult HIV-1 infected cohorts [20,21]. We performed surface staining and intracellular cytokine staining on 17 LTS-NS subjects and 15 LTS-SS subjects, stimulating PBMC with single Gag peptides.

Surface staining of the total CD8+ T cell population revealed a significantly higher frequency of naïve T cells (CCR7+ CD45RA+) in LTS-NS subjects ($p = 0.0066$). We observed a trend towards higher levels of T_{EM} (CCR7−CD45RA−) cells in the LTS-SS group although this was not significant ($p = 0.2$). There was no difference in the levels of T_{CM} (CCR7+ CD45RA−) or T_{EMRA} (CCR7−CD45RA+) cells between the two groups (Figure 1A). We characterized epitope-specific CD8+ T cells for maturation profiles using intracellular cytokine staining. No differences in the maturational profiles of epitope-specific CD8+ T cells between the two groups were observed (Figure 1B).

Striking Differences in CD4+ T cell Maturational Profiles between Progression Groups

We next analyzed the characteristics of CD4+ T cells in these subjects. CD4+ cells were defined as CD3+CD8− cells. In a different panel with all three markers we verified that, on average, 93% of CD3+CD8− cells were CD4+. Remarkable differences in the maturational profiles of CD4+ T cells between the two progression groups were observed. As shown in Figure 2, subjects in the LTS-NS groups had much higher frequencies of naïve and central memory CD4+ T cells, which were highly statistically significant ($p = 0.0005$ and $p<0.0001$). There was no difference in the levels of effector memory CD4+ T cells ($p = 0.984$). Interestingly, subjects in the LTS-SS group had significantly higher levels of T_{EMRA} cells than LTS-NS subjects, which was also highly statistically significant ($p<0.0001$).

Additionally, the levels of T_{NAIVE} cells and T_{CM} cells showed a strong positive correlation with CD4% (Spearman $r = 0.713$ and 0.716, respectively, and $p<0.0001$ for both) and negatively with LVL (Spearman $r = -0.421$, $p = 0.018$; and Spearman $r = -0.731$, $p<0.0001$, respectively) (Figure 3A–D). In contrast, the levels of T_{EMRA} cells were strongly negatively correlated with CD4% (Spearman $r = -0.836$, $p<0.0001$) and positively correlated with LVL (Spearman $r = 0.0026$, $p = 0.0026$) (Figure 3G and H).

In order to further characterize these CD4+ T cells, levels of CD57 expression were also measured. CD57 has been described a marker of T cell senescence [22]. CD57 expression on CD4+ T cells from LTS-SS subjects was much higher than that seen on CD4+ T cells from the LTS-NS group, ($p = 0.0025$) (Figure 4A). The frequency of CD4+ T cells expressing CD57 was also negatively correlated with CD4% (Spearman $r = -0.572$, $p = 0.001$) and positively correlated with LVL (Spearman $r = 0.41$, $p = 0.02$) (Figure 4B and C).

Discussion

Several recent studies have suggested that qualitative characteristics of the HIV-1-specific T cell are associated with protection, viral control, and rate of disease progression [8,20,21,23,24]. To our knowledge this is the first study to compare the qualitative characteristics of total CD8+ and CD4+ as well as HIV-specific T cell responses in perinatally infected children with different levels of disease progression, with a significant finding relating specific CD4+ T cell profiles with disease progression rate. Moreover, unlike previous studies which have focused on individuals of Northern European descent, this work concentrated primarily on African Americans and Hispanics.

The children in this study, all older than 10 years of age and thus considered long-term survivors (LTS), were categorized, based on CD4+ T cell percentage levels, into those with no immune suppression (LTS-NS) and those with severe immune suppression (LTS-SS), based on previously published CDC guidelines [19]. We observed a highly significant increase in the frequency of naïve CD8+ T cells (T_{NAIVE}) in the LTS-NS subjects ($p = 0.0066$), compared to the LTS-SS subjects, but no differences in any other CD8+ T cell subsets. The differentiation profiles of Gag-specific CD8+ T cells were similar between the progression groups.

The most striking finding of this study was the CD4+ T cell differentiation profiles between the two progression groups. Subjects in the LTS-NS group had significantly higher levels of naïve T cells (T_{NAIVE}) and central memory (T_{CM}) CD4+ T cells than LTS-SS children ($= 0.0005$ and $p<0.0001$, respectively). In contrast, children in the LTS-SS group had significantly higher levels of effector memory RA+ (T_{EMRA}) cells ($p<0.0001$). These data suggest that disease progression in these vertically infected younger patients is different than adults and is associated with a shift towards greater T_{EMRA} cell numbers.

The shift towards greater T_{EMRA} cells could represent a disproportionate loss of certain T cell subsets in LTS-SS subjects consistent with published data. A recent study showed that CD4+ cells with the T_{EMRA} phenotype (CCR7−CD45RA+) were more prevalent in HIV-1-infected individuals than in uninfected controls [25]. They described that these cells were resistant to *in vitro* infection by CCR5-tropic strains of HIV-1, despite robust expression of CCR5. Loss of Naïve T cells was also observed in a study of HIV infected infants. In this study, there was an association between rapid disease progression and decreases in naïve cells but with little effect on memory cells. The loss of naïve cells appeared to be mediated through thymic dysfunction [26,27]. Our cohort consists of long term survivors of vertically acquired

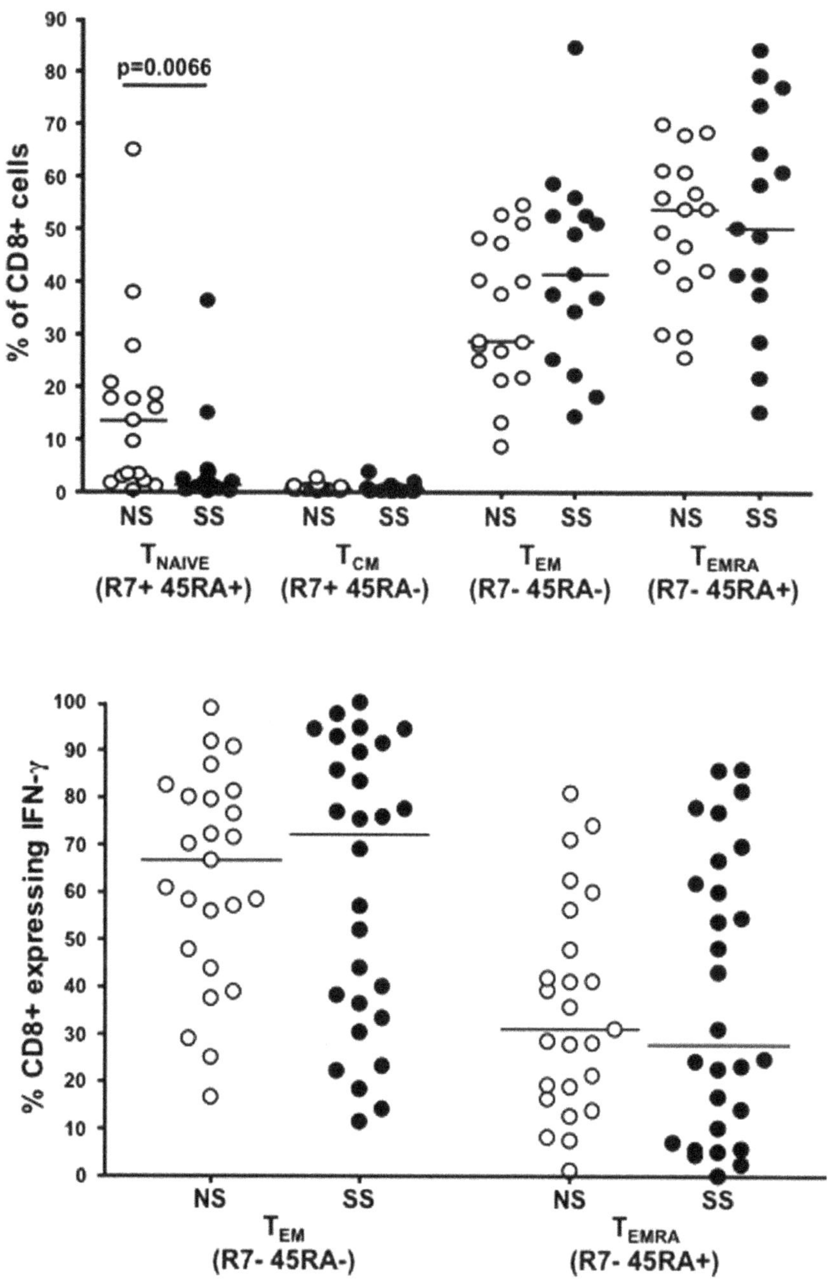

Figure 1. Comparison of differentiation profiles of total CD8+ T cells between progression groups (A) and Comparison of differentiation profiles of Gag-specific effector CD8+ T cells between progression groups (B). We used expression of CCR7 and CD45RA to categorize CD8+ T cells into one of four differentiation phenotypes. Filled circles (●) represent LTS-SS patients and empty circles (○) represent LTS-NS patients. The line in each column represents the median and the differentiation phenotype is beneath each column.

HIV-1 infection who were infected perinatally. The loss of naïve and central memory cells and increased frequency of T_{EMRA} cells could therefore be due to a combination of a greater susceptibility to HIV-1 related cell death, together with thymic dysfunction. Future studies would need to address the relative contributions of these conditions to the observations.

The greater susceptibility of naïve and central memory T cells to loss could potentially be due to effects of chronic immune stimulation from HIV-1. Additional studies would also benefit from analyses looking at cell surface activation markers such as CD38 or HLA-DR. The loss of naïve and central memory T cells, with the accumulation of T_{EMRA} cells, suggests altered T cell maturation kinetics or a change in T_{EMRA} lifespan in progressing subjects. We observed a greater frequency of CD4+CD57+ cells in the LTS-SS group that correlated negatively with CD4% and positively with viremia. CD57 is a marker of senescence. The relationship of the increased CD57+ frequency with other markers of disease progression corroborates the proposed detrimental effect of maturation. This suggests an inability of homeostatic mechanisms to maintain the appropriate proportion of T cell phenotypes necessary for HIV-1 control in progressing subjects and could be related to the accumulation of T_{EMRA} cells.

This study suggests that T cell maturation patterns are significantly different in perinatally HIV-1-infected children with

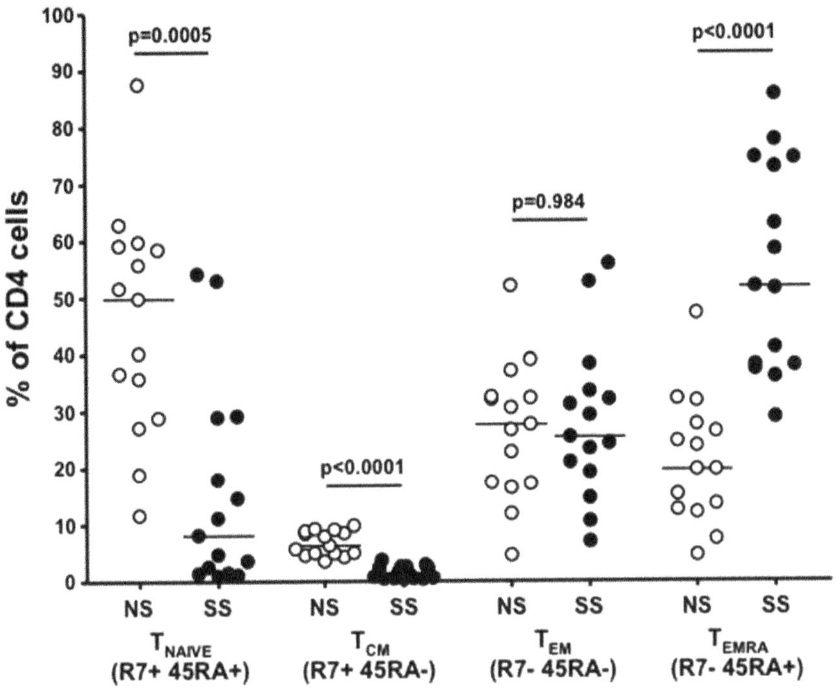

Figure 2. Comparison of differentiation profiles of total CD4 T cells between progression groups. We used expression of CCR7 and CD45RA to categorize CD4 T cells into one of four differentiation phenotypes. Filled circles (●) represent LTS-SS patients and empty circles (○) represent LTS-NS patients. The line in each column represents the median and the differentiation phenotype is beneath each column.

different levels of disease progression, but there are some caveats to be considered. The relatively small number of subjects in the study precludes us from applying these findings to a general pediatric population. The subjects were not all on the same antiretroviral treatment regimens. However, we attempted to minimize these concerns by choosing subjects for the study who: 1) did not receive HAART in the first two years of life; 2) had some levels of ongoing viral replication; and 3) were ARV-experienced, except for two patients. Another equalizing factor is that both groups, as a whole, had generally similar treatment adherence rates. We also cannot be completely confident that the staining protocol does not potentially alter the pattern of staining of CD4+ T cells, which would be avoided by staining antigen specific cells with tetramers. However, few class II tetramers are now available for such studies.

We observed an extremely strong correlation between increased CD4+ T_{EMRA} cells and more severe immunological suppression. Although this suggests that these cells are accumulating during progressive infection, more research into this area is needed. The previously observed resistance of these terminally differentiated cells to R5 tropic strains of HIV-1 is intriguing and may be part of the explanation why these patients are long-term survivors despite persistently low CD4+ T cell levels. These findings could be of importance to the field of pediatric HIV-1 immunology as well as the larger field of HIV-1 vaccine design.

Materials and Methods

Ethics Statement

The research involving human participants reported in this study was approved by the University of California San Francisco (UCSF) and Albert Einstein College of Medicine (AECOM) institutional review boards IRB, with the approval number H11613–19149. Informed written consent was obtained for all subjects. All clinical investigation were conducted according to the principles expressed in the Declaration of Helsinki.

Patient Sample Characteristics

All subjects attended the Pediatric HIV clinic at Jacobi Medical Center in the Bronx, NY. The vast majority of attendees of the Jacobi Pediatric HIV Clinic are either African-American or Hispanic. Stored samples from these patients were selected for this study based on clinical characteristics that allowed them to be classified according to previously published CDC guidelines [19], as explained below. Heparinized whole-blood samples were obtained from 58 subjects after informed consent, based on local Institutional Review Board-approved protocols. Plasma HIV-1 RNA was measured with the Amplicor HIV-1 Monitor with a lower limit of quantification at 50 copies RNA/ml (Roche Diagnostic Systems, Branchburg, NJ).

All subjects were perinatally infected and over 10 years of age, and can thus be defined as long-term survivors (LTS). Since all of the patients were born in an era prior to the availability of pediatric HAART (1996 or before), none of the subjects received potent, suppressive combination therapy during the first two years of life. All of the patients, with the exception of 2 children, were either taking antiretrovirals (ARVs) or were ARV-experienced, at the time of sampling. Additionally, all subjects were viremic at time of sampling and most had variable treatment adherence rates. There were no significant differences in treatment regimen or adherence levels between the two clinical groups.

Clinical Categorization

The general consensus in the pediatric HIV field is that the CD4% value is the most valuable marker of disease progression and is used by the CDC to classify levels of disease status in HIV infected children [19]. In this study, patients were categorized into

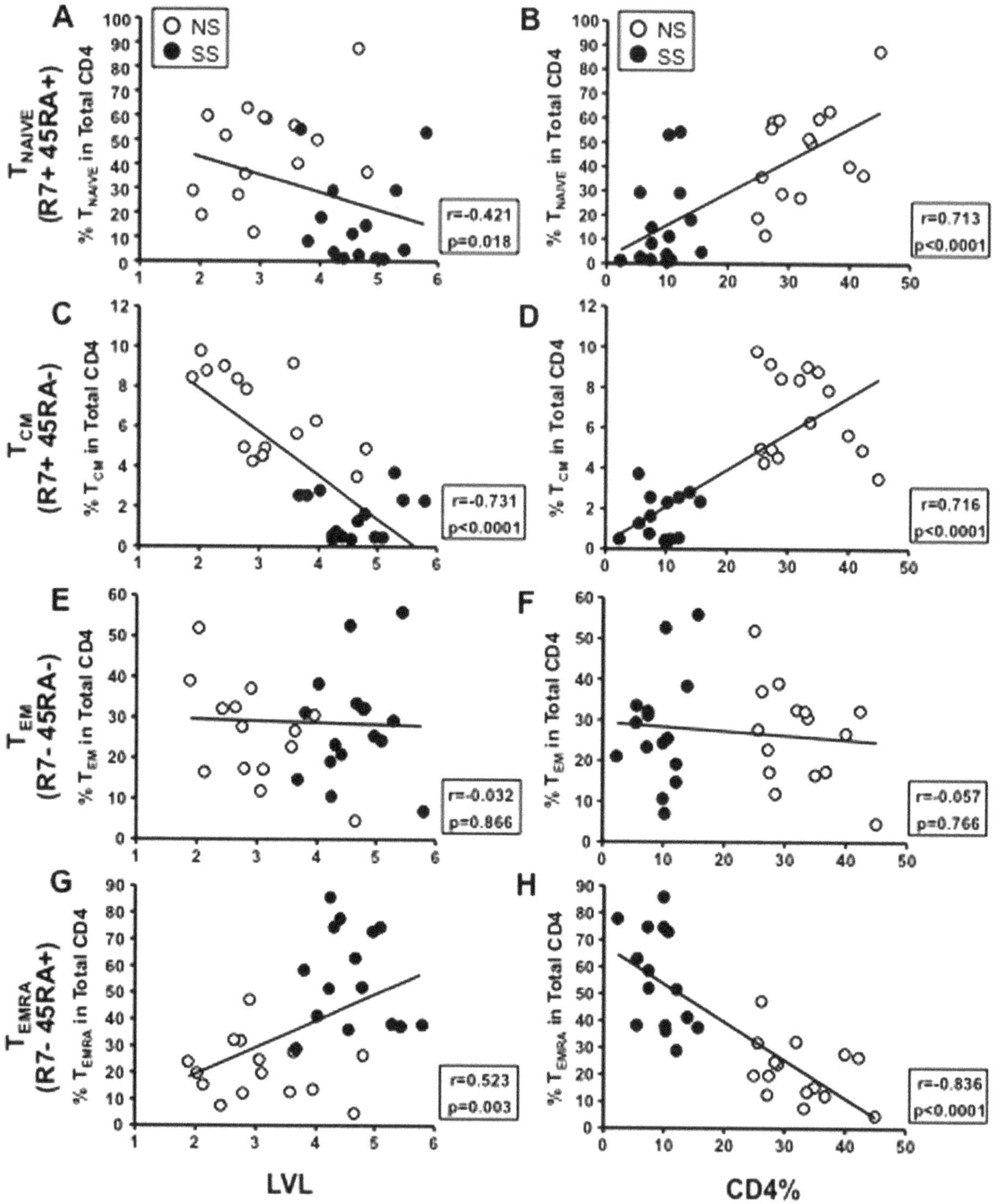

Figure 3. Correlations between frequency of CD4 T cell subsets and clinical characteristics. Log viral load (LVL) versus frequency of CD4 T cell subsets are shown in **A**, **C**, **E**, and **G**. CD4% (of total white blood cells) versus frequency of CD4 T cell subsets are shown in **B**, **D**, **F**, and **H**. The CD4 T cell subset analyzed is at the beginning of each row.

two groups based on CD4% values, according to CDC guidelines [19]. Subjects with a sustained CD4%≥25% were considered LTS with No Evidence of Immune Suppression (LTS-NS). Those with a sustained CD4%≤15% were considered LTS with Severe Immune Suppression (LTS-SS).

Patient histories were used to categorizing patients. Only patients that had always possessed CD4% levels very near or above 25% were considered as an LTS-NS subject. Patients that possessed CD4% levels very near or below 15% for several clinic visits were grouped as an LTS-SS subject. A window was delineated for each patient within which samples were assayed immunologically. We chose a period of time in which samples were available and the patient was as clinically stable as possible, as defined by CD4% and viral loads. We acknowledge that a range

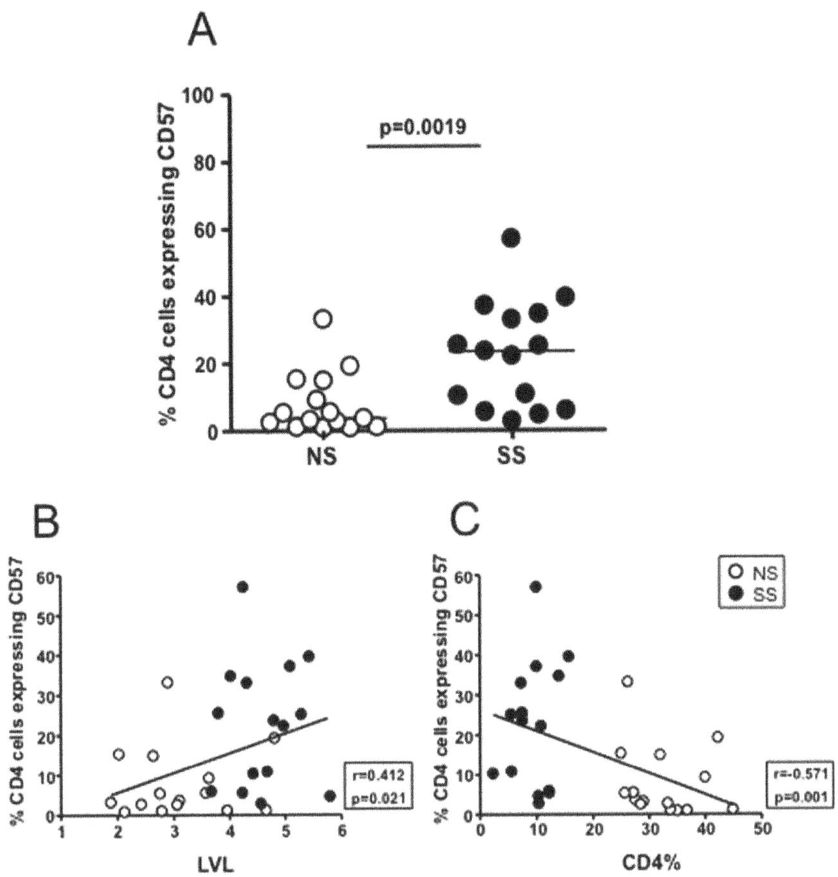

Figure 4. Association between CD57 expression on CD4 T cells and disease progression. A. Comparison of CD57 expression on CD4 T cells between progression groups. **B.** Correlation between log viral load (LVL) and CD57 expression on CD4 T cells. **C.** Correlation between CD4% and expression of CD57 on CD4 T cells.

of immunosuppresion exists within each category, but we have given an overall classification of "no evidence" and "severe" to help distinguish the groups.

Multi-parameter flow cytometry

Single peptides, comprising the HXB2 sequence of Gag (AIDS Research and Reference Reagent Program, NIH), previously identified as containing targeted epitopes were used as the antigenic stimulus (Sharp et al., in preparation). The negative control was media alone and the positive control was Staphylococcal Enterotoxin B (SEB). We also stimulated cultures with a peptide pool consisting of well-identified HLA class I restricted CMV, EBV and Influenza epitopes (CEF) in patients that had previously demonstrated reactivity.

Briefly, cryopreserved PBMC were thawed and cells were stimulated for one hour with either: media alone, antigen, or positive control. The antibody, CD107 α/β-PECy5 was added with stimulation. Brefeldin A (Sigma-Aldrich, St. Louis, MI, USA) was then added at a concentration of 5 µg/ml and cells incubated overnight. The next day, PBMC were washed and stained with antibodies, in combination, against CD4-Alexa700, CD8-Pacific Blue, CD45RA-biotin, CCR7-PECy7, CD57-PECy5, and a live/dead marker emitting in the aqua wavelength for 20 minutes at 4°C. Cells were washed twice and stained with the secondary antibody streptavidin-Qdot655 for 20 minutes at 4°C. Cells were then washed and fixed in 2% paraformaldehyde. The cells were permeabilized using FACS Perm solution (BD Biosciences), washed and stained using antibodies, in combination, against CD3-ECD and IFN-γ-APC for 30 minutes at 25°C. Following staining, the cells were washed, fixed in 1% paraformaldehyde, and collected on a BD LSR-II using FACS DIVA software (BD Biosciences). Data was analyzed using FlowJo (TreeStar).

Gating Strategy

In all analyses a forward scatter (FSC)-height versus FSC-area plot to exclude all cell conjugates was used. Dead cells were then excluded by only gating on cells negative for the live/dead marker. A FSC-area vs. side scatter (SSC)-area plot was used to define the lymphocyte gate. T cells were selected by gating on CD3+ lymphocytes, followed by selection of CD8+ cells by gating on CD3+CD8+ cells. CD4+ cells were defined as CD3+CD8− cells. In panels that contained CD3, CD4, and CD8 antibodies, we verified that, on average, 93% of CD3+CD8− cells were CD4+. IFN-γ+ cells were defined using an APC "fluorescence minus one" (FMO) sample. Quadrant gates were set for expression of CCR7 and CD45RA by using a QDot655 FMO and a PECy7 FMO. IFN-γ+ cells were further analyzed for expression of T-cell memory markers in a CCR7 versus CD45RA.

Statistical Methods

A median (interquartile range) was used as a measure of central tendency for continuous variables. We employed the Mann-Whitney two-tailed t-test for all simple comparisons between two groups. The Spearman Rank correlation test and linear regression analyses were used to explore associations between 2 continuous variables. Differences between categorical data were calculated using Fisher's exact test. We considered a p-value of <0.05 significant. All statistical analyses were performed using the GraphPad Prism 4.03 software package (La Jolla, CA).

Acknowledgments

We thank the patients and their families for participating in this study.

Author Contributions

Conceived and designed the experiments: ERS CBW AAW MGR DFN. Performed the experiments: ERS CBW. Analyzed the data: ERS CBW PJK MGR DFN. Contributed reagents/materials/analysis tools: ERS CBW PJK JA GJF JD AAW MGR DFN. Wrote the paper: ERS CBW PJK AAW MGR DFN.

References

1. Kalams SA, Buchbinder SP, Rosenberg ES, Billingsley JM, Colbert DS, et al. (1999) Association between virus-specific cytotoxic T-lymphocyte and helper responses in human immunodeficiency virus type 1 infection. J Virol 73: 6715–6720.
2. Rosenberg ES, Billingsley JM, Caliendo AM, Boswell SL, Sax PE, et al. (1997) Vigorous HIV-1-specific CD4+ T cell responses associated with control of viremia. Science 278: 1447–1450.
3. Edwards BH, Bansal A, Sabbaj S, Bakari J, Mulligan MJ, et al. (2002) Magnitude of functional CD8+ T-cell responses to the gag protein of human immunodeficiency virus type 1 correlates inversely with viral load in plasma. J Virol 76: 2298–2305.
4. Addo MM, Yu XG, Rathod A, Cohen D, Eldridge RL, et al. (2003) Comprehensive epitope analysis of human immunodeficiency virus type 1 (HIV-1)-specific T-cell responses directed against the entire expressed HIV-1 genome demonstrate broadly directed responses, but no correlation to viral load. J Virol 77: 2081–2092.
5. Cao J, McNevin J, Holte S, Fink L, Corey L, et al. (2003) Comprehensive analysis of human immunodeficiency virus type 1 (HIV-1)-specific gamma interferon-secreting CD8+ T cells in primary HIV-1 infection. J Virol 77: 6867–6878.
6. Champagne P, Ogg GS, King AS, Knabenhans C, Ellefsen K, et al. (2001) Skewed maturation of memory HIV-specific CD8 T lymphocytes. Nature 410: 106–111.
7. Appay V, Dunbar PR, Callan M, Klenerman P, Gillespie GM, et al. (2002) Memory CD8+ T cells vary in differentiation phenotype in different persistent virus infections. Nat Med 8: 379–385.
8. Northfield JW, Loo CP, Barbour JD, Spotts G, Hecht FM, et al. (2007) Human immunodeficiency virus type 1 (HIV-1)-specific CD8+ T(EMRA) cells in early infection are linked to control of HIV-1 viremia and predict the subsequent viral load set point. J Virol 81: 5759–5765.
9. Betts MR, Ambrozak DR, Douek DC, Bonhoeffer S, Brenchley JM, et al. (2001) Analysis of total human immunodeficiency virus (HIV)-specific CD4(+) and CD8(+) T-cell responses: relationship to viral load in untreated HIV infection. J Virol 75: 11983–11991.
10. Teixeira L, Valdez H, McCune JM, Koup RA, Badley AD, et al. (2001) Poor CD4 T cell restoration after suppression of HIV-1 replication may reflect lower thymic function. Aids 15: 1749–1756.
11. Garber DA, Silvestri G, Barry AP, Fedanov A, Kozyr N, et al. (2004) Blockade of T cell costimulation reveals interrelated actions of CD4+ and CD8+ T cells in control of SIV replication. J Clin Invest 113: 836–845.
12. Staprans SI, Barry AP, Silvestri G, Safrit JT, Kozyr N, et al. (2004) Enhanced SIV replication and accelerated progression to AIDS in macaques primed to mount a CD4 T cell response to the SIV envelope protein. Proc Natl Acad Sci U S A 101: 13026–13031.
13. Pitcher CJ, Quittner C, Peterson DM, Connors M, Koup RA, et al. (1999) HIV-1-specific CD4+ T cells are detectable in most individuals with active HIV-1 infection, but decline with prolonged viral suppression. Nat Med 5: 518–525.
14. Bitmansour AD, Douek DC, Maino VC, Picker LJ (2002) Direct ex vivo analysis of human CD4(+) memory T cell activation requirements at the single clonotype level. J Immunol 169: 1207–1218.
15. Okoye A, Meier-Schellersheim M, Brenchley JM, Hagen SI, Walker JM, et al. (2007) Progressive CD4+ central memory T cell decline results in CD4+ effector memory insufficiency and overt disease in chronic SIV infection. J Exp Med 204: 2171–2185.
16. Chomont N, DaFonseca S, Vandergeeten C, Ancuta P, Sekaly RP (2011) Maintenance of CD4+ T-cell memory and HIV persistence: keeping memory, keeping HIV. Curr Opin HIV AIDS 6: 30–36.
17. Younes SA, Trautmann L, Yassine-Diab B, Kalfayan LH, Kernaleguen AE, et al. (2007) The duration of exposure to HIV modulates the breadth and the magnitude of HIV-specific memory CD4+ T cells. J Immunol 178: 788–797.
18. Dion ML, Bordi R, Zeidan J, Asaad R, Boulassel MR, et al. (2007) Slow disease progression and robust therapy-mediated CD4+ T-cell recovery are associated with efficient thymopoiesis during HIV-1 infection. Blood 109: 2912–2920.
19. CDC (1994) 1994 Revised Classification System for Human Immunodeficiency Virus Infection in Children less than 13 Years of Age. MMWR Morb Mortal Wkly Rep 43: 1–10.
20. Addo MM, Draenert R, Rathod A, Verrill CL, Davis BT, et al. (2007) Fully differentiated HIV-1 specific CD8+ T effector cells are more frequently detectable in controlled than in progressive HIV-1 infection. PLoS ONE 2: e321.
21. Hess C, Altfeld M, Thomas SY, Addo MM, Rosenberg ES, et al. (2004) HIV-1 specific CD8+ T cells with an effector phenotype and control of viral replication. Lancet 363: 863–866.
22. Brenchley JM, Karandikar NJ, Betts MR, Ambrozak DR, Hill BJ, et al. (2003) Expression of CD57 defines replicative senescence and antigen-induced apoptotic death of CD8+ T cells. Blood 101: 2711–2720.
23. Betts MR, Nason MC, West SM, De Rosa SC, Migueles SA, et al. (2006) HIV nonprogressors preferentially maintain highly functional HIV-specific CD8+ T cells. Blood 107: 4781–4789.
24. Hansen SG, Vieville C, Whizin N, Coyne-Johnson L, Siess DC, et al. (2009) Effector memory T cell responses are associated with protection of rhesus monkeys from mucosal simian immunodeficiency virus challenge. Nat Med 15: 293–299.
25. Oswald-Richter K, Grill SM, Leelawong M, Tseng M, Kalams SA, et al. (2007) Identification of a CCR5-expressing T cell subset that is resistant to R5-tropic HIV infection. PLoS Pathog 3: e58.
26. Kourtis AP, Ibegbu C, Nahmias AJ, Lee FK, Clark WS, et al. (1996) Early progression of disease in HIV-infected infants with thymus dysfunction. N Engl J Med 335: 1431–1436.
27. Nahmias AJ, Clark WS, Kourtis AP, Lee FK, Cotsonis G, et al. (1998) Thymic dysfunction and time of infection predict mortality in human immunodeficiency virus-infected infants. CDC Perinatal AIDS Collaborative Transmission Study Group. J Infect Dis 178: 680–685.

8

Spatially Explicit Burden Estimates of Malaria in Tanzania: Bayesian Geostatistical Modeling of the Malaria Indicator Survey Data

Laura Gosoniu[1], Amina Msengwa[2], Christian Lengeler[1], Penelope Vounatsou[1]*

1 Department of Public Health and Epidemiology, Swiss Tropical and Public Health Institute, University of Basel, Switzerland, **2** Department of statistics, University of Dar es Salaam, Dar es Salaam, Tanzania

Abstract

A national HIV/AIDS and malaria parasitological survey was carried out in Tanzania in 2007–2008. In this study the parasitological data were analyzed: i) to identify climatic/environmental, socio-economic and interventions factors associated with child malaria risk and ii) to produce a contemporary, high spatial resolution parasitaemia risk map of the country. Bayesian geostatistical models were fitted to assess the association between parasitaemia risk and its determinants. Bayesian kriging was employed to predict malaria risk at unsampled locations across Tanzania and to obtain the uncertainty associated with the predictions. Markov chain Monte Carlo (MCMC) simulation methods were employed for model fit and prediction. Parasitaemia risk estimates were linked to population data and the number of infected children at province level was calculated. Model validation indicated a high predictive ability of the geostatistical model, with 60.00% of the test locations within the 95% credible interval. The results indicate that older children are significantly more likely to test positive for malaria compared with younger children and living in urban areas and better-off households reduces the risk of infection. However, none of the environmental and climatic proxies or the intervention measures were significantly associated with the risk of parasitaemia. Low levels of malaria prevalence were estimated for Zanzibar island. The population-adjusted prevalence ranges from 0.29% in Kaskazini province (Zanzibar island) to 18.65% in Mtwara region. The pattern of predicted malaria risk is similar with the previous maps based on historical data, although the estimates are lower. The predicted maps could be used by decision-makers to allocate resources and target interventions in the regions with highest burden of malaria in order to reduce the disease transmission in the country.

Editor: Georges Snounou, Université Pierre et Marie Curie, France

Funding: This investigation received financial support from the Swiss National Science Foundation Project No. IZLSZ3 122926). The funders had no role in study design, data collection and analysis, decision to publish, or preparation of the manuscript.

Competing Interests: The authors have declared that no competing interests exist.

* E-mail: penelope.vounatsou@unibas.ch

Introduction

Malaria is still a major public health problem in the United Republic of Tanzania, as the leading cause of inpatient and outpatient consultations. Ninety three percent of the population of Tanzania live in areas where malaria is transmitted for at least one month per year. Although Tanzania has been on the forefront in promoting the use of insecticide treated nets (ITNs), there are still between 60000 and 80000 malaria attributable deaths estimated per year, mainly children under the age of five ([1]). The disease is one of the main obstacles to the economical development of the country. The malaria situation in Zanzibar, the group of islands off the north-eastern coast of the Tanzania mainland, is a bit different than the one on the mainland. Over the past decade Zanzibar has reached very low levels of malaria endemicity due to rapidly scaling up of current antimalarial interventions([2]), and it is now one of the regions that is planning to eliminate the disease.

Planning and evaluating cost-effective strategies for the control and even more, the elimination of malaria, requires contemporary, high spatial resolution maps of the disease distribution as well as reliable estimates of the number of infected people. These measures will help tracking the progress and documenting reduction in parasitaemia rates as a result of control. Some earlier attempts to describe the situation of malaria transmission in Tanzania were based on analysis of historical parasite prevalence data ([3],[4]). However, historical field survey data were collected in different seasons and at non-standardized and overlapping age groups of the population. Therefore, accounting for seasonality and adjusting for age become challenging when modeling malaria survey data. The drawbacks of historical malaria survey data have been discussed in more details and addressed previously ([5], [6]). In addition, the estimated parasitaemia risk based on the analysis of historical data may not reflect the current malaria situation since they don't take into account the effect of malaria interventions which increased over the last decade. In addition, a map of endemic malaria distribution in Tanzania (available on MARA ([7]) website) was produced by [8] using spatially interpolated weather station data to define climatic suitability for malaria transmission.

From October 2007 to February 2008, the National Bureau of Statistics (NBS) in collaboration with the Office of the Chief Government Statistician (OCGS), Zanzibar implemented the Tanzania HIV/AIDS and Malaria Indicator Survey (THMIS).

The aims of this survey were to assess the prevalence of HIV infection among Tanzanian adults and the prevalence of malaria infection and anemia among children under five years old. Here Bayesian geostatistical models based on environmental and climatic risk factors were implemented to produce the first contemporary, high spatial resolution parasitaemia risk map and spatially explicit disease burden estimates for Tanzania by analyzing the THMIS malaria data.

Materials and Methods

1.2 THMIS Data

Ethic statement. The survey protocol was submitted to and approved by the National Institute for Medical Research (NIMR). Written informed consent was obtained from the parent or guardian of the child. The statement explained the purpose of the test, how the test would be administered, and advised the parent or guardian that the results would be available as soon as the test was completed. Finally, permission was requested for the test to be carried out.

The THMIS was conducted over a four-month period, from October 2007 until February 2008. A two-stage sampling approach was used to select the surveyed population. In the first stage were selected 475 clusters consisting of enumeration areas defined for the 2002 Population and Housing Census. In particular, 25 sample points were selected in Dar es Salaam, 18 in each of the other 20 regions in the mainland and 18 sample points in each of the 5 regions in Zanzibar. The second stage of selection involved the systematic sampling of households from the clusters. A total of 9144 households throughout Tanzania were sampled, 16 from each sampling point in Dar es Salaam, 18 households per cluster in the other regions in mainland and Pemba and 36 households per sampling unit in Unguja. Further details on the sampling approach can be found in [9]. In the selected households men and female age 15–49 were interviewed individually. Basic demographic information and data on the health status of the person interviewed and other members of the household were collected. In addition, information on the characteristics of the household dwelling, such as source of water, type of toilet facilities, materials used to construct the house and possession of various durable goods were gathered. Based on the household characteristics and household possessions a wealth index was constructed. The THMIS assembled also information on household coverage of malaria interventions such as IRS activities and ownership/use of bednets or ITNs. In addition, blood samples for anemia and malaria testing among children 6–59 months were collected. Although there is a large amount of information on HIV/AIDS knowledge and behavior and HIV prevalence, the analysis of these data is not the focus of this paper. The sampled clusters where parasitaemia prevalence data were collected are shown Figure 1.

1.3 Environmental and climatic data

Transmission of malaria is environmentally driven, therefore climatic and environmental proxies were used as parasitaemia predictors. The following climatic and environmental factors were used in the analysis: land surface temperature (LST), rainfall, normalized difference vegetation index (NDVI), altitude and distance to nearest permanent water body. The sources of these data, as well as the spatial and temporal resolution are shown in Table 1. Further details on the description of the climatic factors are given in [10]. The environmental factors with available temporal resolution (LST, rainfall and NDVI) were acquired for the one year period previous to the survey and annual average of each environmental covariate was calculated and extracted at each data location.

1.4 Statistical modeling

At each location in $S=(s_1,s_2,\ldots,s_n)^T$ let us consider the binary outcome Y_{ij} which takes value 1 or 0 to indicate whether the child j at location s_i was found parasitaemia positive. A logistic regression model was used to relate the outcome to its predictors. The multivariate logistic regression model is given by

$$logit(p_{ij})=\beta_0+\sum_{k=1}^{p}\beta_k X_{ij}^{(k)}, \tag{1}$$

where p_{ij} is the risk of child j at location s_i of having parasitaemia, $X_{ij}=(X_{ij}^{(1)},X_{ij}^{(2)},\ldots,X_{ij}^{(p)})^T$ are the covariates and $\beta=(\beta_0,\beta_1,\beta_2,\ldots,\beta_p)^T$ is the vector of regression coefficients, including the intercept. Preliminary frequentist statistical analysis was performed in Stata version 10.0 (Stata corporation, College Station, TX) to identify the covariates significantly associated with the parasitaemia prevalence and to check for possible nonlinear trends of the relationship between explanatory variables and response variable. To account for the nonlinear relationship between malaria and demographic or environmental and climatic covariates, the continuous variables were categorized, where the cutoffs points were chosen based on outcome-covariate scatter plots.

1.4.1 Bayesian geostatistical modeling. The model described above does not consider the spatial relationship among the parasitaemia survey locations. The standard way of incorporating the geographical dependence in the model is by introducing spatially correlated random effects ϕ_i at every sampled location s_i. Using the geostatistical design described in [11] the underlying spatial process was modeled by the residuals via a multivariate Normal distribution with mean 0 and the covariance matrix Σ, $\phi=(\phi_1,\ldots,\phi_n)^T\sim MVN(0,\Sigma)$. The covariance matrix is defined as a function which represents the decay in correlation between pairs of locations with distance. For this analysis, an exponential correlation function was chosen, that is $\Sigma_{ij}=\sigma^2 exp(-d_{ij}/\rho)$, where ρ describes how fast the spatial correlation declines with distance between locations i and j and σ^2 represents the variance of the spatial process. Measurement error or microscale variations are modeled by the independent and normally distributed random effects $\varepsilon_i\sim N(0,\tau^2)$, where τ^2 is interpreted as a nugget effect. The model in (1) can be written

$$logit(p_{ij})=\beta_0+\sum_{k=1}^{p}\beta_k X_{ij}^{(k)}+\phi_i+\varepsilon_i, \tag{2}$$

This type of hierarchical models are usually fitted within a Bayesian framework because it allows flexible modeling and inference and avoids the computational problems met in likelihood-based fitting. The trade-off for the flexibility of a fully Bayesian approach is the complexity of the model fit. This step is carried out via the implementation of Markov chain Monte Carlo methods. To complete the specification of the Bayesian hierarchical model, prior distributions need to be assigned to the model parameters $\theta=(\beta,\sigma,\rho)$. Further, Bayesian inference is based on the posterior distribution, that is the conditional distribution over parameters given observed data. Non-informative Normal prior distributions were specified for the intercept and the regression coefficients, $p(\beta)=N(0,1000)$. The spatial correlation parameters σ and ρ were assigned an inverse gamma and a gamma prior distribution, respectively, $p(\sigma)=IG(a_1,b_1)$ and $p(\rho)=G(a_2,b_2)$. Non-informative inverse gamma prior distribution was chosen for

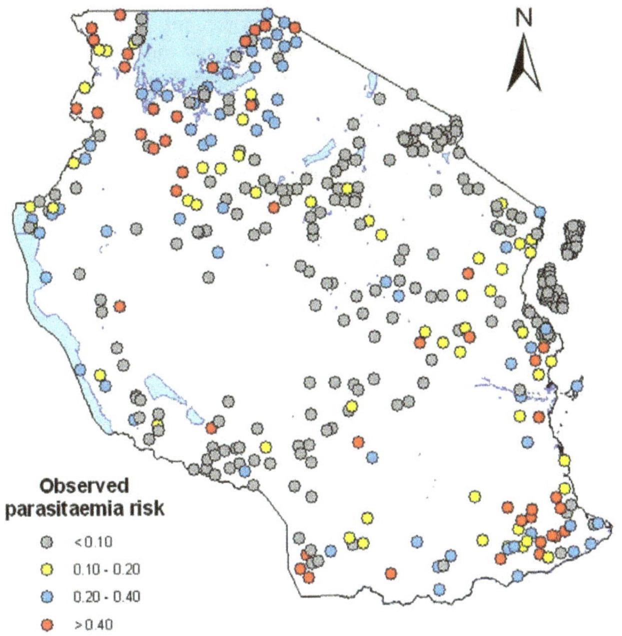

Figure 1. Observed parasitaemia prevalence in children less than 5 years old from the THMIS carried out 465 locations.

the non-spatial variance, $p(\tau^2)=IG(a_3,b_3)$. The values of the parameters a_1,b_1,a_2,b_2,a_3,b_3 were chosen such that the mean of the corresponding distribution is 1 and the variance 100. A two chain sampler of 100000 iterations was run with a burn-in of 10000 iterations and the convergence was assessed by examining the ergodic averages of selected parameters.

Separate geostatistical models were fitted for mainland Tanzania and the two islands covering Zanzibar (Pemba and Unguja). In particular, for each region we fitted Bayesian geostatistical models to assess the effects of interventions after adjusting for climatic and environmental factors and to estimate the disease burden at high spatial resolution. Model A includes as covariates the demographic variables, socio-economic status and malaria interventions, model B includes only the environmental and climatic proxies and model C includes the demographic variables, socio-economic status, malaria interventions and environmental/climatic factors. For each model, a burn-in of 5000 iterations was run. Convergence was assessed by inspection of the ergodic averages for all parameters and was achieved after 100000 iterations for all models. Samples obtained from MCMC are not independent but autocorrelated, therefore a thinning of 10 iterations was used when extracting samples from the posterior distribution. Disease burden estimates were obtained using Bayesian kriging and employing only environmental predictors (model B) because malaria intervention data and wealth index information are not available for the whole country. In particular, predictions were made at 122017 locations covering mainland Tanzania, 204 locations covering Unguja and 125 locations covering Pemba. The Bayesian kriging was implemented using software written by the authors in Fortran 95 (Compaq Visual Fortran Professional 6.6.0) using standard numerical libraries (NAG, The Numerical Algorithms Group Ltd.). The number of children infected with malaria parasites were obtained by combining the number of children with the parasitaemia risk at each of the 122346 locations. The population data were acquired from the International Data Base of the U.S. Census Bureau, Population Division for the year 2006. Although these data are outdated and maybe underestimate the total population in the country, they represent the only source of population data at such small spatial resolution.

To validate model B, which was used to predict parasitaemia risk, model fit was carried out on a randomly selected subset of 299 locations (training set). The remaining 75 locations (test points), comprising a simple random sample, were used for validation. To assess the predictive performance of the model, 11 credible intervals of the posterior predictive distribution at the test locations with probability coverage equal to 5%, 10%, 20%, 30%, 40%, 50%, 60%,70%, 80%, 90% and 100%, respectively were calculated and the percentages of test locations with observed parasitaemia prevalence falling in these intervals were computed.

Results

A total of 6360 children under 5 years old at 465 geo-located clusters had *P. falciparum* parasitaemia results from blood film examination. The prevalence of asymptotic malaria among children in Tanzania was estimated from the pooled data at 13.0% (95% CI: 12.1%–13.8%). In mainland the parasitaemia risk at cluster level ranged from 0.0% to 83.3% with a mean of 15.0%. 87.4% of clusters had malaria risk below 40.0%. The malaria risk in Zanzibar island was much lower, varying from 0.0% to 10.7% in Pemba and 0.0% to 14.3% in Unguja. In terms of malaria

Table 1. Spatial databases used in the analysis.

Factor	Spatial	Temporal	Source
	Resolution	Resolution	
LST	1 km^2	8 days	MODIS
			http://lpdaac.usgs.gov/modis/myd11c1v4.asp
Rainfall	8 km^2	10 days	ADDS
			http://earlywarning.usgs.gov/adds/
NDVI	1 km^2	16 days	MODIS
			http://lpdaac.usgs.gov/modis/mod13q1v4.asp
Altitude	1 km^2	N.A.	USGS-DEM
Permanent water bodies	1 km^2	N.A.	Health Mapper
			http://eros.usgs.gov/products/elevation/dem.html

Table 2. Association of parasitaemia risk with demographic variables, socio-economic status, malaria interventions and environmental/climatic factors in mainland Tanzania resulting from the bivariate and multivariate non-spatial models.

Variable	Bivariate non-spatial model	Multivariate non-spatial model
	OR 95% CI	**OR** 95% CI
Residence (Rural)	1.0	1.0
Urban	0.23 (0.17,0.33)	0.50 (0.34,0.74)
Age (< = 12 months)	1.0	1.0
13–24	1.70 (1.25,2.33)	1.75 (1.27,2.42)
25–36	2.26 (1.67,3.07)	2.49 (1.81,3.42)
37–48	2.28 (1.68,3.11)	2.49 (1.80,3.43)
49–60	2.63 (1.94,3.56)	2.94 (2.14,4.05)
Wealth index (Most poor)	1.0	1.0
Very poor	0.99 (0.81,1.22)	0.89 (0.71,1.10)
Poor	0.87 (0.71,1.07)	0.81 (0.65,1.02)
Less poor	0.52 (0.40,0.66)	0.55 (0.42,0.72)
Least poor	0.15 (0.10,0.24)	0.28 (0.17,0.45)
Having bednet (No)	1.0	1.0
Yes	1.12 (0.96,1.32)	1.03 (0.86,1.23)
IRS (No)	1.0	1.0
Yes	1.19 (0.61,2.32)	1.03 (0.50,2.15)
Altitude (< = 1500 m)	1.0	1.0
1500	0.28 (0.21,0.37)	0.43 (0.30,0.61)
Distance to nearest water body (< = 700 m)	1.0	1.0
700–2500	1.41 (1.09,1.83)	1.43 (1.09,1.89)
2500	1.63 (1.27,2.09)	1.67 (1.28,2.18)
Rainfall (< 15 mm)	1.0	1.0
15–20	2.69 (1.92,3.76)	1.86 (1.30,2.65)
20	4.46 (3.24,6.14)	2.80 (1.99,3.94)
NDVI (< 0.4)	1.0	1.0
0.4–0.6	4.15 (3.25,5.29)	2.70 (2.07,3.51)
0.6	4.42 (3.23,6.05)	2.68 (1.83,3.94)
Day temperature (< 26.0°C)	1.0	1.0
26.0–29.0	2.76 (2.01,3.80)	2.15 (1.53,3.03)
29.0	1.76 (1.30,2.39)	1.65 (1.15,2.38)
Night temperature (< 16.0°C)	1.0	1.0
16.0–20.0	2.12 (1.74,2.59)	1.67 (1.27,2.20)
20.0	1.58 (1.21,2.07)	1.52 (1.08,2.12)

intervention coverage, there is a big discrepancy between mainland and Zanzibar islands. In particular, 61.3% of households in mainland and 93.3% of households in Zanzibar had at least one bednet used for sleeping (p-value < 0.0001). The difference is even bigger when it comes to IRS coverage. In mainland, only 1.2% of household had walls sprayed with insecticide, while in Zanzibar island the proportion was 95.7% (p-value < 0.0001).

The estimates of the effect of demographic, wealth index, malaria interventions and environmental/climatic factors on parasitaemia risk obtained from the bivariate and multivariate non-spatial models in mainland Tanzania are presented in Table 2. The bivariate analyses indicates that in mainland all predictors except malaria interventions were statistical significantly associated with the parasitaemia risk at 5% significance level. In particular, children living in urban areas had significantly lower risk of parasitaemia compared with children in rural areas. A positive relationship with age indicated that the older the child the higher the risk of malaria. As it was expected, the wealth index was negatively associated with the parasitaemia risk, suggesting that children belonging to better-off households had less risk of acquiring malaria. Both malaria intervention variables included in this analysis (bednet ownership and IRS) showed a non-protective effect, although none of them were statistically significant. Altitude was negatively associated with the parasitaemia risk, indicating that children at above 1500 meters had lower odds of malaria. Surprisingly, the odds of malaria for children living further away from water bodies were higher than the odds of children closer to permanent sources of water. The results also

Table 3. Association of parasitaemia risk with demographic variables, socio-economic status, malaria interventions and environmental/climatic factors in mainland Tanzania resulting from the Bayesian geostatistical models.

Variable	Geostatistical model A*		Geostatistical model B**		Geostatistical model C***	
	OR	95% BCI	OR	95% BCI	OR	95% BCI
Residence (Rural)	1.0				1.0	
Urban	0.36	(0.20,0.62)			0.42	(0.24,0.74)
Age (<=12 months)	1.0				1.0	
13–24	1.89	(1.34,2.68)			1.88	(1.33,2.69)
25–36	2.64	(1.88,3.74)			2.64	(1.87,3.74)
37–48	2.63	(1.87,3.72)			2.64	(1.87,3.75)
49–60	3.41	(2.43,4.83)			3.44	(2.43,4.88)
Wealth index (Most poor)	1.0				1.0	
Very poor	1.07	(0.83,1.37)			1.07	(0.83,1.37)
Poor	0.95	(0.73,1.24)			0.95	(0.73,1.24)
Less poor	0.69	(0.50,0.95)			0.70	(0.51,0.96)
Least poor	0.34	(0.20,0.59)			0.37	(0.20,0.63)
Having bednet (No)	1.0				1.0	
Yes	0.95	(0.77,1.16)			0.92	(0.75,1.13)
IRS (No)	1.0				1.0	
Yes	1.42	(0.42,4.28)			1.17	(0.33,3.63)
Altitude (<=1500 m)			1.0		1.0	
1500			0.53	(0.25,1.04)	0.51	(0.25,1.02)
Distance to nearest water body (<=700 m)			1.0		1.0	
700–2500			1.34	(0.82,2.24)	1.35	(0.82,2.23)
2500			1.39	(0.84,2.50)	1.40	(0.86,2.28)
Rainfall (<15 mm)			1.0		1.0	
15–20			0.76	(0.36,1.60)	0.97	(0.48,1.90)
20			1.28	(0.47,2.99)	1.43	(0.63,3.14)
NDVI (<0.4)			1.0		1.0	
0.4–0.6			1.79	(1.13,2.91)	1.47	(0.88,2.45)
0.6			1.90	(0.89,3.89)	1.40	(0.67,2.98)
Day temperature (<26.0°C)			1.0		1.0	
26.0–29.0			2.09	(1.14,3.87)	2.01	(1.13,3.60)
29.0			0.94	(0.49,1.82)	1.07	(0.56,2.03)
Night temperature (<16.0°C)			1.0		1.0	
16.0–20.0			1.46	(0.83,2.63)	1.47	(0.81,2.73)
20.0			1.20	(0.58,2.42)	1.31	(0.61,2.81)

*The model includes only the demographic variables, socio-economic status and malaria interventions as predictors.
**The model includes only the environmental and climatic proxies as predictors.
***The model includes the demographic variables, socio-economic status, malaria interventions and environmental/climatic factors as predictors.

suggest that the malaria odds are increasing with an increase in rainfall, vegetation index, day and night temperature. In Pemba, the relationship between parasitaemia and age and wealth index is not monotone, as in mainland. In addition, we observe a protective effect of bednets, which is not significant. Bivariate analysis suggested that in Unguja none of the covariates under study were significantly associated with parasitaemia prevalence.

Table 3 presents the effect of residence, age, wealth index, malaria interventions and environmental/climatic factors on parasitaemia risk in mainland. These estimates were obtained by fitting Bayesian geostatistical models described in section 2.3.1. After taking into account the spatial correlation, residence (living in urban area has a protective effect), age (older children are more likely than younger children to test positive for malaria) and wealth index (living in better-off households has a protective effect) remained significantly associated with malaria. This was not the case for the environmental and climatic proxies. When all covariates were included in the model, only residence, age, wealth index (less poor, least poor) remained statistically significant associated with parasitaemia risk in mainland Tanzania (Table 3).

Posterior estimates of the spatial parameters (spatial variance and decay parameter) and the non-spatial variance are presented

Table 4. Posterior estimates of spatial parameters.

Spatial parameter	Tanzania		Pemba		Unguja	
	Median	95% BCI[a]	Median	95% BCI[a]	Median	95% BCI[a]
σ^2	1.74	(0.63, 148.4)	3.23	(0.48, 40.5)	2.89	(0.41, 95.68)
τ^2	0.59	(0.22, 0.98)	1.47	(0.28, 21.65)	1.49	(0.29, 31.5)
range[b]	206.25	(124.53, 370.79)	1.05	(0.52, 21.22)	0.67	(0.34, 17.41)

[a]: Bayesian confidence intervals.
[b]: Based on the decay parameter ρ, the range parameter $3/\rho$ (in km) is calculated.

in Table 4. In all three areas the spatial variance was significantly larger than the non-spatial variance. The estimates of the range parameter suggest a strong spatial correlation in mainland and a weak spatial correlation in Pemba and Unguja.

Figure 2 shows the prediction performance of model B via proportion of test locations with malaria prevalence falling into credible intervals of coverage ranging from 5% to 100%. Based on these results we can state that the model is fairly accurate, with 4%, 53% and 85.33% of the test locations within the 5%, 90% and 100% credible interval respectivelly.

The map of predicted parasitaemia risk for the United Republic of Tanzania is shown in Figure 3. The risk of malaria varies from 0.1% to 38.9%, with a median of 4.9%. High levels of prevalence (>20%) were predicted in the north of the country, the area around Lake Victroia (regions Kagera, Mara and Shinyanga) as well as in the south of the country (provinces Pwani, Lindi, Mtwara and Ruvuma). Low levels of parasitaemia risk (<5%) are observed in the central part of the country, north-east and south-west and the island of Zanzibar. The lower (2.5%) and upper (97.5%) percentiles of the posterior distribution corresponding to the predicted malaria risk are depicted in Figure 4.

Figure 5 shows the predicted number of children with malaria parasites in the United Republic of Tanzania. The estimates of number of children <5 with malaria parasites at the regional level are presented in Table 5. We observe that both before and after adjusting for population distribution, Kaskazini region in Unguja had the lowest risk of malaria and Mtwara region in mainland had the highest risk.

Discussion

The parasitaemia survey of the 2007–08 THMIS was designed to provide an estimate of the malaria prevalence among children under five and to measure malaria prevention and treatment outcomes including possession and use of ITNs and IRS activities in the United Republic of Tanzania. Parasitaemia data of this survey were modeled within a spatial context to identify predictors significantly associated with malaria and to produce the 2008 malaria risk map as well as the map of infected children under five in the United Republic of Tanzania. The geostatistical model had a high predictive ability as shown by the high percentage of test locations with observed parasitaemia prevalence falling in the

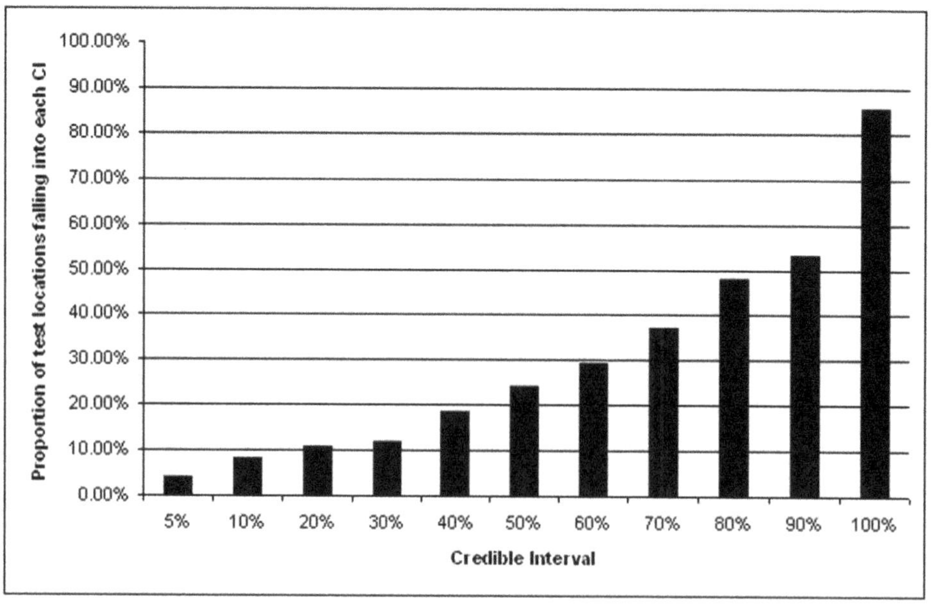

Figure 2. Percentage of test locations with observed malaria prevalence falling within the 5%, 10%, 20%, 30%, 40%, 50%, 60%, 70%, 80%, 90% and 100% credible intervals of the posterior predictive distribution.

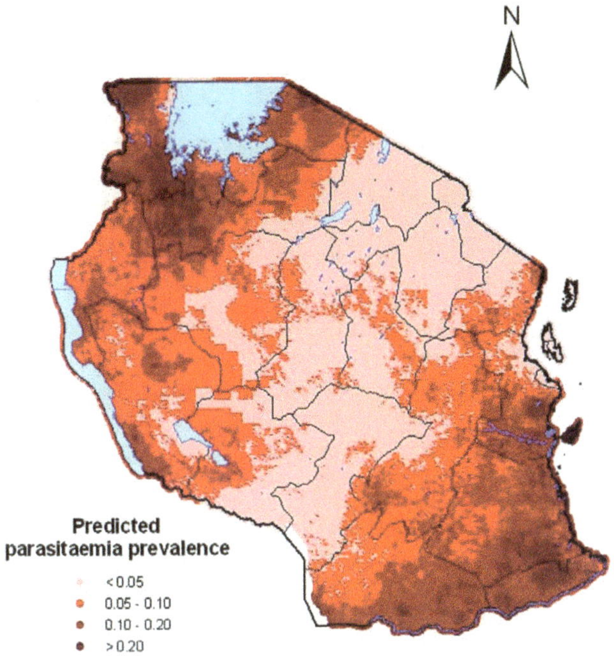

Figure 3. Smooth map of the parasitaemia risk in children <5 years in Tanzania.

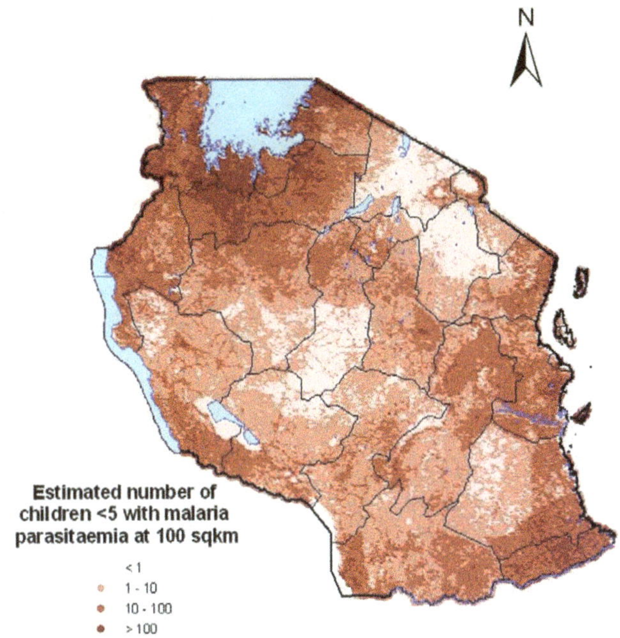

Figure 5. Estimated number of children <5 years infected with malaria parasite in Tanzania.

credible intervals. Previous efforts ([12], [3],[4]) have been made to map malaria prevalence in Tanzania, by collecting and analyzing historical survey data. The risk map presented here depicts with high-fidelity the contemporary situation of malaria in the country and could be used as part of monitoring and evaluation of malaria situation and ongoing interventions in the country.

Compared to the distribution maps based on historical data([3],[4]), our malaria risk map shows an overall lower prevalence over the country. The malaria distribution map shows very low levels of prevalence (<0.05%) on the island of Zanzibar. This could be explained by the increase in coverage levels of interventions which significantly reduced the burden of disease [13]. This type of interventions should be emulated in mainland Tanzania, especially in the areas of high risk (provinces Kagera, Mara, Shinyanga, Pwani, Lindi, Mtwara and Ruvuma). Although we observe a decrease in malaria prevalence over the last years, the magnitude of the decline is not clear in the absence of a baseline map. There are, however, evidences from other studies such as the National Malaria Control Programme (NMCP) survey carried out in 21 districts which shows a decline of 30% in under-five malaria risk between 2006 and 2008. In Ifakara and Rufiji Demographic Surveillance System (DSS) all-age malaria preva-

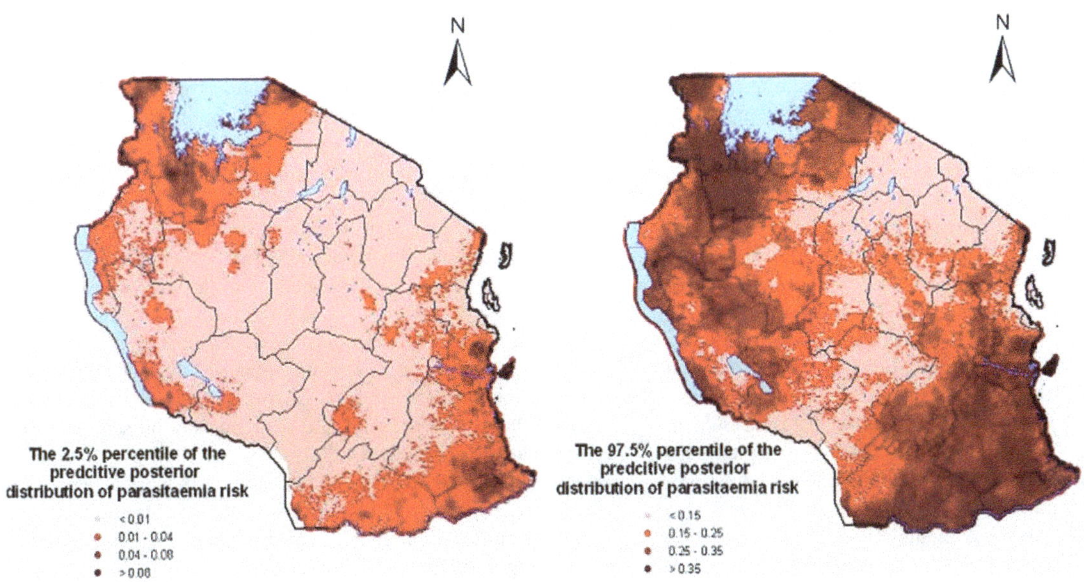

Figure 4. The 2.5% (left) and 97.5% (right) percentiles of the predicted posterior distribution for the parasitaemia prevalence.

Table 5. Estimates of the number of children less than 5 years old with malaria parasites at regional level.

Region	Number of children <5	Infected children	95%CI	Model-based prevalence	Model-based prevalence adjusted for population
Arusha	243725	1694	(200,11362)	1.11%	0.70%
Dar-Es-Salaam	422267	6203	(2180,15486)	3.05%	1.47%
Dodoma	287515	6895	(849,37505)	2.70%	2.40%
Iringa	251918	5374	(610,30768)	2.14%	2.13%
Kagera	349344	58494	(13291,122501)	17.68%	16.74%
Kaskazini-Pemba	31049	366	(105,1152)	1.04%	1.18%
Kaskazini-Unguja	25086	73	(16,263)	0.32%	0.29%
Kigoma	286895	24568	(4423,79297)	7.78%	8.56%
Kilimanjaro	216248	1287	(162,8223)	0.60%	0.59%
Kusini Unguja	14436	163	(41,595)	0.99%	1.13%
Kusini-Pemba	29202	263	(81,864)	0.77%	0.90%
Lindi	130174	22810	(5931,48259)	12.82%	17.52%
Manyara	170711	2535	(328,14111)	1.37%	1.49%
Mara	232267	36158	(12153,19547)	11.26%	15.57%
Mbeya	349050	9053	(1186,45019)	3.47%	2.59%
Mjini-Magharibi	44467	386	(127,1035)	0.76%	0.87%
Morogoro	304225	17724	(2621,72404)	6.01%	5.83%
Mtwara	192776	35946	(10332,71287)	17.96%	18.65%
Mwanza	448578	55631	(13867,130405)	13.13%	12.40%
Pwani	155518	17365	(4362,43447)	11.10%	11.17%
Rukwa	192567	13998	(2529,48138)	6.62%	7.27%
Ruvuma	193856	18826	(3478,55652)	10.64%	9.71%
Shinyanga	492062	56444	(12798,144062)	10.97%	11.47%
Singida	191261	4438	(596,24707)	2.21%	2.32%
Tabora	288518	12991	(2090,53399)	4.82%	4.50%
Tanga	265337	9591	(1671,37409)	4.44%	3.61%
TOTAL	5809052	419277	(96028,1170757)	5.99%	7.22%

lence has dropped 50%–60% between the years 2000 and 2008 (Impact and ALIVE projects, Ifakara Health Institute, unpublished). These reports are also supported by reduction in the intensity of malaria transmission by about 80% between 1990 and 2001–2003 ([14]) due mainly to increase of bednets and ITNs use. A comprehensive review of the impact of malaria control in Tanzania can be found in [15] who concluded that malaria is "down but not out".

Intervention measures (bednet, IRS) seem to have no statistically significant effect on malaria risk. These results could be explained, on one hand, by the fact that only data on bednet ownership/use were collected, without distinguishing between treated and untreated nets. Since untreated nets are less effective than treated ones ([16]), this had certainly influence the results of the risk factor analysis. On the other hand, usage of mosquito nets, especially by children is very important, but not all owned bednets were also used. The other important factor is that the IRS coverage was very low for the mainland (1.12%), therefore it is difficult to observe a significant effect, especially if the implementation of the intervention is not fully correct. The absence of significant association between intervention measures and malaria risk may be explained by other factors such as indication bias (children living in high risk areas use more frequently the intervenition measures), exophilic behavior of vectors, resistance of vectors to the insecticides and lack of efficacy of these interventions.

In the multivariate non-spatial model for mainland Tanzania demographic (residence and age), wealth index and environmental covariates were all significant. However, in the Bayesian geostatistical model, the environmental factors did not remain significant. This could be explained by other unmeasured factors such as: access to health care, deforestation (especially the Lake Victoria shores areas), irrigation, swamp draining, etc. Information on some of these factors may be obtained from remote sensing sources. However, information on health related factors would require collection of national and regional data on such variables at high spatial resolution. We observe that in Zanzibar none of the covariates included in the analysis were significantly associated with malaria risk. This is not surprising considering the high level of malaria control implemented on the islands, which counteracted the environmental and climatic effects.

Additional nationally representative surveys were carried out in Tanzania during 2008, namely the NMCP malaria indicator survey (June–July) and the Tanzania National Insecticide Treated

Nets Programme (NATNETS) (July–September). Although the three surveys differ in timing and sampling methods, one could compile the data sets and check if the model-based predictions are more accurate, especially in areas where our map shows high uncertainty. If the disease burden estimates would be similar, one could suggest optimizing the resource allocation for conducting a single national survey, instead of three.

Acknowledgments

We would like to thank MEASURE DHS for providing the data.

Author Contributions

Conceived and designed the experiments: LG PV. Analyzed the data: LG. Contributed reagents/materials/analysis tools: LG PV AM CL. Wrote the paper: LG.

References

1. National malaria medium term strategic plan 2002–2007. WHO website. Available: http://www.rbm.who.int/countryaction/nsp/tanzania.pdf http://www.rbm.who.int/countryaction/nsp/tanzania.pdf. Accessed 2012 April 25.
2. Global malaria control and elimination: report of a technical review. WHO website. Available: http://www.who.int/malaria/publications/atoz/9789241596756/en/index.html http://www.who.int/malaria/publications/atoz/9789241596756/en/index.html. Accessed 2012 April 16.
3. Hay SI, Guerra CA, Gething PW, Patil AP, Tatem AJ, et al. (2009) A world malaria map: Plasmodium falciparum endemicity in 2007. PLoS Medicine 6(3): e1000048.
4. Msengwa A (2010) Statistical Modeling and Analysis of Malaria Risk and Child Mortality in Tanzania. Doctorial Thesis, University of Dar es Salaam.
5. Gemperli A, Sogoba N, Fondjo E, Mabaso M, Bagayoko M, et al. (2006) Mapping Malaria Transmission in West- and Central Africa. Tropical Medicine and International Health, 11(7): 1032–1046.
6. Gosoniu L (2007) Development of Bayesian geostatistical models with applications in malaria epidemiology. Doctoral Dissertation, Swiss Tropical and Public Health Institute, University of Basel.
7. MARA/ARMA (1998) Towards an Atlas of Malaria Risk in Africa. First technical report of the MARA/ARMA collaboration. MARA website. Available: http://www.mara.org.za/ http://www.mara.org.za/. Accessed 2012 April 16.
8. Craig MH, Snow RW, Le Sueur D (1999) A climate-based distribution model of malaria transmission in sub-Saharan Africa. Parasitology Today 15: 105–111.
9. Tanzania HIV/AIDS and Malaria Indicator Survey 2007–08. Final Report. Measure DHS website. Available: http://www.measuredhs.com/publications/publication-AIS6-AIS-Final-Reports.cfm http://www.measuredhs.com/publications/publication-AIS6-AIS-Final-Reports.cfm. Accessed 2012 April 16.
10. Gosoniu L, Veta AM, Vounatsou P (2010) Bayesian Geostatsistical Modeling of Malaria Indicator Survey in Angola. PLoS ONE 5(3): e9322. doi:10.1371/journal.pone.0009322.
11. Diggle PJ, Tawn JA (1998) Model-based geostatistics. Applied Statistics 47: 299–350.
12. Le Sueur D, Binka F, Lengelerc C, de Savigny D, Teuscher T, et al. (1998) An Atlas of Malaria in Africa. Cambridge, United Kingdom: Medimedia Ltd. 19(2): 23–24.
13. Ministry of Health and Social Welfare (2006) Zanzibar Malaria Control Program (ZMCP) Annual Report Ministry of Health and Social Welfare, Revolutionary Government of Zanzibar.
14. Killeen GF, Smith TA, Ferguson HM, Mshinda H, Abdulla S, et al. (2007) Preventing childhood malaria in Africa by protecting adults from mosquitoes with insecticide-treated nets. PLoS Medicine 4: e229.
15. Smithson P (2009) Down but not out. The impact of malaria control in Tanzania Ifakara Health Institute, Spotlight, Issue 2.
16. Lengeler C (2004) Insecticide-treated bed nets and curtains for preventing malaria (Cochrane Review). The Cochrane Database of Systematic Reviews, Issue 2.

9

Features and Prognosis of Severe Malaria Caused by *Plasmodium falciparum*, *Plasmodium vivax* and Mixed *Plasmodium* Species in Papua New Guinean Children

Laurens Manning[1], Moses Laman[1,2], Irwin Law[2¤a], Cathy Bona[2], Susan Aipit[2], David Teine[2], Jonathan Warrell[2], Anna Rosanas-Urgell[2], Enmoore Lin[2], Benson Kiniboro[2], John Vince[3], Ilomo Hwaiwhanje[4], Harin Karunajeewa[1¤b], Pascal Michon[2¤c], Peter Siba[2], Ivo Mueller[2¤d¤e❧], Timothy M. E. Davis[1*❧]

1 School of Medicine and Pharmacology, University of Western Australia, Fremantle Hospital, Fremantle, Western Australia, Australia, **2** Papua New Guinea Institute of Medical Research, Madang, Madang Province, Papua New Guinea, **3** School of Medicine and Health Sciences, University of Papua New Guinea, Boroko, Port Moresby, Papua New Guinea, **4** Department of Pediatrics, Goroka Base Hospital, Goroka, Eastern Highlands Province, Papua New Guinea

Abstract

Background: Mortality from severe pediatric falciparum malaria appears low in Oceania but *Plasmodium vivax* is increasingly recognized as a cause of complications and death. The features and prognosis of mixed *Plasmodium* species infections are poorly characterized. Detailed prospective studies that include accurate malaria diagnosis and detection of co-morbidities are lacking.

Methods and Findings: We followed 340 Papua New Guinean (PNG) children with PCR-confirmed severe malaria (77.1% *P. falciparum*, 7.9% *P. vivax*, 14.7% *P. falciparum/vivax*) hospitalized over a 3-year period. Bacterial cultures were performed to identify co-incident sepsis. Clinical management was under national guidelines. Of 262 children with severe falciparum malaria, 30.9%, 24.8% and 23.2% had impaired consciousness, severe anemia, and metabolic acidosis/hyperlactatemia, respectively. Two (0.8%) presented with hypoglycemia, seven (2.7%) were discharged with neurologic impairment, and one child died (0.4%). The 27 severe vivax malaria cases presented with similar phenotypic features to the falciparum malaria cases but respiratory distress was five times more common ($P = 0.001$); one child died (3.7%). The 50 children with *P. falciparum/vivax* infections shared phenotypic features of mono-species infections, but were more likely to present in deep coma and had the highest mortality (8.0%; $P = 0.003$ vs falciparum malaria). Overall, bacterial cultures were positive in only two non-fatal cases. 83.6% of the children had alpha-thalassemia trait and seven with coma/impaired consciousness had South Asian ovalocytosis (SAO).

Conclusions: The low mortality from severe falciparum malaria in PNG children may reflect protective genetic factors other than alpha-thalassemia trait/SAO, good nutrition, and/or infrequent co-incident sepsis. Severe vivax malaria had similar features but severe *P. falciparum/vivax* infections were associated with the most severe phenotype and worst prognosis.

Editor: Jose Antonio Stoute, Pennsylvania State University College of Medicine, United States of America

Funding: This study was funded by a National Health and Medical Research Council (NHMRC) grant (#513782). The authors also acknowledge support from the MalariaGen Genomic Epidemiology Network. ML was supported by a Fogarty Foundation scholarship, LM by a Basser scholarship from the Royal Australian College of Physicians and an NHMRC scholarship, and TMED by an NHMRC Practitioner Fellowship. The funders had no role in study design, data collection and analysis, decision to publish, or preparation of the manuscript.

Competing Interests: The authors have declared that no competing interests exist.

* E-mail: tdavis@cyllene.uwa.edu.au

❧ These authors contributed equally to this work.

¤a Current address: National Tuberculosis Programme, Vientiane, Laos
¤b Current address: Western Health, Footscray, Victoria, Australia
¤c Current address: Faculty of Health Sciences, Divine Word University, Madang, Madang Province, Papua New Guinea
¤d Current address: Infection and Immunity Division, Walter and Eliza Hall Institute, Parkville, Victoria, Australia
¤e Current address: Center de Recerca en Salut Internacional de Barcelona (CRESIB), Barcelona, Spain

Introduction

The features and prognosis of severe pediatric falciparum malaria have been characterized in observational and intervention studies from sub-Saharan Africa [1–4]. Equivalent studies in other epidemiologic contexts are fewer but important differences have emerged. There is some evidence that mortality from severe *Plasmodium falciparum* infections in children is relatively low in the Oceania region [5–7], perhaps due to the acquisition of cross-species functional immunity from greater exposure to *P. vivax* in early childhood. Nevertheless, *P. vivax* is itself increasingly recognized as a cause of both complications similar to those seen in falciparum malaria and death [8]. In the case of mixed *Plasmodium* species infections (commonly *P. falciparum/vivax*), there are reports of reduced [9,10], equivalent [11,12] and increased [12] morbidity relative to *P. falciparum* mono-infections.

The incidence of complications and death from severe malaria will depend on selection/recruitment strategies, sensitivity of malaria diagnosis/speciation, definitions of severity, inpatient management including identification of co-incident disease, and social, cultural and genetic factors that can influence presentation and clinical course. Apparent inconsistencies between published studies may reflect differences in one or more such factors. The characteristics and outcome of severe malaria are, therefore, best assessed prospectively, in a representative, ethnically homogeneous sample, and with clinical and laboratory data sufficient both to allow accurate diagnosis [13] and the detection of important co-morbidities such as sepsis [14].

We have carried out such a study in children in coastal Papua New Guinea (PNG) presenting with severe malarial illness, a setting in which a high prevalence of alpha-thalassemia and South Asian ovalocytosis (SAO) implies that malaria has had a strong selective effect [15–17]. We hypothesized that i) severe falciparum malaria has a low mortality relative to African studies as found previously in simple observational studies [5–7,18], and that ii) severe *P. vivax* and mixed *P. falciparum/vivax* malaria, although less common than that caused by *P. falciparum*, have a similar spectrum of clinical disease and prognosis.

Methods

Study sites and local malaria epidemiology

The present study was conducted in Madang and Sepik Provinces on the northern PNG coast where most of the population are subsistence farmers and their families. The annual entomological inoculation rate (EIR) for Madang Province has recently been estimated at 37 for *P. falciparum* and 24 for *P. vivax* [19]. At the Sepik study site, the EIR is 35 for *P. falciparum* and 12 for *P. vivax* [20]. In healthy, asymptomatic Madang children aged 1–10 years, the spleen rate is 13% and the prevalence of parasitemia by microscopy is 8.2% for *P. falciparum* (median [interquartile range (IQR)] 1360 [453–2881]/μL) and 14.1% (348 [226–727]/μL) for *P. vivax* [21]. Approximately 90% of local children have alpha-thalassemia trait [15]. The national human immunodeficiency virus (HIV) seroprevalence is 0.9% [22].

Ethics statement

The present study was approved by the PNG Institute of Medical Research Institutional Review Board and the Medical Research Advisory Committee of the PNG Health Department, and conducted according to the principles of the Declaration of Helsinki. Written informed consent was obtained from parent(s)/guardian(s) before recruitment.

Patients

Between October 2006 and December 2009, all children aged 0.5–10 years admitted to Modilon Hospital, the provincial hospital to which the majority of children with severe illness are referred, were assessed for recruitment to an observational study of severe pediatric illness. Inclusion criteria included any of: i) impaired consciousness/coma (Blantyre Coma Score (BCS)<5 [23]), ii) prostration (inability to sit/stand unaided), iii) multiple seizures, iv) hyperlactatemia (blood lactate>5 mmol/L), v) severe anemia (hemoglobin<50 g/L), vi) dark urine, vii) hypoglycemia (blood glucose≤2.2 mmol/L), viii) jaundice, ix) respiratory distress, x) persistent vomiting, xi) abnormal bleeding or xii) signs of shock. These criteria reflect the World Health Organization (WHO) definition of severe malarial illness [13]. All severely-ill blood slide-positive children were considered for recruitment but only those in whom *Plasmodium* species were detected by nested polymerase chain reaction (nPCR) were included in the present analyses. The final speciation as a mono- or mixed infection was based on the nPCR result.

Clinical assessment and management

After recruitment, a standardized case report form that recorded demographic and medical data was completed [24]. This included details of immunizations, past medical history and recent treatment with antimalarial drugs and antibiotics, as documented in each child's hand-held medical record book. Trained study nurses carried out clinical assessments on admission and an additional detailed neurological examination was performed by study clinicians (LM, ML) on all children admitted with a BCS≤4, regardless of the time of admission. Weekly bedside teaching by the study clinicians was conducted to ensure consistency of clinical assessment by study nurses.

A BCS≤2 was considered deep coma and a BCS≤4 as impaired consciousness at 0.5, 1 or 6 hours after correction of hypoglycemia, a seizure or parenteral anticonvulsant therapy, respectively. Respiratory distress was considered present if the child had i) deep breathing, ii) inter-costal in-drawing, iii) subcostal recession, iv) persistent alar flaring, v) tracheal tug, and/or vi) respiratory rate>60/minute. Due to variable availability and safety concerns, chest radiography was performed in a minority of children with respiratory symptoms. Inpatient management, including the decision to perform lumbar puncture (LP), was co-ordinated by attending ward clinicians under PNG national guidelines [25] and included intravenous dextrose/saline and antibiotics (chloramphenicol 25 mg/kg by intramuscular injection 6-hourly), intramuscular artemether (3.2 mg/kg on admission and 1.6 mg/kg daily until oral antimalarial therapy could be tolerated), and blood transfusion if required (in the absence of cardiovascular compromise, at a hemoglobin<40 g/L). Each child was reviewed at least daily until discharge/death. At discharge and, where possible, at the child's home two months post-discharge, the presence of residual neurologic deficits was assessed.

Laboratory Procedures

A baseline venous blood sample was taken for microscopy and rapid diagnostic testing (RDT) (ICT Diagnostics, Brookvale, Australia). Giemsa-stained thick blood smears were examined and the parasitemia quantified independently by two skilled microscopists with discrepancies adjudicated by a third microscopist [26]. Parasite densities were calculated from the number of parasites per 200 white cells and an assumed total peripheral white cell count of 8,000/μL. The final density was the geometric mean of the two values [26]. Additional on-site tests comprised whole blood glucose (Hemocue, Ängelholm, Sweden) and lactate (Lactate Pro, Arkray, Japan), and a full blood count (Coulter Ac·T diff, Beckman Coulter, Brea, USA).

When sufficient blood was available from the admission venepuncture after the above tests, 1–3 mL was placed in Bactec™ Peds Plus™/F bottles (Becton Dickinson, Franklin, USA) and incubated using an automated Bactec™ system. Cerebrospinal fluid (CSF) obtained at LP was examined macroscopically and microscopically [24], and semi-quantitative glucose and protein concentrations obtained by urine dipstick (Acon® Laboratories, San Diego, USA) [27]. If>10 white blood cells/mm^3 were present, CSF was incubated on chocolate agar for 3 days. Bacterial isolates from blood/CSF cultures were identified using standard procedures [24]. Coagulase-negative staphylococci, *Corynebacterium* and *Bacillus spp.* were considered contaminants. The remaining baseline blood sample was centrifuged promptly and separated plasma and erythrocytes stored at $-70°C$ and $-20°C$, respectively.

Additional laboratory tests not necessary for initial clinical management were performed subsequently and included i) plasma electrolytes, urea, creatinine, alanine aminotransferase (ALT), total bilirubin, C-reactive protein (CRP) and creatine kinase (COBAS INTEGRA 800, Roche Diagnostics, Mannheim, Germany), ii) *Plasmodium* speciation by nPCR [28] after parasite DNA extraction (QIAamp 96 DNA Blood Mini Kit, QIAGEN, Valencia, CA) and iii) genetic testing for alpha-thalassemia (3.7 kb and 4.2 kb deletions) and SAO (SLC4A1Δ27) mutations after host DNA extraction [29,30]. Serologic testing for HIV was not routinely performed.

Reference intervals for laboratory tests were determined from 327 healthy Melanesian children who were age- and sex-matched to the present children [21]. Metabolic acidosis was defined as a plasma bicarbonate<12.2 mmol/L, hyperbilirubinemia as a plasma bilirubin>35 μmol/L, an acute inflammatory response as a plasma CRP>64 mg/L (twice the upper limit of the reference interval), and significant liver inflammation as a plasma ALT>90 IU/mL. Schwartz's formula was used to estimate creatinine clearance (CrCl) [31], with impaired renal function defined as a CrCl<75 mL/min.

Prospective population-based study

To compare the proportions of the present hospitalized cases by *Plasmodium* species with those of community-acquired malaria in a similar epidemiologic situation, we used data from 264 children aged 1–4 years from the Ilaita area of neighbouring East Sepik Province who were followed with fortnightly active morbidity assessment and passive case detection at a local health center between April 2006 and August 2007 [32]. At each visit, an RDT was performed to guide treatment, and blood slides and erythrocytes were retained for diagnostic confirmation by microscopy and PCR, respectively. When a child presented with severe illness, a detailed adverse event report was completed. A consensus determination of incident cases of WHO-defined severe malaria [13] was performed by study clinicians (LM, TMED). The denominator for severe malaria incidence was the total at-risk exposure, regardless of antimalarial therapy.

Data analysis

Summary data are presented as median and [IQR]. Comparisons of variables between groups were by parametric or non-parametric tests as appropriate, with *post hoc* two-group comparisons by Dunn's test for continuous and Bonferroni's correction for categorical variables. Crude odds ratios (ORs) for the observed frequencies of overlapping clinical phenotypes were calculated using 2×2 contingency tables. Multivariate analysis was performed using backward stepwise logistic regression. Variables other than age were entered based on biological plausibility and $P<0.20$ on univariate regression analysis and the most parsimonious model chosen using Aikake's Information Criterion. A two-tailed significance level of $P<0.05$ was used throughout.

Results

During the study, 3,019 of 3,181(94.9%) hospitalized children aged between 6 months and 10 years were screened for inclusion to the study (see Figure 1). Of 353 with presumptive severe malaria based on microscopy, 13 were excluded because *Plasmodium* DNA was undetectable by nPCR. The remaining 340 children had a median age of 40 [29–55] months and 189 (55.6%) were males. In most cases (87.1%), both parents were from Madang or East Sepik provinces, with the rest from other parts of PNG. Based on clinical features, blood film microscopy and nPCR, there were 262 severely-ill children with *P. falciparum* (77.1%), 27 with *P. vivax* (7.9%), 50 with mixed *P. falciparum/vivax* (14.7%) and one with mixed *P. falciparum/malariae* (0.3%; see Table 1).

Of the sample of 340 children, 19.5%, 5.3% and 5.3%, respectively, had been treated with oral, parenteral or oral plus parenteral antimalarial therapy before admission. Prior treatment was associated with a lower parasite density in children with *P. falciparum* mono-infections (median [IQR] 13,347 [1,784-80,560] vs 68,860 [11,197-171,929] in untreated children, $P<0.001$) but not in children with *P. vivax* mono-infections. For *P. falciparum* mono-infections by nPCR, there was 98.5% concordance with microscopy; two cases were diagnosed as *P. vivax* and two as *P. falciparum/vivax*. For *P. vivax* mono-infections by nPCR, there was 88.9% concordance with microscopy; three cases were diagnosed as *P. falciparum* mono-infections. Six of these seven discordant results were in patients with low parasite densities (<220/μL). For mixed *P. falciparum/vivax* infections, concordance was only 16%, with 68% diagnosed as *P. falciparum* and 16% as *P. vivax* mono-infections by microscopy.

Presenting features

Of 262 children with severe *P. falciparum* mono-infections, 81 (30.9%), 65 (24.8%) and 61 (23.2%) had impaired consciousness, severe anemia, and metabolic acidosis/hyper-lactatemia, respectively (see Figure 2). There were fewer children with the overlap syndrome of impaired consciousness and severe anemia than expected by chance alone (OR and 95% confidence intervals (CI) 0.37 (0.18–0.75), $P=0.005$) and a greater than expected frequency of impaired consciousness plus acidosis (OR 2.1 (1.1–3.7), $P=0.02$). Severe anemia plus acidosis occurred at expected frequency (OR 1.2 (0.6–1.9), $P=0.61$). There were 7 children with all three phenotypes. Only two had hypoglycemia on admission.

Eight children with severe vivax malaria (29.6%) presented with impaired consciousness or deep coma, three (11.1%) with severe anemia, and five (18.5%) with metabolic acidosis or hyperlactatemia. Children with severe vivax malaria had higher median hemoglobin concentrations, smaller spleens, higher median plasma sodium concentrations, and lower median plasma bilirubin and CRP concentrations than children with severe falciparum malaria (see Table 1). After adjustment for the binary variables hyperlactatemia and severe anemia, the proportion of children with respiratory distress was five times that in the severe falciparum malaria group (odds ratio [95% confidence interval] 5.04 [1.84–13.2], $P=0.001$). There were no other statistically significant differences between the presenting features of severe malaria caused by *P. vivax* or *P. falciparum*.

When compared to those with severe falciparum malaria, children with *P. falciparum/vivax* had a higher median respiratory rate ($P=0.014$), a lower BCS ($P=0.018$) and a greater proportion with deep coma ($P=0.030$; see Table 1). In parallel with the severe *P. falciparum* cases, these children had lower median hemoglobin and serum sodium concentrations, and a higher median plasma bilirubin, than the severe vivax malaria cases. The 5 year-old child with *P. falciparum/malariae* presented with fever, abdominal pain and features of nephrotic syndrome secondary to chronic *P. malariae* infection.

Clinical course

Most children responded to antimalarial/supportive therapy and were discharged well, including the two hypoglycemic

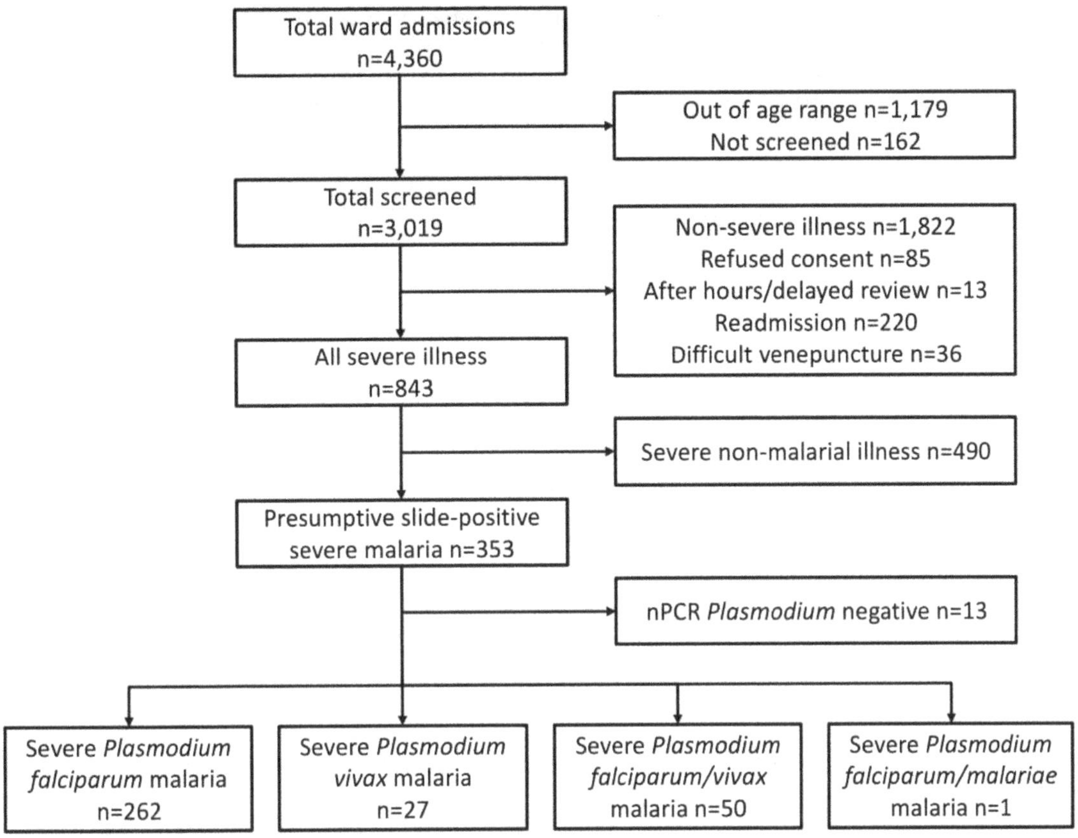

Figure 1. Consort diagram outlining categorization of children presenting to Modilon Hospital, Madang Province, during the study period. Severe malaria cases were identified by clinical and laboratory features at presentation including blood film microscopy, and subsequent nPCR for *Plasmodium* speciation.

children and the child with *P. falciparum/malariae* malaria. Blood cultures were performed in 258 (75.9%) with contaminants identified in 13 (5.0%). Only two significant isolates were obtained, a non-albicans *Candida* from an admission blood culture from an immuno-competent child and a *Klebsiella pneumoniae* from a child after a week of inpatient treatment for severe malaria. Both children were treated with appropriate antimicrobial therapy and discharged well. A LP was performed in 129 children of whom 11 had>10 white blood cells/µL CSF. Routine bacterial culture, bacterial antigen testing, and India ink staining for *Cryptococcus gattii*, were negative in all cases.

Six children (1.8%) died - one with falciparum (0.4%), one with vivax (3.7%) and four with mixed-species infection (8.0%) - all within 12 hours of admission. The child with falciparum malaria presented deeply comatose and died of cardio-respiratory failure. The fatal *P. vivax* case was a previously well child who presented with breathlessness, and abdominal/lower limb swelling. She had severe respiratory distress, a raised jugular venous pressure and an oxygen saturation of 92% despite supplementary oxygen. Her hemoglobin and blood lactate were 41 g/L and 2.7 mmol/L, respectively. A clinical diagnosis of pericardial effusion with cardiac tamponade was made and she had a cardio-respiratory arrest during attempted pericardiocentesis. Subsequent biochemical analysis revealed renal failure (serum creatinine 460 µmol/L), acidosis and hyperkalemia. The children with mixed *P. falciparum/vivax* infections had the greatest mortality ($P = 0.003$ vs falciparum malaria). Of these four deaths, three were due to cerebral malaria. The fourth child had a hemoglobin concentration of 19 g/L and suffered a cardio-respiratory arrest before blood transfusion could be arranged.

Eight children (2.4%), seven with *P. falciparum* and one with *P. falciparum/vivax*, were discharged with neurologic impairment; three with deep coma on admission developed cortical blindness and five had motor deficits ranging from mild ataxia to spastic quadriparesis. Only two of these eight children had persistent neurologic deficits at follow-up two months later. Another child who recovered from severe vivax malaria with respiratory distress died between discharge and follow-up. When admitted, he had clinical signs of severe pulmonary hypertension and a prior history of echocardiographically confirmed cyanotic heart disease.

The genetic deletion causing SAO was present in 17 of 320 (5.3%) children, including 1, 2 and 14 with severe disease due to *P. vivax*, mixed *P. falciparum/vivax* and *P. falciparum*, respectively. Three children with SAO deletions presented with deep coma (BCS of 1, 2 and 2, respectively) and a further four with impaired consciousness. At least one alpha-thalassemia deletion was observed in 83.6% of the children with severe malaria (see Table 1).

Population-based rates of severe malaria

Episodes of malaria during a total of 247 person-years of follow-up in the East Sepik cohort study [32] are summarized in Table 2. The data show that the risk of a severe compared with an uncomplicated *P. falciparum/vivax* infection is similar to that with *P. falciparum* alone (3.4% vs 4.2%, $P = 0.81$ by Fisher's exact test) but greater than with *P. vivax* alone (3.4% vs 0.9%, $P = 0.035$). The

Table 1. Baseline clinical and laboratory data for children with severe malaria categorized by *Plasmodium* species.

	Plasmodium falciparum (n = 262)	*Plasmodium vivax* (n = 27)	*Plasmodium falciparum/vivax* (n = 50)	*P*-value*
Age (months)	42 [30–57]	33 [26–61]	36 [29–48]	0.25
Male sex (%)	58.5	55.6	42.0	0.17
Axillary temperature (°C)	37.9 [37.2–38.7]	37.6 [36.9–38.8]	38.0 [37.0–38.4]	0.28
Pulse rate (/minute)	132 [117–145]	133 [119–146]	139 [121–149]	0.37
Respiratory rate (/minute)	32 [28–38][a]	36 [31.5–43]	38 [31–48]	0.014
Respiratory distress (%)	9.9[b]	29.6	22.0	0.002
Oxygen saturation (%)	98 [97–99]	98 [96.5–98.5]	99 [97–100]	0.049
Spleen size (cm)	2 [0–4]	0 [0–2][c]	3 [0–5.3]	0.021
Blantyre Coma Score	5 [4–5][a]	5 [4–5]	4.5 [3–5]	0.018
Impaired consciousness (3–4; %)	20.6	22.2	28.0	<0.0001
Deep coma (≤2; %)	10.3	3.7	22.0	
Multiple/complex fits (%)	21.8	25.9	22.0	0.88
Hemoglobin (g/L)	77 [50–94][b]	95 [77–105][c]	73 [50–92]	0.015
Severe anemia (<50 g/L, %)	24.9	11.1	24.0	0.28
Leukocyte count ($\times 10^9$/L)	8.4 [6.0–12.5]	9 [6.6–12.8]	9.0 [7.1–12.3]	0.67
Platelet count ($\times 10^9$/L)	101 [56–167]	147 [96.5–204]	127 [71–199]	0.07
Blood lactate (mmol/L)	2.9 [2–4.3]	2.7 [2.0–3.6]	3 [2.1–5.3]	0.63
Hyperlactatemia (>5.0 mmol/L, %)	17.6	7.4	28.0	0.07
Plasma bicarbonate (mmol/L)	16.2 [13.8–18.4]	14.9 [13.7–16.4]	15.1 [13.7–17.4]	0.08
Metabolic acidosis (<12.2 mmol/L, %)	11.6	11.1	16.0	0.68
Blood glucose (mmol/L)	7.6 [6.3–9.1]	7.9 [6–10.5]	7.5 [6.6–9.1]	0.83
Plasma sodium (mmol/L)	129 [127–132][b]	132 [130–134][c]	129 [126–132]	0.007
Plasma creatinine (μmol/L)	26 [21–33]	27 [21–35]	24 [19–32]	0.27
Creatinine clearance (ml/min/1.73 m^2)	166 [140–199]	158 [123–191]	179 [148–212]	0.16
Renal impairment (<75 ml/min/1.73 m^2, %)	3.2	3.7	6.0	0.60
Plasma bilirubin (μmol/L)	11.3 [7.2–22][b]	5.7 [4.1–14][c]	10.0 [6.5–26.5]	0.002
Hyperbilirubinemia (>35 μmol/L, %)	10.5	0.0	14.6	0.13
Plasma C-reactive protein (mg/dL)	99 [51–154][b]	41 [16–81]	72 [23–147]	<0.0001
Plasma C-reactive protein>64 mg/L (%)	70.0[b]	37.0	53.2	0.001
Plasma creatine kinase (IU/mL)	67 [17–405]	66 [25–284]	59 [25–592]	0.87
Plasma creatine kinase>2000 IU/mL (%)	9.3	3.8	12.8	0.45
P. falciparum density (parasites/μL)	50061 [4817–130344]	0 [0-0]	18715 [155–126894]	0.07[#]
Hyperparasitemia (>100,000/μL, %)	32.1		32.0	1.0
P. vivax density(parasites/μL)	0 [0-0]	1298 [164–4408]	0 [0–107]	<0.0001
South Asian ovalocytosis (SLC4A1Δ27, %)	5.7	3.8	4.3	0.87
Alpha thalassemia (3.7 or 4.2 kb deletions, wt/wt, α^{del}/wt, $\alpha^{del}/\alpha^{del}$, %)	16.2/38.2/45.6	21.7/34.8/43.5	14.6/36.6/48.8	0.95

Data are, unless otherwise stated, median and [inter-quartile range].
[a]*P*<0.05 for post-test comparison between *P. falciparum* vs *P. falciparum/vivax*;
[b]*P*<0.05 for post-test comparison between *P. falciparum* vs *P. vivax*;
[c]*P*<0.05 for post-test comparison between *P. vivax* vs *P. falciparum/vivax*;
*Kruskal-Wallis or Chi-squared test;
[#]Mann-Whitney test for *P. falciparum* vs *P. falciparum/vivax*; wt, wildtype; α^{del}/wt, heterozygous for either 3.7 or 4.2 kb deletions; $\alpha^{del}/\alpha^{del}$, homozygous or compound heterozygous for either 3.7 or 4.2 kb deletion.

main manifestations of severe malaria in the 30 children were severe anemia (46.7%) and multiple convulsions (36.7%). Two children with severe falciparum malaria died, one from cardio-respiratory failure secondary to severe anemia (hemoglobin 16 g/L). The other was an anemic child (hemoglobin 63 g/L) with *P. falciparum* whose condition deteriorated after outpatient antimalarial treatment and who died 6 hours later.

Discussion

The present study confirms that, although severe *P. falciparum* malaria in Melanesian children presents with the same phenotypes as those in African children, the mortality is low (<1%) in a hospital setting. The relatively few cases of severe vivax malaria in our series exhibited presenting features that were similar to those

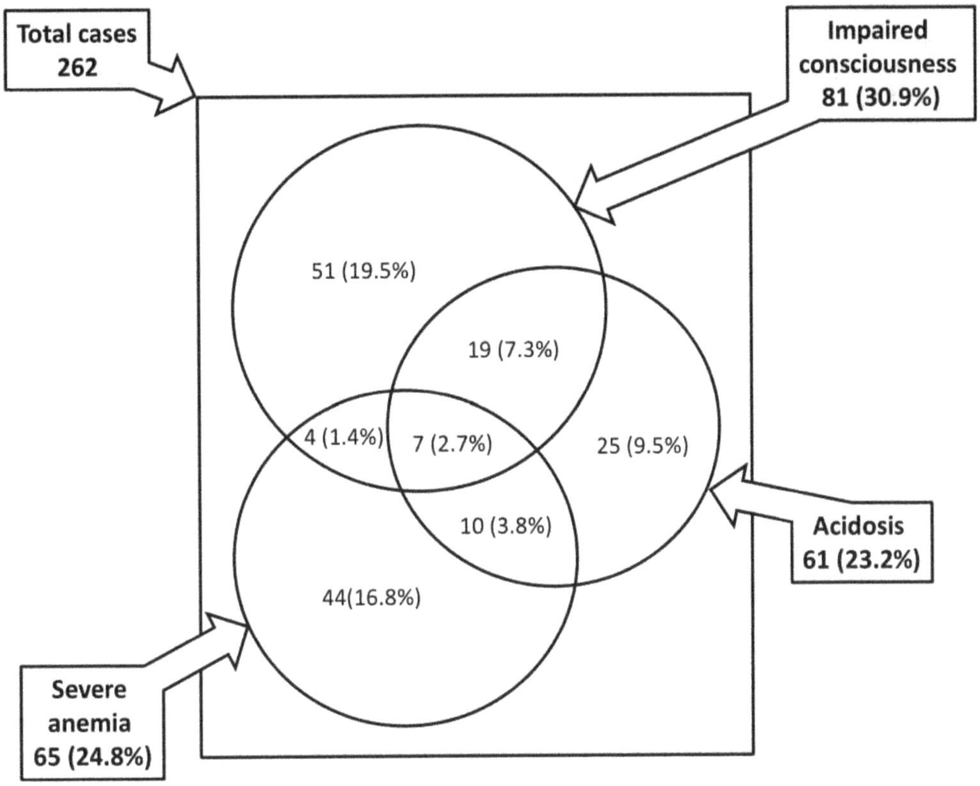

Figure 2. Overlapping clinical phenotypes of severe malaria caused by *Plasmodium falciparum*.

in the children with severe *P. falciparum* malaria but with a higher likelihood of respiratory distress. Severe mixed *P. falciparum/vivax* infections were greater in number than the vivax malaria cases. These children also had comparable admission clinical/laboratory findings to those of the patients with severe falciparum and vivax malaria, but their subsequent mortality was the highest of the three groups. These observations confirm and extend data relating to severe malaria in an area of intense transmission of multiple *Plasmodium* species, especially in relation to mixed-species infections.

Our children with severe falciparum malaria had rates of impaired consciousness, acidosis, anemia, and combinations of these, that were similar to those reported in African studies [1–4,33–35]. Impaired consciousness was more often associated with acidosis than severe anemia, again paralleling African data [1]. We had two cases of hypoglycemia, a prevalence of 0.8%. In the recent large-scale African Quinine Artesunate Malaria Trial (AQUAMAT) [36], 10% of children were hypoglycemic at recruitment. This suggests that the nutritional status of our children, including hepatic glycogen reserves (which may reflect differences in duration and/or severity of illness), was better than in African children. Alternatively, a proportion of the patients had received quinine prior to recruitment to AQUAMAT with the risk of attendant hyperinsulinemia [37]. There may also be genetic differences in glucose metabolism between African and Melanesian populations that account for differences in hypoglycemia risk.

Table 2. Uncomplicated and severe malaria numbers, and incidence of severe malaria, by infecting *Plasmodium* species from a longitudinal surveillance study of 264 children followed over 17 months in neighbouring East Sepik Province.

Plasmodium species	Uncomplicated malaria (n)	Severe malaria (n)	Severe malaria (%)	Incidence of severe malaria per 1,000 person-years at risk
falciparum	483	21	4.2[†]	81.8
vivax	461	4	0.9	16.1
falciparum/vivax	140	5	3.4[†]	20.2
Other*	50	0	0	0
Total	1134	30	2.6 (1.8–3.8)[¶]	121 (82–173)[¶]

Data are from Lin *et al.* [32].
*Single or mixed infections with *P. malariae* or *P. ovale*;
[¶](95% confidence intervals);
[†]$P<0.05$ vs *P. vivax*.

Case fatality rates in African children with severe falciparum malaria lie between 3% and 50% [1–4]. Our results are consistent with other Melanesian studies in showing lower mortality [5,6,18]. This difference could reflect protective genetic factors, relatively infrequent hypoglycemia and bacteremia, and/or better access to quality healthcare. We found alpha-thalassemia deletions in 83.6% of our children, a lower percentage than the 97% found in the general Madang population, and 5.3% had SAO deletions reflecting the results of previous studies in the province [16,17]. These polymorphisms have previously been shown to be protective against complications of malaria [15–17,38,39], including near complete protection for SAO against cerebral malaria [16,38]. Although our study was not designed to assess such a protective effect, the observation that three children with cerebral malaria had the SAO deletion, as did a further four children with impaired consciousness, contrasts with previous studies. This finding suggests that unrecognized favourable genetic traits other than SAO and alpha-thalassemia have emerged through strong selection pressure which might help explain the low mortality observed in our children.

African studies show hypoglycemia-associated mortality of >50% [34], but neither of our two hypoglycemic children died. Similarly, invasive bacterial disease has been detected in 5–8% of African children with severe malaria, especially non-typhoidal *Salmonellae* infection that substantially increase mortality [14], but there was a much lower rate in our cohort. Most of our children had blood cultures performed with an acceptable contamination rate. While we identified invasive bacterial isolates from children severe non-malarial disease (data not shown), only two significant pathogens were obtained from our children with severe malaria. Unregulated antibiotic access is widespread in PNG, but only 8.4% and 7.6%, respectively, had documented amoxicillin or chloramphenicol treatment before admission suggesting that prior antibiotic therapy was not responsible. In addition, no *Salmonellae* were isolated from the present or other children with severe non-malarial disease studied contemporaneously (data not shown). All our children were treated empirically with intramuscular artemether, parenteral chloramphenicol and other supportive therapy [25], and prompt access to good quality standard treatment may also have contributed to their relatively low mortality. Nevertheless, children in the AQUAMAT study had similar management but even those treated with artesunate rather than quinine had a mortality of 8.5% [36].

Severe vivax malaria has been associated with a wide variety of clinical manifestations in adults and children that include severe anemia, altered consciousness, respiratory distress, jaundice, thrombocytopenia, acidosis and renal failure [8,12,40–44]. There are, however, large between-study differences in the frequency of individual presenting features. This reflects, in part, the fact that few studies have involved prospective collection of clinical and laboratory data sufficient to capture the broad range of features of severe malaria, exclude other causes of severe illness and confirm *Plasmodium* speciation using molecular methods.

A case in point is respiratory distress. In one of two recent prospective studies of severe pediatric *P. vivax* infection from the island of New Guinea [12], children had a limited clinical assessment that included respiratory rate and oxygen saturation. These two features were used to define respiratory distress that was present in approximately 5% of children with severe *P. vivax* malaria. In the second study, which involved prospective community-based morbidity surveillance [41], respiratory distress defined as a respiratory rate>40–50/minute in the presence of chest in-drawing or a history of breathlessness was present in 60.5% of 86 children identified with severe vivax malaria over 8 years. Our prevalence of respiratory distress, based on well-defined specific criteria including a higher respiratory rate threshold, was intermediate between these two figures. Consistent with the other PNG study [41] but not the study from southern Papua [12], respiratory distress was more common in our *P. vivax* cases than those with *P. falciparum*. Acute respiratory distress syndrome (ARDS), interstitial pneumonia and pulmonary oedema can complicate vivax malaria in adults [8]. Since *P. vivax*-infected erythrocytes can bind to cells expressing endothelial receptors known to mediate the cytoadhesion of *P. falciparum* [45], this could reflect parasite microvascular sequestration [46] which may be prominent in the pulmonary capillary bed [47]. This phenomenon may have contributed to respiratory distress in the child with cyanotic heart disease, but there is also evidence that such children may be at increased risk of other manifestations of severe malaria including altered consciousness [48].

There was a single death from *P. vivax* malaria in our cohort. Although this child died during attempted pericardiocentesis, she had severe anemia, respiratory distress, renal impairment and acidosis. In the larger observational study from southern Papua [12] that revealed a case fatality rate for severe vivax malaria in young children (approaching 2%) comparable to that in the present study (3.7%), these presenting features were strongly predictive of death. In a retrospective study from north-eastern Indonesian Papua [11], the overall death rate for severe vivax malaria was 25% in 36 cases. The mortality from severe infections (*P. falciparum* or *vivax*) was lower in children than adults but no pediatric-specific vivax malaria mortality data were reported in this study or a previous prospective observational study from PNG [41].

Our children with severe mixed *P. falciparum/vivax* infections had clinical and laboratory features that were mostly similar to those of the severe falciparum cases despite generally lower *P. falciparum* parasitemias. The exceptions were a higher baseline respiratory rate and a lower BCS. These features suggest that the children in this group were the most severely ill, at risk of the pathophysiologic effects of both parasite species with the possibility that *P. vivax* microvascular cytoadherence as observed in lung [47] and spleen [46] might also occur in the brain.

Other studies have found that, in contrast to the present data, severe anemia is less common in severe *P. falciparum/vivax* infections than severe falciparum or vivax malaria [12], that mixed infections are more likely than *P. vivax* infections to be associated with respiratory distress [41], and that coma is least likely in mixed infections [41]. These apparent inconsistencies may reflect between-study differences in patient selection, definitions of complications, and the availability and quality of clinical/laboratory data including accurate microscopy and/or molecular confirmation of *Plasmodium* species. Nevertheless, our data indicate that WHO criteria for severe malaria [13] that are based on studies of *P. falciparum* encompass the spectrum of severe infections caused by *P. vivax* with or without co-incident *P. falciparum*.

Although from a study with a different design, the community-based longitudinal data from a cohort of similarly aged East Sepik children who had similar red-cell polymorphisms and who were from an area of comparable malaria transmission [32], suggest that both *P. falciparum* mono-infections and *P. falciparum/vivax* infections in a PNG child are more likely to progress to severe disease than *P. vivax* mono-infections. Indeed, the numbers of severe cases in these categories (21, 5 and 4, respectively) were consistent those of the present study (262, 50 and 27), suggesting that our hospitalized patients were representative of malaria in the community. The mortality in our series was greatest in severe *P. falciparum/vivax* infections, consistent with the presenting clinical and laboratory features of these children. In the two other studies with mortality data [11,12], there was no significant difference between mixed and single-species infections but no pediatric-specific outcomes were included. Thus, our data are the first to suggest that mixed-species infections carry an adverse prognosis in children.

Our study had limitations. It is possible that the most severely ill children in the study catchment area die before they can be transferred for inpatient care, thus compromising the representative nature of our sample. Due mainly to issues with obtaining a sufficient volume of blood from a small, distressed and severely ill child, we could not exclude bacteremia in every case, while diagnostic tests for viral and fungal pathogens were not possible in this clinical setting. Obtaining *post mortem* tissue samples that may have clarified underlying pathology is culturally problematic in PNG.

The strengths of the present study were its prospective standardized data collection, the use of nPCR as a way of compensating for the known limitations of microscopy, and the availability of bacteriology facilities that enabled detection of common invasive bacterial infections. Such a rigorous approach has been used in few previous descriptive studies of severe childhood malaria. Our data confirm the lack of sensitivity of microscopy in identifying mixed species infections [49,50], with low-level *P. vivax* densities that can be missed by microscopy in this situation probably reflecting density dependent cross-species regulation [51]. Although nPCR is not a quantitative test and the relative contribution of each species to the overall parasitemia remains uncertain, microscopic misdiagnosis of mixed infections in previous studies may have obscured the association with more severe disease observed in the present patients. Given the presenting features and clinical course of our patients, it is unlikely that there were significant numbers of cases with diagnoses that would have been identified by specialized serologic and other tests. Indeed, in the case of encephalitis, more than one third of cases remain undiagnosed in a resource-rich healthcare setting [52]. It has been suggested that parasite density thresholds are employed in areas where asymptomatic parasitemia is common in otherwise healthy children [53,54]. While the severe malaria-attributable fraction or diagnostic specificity increases with higher parasitemia, sensitivity is reduced. The choice of threshold will depend on factors such as local transmission, age-dependent malarial immunity and genetic factors modulating infection severity.

The present study of well-characterized children from an area of intense transmission of multiple *Plasmodium* species has identified significant differences between the presentation and outcome of severe *P. falciparum*, *vivax* and *falciparum/vivax* infections in PNG. The low mortality observed for severe falciparum malaria does not appear related to high endemicity of *P. vivax* but may reflect protective genetic factors, better prior nutrition, and/or less exposure/susceptibility to secondary bacterial infection than in African children. Severe vivax malaria presents with features seen in severe *P. falciparum* infections but respiratory distress is more prominent, suggesting preferential cytoadherence of this parasite within the lung microvasculature. Severe *P. falciparum/vivax* infections in PNG children appear to have the worst prognosis, perhaps because they share the adverse presenting features of the respective mono-infections. These findings provide impetus for further research on the pathogenic potential of *P. vivax* infections when this parasite is present alone and especially in combination with other *Plasmodium* species.

Acknowledgments

The authors gratefully acknowledge the assistance of staff on the Pediatric Ward at Modilon Hospital, the Papua New Guinea Institute of Medical Research staff at Modilon Hospital and the Yagaum campus, and the patients and their families for their participation.

Author Contributions

Conceived and designed the experiments: TD HK JV PS IM. Performed the experiments: LM ML IL CB SA DT JW AR-U EL BK PM IH. Analyzed the data: LM ML IM TD. Wrote the paper: LM TD IM.

References

1. Marsh K, Forster D, Waruiru C, Mwangi I, Winstanley M, et al. (1995) Indicators of life-threatening malaria in African children. N Engl J Med 332: 1399–1404.
2. Mockenhaupt FP, Ehrhardt S, Burkhardt J, Bosomtwe SY, Laryea S, et al. (2004) Manifestation and outcome of severe malaria in children in northern Ghana. Am J Trop Med Hyg 71: 167–172.
3. Schapira A, Solomon T, Julien M, Macome A, Parmar N, et al. (1993) Comparison of intramuscular and intravenous quinine for the treatment of severe and complicated malaria in children. Trans R Soc Trop Med Hyg 87: 299–302.
4. Imbert P, Gerardin P, Rogier C, Ka AS, Jouvencel P, et al. (2002) Severe falciparum malaria in children: a comparative study of 1990 and 2000 WHO criteria for clinical presentation, prognosis and intensive care in Dakar, Senegal. Trans R Soc Trop Med Hyg 96: 278–281.
5. Allen SJ, O'Donnell A, Alexander ND, Clegg JB (1996) Severe malaria in children in Papua New Guinea. QJM 89: 779–788.
6. Maitland K, Williams TN, Peto TE, Day KP, Clegg JB, et al. (1997) Absence of malaria-specific mortality in children in an area of hyperendemic malaria. Trans R Soc Trop Med Hyg 91: 562–566.
7. Stace J, Bilton P, Coates K, Stace N (1982) Cerebral malaria in children: a retrospective study of admissions to Madang Hospital, 1980. P N G Med J 25: 230–234.
8. Price RN, Douglas NM, Anstey NM (2009) New developments in *Plasmodium vivax* malaria: severe disease and the rise of chloroquine resistance. Curr Opin Infect Dis 22: 430–435.
9. Luxemburger C, Ricci F, Nosten F, Raimond D, Bathet S, et al. (1997) The epidemiology of severe malaria in an area of low transmission in Thailand. Trans R Soc Trop Med Hyg 91: 256–262.
10. Price RN, Simpson JA, Nosten F, Luxemburger C, Hkirjaroen L, et al. (2001) Factors contributing to anemia after uncomplicated falciparum malaria. Am J Trop Med Hyg 65: 614–622.
11. Barcus MJ, Basri H, Picarima H, Manyakori C, Sekartuti, et al. (2007) Demographic risk factors for severe and fatal vivax and falciparum malaria among hospital admissions in northeastern Indonesian Papua. Am J Trop Med Hyg 77: 984–991.
12. Tjitra E, Anstey NM, Sugiarto P, Warikar N, Kenangalem E, et al. (2008) Multidrug-resistant *Plasmodium vivax* associated with severe and fatal malaria: a prospective study in Papua, Indonesia. PLoS Med 5: e128.
13. WHO (2000) Severe falciparum malaria. Trans R Soc Trop Med Hyg 94 Suppl 1: S1–90.
14. Berkley J, Mwarumba S, Bramham K, Lowe B, Marsh K (1999) Bacteraemia complicating severe malaria in children. Trans R Soc Trop Med Hyg 93: 283–286.
15. Yenchitsomanus PT, Summers KM, Bhatia KK, Cattani J, Board PG (1985) Extremely high frequencies of alpha-globin gene deletion in Madang and on Kar Kar Island, Papua New Guinea. Am J Hum Genet 37: 778–784.
16. Allen SJ, O'Donnell A, Alexander ND, Mgone CS, Peto TE, et al. (1999) Prevention of cerebral malaria in children in Papua New Guinea by southeast Asian ovalocytosis band 3. Am J Trop Med Hyg 60: 1056–1060.
17. Allen SJ, O'Donnell A, Alexander ND, Alpers MP, Peto TE, et al. (1997) alpha+-Thalassemia protects children against disease caused by other infections as well as malaria. Proc Natl Acad Sci U S A 94: 14736–14741.
18. Karunajeewa HA, Reeder J, Lorry K, Dabod E, Hamzah J, et al. (2006) Artesunate suppositories versus intramuscular artemether for treatment of severe malaria in children in Papua New Guinea. Antimicrob Agents Chemother 50: 968–974.
19. Michon P, Cole-Tobian JL, Dabod E, Schoepflin S, Igu J, et al. (2007) The risk of malarial infections and disease in Papua New Guinean children. Am J Trop Med Hyg 76: 997–1008.
20. Smith T, Hii JL, Genton B, Muller I, Booth M, et al. (2001) Associations of peak shifts in age–prevalence for human malarias with bednet coverage. Trans R Soc Trop Med Hyg 95: 1–6.

21. Manning L, Laman M, Townsend MA, Chubb SP, Siba PM, et al. (2011) Reference intervals for common laboratory tests in melanesian children. Am J Trop Med Hyg 85: 50–54.
22. UNAIDS (2010) Global Report Fact Sheet - Oceania. http://www.unaids.org/en/media/unaids/contentassets/documents/factsheet2010/20101123_FS_oceania_em_en.pdf. Accessed October 2011.
23. Molyneux ME, Taylor TE, Wirima JJ, Borgstein A (1989) Clinical features and prognostic indicators in paediatric cerebral malaria: a study of 131 comatose Malawian children. Q J Med 71: 441–459.
24. Laman M, Manning L, Hwaiwhange I, Vince J, Aipit S, et al. (2010) Lumbar puncture in children from an area of malaria endemicity who present with a febrile seizure. Clin Infect Dis 51: 534–540.
25. Paediatrics Society of PNG (2005) Standard treatment for common illnesses of children in PNG. .
26. Karunajeewa HA, Mueller I, Senn M, Lin E, Law I, et al. (2008) A trial of combination antimalarial therapies in children from Papua New Guinea. N Engl J Med 359: 2545–2557.
27. Moosa AA, Quortum HA, Ibrahim MD (1995) Rapid diagnosis of bacterial meningitis with reagent strips. Lancet 345: 1290–1291.
28. Snounou G, Viriyakosol S, Jarra W, Thaithong S, Brown KN (1993) Identification of the four human malaria parasite species in field samples by the polymerase chain reaction and detection of a high prevalence of mixed infections. Mol Biochem Parasitol 58: 283–292.
29. Imrie H, Fowkes FJ, Michon P, Tavul L, Hume JC, et al. (2006) Haptoglobin levels are associated with haptoglobin genotype and alpha+ -thalassemia in a malaria-endemic area. Am J Trop Med Hyg 74: 965–971.
30. Jarolim P, Palek J, Amato D, Hassan K, Sapak P, et al. (1991) Deletion in erythrocyte band 3 gene in malaria-resistant Southeast Asian ovalocytosis. Proc Natl Acad Sci U S A 88: 11022–11026.
31. Schwartz GJ, Haycock GB, Edelmann CM, Jr., Spitzer A (1976) A simple estimate of glomerular filtration rate in children derived from body length and plasma creatinine. Pediatrics 58: 259–263.
32. Lin E, Kiniboro B, Gray L, Dobbie S, Robinson L, et al. (2010) Differential patterns of infection and disease with *P. falciparum* and *P. vivax* in young Papua New Guinean children. PLoS One 5: e9047.
33. Dzeing-Ella A, Nze Obiang PC, Tchoua R, Planche T, Mboza B, et al. (2005) Severe falciparum malaria in Gabonese children: clinical and laboratory features. Malar J 4: 1.
34. White NJ, Waller D, Crawley J, Nosten F, Chapman D, et al. (1992) Comparison of artemether and chloroquine for severe malaria in Gambian children. Lancet 339: 317–321.
35. Ranque S, Poudiougou B, Traore A, Keita M, Oumar AA, et al. (2008) Life-threatening malaria in African children: a prospective study in a mesoendemic urban setting. Pediatr Infect Dis J 27: 130–135.
36. Dondorp AM, Fanello CI, Hendriksen IC, Gomes E, Seni A, et al. (2010) Artesunate versus quinine in the treatment of severe falciparum malaria in African children (AQUAMAT): an open-label, randomised trial. Lancet 376: 1647–1657.
37. Davis TM (1997) Antimalarial drugs and glucose metabolism. Br J Clin Pharmacol 44: 1–7.
38. Genton B, al-Yaman F, Mgone CS, Alexander N, Paniu MM, et al. (1995) Ovalocytosis and cerebral malaria. Nature 378: 564–565.
39. Mockenhaupt FP, Ehrhardt S, Gellert S, Otchwemah RN, Dietz E, et al. (2004) Alpha(+)-thalassemia protects African children from severe malaria. Blood 104: 2003–2006.
40. Lacerda MV, Alexandre MA, Santos PD, Arcanjo AR, Alecrim WD, et al. (2004) Idiopathic thrombocytopenic purpura due to vivax malaria in the Brazilian Amazon. Acta Trop 90: 187–190.
41. Genton B, D'Acremont V, Rare L, Baea K, Reeder JC, et al. (2008) *Plasmodium vivax* and mixed infections are associated with severe malaria in children: a prospective cohort study from Papua New Guinea. PLoS Med 5: e127.
42. Kochar DK, Das A, Kochar SK, Saxena V, Sirohi P, et al. (2009) Severe *Plasmodium vivax* malaria: a report on serial cases from Bikaner in northwestern India. Am J Trop Med Hyg 80: 194–198.
43. Alexandre MA, Ferreira CO, Siqueira AM, Magalhaes BL, Mourao MP, et al. (2010) Severe *Plasmodium vivax* malaria, Brazilian Amazon. Emerg Infect Dis 16: 1611–1614.
44. Kochar DK, Tanwar GS, Khatri PC, Kochar SK, Sengar GS, et al. (2010) Clinical features of children hospitalized with malaria - a study from Bikaner, northwest India. Am J Trop Med Hyg 83: 981–989.
45. Carvalho BO, Lopes SC, Nogueira PA, Orlandi PP, Bargieri DY, et al. (2010) On the cytoadhesion of *Plasmodium vivax*-infected erythrocytes. J Infect Dis 202: 638–647.
46. Fernandez-Becerra C, Yamamoto MM, Vencio RZ, Lacerda M, Rosanas-Urgell A, et al. (2009) *Plasmodium vivax* and the importance of the subtelomeric multigene vir superfamily. Trends Parasitol 25: 44–51.
47. Anstey NM, Handojo T, Pain MC, Kenangalem E, Tjitra E, et al. (2007) Lung injury in vivax malaria: pathophysiological evidence for pulmonary vascular sequestration and posttreatment alveolar-capillary inflammation. J Infect Dis 195: 589–596.
48. Okeniyi J, Kuti B (2008) Cerebral malaria in children with cyanotic heart diseases: the need for a closer look. Congenit Heart Dis 3: 73–76.
49. Ohrt C, Purnomo, Sutamihardja MA, Tang D, Kain KC (2002) Impact of microscopy error on estimates of protective efficacy in malaria-prevention trials. J Infect Dis 186: 540–546.
50. Zimmerman PA, Mehlotra RK, Kasehagen LJ, Kazura JW (2004) Why do we need to know more about mixed *Plasmodium* species infections in humans? Trends Parasitol 20: 440–447.
51. Bruce MC, Donnelly CA, Alpers MP, Galinski MR, Barnwell JW, et al. (2000) Cross-species interactions between malaria parasites in humans. Science 287: 845–848.
52. Granerod J, Ambrose HE, Davies NW, Clewley JP, Walsh AL, et al. (2010) Causes of encephalitis and differences in their clinical presentations in England: a multicentre, population-based prospective study. Lancet Infect Dis 10: 835–844.
53. Bejon P, Berkley JA, Mwangi T, Ogada E, Mwangi I, et al. (2007) Defining childhood severe falciparum malaria for intervention studies. PLoS Med 4: e251.
54. Schellenberg JR, Smith T, Alonso PL, Hayes RJ (1994) What is clinical malaria? Finding case definitions for field research in highly endemic areas. Parasitol Today 10: 439–442.

10

Variability in Pediatric Infectious Disease Consultants' Recommendations for Management of Community-Acquired Pneumonia

Adam L. Hersh[1]*, Daniel J. Shapiro[2], Jason G. Newland[3], Philip M. Polgreen[4], Susan E. Beekmann[4], Samir S. Shah[5,6]

1 Pediatric Infectious Diseases, University of Utah, Salt Lake City, Utah, United States of America, **2** Institute for Health Policy Studies, University of California San Francisco, San Francisco, California, United States of America, **3** Children's Mercy Hospital and Clinics, Kansas City, Missouri, United States of America, **4** University of Iowa Carver College of Medicine, Iowa City, Iowa, United States of America, **5** Departments of Pediatrics and Biostatistics and Epidemiology, and the Center for Clinical Epidemiology and Biostatistics, University of Pennsylvania School of Medicine, Philadelphia, Pennsylvania, United States of America, **6** Division of Infectious Diseases, Center for Pediatric Clinical Effectiveness, The Children's Hospital of Philadelphia, Philadelphia, Pennsylvania, United States of America

Abstract

Background: Community-acquired pneumonia (CAP) is a common childhood infection. CAP complications, such as parapneumonic empyema (PPE), are increasing and are frequently caused by antibiotic-resistant organisms. No clinical guidelines currently exist for management of pediatric CAP and no published data exist about variations in antibiotic prescribing patterns. Our objectives were to describe variation in CAP clinical management for hospitalized children by pediatric infectious disease consultants and to examine associations between recommended antibiotic regimens and local antibiotic resistance levels.

Methods: We surveyed pediatric members of the Emerging Infections Network, which consists of 259 pediatric infectious disease physicians. Participants responded regarding their recommended empiric antibiotic regimens for hospitalized children with CAP with and without PPE and their recommendations for duration of therapy. Participants also provided information about the prevalence of penicillin non-susceptible *S. pneumoniae* and methicillin-resistant *S. aureus* (MRSA) in their community.

Results: We received 148 responses (57%). For uncomplicated CAP, respondents were divided between recommending beta-lactams alone (55%) versus beta-lactams in combination with another class (40%). For PPE, most recommended a combination of a beta-lactam plus an anti-MRSA agent, however, they were divided between clindamycin (44%) and vancomycin (57%). The relationship between reported antibiotic resistance and empiric regimen was mixed. We found no relationship between aminopenicillin use and prevalence of penicillin non-susecpetible *S. pneumoniae* or clindamycin use and clindamycin resistance, however, respondents were more likely to recommend an anti-MRSA agent when MRSA prevalence increased.

Conclusions: Substantial variability exists in recommendations for CAP management. Development of clinical guidelines via antimicrobial stewardship programs and dissemination of data about local antibiotic resistance patterns represent opportunities to improve care.

Editor: Brad Spellberg, Los Angeles Biomedical Research Institute, United States of America

Funding: This study was supported by grant/cooperative agreement number U50 CCU112346 from the Centers for Disease Control and Prevention (CDC). The funders had no role in study design, data collection and analysis, decision to publish, or preparation of the manuscript.

Competing Interests: The authors have declared that no competing interests exist.

* E-mail: adam.hersh@hsc.utah.edu

Introduction

Community acquired pneumonia (CAP) is a common serious infection in childhood, accounting for over 150,000 hospitalizations each year in the US [1]. Despite its importance, no national clinical guidelines currently exist for the management of pediatric CAP. Recent evidence indicates that overall antibiotic utilization for hospitalized children varies widely across hospitals [2], although the extent to which this variation exists for individual conditions, such as CAP, remains unknown.

CAP-associated complications, such parapneumonic empyema (PPE), have increased in recent years [1,3,4]. Antibiotic-resistant organisms, especially *Staphylococcus aureus* and *Streptococcus pneumoniae* are important causes of CAP and PPE. Resistance patterns for these organisms vary widely throughout the United States [5,6,7,8]. The extent to which antibiotic recommendations for pneumonia reflect local resistance patterns for these organisms is unknown. For instance, it is unknown whether clindamycin and vancomycin, which have activity against methicillin-resistant *S. aureus* (MRSA), are recommended more frequently for PPE in communities where MRSA prevalence is higher. Delays in matching the antibiotic spectrum to the causative bacteria is clinically relevant for CAP [9,10].

Infectious disease consultants are frequently involved in the care of children with CAP and local guideline development for the management of CAP. Additionally, interventions such as antimicrobial stewardship programs (ASPs, hospital-based interventions where antimicrobial prescribing is monitored and physicians receive feedback), and unit- or disease-specific antibiograms provide assistance to physicians in selecting the optimal empiric antibiotic and are typically led by infectious disease consultants [11,12,13,14]. The objectives of this study were to describe variation in the clinical management by pediatric infectious diseases consultants for hospitalized children with CAP and to examine the associations between infectious disease consultants' recommended antibiotic regimens, reported antibiotic resistance levels in their communities, and the presence of ASPs.

Materials and Methods

Ethics Statement

This study was determined to be exempt from review by the University of Iowa Institutional Review Board and is not considered to be human subjects research.

Study design

We conducted a survey of pediatric infectious diseases consultants during Fall 2009 regarding their management recommendations for pediatric CAP and the reported prevalence of antibiotic resistance among *S. pneumoniae* and *S. aureus* in their community. All survey questions related to hospitalized children ages 1–18 years, with no known underlying medical conditions predisposing them to severe or recurrent pneumonia. Respondents completed an electronic or paper data entry form. Non-respondents received up to 2 follow-up queries.

Data Source

The data source was the pediatric members of the Emerging Infections Network which consists of 259 pediatric infectious diseases physicians throughout North America. Membership is drawn from the Pediatric Infectious Diseases Society and the Infectious Diseases Society of America and includes physicians from 44 states and 3 Canadian Provinces. EIN members represent over 50% of the children's hospitals in the United States [15].

Survey Questions

The EIN maintains demographic data on individual members including years of practice, geographic region and practice setting. For this survey we ascertained supplementary information including the type of hospital with which the respondent is primarily affiliated (freestanding children's hospital, children's hospital within a hospital and general hospital with pediatric beds) and whether or not the hospital has housestaff, whether the hospital has an antimicrobial stewardship program, and whether there is a clinical guideline or pathway for CAP.

To address the first objective, survey respondents were asked to select the specific antibiotic agent or combination of agents that they recommended for children hospitalized for CAP, distinguishing between uncomplicated and PPE cases. We defined uncomplicated CAP by the presence of a focal consolidation and PPE by the presence of a focal consolidation plus empyema. For each case, respondents selected among one or more of the following agents: ampicillin, ampicillin/sulbactam, 2nd/3rd generation cephalosporins, azithromycin, vancomycin, clindamycin and linezolid. For subsequent analyses, we categorized ampicillin, ampicillin/sulbactam and cephalosporins as beta-lactam antibiotics and vancomycin, clindamycin and linezolid as anti-MRSA antibiotics. Respondents were also asked to select the duration of antibiotic therapy they recommend for uncomplicated and PPE cases. Respondents selected among the following categories: 3–5 days; 6–7 days; 8–10 days; 11–14 days; 15–21 days; >21 days.

To collect data for the second objective, respondents were asked to estimate the resistance levels among isolates in their hospital for *S. pneumoniae* and *S. aureus*. To characterize *S. pneumoniae*, they indicated the percentage of isolates with intermediate susceptibility to penicillin (defined as mean inhibitory concentration (MIC) of 4 μg/mL) and penicillin resistance (defined as an MIC of ≥8 μg/mL). To characterize *S. aureus*, they indicated the percentage of all *S. aureus* isolates that are MRSA and the percentage of MRSA isolates that are resistant to clindamycin (including by D-test). For all three estimates, they selected among the following categories: <10%; 10–25%; 26–50%; and >50%.

Analysis

We used descriptive statistics to describe variations in the recommended empiric antibiotic regimens, andrecommended treatment durations. We performed a chi-square test for linear trend to determine whether there was an association between respondents' recommended antibiotic regimens and their estimates for resistance levels. Specifically, we hypothesized that respondents that reported a lower percentage of penicillin non-susceptible isolates (intermediate plus resistant) would be more likely to recommend an aminopenicillin-containing antibiotic (e.g. ampicillin or ampicillin/sulbactam) in their empiric regimen for uncomplicated CAP. We also hypothesized that respondents reporting a higher reported percentage of MRSA among *S. aureus* isolates would be more likely to include an anti-MRSA agent in their empiric regimen for PPE. Additionally, we hypothesized that among those who included an anti-MRSA agent for PPE, those with higher reported clindamycin resistance would be less likely to select clindamycin (as opposed to vancomycin or linezolid).

Because any observed relationships between antibiotic regimens and reported resistance levels could be subject to confounding, we conducted multivariable analysis using logistic regression to examine the association of other factors, besides resistance, with antibiotic recommendations using data from the survey. Specifically, we developed a model for the relationship between reported resistance for *S. pneumoniae* and aminopencillin use for uncomoplicated CAP and reported clindamycin resistance and clindamycin selection for PPE. To identify variables for inclusion in the model, we first examined the bivariate associations between independent and dependent variables. The independent variables considered for inclusion in the models were hospital type (freestanding children's, children's hospital within a hospital or pediatric ward); whether or not the hospital has housestaff; geographic region; presence of an ASP; presence of a CAP clinical guideline; and reported resistance levels for penicillin, MRSA and clindamycin. The dependent variables for the two models were aminopenicillins for uncomplicated CAP and clindamycin for PPE. In the final models we included variables with a bivariate association of $p < 0.2$. For certain variables where we hypothesized that a relationship might exist (e.g. ASP and CAP clinical guideline) we tested the model outcome by forcing the variable into the model even if the bivariate association was below 0.2. All analyses were conducted using STATA 11 (STATA CORP, College Station, TX).

Results

We received responses from 148 out of 259 members for an overall response rate of 57%. We found no differences between respondents and non-respondents in terms of their employment settings, the region of the country where they practiced, or their total years of experience. Seven respondents did not provide inpatient clinical care, leaving 141 respondents for subsequent analysis. Among these, 48% reported having an ASP at their institution and 34% reported having a clinical pathway or guideline for CAP.

Antibiotic regimens for uncomplicated CAP

There was considerable variation in the categories of recommended regimens for uncomplicated CAP (Table 1). Data were available from all 141 respondents. Most respondents (95%) recommended a beta-lactam, although they were divided among those recommending a beta-lactam alone and those recommending a beta-lactam in combination with another antibiotic category. Azithromycin was recommended only in the context of combination therapy (Table 1). An anti-MRSA regimen was recommended in 20% of cases, typically in combination with beta-lactam therapy.

Antibiotic regimens for PPE

For PPE, there was similar variability in terms of the antibiotic categories included in the recommended regimens (Table 1); 1 respondent did not include antibiotic recommendations for PPE, leaving 140 respondents for analysis. Most (90%; 127/140) recommended including an anti-MRSA antibiotic in their empiric regimen, typically in combination with a beta-lactam antibiotic with or without concomitant macrolide therapy. Only 7% (10/140) recommended a beta-lactam alone and 3% (4/140) recommended a beta-lactam plus azithromycin.

Antibiotic selection within categories

In addition to variation in the antibiotic categories that were recommended, there was variation within categories in terms of the specific agents recommended. For beta-lactams, 74% (105/141) of respondents recommended a cephalosporin for uncomplicated CAP while 95% (133/140) recommended a cephalosporin for PPE. Aminopencillins were recommended for uncomplicated CAP by 25% (35/141) of respondents. For anti-MRSA agents, further variation was noted. For uncomplicated cases, clindamycin was recommended by 86% (24/28) of respondents and vancomycin by 14% (4/28) of those recommending this category. For PPE, clindamycin was included in the recommended anti-MRSA regimen by 44% (55/126) of respondents, vancomycin by 57% (72/126) and linezolid by 4% (5/126). This sums to >100% due to 6 respondents recommending multiple anti-MRSA agents concurrently.

Table 1. Empiric antibiotic regimens recommended for uncomplicated pneumonia and PPE.

	Uncomplicated (%, N = 141)	PPE (%, N = 140)
Beta-lactam Alone	77 (55)	10 (7)
Beta-lactam in combination	57 (40)	127 (90)
Beta lactam+macrolide	*36 (26)*	*4 (3)*
Beta lactam+anti-mrsa	*20 (14)*	*99 (71)*
Beta lactam+anti-mrsa+macrolide	*1 (1)*	*24 (17)*
Anti-mrsa alone	5 (4)	1(1)
Anti-mrsa+macrolide	2 (1)	2 (1)

PPE, parapneumonic empyema.
MRSA, methicillin-resistant *S. aureus*.

Duration of therapy

Overall, respondents generally recommended longer duration for PPE than for uncomplicated cases (Figure 1). For uncomplicated cases, 140 respondents provided data for duration and only 10% (14/140) recommended a duration of 7 days or less. The most common duration was 8–10 days, recommended by 56% (78/140). For PPE, 138 respondents provided data and 35% (48/138) recommended 11–14 days, 41% (57/138) recommended 15–21 days and 17% (24/138) recommended >21 days. We found no associations between treatment duration and antibiotic regimens, reported MRSA prevalence, the presence of a clinical guideline or ASP or years of experience for either uncomplicated CAP or PPE.

Relationship between reported antibiotic resistance and antibiotic recommendations

Aminopenicillins for uncomplicated CAP. 127 respondents provided data on *S. pneumoniae* resistance. Among these, 27 (21%) recommended either ampicillin or ampicillin/sulbactam as the sole agent for uncomplicated CAP while 100 recommended another regimen. The percentage of respondents recommending aminopenicillins did not increase as the reported prevalence of penicillin non-susceptible pneumococci decreased. Aminopenicillins were recommended in 26% of cases where the reported prevalence of penicillin non-susceptible pneumococci was <10% and 25% of cases where the prevalence of penicillin non-susceptible pneumococci was 26%–50% (p-value for trend = 0.46). Only 4 respondents reported prevalence >50% for *S. pneumoniae* non-susceptibility and none recommended aminopenicillins. In multivariable analysis, based on bivariate associations, geographic region, reported prevalence of penicillin non-susceptible pneumococci, presence of ASP and CAP clinical guideline were included in the model. None of these variables were independently associated with recommending aminopenicillins.

Anti-MRSA agents. There were 135 respondents who provided data on MRSA prevalence and empiric antibiotic recommendations for uncomplicated CAP and 134 for PPE. In contrast to penicillin non-susceptible pneumococci, we observed an increasing percentage of respondents who recommended anti-MRSA agents across the increasing levels of reported MRSA prevalence for uncomplicated CAP and PPE (Figure 2). For uncomplicated CAP,

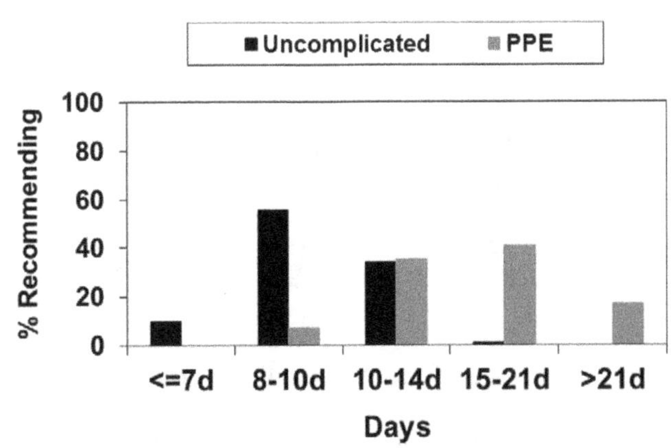

Figure 1. Recommended duration of therapy for uncomplicated CAP (N = 140) and PPE (N = 138). CAP, community-acquired pneumonia; PPE, parapneumonic empyema.

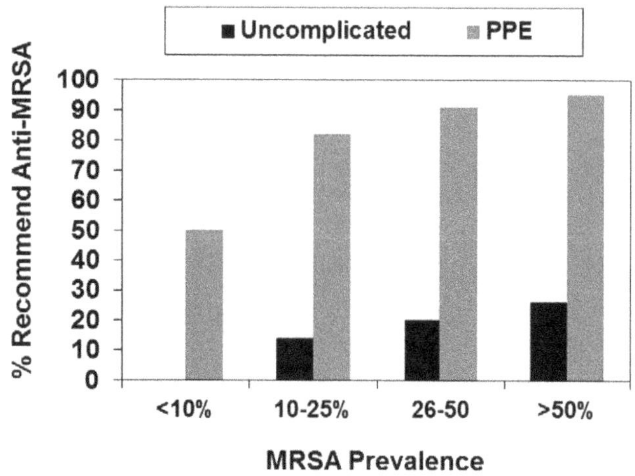

Figure 2. Percentage of respondents who recommended an anti-MRSA agent for uncomplicated CAP (N = 135) and PPE (N = 134) across a range of reported MRSA prevalence levels in their community. MRSA, methicillin-resistant *S. aureus*; CAP, community-acquired pneumonia; PPE, parapneumonic empyema.

the percentage increased from 0% of respondents recommending anti-MRSA agents who reported MRSA prevalence <10% to 26% of those who reported MRSA prevalence >50% (p trend = 0.14). For PPE, the percentage increased from 50% of respondents who reported MRSA prevalence <10% to 94% of respondents who reported MRSA prevalence >50% (p trend = 0.01).

Selection of clindamycin for an anti-MRSA agent

There were 27 respondents who selected an anti-MRSA agent for uncomplicated CAP and provided data on clindamycin resistance and 117 for PPE. Overall, we found no direct relationship between the selection of clindamycin as an anti-MRSA agent and the reported level of clindamycin resistance (Figure 3). For uncomplicated CAP, examining this relationship is somewhat limited due to the fact that clindamycin was the anti-MRSA agent recommended by 86% of respondents. There was a trend towards a decline in the percentage of respondents who selected clindamycin as reported clindamycin resistance increased, declining from 100% among those reporting clindamycin resistance <10% to 67% among those reporting clindamycin resistance 25–50% (p trend = 0.06), however, selection of clindamycin remained high overall. For PPE, the percentage recommending clindamycin as the anti-MRSA agent was unchanged as reported clindamycin resistance increased, ranging from 38%–41% across all levels (p trend = 0.86).

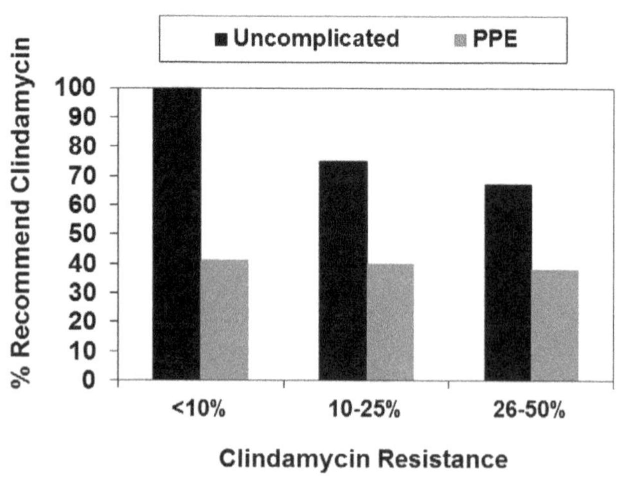

Figure 3. Percentage of respondents who recommended clindamycin as an anti-MRSA agent for uncomplicated CAP (N = 27) and PPE (N = 117) across a range of reported clindamycin resistance levels. MRSA, methicillin-resistant *S. aureus*; CAP, community-acquired pneumonia; PPE, parapneumonic empyema.

Because reported clindamycin resistance did not seem to have a strong influence on selection of clindamycin versus another anti-MRSA agent, especially for PPE, we developed a multivariable logistic model to assess whether any other factors were associated specifically with recommending clindamycin for PPE. Based on bivariate associations, the variables included in the model included reported MRSA prevalence and clindamycin resistance, practicing at a teaching hospital, the presence of a clinical pathway for pneumonia and the number of years of clinical experience in infectious disease. The only factor that was independently associated with recommending clindamycin was years of experience. Compared with those with >15 years of experience, the odds of recommending clindamcyin as an anti-MRSA agent for PPE (as opposed to vancomycin or linezolid) was substantially greater for those with <5 years (OR 7.8; 95% CI 1.9–31.3) and 5–15 years (OR 6.4; 95% CI 1.6–25.3). These results were unchanged when presence of an ASP was forced into the model.

Discussion

Our study has two important findings. First, we found evidence that substantial variation exists in the recommendations for CAP management from pediatric infectious diseases consultants, including the empiric antibiotic regimens and duration of therapy. Second, we found that differences in reported local antibiotic resistance patterns do not fully account for variations in antibiotic prescribing recommendations.

There are currently no national clinical guidelines for pediatric CAP, although 33% of our respondents indicated that they had a guideline established at their hospital. While the existence of a local guideline could reduce variation within an individual institution, the lack of association between the presence of a guideline and any of the practice patterns we examined (e.g. aminopenicillins for uncomplicated CAP) suggests that existing CAP guidelines are not uniform. Some of the variation we observed may reflect local factors that differ between hospitals including resistance patterns or formulary differences. It is likely, however, that much of the variation in terms of recommended antibiotics and treatment duration simply reflects a lack of consensus, due in part to limited evidence. A recently developed CAP clinical guideline from the Infectious Diseases Society of America (IDSA) has the potential to improve clinical practice and reduce variation.

CAP is a model condition for the development of clinical guidelines and ASP interventions considering that it is a common condition, has geographic variation in etiology and resistance and the potential for significant practice pattern variation. Empiric prescribing practices need to be individualized to account for each institution's local antibiotic resistance patterns. Additionally, treatment of CAP, especially PPE, is made more challenging by the fact that cultures are frequently negative, although newer molecular methods are promising [16]. The development and dissemination of clinical guidelines as well as antibiograms to assist with clinical decision making are important ASP functions [14].

Although antibiograms that are tailored to specific patient populations with specific conditions (e.g. pneumonia) have the potential to improve empiric antibiotic prescribing, they may not be easily accessible or widely used [17]. Furthermore, ASPs and guidelines can emphasize the importance of viral testing for patients with CAP, as certain viral infections such as influenza are associated with higher rates of CAP complications and differences in the etiology of bacterial co-infection [18]. Previous studies indicate that many pediatric institutions do not have ASPs and that existing ASPs have substantial deficiencies [15]. Improving the extent to which unit and condition specific antibiograms are made accessible to providers is a key area for ASP to support front-line prescribing physicians [11,12]. Our findings that ASPs and CAP guidelines were not associated with differences in treatment recommendations suggest that opportunities exist for these interventions to focus on enhancing the treatment of CAP with narrower spectrum antibiotic alternatives (e.g. ampicillin) and the extent to which treatment recommendations match local resistance patterns.

We were surprised to find no relationship between recommending clindamycin for PPE and reported clindamycin resistance. In particular, many respondents noted that they would recommend clindamycin despite noting relatively high levels of resistance in their community. There are several potential explanations for this result. A lack of reliable susceptibility data from antibiograms is one possibility. Another is that other factors favoring clindamycin relative to vancomycin, such as the availability of an oral formulation and that therapeutic drug monitoring is not necessary, are more important drivers for ID consultants' recommendations. A previous study suggested that ID consultants do not rank antibiotic resistance among the most important factors influencing their prescribing decisions [19]. It may also be that some respondents who prescribe clindamycin in settings where resistance was reportedly high feel that *S. aureus* is an uncommon cause of complicated CAP and thus the risk of a susceptibility mismatch is low. We did, however, observe a relationship between higher reported MRSA prevalence and more recommendations for anti-MRSA agents, indicating that respondents accounted for it as an important pathogen.

Unlike the association between antibiotic selection and MRSA prevalence, we did not observe a relationship between antibiotic selection and resistance in the case of aminopenicillins and the reported prevalence of penicillin non-susceptible *S. pneumoniae*. As with selecting clindamycin for MRSA, other factors besides resistance may contribute to physician preferences. In this instance, some physicians may find aminopenicillins less attractive than cephalosporins because of greater dosing frequency [20], even with low prevalence of penicillin non-susceptible *S. pneumoniae*. At the same time, evidence supports the use of aminopenicillins for treatment of CAP, even in the setting of relative resistance [21,22,23], which may explain why some respondents were comfortable prescribing this class with in this context.

We found that respondents with fewer years of clinical experience were far more likely to prescribe clindamycin for PPE than those with more clinical experience. A potential explanation for this finding is that respondents who completed training more recently may have more readily adopted practice patterns reflecting the emergence of the USA300 strain of community-associated MRSA, which is frequently susceptible to clindamycin [24].

We are not aware of any other studies that have explicitly examined the relationship between reported antibiotic resistance and antibiotic selection. Our findings indicate that many factors contribute to antibiotic selection, and perceived levels of antibiotic resistance is not necessarily the primary one. Nonetheless, our findings with respect to recommendations for clindamycin do raise some concerns. Use of clindamycin for treatment of pediatric MRSA infections has increased dramatically nationwide [25]. Because there may be seasonal, institutional and geographic variation in the organisms that cause uncomplicated and complicated CAP, combined with variation in resistance patterns, it is imperative that physicians have access to updated epidemiologic data for their community. Indeed, over 80% of our respondents indicated that they desired more information about local antibiotic resistance rates to assist in empiric prescribing decisions.

We observed variation in recommendations for macrolides. Monotherapy with a macrolide was not recommended by any respondents, even for uncomplicated CAP, presumably as a reflection of *S. pneumoniae* resistance. Although IDSA guidelines for the treatment of adult CAP recommend empiric therapy targeting atypical pathogens [26], evidence favoring use of macrolides to target these organisms (especially *Mycoplasma pneumoniae*) for treatment of pediatric CAP is not convincing [27].

There are several limitations to our study. Because the data are derived from a survey and not from an administrative database or chart review, the respondents' reported practices might not match their actual practices. Infectious diseases physicians are not usually the primary prescribers for children with CAP, however, they do frequently contribute to guidelines and local practice consensus. Physicians may have different antibiotic prescribing practices for pediatric CAP for patients in different age groups (e.g. <1–5 years and >5 years) which was not captured by this survey. Our analysis of resistance was based on respondents' report rather than antibiogram data and thus may not reflect actual epidemiology. However, the relationship between what respondents believe the resistance patterns to be to their and their practice patterns is likely a more important driver of practice.

We found that substantial variation exists among pediatric infectious disease consultants in their recommendations for empiric antibiotic regimens for pneumonia and that this variation is only partly related to reported local antibiotic resistance patterns. One area highlighted by our findings is that greater dissemination improvements to resources about the epidemiology of local resistance patterns may assist physicians in their selection of empiric antibiotic regimens for CAP or other conditions where antibiotic resistance is common.

Author Contributions

Conceived and designed the experiments: ALH JGN PMP SEB SSS. Performed the experiments: ALH JGN PMP SEB SSS. Analyzed the data: ALH DJS. Wrote the paper: ALH. Critical revision of manuscript: DJS JGN PMP SEB SSS.

References

1. Lee GE, Lorch SA, Sheffler-Collins S, Kronman MP, Shah SS (2010) National hospitalization trends for pediatric pneumonia and associated complications. Pediatrics 126: 204–213.
2. Gerber JS, Newland JG, Coffin SE, Hall M, Thurm C, et al. (2010) Variability in Antibiotic Use at Children's Hospitals. Pediatrics.
3. Grijalva CG, Nuorti JP, Zhu Y, Griffin MR (2010) Increasing incidence of empyema complicating childhood community-acquired pneumonia in the United States. Clin Infect Dis 50: 805–813.
4. Li ST, Tancredi DJ (2010) Empyema hospitalizations increased in US children despite pneumococcal conjugate vaccine. Pediatrics 125: 26–33.

5. Centers for Disease Control and Prevention, Active Bacterial Core Surveillance. Available: http://www.cdc.gov/abcs/reports-findings/surv-reports.html. Accessed 2010 Nov 10.
6. Liu C, Bayer A, Cosgrove SE, Daum RS, Fridkin SK, et al. (2011) Clinical practice guidelines by the infectious diseases society of america for the treatment of methicillin-resistant Staphylococcus aureus infections in adults and children. Clin Infect Dis 52: e18–55.
7. Schultz KD, Fan LL, Pinsky J, Ochoa L, Smith EO, et al. (2004) The changing face of pleural empyemas in children: epidemiology and management. Pediatrics 113: 1735–1740.
8. Byington CL, Korgenski K, Daly J, Ampofo K, Pavia A, et al. (2006) Impact of the pneumococcal conjugate vaccine on pneumococcal parapneumonic empyema. Pediatr Infect Dis J 25: 250–254.
9. Kollef MH (2008) Broad-spectrum antimicrobials and the treatment of serious bacterial infections: getting it right up front. Clin Infect Dis 47 Suppl 1: S3–13.
10. Muszynski JA, Knatz NL, Sargel CL, Fernandez SA, Marquardt DJ, et al. (2010) Timing of Correct Parenteral Antibiotic Initiation and Outcomes From Severe Bacterial Community-acquired Pneumonia in Children. Pediatr Infect Dis J.
11. Patel SJ, Rosen E, Zaoutis T, Prasad P, Saiman L (2010) Neonatologists' perceptions of antimicrobial resistance and stewardship in neonatal intensive care units. Infect Control Hosp Epidemiol 31: 1298–1300.
12. Pogue JM, Alaniz C, Carver PL, Pleva M, Newton D, et al. (2011) Role of Unit-Specific Combination Antibiograms for Improving the Selection of Appropriate Empiric Therapy for Gram-Negative Pneumonia. Infect Control Hosp Epidemiol 32: 289–292.
13. Newland JG, Hersh AL (2010) Purpose and design of antimicrobial stewardship programs in pediatrics. Pediatr Infect Dis J 29: 862–863.
14. Dellit TH, Owens RC, McGowan JE, Jr., Gerding DN, Weinstein RA, et al. (2007) Infectious Diseases Society of America and the Society for Healthcare Epidemiology of America guidelines for developing an institutional program to enhance antimicrobial stewardship. Clin Infect Dis 44: 159–177.
15. Hersh AL, Beekmann SE, Polgreen PM, Zaoutis TE, Newland JG (2009) Antimicrobial stewardship programs in pediatrics. Infect Control Hosp Epidemiol 30: 1211–1217.
16. Blaschke AJ, Heyrend C, Byington CL, Obando I, Vazquez-Barba I, et al. (2010) Molecular Analysis Improves Pathogen Identification and Epidemiologic Study of Pediatric Parapneumonic Empyema. Pediatr Infect Dis J.
17. Mermel LA, Jefferson J, Devolve J (2008) Knowledge and use of cumulative antimicrobial susceptibility data at a university teaching hospital. Clin Infect Dis 46: 1789.
18. Williams DJ, Hall M, Brogan TV, Farris RW, Myers AL, et al. (2011) Influenza Coinfection and Outcomes in Children With Complicated Pneumonia. Arch Pediatr Adolesc Med.
19. Metlay JP, Shea JA, Crossette LB, Asch DA (2002) Tensions in antibiotic prescribing: pitting social concerns against the interests of individual patients. J Gen Intern Med 17: 87–94.
20. Rosen J, Beekmann S, Polgreen P, Moore M (2010) Barriers to intravenous penicillin use for treatment of nonmeningitis pneumococcal disease. J Clin Microbiol 48: 3372–3374.
21. Cardoso MR, Nascimento-Carvalho CM, Ferrero F, Berezin EN, Ruvinsky R, et al. (2008) Penicillin-resistant pneumococcus and risk of treatment failure in pneumonia. Arch Dis Child 93: 221–225.
22. Furuno JP, Metlay JP, Harnett JP, Wilson J, Langenberg P, et al. (2006) Population antibiotic susceptibility for Streptococcus pneumoniae and treatment outcomes in common respiratory tract infections. Pharmacoepidemiol Drug Saf 15: 1–9.
23. Yu VL, Chiou CC, Feldman C, Ortqvist A, Rello J, et al. (2003) An international prospective study of pneumococcal bacteremia: correlation with in vitro resistance, antibiotics administered, and clinical outcome. Clin Infect Dis 37: 230–237.
24. Kaplan SL (2005) Treatment of community-associated methicillin-resistant Staphylococcus aureus infections. Pediatr Infect Dis J 24: 457–458.
25. Herigon JC, Hersh AL, Gerber JS, Zaoutis TE, Newland JG (2010) Antibiotic management of Staphylococcus aureus infections in US children's hospitals, 1999–2008. Pediatrics 125: e1294–1300.
26. Mandell LA, Wunderink RG, Anzueto A, Bartlett JG, Campbell GD, et al. (2007) Infectious Diseases Society of America/American Thoracic Society consensus guidelines on the management of community-acquired pneumonia in adults. Clin Infect Dis 44 Suppl 2: S27–72.
27. Mulholland S, Gavranich JB, Chang AB (2010) Antibiotics for community-acquired lower respiratory tract infections secondary to Mycoplasma pneumoniae in children. Cochrane Database Syst Rev: CD004875.

11

Treatment of Hepatitis C in Children

Jia Hu[1]*, Karen Doucette[2], Lisa Hartling[1,3], Lisa Tjosvold[1,3], Joan Robinson[1]*

1 Department of Pediatrics, University of Alberta, Edmonton, Canada, 2 Department of Medicine, University of Alberta, Edmonton, Canada, 3 Alberta Research Centre for Health Evidence, University of Alberta, Edmonton, Canada

Abstract

Background: Current guidelines recommend children be treated for hepatitis C virus (HCV) using the same principles applied in adults. There are however few published studies which assess the efficacy and safety of HCV therapy in children.

Methodology/Principal Findings: A systematic review of the literature was completed for studies of any design that evaluated HCV therapy in children. The primary outcome was sustained virologic response (SVR), with sub-group analysis of response rates by genotype. There were 4 randomized controlled trials (RCTs) and 31 non-randomized studies, all involving interferon, pegylated interferon (PEG-IFN), or combinations of these drugs with ribavirin. The SVR rate could not be directly compared as the populations and interventions differed across studies. Genotype was not reported or differed substantially from study to study. The overall SVR rate for PEG-IFN and ribavirin ranged from 30 to 100% which is comparable to the rate in adults. Similar to adults, the SVR rates were significantly higher in children with genotype 2 or 3 compared to genotype 1. Adverse effects were primarily flu-like symptoms and neutropenia. There were insufficient data to assess the applicability of the week 12 stop rule (stopping therapy at week 12 if there is less than a 2 log drop in HCV RNA) or the efficacy of shortening therapy to 24 weeks in children with genotype 2 and 3.

Conclusions/Significance: Current guidelines for the treatment of HCV in children are based on limited data. Further research is needed to define the optimal therapy for HCV in children.

Editor: Wen-Liang Zhou, Sun Yat-Sen University, China

Funding: The authors have no support or funding to report.

Competing Interests: The authors have declared that no competing interests exist.

* E-mail: jr3@ualberta.ca (JLR); jh11@ualberta.ca (JH)

Introduction

Treatment guidelines for hepatitis C virus (HCV) infection in adults are based on a large body of published natural history studies and randomized controlled trials (RCTs). There is a relative paucity of data regarding the impact of HCV on the morbidity and mortality of infected children and few published studies which assess the efficacy and safety of HCV therapy in children. Despite this, current guidelines recommend children be assessed and treated for HCV in a similar manner to adults [1].

The prevalence of HCV infection in children varies widely by country, ranging from 0% in Japan and 0.4% in Italy to up to 14.5% in Cameroon.[2,3,4] A study performed in the early 1990s in the United States documented HCV antibodies in 0.2% of children aged 6 to 12 and 0.4% of children aged 12 to 19 [5]. It is estimated that 75–80% of children who are antibody positive are also HCV RNA positive [5].

The natural history of HCV in children is not completely understood. However, compared to adult infection, spontaneous clearance is more common and both fulminant hepatitis and progression of chronic infection to advanced fibrosis and cirrhosis are less likely [6,7,8,9,10,11]. Despite the overall more favorable prognosis than in adults, approximately 4 to 6% of children with chronic HCV infection have evidence of advanced fibrosis or cirrhosis on liver biopsy [11,12], and 4 to 5 children each year undergo liver transplantation in the United States for end-stage liver disease as a consequence of HCV [13].

Despite the significant number of children infected with HCV, and a clear subset of those who may benefit from HCV therapy, there is little consensus on when or how to optimally treat children with HCV infection. A previous meta-analysis examining interferon monotherapy for pediatric HCV concluded that the sustained virologic response (SVR) was higher and that therapy was better tolerated than in adults [14]. Combination therapy with pegylated interferon (PEG-IFN) and ribavirin has been shown to be superior to standard interferon monotherapy or combination therapy with interferon and ribavirin and is the current gold standard for HCV therapy in adults [1,15,16] but there is a paucity of pediatric RCTs of this therapy.

This paper represents a comprehensive and systematic review of evidence specific to children for the treatment of HCV infection. The primary aim was to determine if there is sufficient evidence to recommend any ways in which the approach to therapy of children with HCV should differ from the approach in adults. A secondary aim was to use this data to serve as a basis to identify priority areas for future research.

Methods

Searching

A medical research librarian conducted comprehensive searches in the following electronic databases: Medline® (1950-April Week 2 2009), Embase (1980 to 2009 Week 16), EBM Reviews – Cochrane Central Register of Controlled Trials (1st Quarter 2009), Web of Science® (1900–2009), Scopus® (1966–2009), LILACS (1982–2009), Biosis Previews® (1926–2009), Proquest Dissertations and Theses (1900–2009) and the ARIF Reviews Database (1996–2009). No language restrictions were applied. Search strategies were modified to accommodate the controlled vocabulary and search language of each database. The search strategy for Medline appears in Appendix S1. Search strategies for the other databases are available from the corresponding author.

Unpublished studies were identified by hand searching the following conference proceedings: North American and European Societies of Pediatric Gastroenterology and Nutrition (2007–2009), American Association for the Study of Liver Diseases (2006–2009), American Gastroenterology Association (2006–2010), European Association for the Study of the Liver (2007–2010). Ongoing studies were identified through searches of UMIN-CTR, Current Controlled Trials and Clinical Trials.gov. Studies were also located by scanning reference lists of existing systematic reviews and included studies

Study Selection and Characteristics

The title and abstracts of studies identified by the search were screened for potential relevance. The full text of all potentially relevant studies was reviewed to determine if they fulfilled the eligibility criteria. Studies were included if: 1) they included only children (≤18 years of age) or presented data separately for children; 2) HCV infection was confirmed by detection of HCV RNA; 3) details of the treatment regimen were provided; and 4) data were provided for the sustained virologic response (SVR, defined as a negative HCV RNA at least 24 weeks after cessation of therapy) which was the outcome of interest. All interventions for the treatment of HCV were included, as were all comparisons. We anticipated that there would be a small number of RCTs meeting our inclusion criteria; therefore, we chose to include studies of any design that reported the efficacy or effectiveness of treatment in a cohort of children infected with HCV.

Validity assessment of randomized controlled trials

All relevant RCTs were assessed for risk of bias independently by two reviewers (JH, LH) using the Cochrane Risk of Bias (RoB) tool. The Cochrane RoB tool evaluates six domains including: sequence generation, allocation concealment, blinding, missing outcome data, selective outcome reporting, and "other sources of bias." Disagreements were resolved through discussion.

Data abstraction

An electronic data extraction form was developed in MS Excel a priori and used for data entry. Extracted items included characteristics of the study population and intervention and control groups, inclusion and exclusion criteria, treatments given, SVR, and adverse effects. Data from RCTs was extracted by a single reviewer and checked by a second reviewer. Authors of RCTs with missing data were contacted for details.

Quantitative data synthesis

There was significant clinical and methodological heterogeneity across studies in terms of the interventions, comparisons, and study designs. Therefore, meta-analysis was not appropriate. We described the studies qualitatively and present detailed results in evidence tables. The results are presented by study design, i.e., RCTs and non-randomized studies with separate analysis for genotype 1 versus other genotypes where specified.

Results

Flow of included studies

The comprehensive literature search returned a total of 1914 articles (Figure 1). Of these, 4 met the inclusion criteria as RCTs while 31 met the inclusion criteria as non-randomized studies.

Study Characteristics - Randomized Controlled Trials

Among the four relevant RCTs, three were peer-reviewed manuscripts and one was an abstract presented at the 2008 Annual Meeting of the American Association for the Study of Liver Diseases (Table 1). Three included only pediatric populations [17,18,19] while one had a mixed pediatric-adult population [20]. All four RCTs were deemed to have an unclear risk of bias based on the Cochrane Risk of Bias tool. The RCT by Schwarz et al. [19] appeared to be the most methodologically rigorous but was still rated unclear since only the study protocol and abstract were available for assessment. Sequence generation and allocation concealment were generally poorly described. Inappropriate sequence generation and inadequate allocation concealment can result in overestimates of treatment effects.

Quantitative Data Synthesis - Randomized Controlled Trials

Two studies conducted in Italy were both published in 1995, and randomized children up to 14 years of age with biopsy-proven

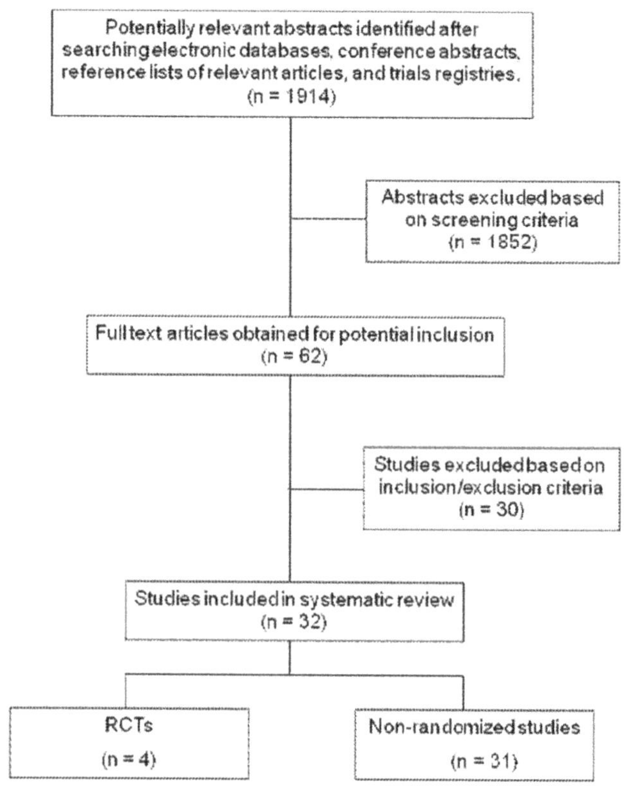

Figure 1. Systematic review process flowchart.

Table 1. Study design of randomized controlled trials of pediatric HCV therapy.

Author/Year/ Country	Entry criteria	Group A Characteristics	Group B Characteristics	Group A Treatment	Group B Treatment
1. Iorio 1995, Italy [18]	Children with HCV attending liver diseases clinic 1 to 14 years of age with chronic hepatitis on biopsy, elevated ALT for at least 6 months, and anti-HCV antibodies	7 males, 4 females; 7 genotype 1, 5 non-genotype 1	4 males, 6 females; 7 genotype 1, 3 non-genotype 1	Interferon alfa, 3 MU/m^2times weekly for 12 months	No treatment
2. Bortolotti, 1995, Italy [17]	Children with HCV 2 to 14 years of age with chronic hepatitis on biopsy, elevated ALT for at least 6 months, and anti-HCV antibodies	7 males, 7 females; 7 genotype 1, 7 non-genotype 1	5 males, 8 females; 6 genotype 1, 8 non-genotype 1	Interferon alfa-2b 5 MU/m^2 3 times weekly for 12 months	No treatment
3. Fried 2002, USA [20]	Adolescents with HCV and haemophilia 13 to 17 years of ages and with detectable HCV-RNA	17 adolescents; All infected by transfusion	20 adolescents; All infected by transfusion	Interferon alfa-2b 3 MU/m^2 3 times weekly + 1000 mg ribavirin daily for 48 weeks	Interferon alfa-2b 3 MU/m^2 3 times weekly for 48 weeks
4. Schwarz 2008, USA [19]	Children with HCV 5 to 17 years of age with chronic hepatitis on biopsy and detectable HCV-RNA	34 males, 21 females; 44 genotype 1; 11 non-genotype 1	29 males, 30 females; 48 genotype 1; 11 non-genotype 1	PEG-IFN alfa-2a 180 micrograms/1.73 m^2 + ribavirin 15/mg/kg/day for 48 weeks	PEG-IFN alfa-2a 180 micrograms/1.73 m^2 for 48 weeks

chronic hepatitis and elevated ALT to interferon (using different regimens in each study as shown in Table 1) versus no treatment for 12 months. Iorio et al. found that 5 of 11 (45%) treated patients and 1 of 11 controls (9%) achieved a SVR [18] (Table 2). These results were borderline statistically significant ($p = 0.056$), likely due to the small numbers of patients. Bortolotti et al. reported that SVR was achieved in 9 of 13 (69%) treated patients and 0 of 13 controls ($p<0.001$) [17]. Almost all treated patients had flu-like symptoms, and doses of interferon were decreased in 7 of 25 children (28%) due to neutropenia. Therapy was stopped in 3 other children for ALT flares.

Fried et al. studied a mixed pediatric-adult population at US hemophiliac clinics [20]. Viremic subjects aged 13 years and older were randomized to interferon alfa-2b and ribavirin versus interferon monotherapy for 48 weeks. The only outcome data provided for adolescents was a SVR in 10 of 17 (59%) in those on combination therapy. The authors were contacted and were not able to provide SVR rates in adolescents on monotherapy, but pointed out that only 6 of 57 adults and adolescents combined (11%) achieved SVR on monotherapy.

A fourth RCT by Schwarz et al. randomized children with biopsy-proven chronic hepatitis and viremia in Europe, the US, and South America to PEG-IFN alfa-2a 180ug/1.73m2/week and ribavirin 15 mg/kg/day versus PEG-IFN alfa- 2a monotherapy for 48 weeks [19]. Data was extracted from an abstract published in 2008. SVR was achieved in 29 of 55 (53%) children on combination therapy and in 12 of 59 (21%) on monotherapy ($p<0.001$). Four percent of children on combination therapy and 7% on monotherapy required early discontinuation, presumably due to adverse events, while 51% on combination therapy and 54% on monotherapy required dose reduction. An abstract from this study described one child with ischemic retinopathy, one with uveitis, and one with transient monocular blindness that the authors attributed to PEG-IFN [21]. The presence of autoantibodies did not alter the SVR rate [22].

Among the four RCTs, viral genotype was only mentioned in the Schwarz study with SVR being 80% in those with non-genotype 1 on combination therapy versus 36% on monotherapy. SVR for those with genotype 1 was 47% on combination therapy versus 18% on monotherapy.

Table 2. Outcome of randomized controlled trials of pediatric HCV therapy.

Author/Year/ Country	Group A Therapy Incomplete	Group B Therapy Incomplete	Group A SVR	Group B SVR	Group A Adverse Effects	Group B Adverse Effects
1. Iorio 1995, Italy	Discontinued in 1 child in first month from ALT flare-up and in 5 others at 6 months since no response in ALT	Not applicable as no therapy given	5 of 11 (45%) at 30 months	1 of 11 (9%) at 30 months	Transient influenza-like syndrome in all patients; other symptoms included anorexia, asthenia, irritability, headache, abdominal pain, and leukopenia	Not reported
2. Bortolotti, 1995, Italy	Discontinued in 2 children from ALT flare-up, in 1 child from febrile seizure, and 1 since no response in ALT	Not applicable as no therapy given	9 of 13 (69%) at 24 months	0 of 13 (0%) at 24 months	Transient influenza-like syndrome in all patients; Other symptoms included pruritus, weight loss, and leukopenia	Not reported
3. Fried 2002, USA	Not reported	Not reported	10 of 17 (59%) at 72 weeks	Not reported	Not reported	Not reported
4. Schwarz 2008, USA	Discontinued in 2 children	Discontinued in 4 children	29 of 55 (53%) at 72 weeks	15 of 59 (21%) at 72 weeks	Not reported	Not reported

Study Characteristics - Non-randomized Studies

Thirty-one non-randomized studies met the inclusion criteria (Table S1). Full manuscripts were available for 26 of these studies; the others were only available in abstract form. One study had a comparison group: interferon/ribavarin combination therapy versus interferon monotherapy [23]. The remaining studies were uncontrolled before-after studies; therefore, 32 treatment groups were available for analysis.

The studies were published between 1992 and 2010. The number of participants ranged from 8 to 151 (median: 24). All studies described one of the following four therapies in various standardized doses, most commonly 3 or 5 MU/m^2 interferon thrice weekly or PEG-IFN alfa-2b 1.0 to 1.5 ug/kg/week and 15 mg/kg/day ribavirin:

1) Interferon monotherapy – 16 treatment groups
2) PEG-IFN monotherapy – 1 treatment group
3) Interferon + ribavarin combination therapy – 6 treatment groups
4) PEG-IFN + ribavarin combination therapy – 9 treatment groups

Quantitative Data Synthesis - Non-randomized Studies

Among the 16 interferon monotherapy therapy groups, SVR ranged from 0% to 76% (median: 37%) with 122 of 342 children (36%) achieving SVR (Figure 2). In the only study of PEG-IFN monotherapy, 6 of 14 children (43%) achieved SVR [24]. Among the 6 interferon/ribavarin combination therapy groups, SVR ranged from 27% to 64% (median: 48%) with 109 of 233 children (49%) achieving SVR (Figure 3). Among the 9 PEG-IFN/ribavarin combination therapy groups, SVR ranged from 30% to 100% (median: 63%) with 341 of 493 children (69%) achieving SVR (Figure 4).

Many of the interferon monotherapy studies did not report viral genotypes. For the interferon/ribavirin case series, the SVR for genotype 1 ranged from 27% to 53% (median: 40%). Only two patients among the interferon/ribavirin case series were reported to have genotype 4, and neither of them responded to therapy. The SVR for genotypes 2 and 3, which respond more favorably to treatment than genotypes 1 or 4, was reported in three studies as 84%, 100%, and 100%.

For the PEG-IFN/ribavirin case series where the genotype was specified, the SVR for genotype 1 ranged from 22% to 100% (median: 51%) with a combined response of 215/342 (51%) (Table S1). For genotype 2 or 3, 53 of 54 patients responded (98%) and for genotype 4, 9 of 12 patients responded in one study (75%) and 80% of patients responded in another study (number of patients not provided).

Figure 5 shows the SVR in all non-randomized and RCTs combined, showing improved results with PEG-IFN/ribavirin (statistics not applied as most studies not randomized).

Discussion

Interferon monotherapy was the initial therapy studied for pediatric HCV infection and was the focus of 16 studies published between 1992 and 2003. Multiple dosing regimens of interferon were studied with the most common being thrice weekly interferon-alfa for a minimum of 22 weeks. A range of SVR from 0 to 76% from non-randomized studies and a SVR of 45%[18] and 69% [17] from RCTs was reported. There was only one study of PEG-IFN monotherapy with a 43% SVR [24]. Adding ribavirin to interferon was reported in 8 studies published from 2000 to 2007 with a range in SVR from 27% to 64% for the non-randomized studies and SVR of 59% for the RCT [20].These therapies are no longer used as standard therapy for adults and are unlikely to be studied further in children, especially since IFN

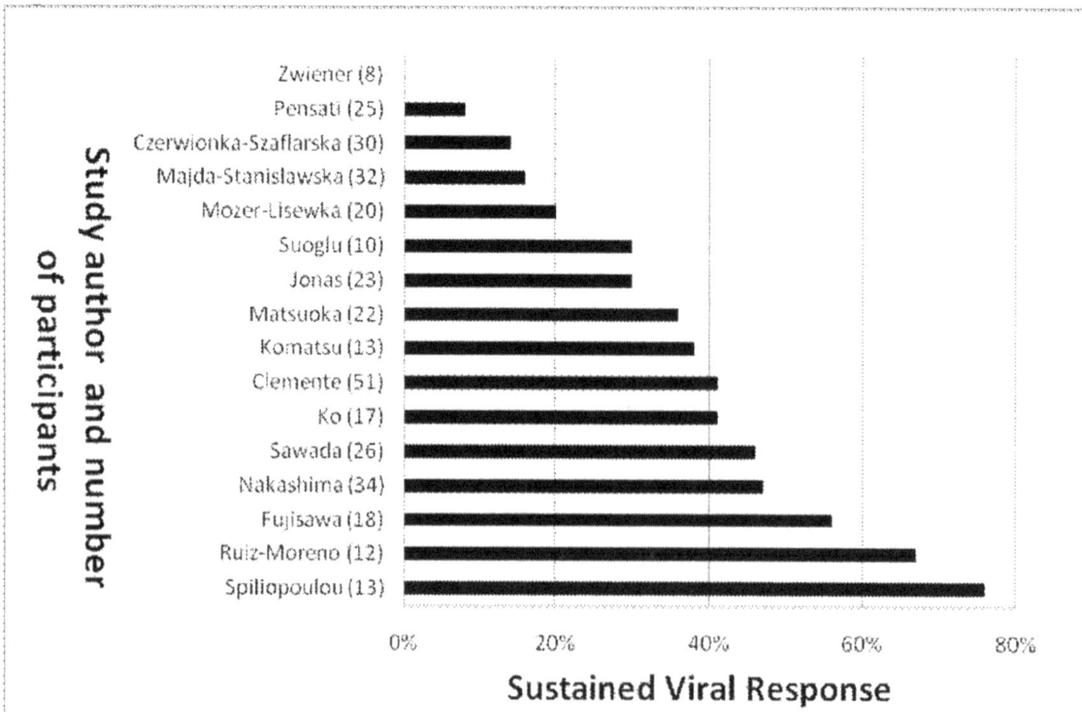

Figure 2. SVR of interferon monotherapy in non-randomized studies.

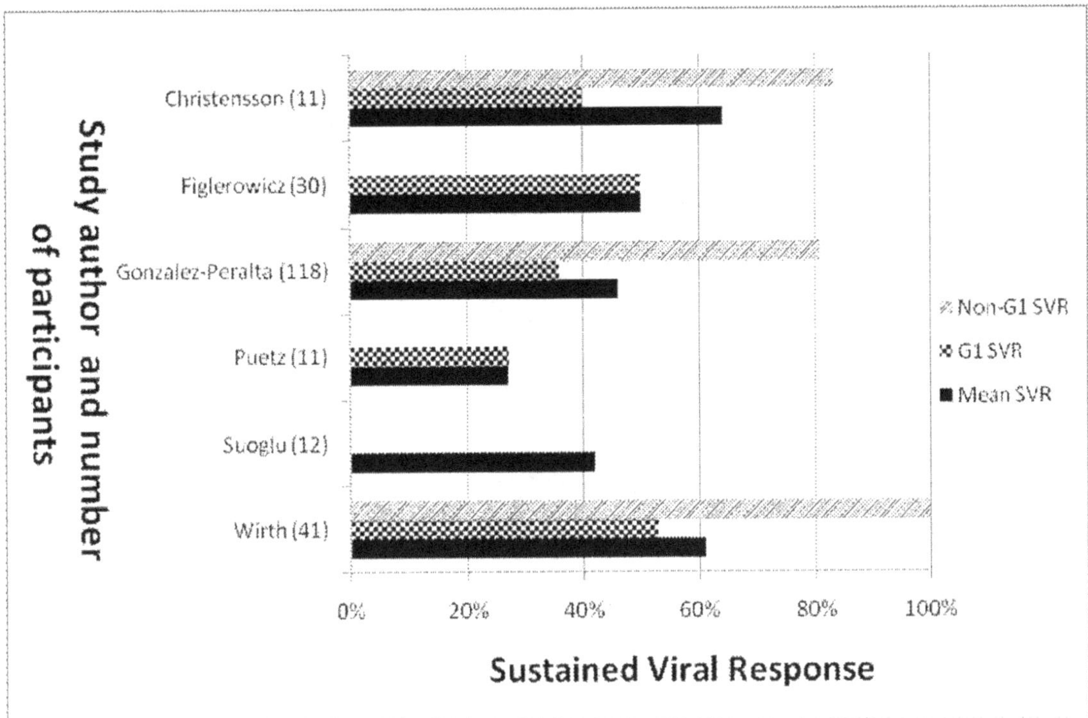

Figure 3. SVR by genotype of interferon/ribavirin therapy in non-randomized studies. Note the Suoglu study did not report data on genotype and all patients in the Puetz and Figlerowicz studies were infected with genotype 1.

requires thrice weekly injections versus weekly injections with PEG-IFN. Nonetheless, data on response rates is potentially useful in situations where children do not tolerate newer therapies.

The current standard of care for adults with chronic HCV is combination therapy with PEG-IFN and ribavirin [1,15,16]. PEG-IFN alfa-2b is approved by the US Food and Drug Administration

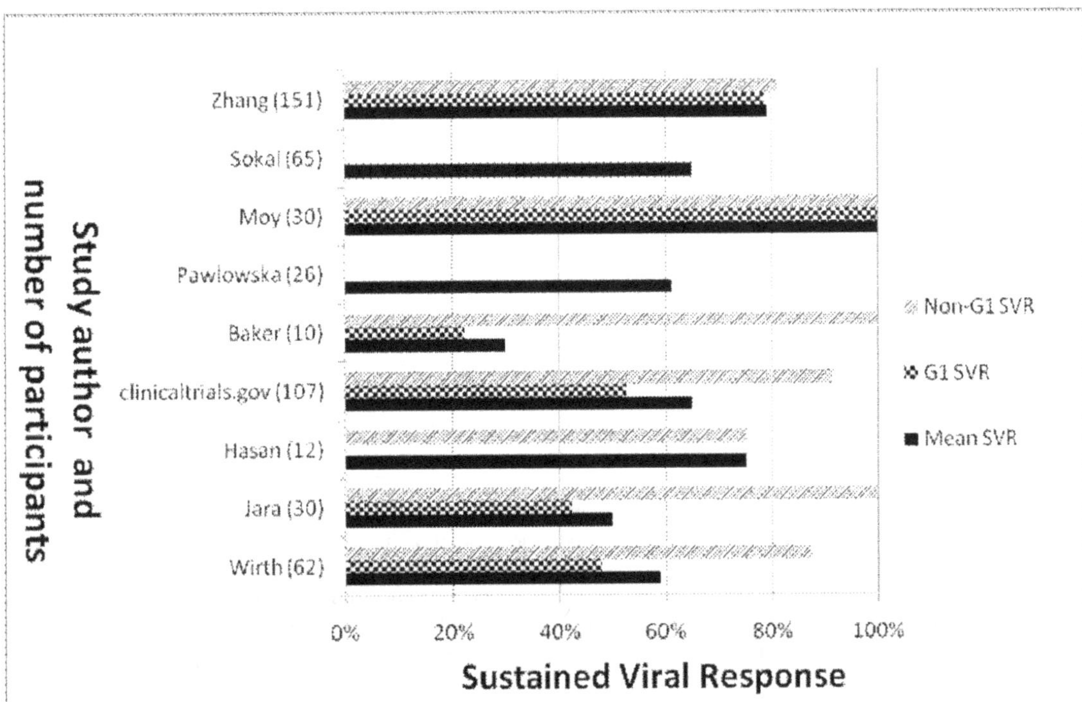

Figure 4. SVR by genotype of PEG-IFN/ribavirin therapy in non-randomized studies. Note all patients in the Hasan study were infected with genotype 4 and genotype 1 vs. non-genotype 1 SVR was not reported for the Pawlowska and Sokal studies.

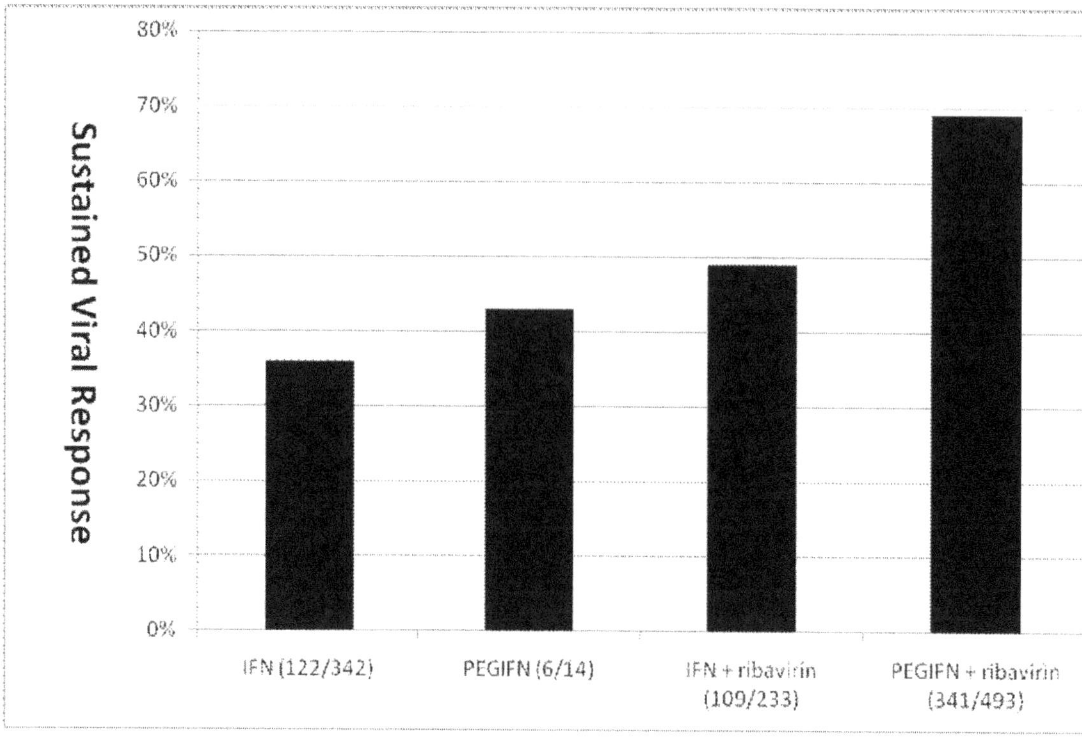

Figure 5. SVR and aggregate number of patients included and who achieved SVR by treatment class.

(FDA) for children aged 3 years and older and by the European Medicines Agency with approval of PEG-IFN alfa-2a by the FDA anticipated to occur soon. In adults, a recent large multicenter RCT demonstrated no significant difference in the SVR rate between the two available peginterferon-ribavirin regimens [25].

There were 9 pediatric non-randomized studies of PEG-IFN with ribavirin with a range in SVR from 30% to 100%. The only RCT described a 53% SVR [19]. This is certainly no better in comparison to the 45% to 69% [17,18] and 59% [20] SVR rates achieved with interferon monotherapy and combination interferon and ribavirin respectively in RCTs. However, comparison between trials is clearly flawed given differences in the populations studied and in particular the lack of comprehensive genotype-specific outcomes.

The vast majority of children will tolerate PEG-IFN and ribavirin. Although over half the children in the RCT required dose reduction of PEG-IFN, it is recognized that dose reduction was more common in adult trials than it is in clinical practice. The majority of adverse effects were mild to moderate and the rates of discontinuation of therapy were low in all groups studied.

As with adult HCV infection, genotype 1 is associated with a lower response rate to all therapies than is genotype 2 or 3 in children. In adults, response to therapy with genotype 4 is lower than with genotype 2 or 3, but there is insufficient pediatric data to be certain the same principle applies. The proportion of children with genotype 1 was 81% in the PEG-IFN ribavirin study [19] versus 70% in the interferon and ribavirin RCT [20] and an average of 54% in the two interferon monotherapy RCTs [17,18]. The relatively low percentage of children with genotype 1 in the earlier RCTs may account for the surprisingly high SVRs. The efficacy of PEG-IFN and ribavirin in children seems comparable to adults with a SVR of 42% to 46% in adults (versus 47% in the pediatric RCT) in genotype 1 [15,16], and 76% to 82% in genotype 2 or 3 in adults (versus 80% for non-genotype 1 in the pediatric RCT). Based on adult data, African-American ethnicity is also a risk factor for poor response [26]. Because this was recognized only recently, a minority of pediatric RCTs or case series report ethnicity.

In adults, 24 weeks of therapy for genotype 2 or 3 has been shown to be equivalent to 48 weeks [27]. Currently 48 weeks of therapy is recommended for all children in American Association for Study of Liver Disease guidelines regardless of genotype [1] but a recent small study demonstrated SVR in 16 or 18 children treated for 24 weeks with genotype 2 or 3 [28]. In adults, failure to achieve an early virologic response, as defined by at least a 2 $\log_{10}$ drop in HCV RNA at week 12 from baseline, is associated with non-response [29] and therapy is discontinued. It remains to be determined if this week 12 stopping rule applies to pediatric patients.

The current study did not address routine follow-up for children with HCV infection or when treatment of HCV should be commenced. It would seem logical to perform clinical follow-up with measurement of aminotransferases every 3 to 6 months in children who remain well. However, given the fact that about one-quarter of adults with significant fibrosis have normal aminotransferases [1], it remains very controversial if a liver biopsy should routinely be performed in children after an arbitrary time period, such as 10 years of HCV infection, even with normal aminotransferases. Transient elastography (FibroScan ®, Echo-Sens, Paris, France) may ultimately prove useful as a non-invasive test to identify children who are likely to have fibrosis on biopsy but this requires further study.

For genotype 1 HCV, new therapies with higher efficacy rates [30,31]are likely to be licensed soon. We therefore would advise delaying therapy for genotype 1 HCV unless a biopsy shows significant fibrosis, or the parent or child is very insistent on proceeding. It remains controversial if patients with genotypes 2 or 3 who are likely to be compliant and to tolerate therapy should all be treated with PEG-IFN and ribavirin without a biopsy since the response rate is over 80% in adults [1] and there are no new therapies on the horizon. If the decision is made to treat children with these genotyopes, it would seem reasonable to proceed without a biopsy. For children over 2 years of age with significant fibrosis from any genotype, treatment with weight-adjusted doses of PEG-IFN and ribavirin should be offered, avoiding therapy in younger children because of the risk of neurotoxicity from interferon [32]. The decision of when to start therapy must account for the estimated or known duration of infection, genotype, degree of fibrosis (particularly in genotype 1), comorbidities, predicted compliance, expected adverse events and anticipated interference with home life, school and extra-curricular activities. Topical anesthetic creams should be considered for children with needle phobia. Despite an absence of data, we recommend using the adult early stopping rules for rapid responders and non-responders. Monitoring during therapy should follow adult guidelines [1]. These do not currently recommend routine ophthalmologic assessments. More pediatric data is required to determine if this could prevent any long-term morbidity.

Previous studies have suggested that low baseline serum HCV RNA predicts successful therapy, and that there is no correlation between response and pretreatment serum aminotransferase levels [33]. Recently, a genetic polymorphism near the *IL28B* gene on chromosome 19 has been found to be highly predictive of viral clearance with PEG-IFN and ribavirin, which explains some of the association between response rate and ethnicity [34]. A limitation of the current study is that patients could not be stratified by this polymorphism, age, ethnicity, mode of infection, pretreatment serum aminotransferase levels, pretreatment serum HCV RNA levels, or results of liver histology. Future studies should report these features for all patients in addition to genotype. It would also be useful to document if there is any risk of later relapse in children who attain a SVR.

Newer therapies are on the horizon. Phase 3 trials have been completed in adults with genotype 1 HCV using triple combination PEG-IFN, ribavirin and the protease inhibitors telapravir or boceprevir. There is a clear benefit over combination PEG-IFN and ribavirin, increasing the SVR from 38% to 41% with dual therapy up to 67% to 75% with triple therapy [30,31]. It will be vital to collect data on the safety and efficacy of these novel combination therapies in children. Long-term follow up studies are also needed to determine the incidence and sequelae of potential neurotoxicity from PEG-INF in children and the impact of therapy on morbidity and mortality.

Author Contributions

Conceived and designed the experiments: JH LH JR. Performed the experiments: JH LH LT. Analyzed the data: JH. Wrote the paper: JH KD LH JR.

References

1. Ghany MG, Strader DB, Thomas DL, Seeff LB (2009) Diagnosis, management, and treatment of hepatitis C: an update. Hepatology 49: 1335–1374.
2. Gessoni G, Manoni F (1993) Prevalence of anti-hepatitis C virus antibodies among teenagers in the Venetian area: a seroepidemiological study. Eur J Med 2: 79–82.
3. Ngatchu T, Stroffolini T, Rapicetta M, Chionne P, Lantum D, et al. (1992) Seroprevalence of anti-HCV in an urban child population: a pilot survey in a developing area, Cameroon. J Trop Med Hyg 95: 57–61.
4. Tanaka E, Kiyosawa K, Sodeyama T, Hayata T, Ohike Y, et al. (1992) Prevalence of antibody to hepatitis C virus in Japanese schoolchildren: comparison with adult blood donors. Am J Trop Med Hyg 46: 460–464.
5. Alter MJ, Kruszon-Moran D, Nainan OV, McQuillan GM, Gao F, et al. (1999) The prevalence of hepatitis C virus infection in the United States, 1988 through 1994. N Engl J Med 341: 556–562.
6. Jonas MM, Baron MJ, Bresee JS, Schneider LC (1996) Clinical and virologic features of hepatitis C virus infection associated with intravenous immunoglobulin. Pediatrics 98: 211–215.
7. Stephenne X, Sokal EM (2002) Hepatitis C in children and adolescents: mode of acquisition, natural history and treatment. Acta Gastroenterol Belg 65: 95–98.
8. Tovo PA, Pembrey LJ, Newell ML (2000) Persistence rate and progression of vertically acquired hepatitis C infection. European Paediatric Hepatitis C Virus Infection. J Infect Dis 181: 419–424.
9. Jara P, Resti M, Hierro L, Giacchino R, Barbera C, et al. (2003) Chronic hepatitis C virus infection in childhood: clinical patterns and evolution in 224 white children. Clin Infect Dis 36: 275–280.
10. Iorio R, Giannattasio A, Sepe A, Terracciano LM, Vecchione R, et al. (2005) Chronic hepatitis C in childhood: an 18-year experience. Clin Infect Dis 41: 1431–1437.
11. Goodman ZD, Makhlouf HR, Liu L, Balistreri W, Gonzalez-Peralta RP, et al. (2008) Pathology of chronic hepatitis C in children: liver biopsy findings in the Peds-C Trial. Hepatology 47: 836–843.
12. Guido M, Bortolotti F, Leandro G, Jara P, Hierro L, et al. (2003) Fibrosis in chronic hepatitis C acquired in infancy: is it only a matter of time? Am J Gastroenterol 98: 660–663.
13. Barshes NR, Udell IW, Lee TC, O'Mahony CA, Karpen SJ, et al. (2006) The natural history of hepatitis C virus in pediatric liver transplant recipients. Liver Transpl 12: 1119–1123.
14. Jacobson KR, Murray K, Zellos A, Schwarz KB (2002) An analysis of published trials of interferon monotherapy in children with chronic hepatitis C. J Pediatr Gastroenterol Nutr 34: 52–58.
15. Fried MW, Shiffman ML, Reddy KR, Smith C, Marinos G, et al. (2002) Peginterferon alfa-2a plus ribavirin for chronic hepatitis C virus infection. N Engl J Med 347: 975–982.
16. Manns MP, McHutchison JG, Gordon SC, Rustgi VK, Shiffman M, et al. (2001) Peginterferon alfa-2b plus ribavirin compared with interferon alfa-2b plus ribavirin for initial treatment of chronic hepatitis C: a randomised trial. Lancet 358: 958–965.
17. Bortolotti F, Giacchino R, Vajro P, Barbera C, Crivellaro C, et al. (1995) Recombinant interferon-alfa therapy in children with chronic hepatitis C. Hepatology 22: 1623–1627.
18. Iorio R, Pensati P, Porzio S, Vegnente A (1995) Is alpha-interferon treatment useful in children with non-B, non-C chronic hepatitis? J Hepatol 23: 761–762.
19. Schwarz KB, Gonzalez-Peralta RP, Murray K, Molleston JP, Haber B, et al. (2008) Peginterferon with or without ribavirin for chronic hepatitis C in children and adolescents: final results of the PEDS-C trial. Hepatology 48: 418A.
20. Fried MW, Peter J, Hoots K, Gaglio PJ, Talbut D, et al. (2002) Hepatitis C in adults and adolescents with hemophilia: a randomized, controlled trial of interferon alfa-2b and ribavirin. Hepatology 36: 967–972.
21. Narkewicz M, Rosenthal P, Schwarz KB, Drack A, Margolis T, et al. Ophthalmologic complications in children with chronic hepatitis C treated with pegylated interferon; 2008; San Diego, CA.
22. Molleston JP, Schwarz KB, Barton BA, Gonzalez-Peralta RP, Narkewicz MR, et al. (2009) Autoantibodies and autoimmune disease during the Peds-C trial. J Pediatr Gastroenterol Nutr 49(suppl 1): E73.
23. Suoglu DO, Elkabes B, Sokucu S, Saner G (2002) Does interferon and ribavirin combination therapy increase the rate of treatment response in children with hepatitis C? J Pediatr Gastroenterol Nutr 34: 199–206.
24. Schwarz KB, Mohan P, Narkewicz MR, Molleston JP, Nash SR, et al. (2006) Safety, efficacy and pharmacokinetics of peginterferon alpha2a (40 kd) in children with chronic hepatitis C. J Pediatr Gastroenterol Nutr 43: 499–505.
25. McHutchison JG, Lawitz EJ, Shiffman ML, Muir AJ, Galler GW, et al. (2009) Peginterferon alfa-2b or alfa-2a with ribavirin for treatment of hepatitis C infection. N Engl J Med 361: 580–593.
26. Conjeevaram HS, Fried MW, Jeffers LJ, Terrault NA, Wiley-Lucas TE, et al. (2006) Peginterferon and ribavirin treatment in African American and Caucasian American patients with hepatitis C genotype 1. Gastroenterology 131: 470–477.
27. Hadziyannis SJ, Sette H, Jr., Morgan TR, Balan V, Diago M, et al. (2004) Peginterferon-alpha2a and ribavirin combination therapy in chronic hepatitis C:

a randomized study of treatment duration and ribavirin dose. Ann Intern Med 140: 346–355.

28. Sokal EM, Bourgois A, Stephenne X, Silveira T, Porta G, et al. Peginterferon alfa-2a plus ribavirin for chronic hepatitis C virus infection in children and adolescents. J Hepatol 52: 827–831.
29. Davis GL, Wong JB, McHutchison JG, Manns MP, Harvey J, et al. (2003) Early virologic response to treatment with peginterferon alfa-2b plus ribavirin in patients with chronic hepatitis C. Hepatology 38: 645–652.
30. Kwo P, Lawitz E, McCone J (2009, Abstract 4) HCV SPRINT-1 Final Results: SVR 24 from a Phase 2 Study of Boceprevir Plus PegIntron (Peginterferon Alfa-2b)/Ribavirin in Treatment-Naive Subjects with Genotype-1 Chronic Hepatitis C. Copenhagen, Denmark: EASL.
31. McHutchison JG, Everson GT, Gordon SC, Jacobson IM, Sulkowski M, et al. (2009) Telaprevir with peginterferon and ribavirin for chronic HCV genotype 1 infection. N Engl J Med 360: 1827–1838.
32. Katz JA, Mahoney DH, Steuber CP, Fernbach DJ (1988) Human leukocyte alpha interferon-induced transient neurotoxicity in children. Invest New Drugs 6: 115–120.
33. Mohan N, Gonzalez-Peralta RP, Fujisawa T, Chang MH, Heller S, et al. Chronic hepatitis C virus infection in children. J Pediatr Gastroenterol Nutr 50: 123–131.
34. Ge D, Fellay J, Thompson AJ, Simon JS, Shianna KV, et al. (2009) Genetic variation in IL28B predicts hepatitis C treatment-induced viral clearance. Nature 461: 399–401.
35. Clemente MG, Congia M, Lai ME, Lilliu F, Lampis R, et al. (1994) Effect of iron overload on the response to recombinant interferon-alfa treatment in transfusion-dependent patients with thalassemia major and chronic hepatitis C. J Pediatr 125: 123–128.
36. Czerwionka-Szaflarska M, Chrobot A, Szaflarska-Szczepanik A (2000) Studies of the effectiveness of interferon alpha treatment for chronic hepatitis C in children. Med Sci Monit 6: 964–970.
37. Fujisawa T, Inui A, Ohkawa T, Komatsu H, Miyakawa Y, et al. (1995) Response to interferon therapy in children with chronic hepatitis C. J Pediatr 127: 660–662.
38. Jonas MM, Ott MJ, Nelson SP, Badizadegan K, Perez-Atayde AR (1998) Interferon-alpha treatment of chronic hepatitis C virus infection in children. Pediatr Infect Dis J 17: 241–246.
39. Ko JS, Choe YH, Kim EJ, Lee EH, Jang JJ, et al. (2001) Interferon-alpha treatment of chronic hepatitis C in children with hemophilia. J Pediatr Gastroenterol Nutr 32: 41–44.
40. Komatsu H, Fujisawa T, Inui A, Miyakawa Y, Onoue M, et al. (1996) Efficacy of interferon in treating chronic hepatitis C in children with a history of acute leukemia. Blood 87: 4072–4075.
41. Majda-Stanislawska E, Szaflik I, Omulecka A (2000) Interferon alpha for eradication of HCV and remission of chronic hepatitis in children. Med Sci Monit 6: 1142–1147.
42. Matsuoka S, Mori K, Nakano O, Yuasa Y, Taguchi Y, et al. (1997) Efficacy of interferons in treating children with chronic hepatitis C. Eur J Pediatr 156: 704–708.
43. Mozer-Lisewska I, Sluzewski W, Ali Youseif K, Figlerowicz M, Kowala-Piaskowska A (2003) Virus genotype 1b and long-term response to interferon alpha monotherapy in children with chronic hepatitis C. Eur J Pediatr 162: 755–759.
44. Nakashima E, Fujisawa T, Kimura A, Kage M, Yamato Y, et al. (2003) Efficacy of interferon-alpha treatment in Japanese children with chronic hepatitis C. J Gastroenterol Hepatol 18: 411–414.
45. Pensati P, Iorio R, Botta S, Tuccillo C, Donetto S, et al. (1999) Low virological response to interferon in children with chronic hepatitis C. J Hepatol 31: 604–611.
46. Ruiz-Moreno M, Rua MJ, Castillo I, Garcia-Novo MD, Santos M, et al. (1992) Treatment of children with chronic hepatitis C with recombinant interferon-alpha: a pilot study. Hepatology 16: 882–885.
47. Sawada A, Tajiri H, Kozaiwa K, Guo W, Tada K, et al. (1998) Favorable response to lymphoblastoid interferon-alpha in children with chronic hepatitis C. J Hepatol 28: 184–188.
48. Spiliopoulou I, Repanti M, Katinakis S, Karana-Ginopoulou A, Papanastasiou DA (1999) Response to interferon alfa-2b therapy in muti-transfused children with beta-thalassemia and chronic hepatitis C. Eur J Clin Microbiol Infect Dis 18: 709–715.
49. Zwiener RJ, Fielman BA, Cochran C, Rogers BB, Dawson DB, et al. (1996) Interferon-alpha-2b treatment of chronic hepatitis C in children with hemophilia. Pediatr Infect Dis J 15: 906–908.
50. Christensson B, Wiebe T, Akesson A, Widell A (2000) Interferon-alpha and ribavirin treatment of hepatitis C in children with malignancy in remission. Clin Infect Dis 30: 585–586.
51. Figlerowicz M, Sluzewski W, Kowala-Piaskowska A, Mozer-Lisewska I (2004) Interferon alpha and ribavirin in the treatment of children with chronic hepatitis C. Eur J Pediatr 163: 265–267.
52. Gonzalez-Peralta RP, Kelly DA, Haber B, Molleston J, Murray KF, et al. (2005) Interferon alfa-2b in combination with ribavirin for the treatment of chronic hepatitis C in children: efficacy, safety, and pharmacokinetics. Hepatology 42: 1010–1018.
53. Puetz J, Thrower M, Kane R, Bouhasin J (2004) Combination therapy with ribavirin and interferon in a cohort of children with hepatitis C and haemophilia followed at a pediatric haemophilia treatment center. Haemophilia 10: 87–93.
54. Wirth S, Lang T, Gehring S, Gerner P (2002) Recombinant alfa-interferon plus ribavirin therapy in children and adolescents with chronic hepatitis C. Hepatology 36: 1280–1284.
55. Baker RD, Dee D, Baker SS (2007) Response to pegylated interferon alpha-2b and ribavirin in children with chronic hepatitis C. J Clin Gastroenterol 41: 111–114.
56. Jara P, Hierro L, de la Vega A, Diaz C, Camarena C, et al. (2008) Efficacy and safety of peginterferon-alpha2b and ribavirin combination therapy in children with chronic hepatitis C infection. Pediatr Infect Dis J 27: 142–148.
57. Wirth S, Pieper-Boustani H, Lang T, Ballauff A, Kullmer U, et al. (2005) Peginterferon alfa-2b plus ribavirin treatment in children and adolescents with chronic hepatitis C. Hepatology 41: 1013–1018.
58. Hasan F, Alsarraf K, Qabandi W (2006) Pegylated interferon alfa-2b plus ribavirin for the treatment of chronic hepatitis C genotype 4 in adolescents: a pilot study. Gastroenterology 130: A840.
59. (2009) Assessment of the Safety, Efficacy, Tolerability and Pharmacokinetics of PEG-Intron® Plus REBETOL® in Pediatric Patients With Chronic Hepatitis C.
60. Pawlowska M, Halota W (2009) Pegylated interferon alpha-2a and ribavirin in the treatment of children with chronic hepatitis C. Chicago, Illinois: American Gastroenterology Association Digestive Diseases Week. Abstract 1790.
61. Moy LC, Levine JJ (2009) Chronic hepatitis C in children: response to treatment. Chicago, Illinois: American Gastroenterology Association Digestive Diseases Week. Abstract T1131.
62. Zhang H (2009) Preliminary observational study on efficacy and tolerability of Peg-IFN in 151 pediatric and adolescent chronic hepatitis C patients. Boston, MA: Annual General Meeting of the American Association for the Study of Liver Diseases. Abstract 969.

12

Spread of Epidemic MRSA-ST5-IV Clone Encoding PVL as a Major Cause of Community Onset Staphylococcal Infections in Argentinean Children

Claudia Sola[1], Hugo Paganini[2†], Ana L. Egea[1], Alejandro J. Moyano[1], Analia Garnero[3], Ines Kevric[1], Catalina Culasso[3] , Ana Vindel[4], Study Group of CA-MRSA in Children, Argentina-2007 , Horacio Lopardo[2], José L. Bocco[1]*

1 Centro de Investigaciones en Bioquímica Clínica e Inmunología (CIBICI-CONICET), Departamento de Bioquímica Clínica; Facultad de Ciencias Químicas, Universidad Nacional de Córdoba, Córdoba, Argentina, **2** Hospital de Pediatría "Prof. Dr.Juan P. Garrahan", Autonomous city of Buenos Aires (ACBA), Argentina, **3** Hospital de Niños de la Santísima Trinidad de Córdoba, Córdoba, Argentina, **4** Laboratorio de Infecciones Nosocomiales, Instituto de Salud Carlos III, Centro Nacional de Microbiología, Majadahonda, Madrid, Spain

Abstract

Background: Community-associated methicillin-resistant *Staphylococcus aureus*-(CA-MRSA) strains have emerged in Argentina. We investigated the clinical and molecular evolution of community-onset MRSA infections (CO-MRSA) in children of Córdoba, Argentina, 2005–2008. Additionally, data from 2007 were compared with the epidemiology of these infections in other regions of the country.

Methodology/Principal Findings: Two datasets were used: *i)* lab-based prospective surveillance of CA-MRSA isolates from 3 Córdoba pediatric hospitals-(CBAH1-H3) in 2007–2008 (compared to previously published data of 2005) and *ii)* a sampling of CO-MRSA from a study involving both, healthcare-associated community-onset-(HACO) infections in children with risk-factors for healthcare-associated infections-(HRFs), and CA-MRSA infections in patients without HRFs detected in multiple centers of Argentina in 2007. Molecular typing was performed on the CA-MRSA-(n: 99) isolates from the CBAH1-H3-dataset and on the HACO-MRSA-(n: 51) and CA-MRSA-(n: 213) isolates from other regions. Between 2005–2008, the annual proportion of CA-MRSA/CA-*S. aureus* in Córdoba hospitals increased from 25% to 49%, $P<0.01$. Total CA-MRSA infections increased 3.6 fold-(5.1 to 18.6 cases/100,000 annual-visits, $P<0.0001$), associated with an important increase of invasive CA-MRSA infections-(8.5 fold). In all regions analyzed, a single genotype prevailed in both CA-MRSA (82%) and HACO-MRSA(57%), which showed pulsed-field-gel electrophoresis-(PFGE)-type-"I", sequence-type-5-(ST5), SCC*mec*-type-IVa, *spa*-t311, and was positive for PVL. The second clone, pulsotype-N/ST30/CC30/SCC*mec*IVc/t019/PVL$^+$, accounted for 11.5% of total CA-MRSA infections. Importantly, the first 4 isolates of Argentina belonging to South American-USA300 clone-(USA300/ST8/CC8/SCC*mec*IVc/t008/PVL$^+$/ACME$^-$) were detected. We also demonstrated that a HA-MRSA clone-(pulsotype-C/ST100/CC5) caused 2% and 10% of CA-MRSA and HACO-MRSA infections respectively and was associated with a SCC*mec* type closely related to SCC*mec*IV(2B&5).

Conclusions/Significance: The dissemination of epidemic MRSA clone, ST5-IV-PVL$^+$ was the main cause of increasing staphylococcal community-onset infections in Argentinean children (2003–2008), conversely to other countries. The predominance of this clone, which has capacity to express the h-VISA phenotype, in healthcare-associated community-onset cases suggests that it has infiltrated into hospital-settings.

Editor: Laurence Van Melderen, Universite Libre de Bruxelles, Belgium

Funding: This work was supported by the National Council for Scientific Research and Technology of Argentina (CONICET-PIP-2009-2011 to CS), Agencia Nacional de Promoción Científica y Tecnológica (ANPCyT – PICT 07-01630 to JLB) and Secretaría de Ciencia y Técnica–Universidad Nacional de Córdoba (SECyT-UNC). The funders had no role in study design, data collection and analysis, decision to publish, or preparation of the manuscript.

Competing Interests: The authors and the Members of the Study Group of CA-MRSA in Children, Argentina-2007, have declared that no competing interests exist.

* E-mail: jbocco@fcq.unc.edu.ar

† Deceased.

¶ Membership of the Study Group of CA-MRSA in Children, Argentina-2007 is provided in the Acknowledgments.

Introduction

Methicillin resistant *Staphylococcus aureus* (MRSA) infection has traditionally been associated with healthcare settings (HA-MRSA) until its emergence in the community during late 1990's. This global phenomenon was caused by strains of community-associated methicillin-resistant *Staphylococcus aureus* (CA-MRSA) that emerged from some major genetic lineages, commonly designated by their multilocus sequence type (MLST) or by their pulsed field gel electrophoresis (PFGE) pattern (ST1, ST8-USA300, ST30, ST59, ST93 and ST80),with a specific geographical pattern. These strains are frequently non-multiresistant to antibiotics; most of them harbor the staphylococcal cassette chromosome *mec* (SCC*mec*) type IV(2B) or V(5C2) and the

Panton-Valentine leukocidin (PVL) genes [1–3]. Purulent skin and soft tissue infections are the most common clinical manifestations of CA-MRSA, although increasing reports of serious infections in children with high mortality rates have raised concern during recent years [4,5]. Vancomycin has been the mainstay of treatment for this type of infections and the emergence of resistance is worrying [6,7]. Importantly, CA-MRSA strains have entered the healthcare settings; hence, in some countries, strains of both, CA-MRSA and HA-MRSA circulate in hospitals and communities, causing infections of healthcare or community onset (HO and CO, respectively) [8–10].

In Latin America, three PVL-positive epidemic CA-MRSA clones have been described: *i)* MRSA ST30-IV clone [11], *ii)* MRSA ST5-IV clone [12,13] and *iii)* MRSA ST8-IV clone [14]. The first two were detected in southern areas of South America and the third one in the North.

Epidemiological surveillance for MRSA in Córdoba, Argentina, revealed the emergence of ST5-IV-PVL$^+$ genotype as the most prevalent (89%) CA-MRSA clone in 2005. This clone had displaced in the community setting an "escaped" HA-MRSA clone, which was non-multiresistant to antibiotics, lacked the *pvl* genes and was characterized as ST100 associated with a SCC*mec* related to IVc [12,15]. Prospective surveillance of community onset *S. aureus* infections in children from Argentina during 2007, detected a prevalence of 62% (281/447 CA-*S. aureus*) of CA-MRSA infections; 38% of which were invasive infections [16].

A paucity of data about molecular epidemiology of CA-MRSA infections from South America is a current problem and therefore, it is difficult to follow evolving trends [17–19].

Herein, we report the molecular evolution and antimicrobial resistance profiles of MRSA strains in the community along with the clinical characteristics of these infections in children of Córdoba-Argentina between 2003 and 2008.

We also compared the clinical and molecular epidemiology of CO-MRSA infections in children with risk factors for healthcare-associated infections (HRFs), (healthcare-associated, community-onset infections [HACO]), and in patients without HRFs (CA-MRSA infections), from multiple centers of central, eastern and northern regions of Argentina during 2007.

Materials and Methods

Ethics statement

This study was reviewed and approved by the institutional Ethical Review Board of each Hospital: Hospital de Pediatría Prof. Dr. Juan P. Garrahan; Hospital General de Niños Dr. Pedro de Elizalde; Hospital de Niños Dr. O. Alassia, Santa Fe; Hospital de Niños de San Justo; Hospital Juan Pablo II, Corrientes; Hospital de Niños J. Vilela, Santa Fe; Hospital Pediátrico Dr. A.L. Castelán, Chaco; Hospital Materno Infantil de Mar del Plata Don Victorio Tetamanti, Hospital de Niños de la Santísima Trinidad de Córdoba, Hospital Infantil Municipal de Córdoba; Hospital Pediátrico del Niño Jesús de Córdoba. Written informed consent was obtained from each child's parents for review of the medical information and characterizations of the responsible isolates. However, for the aims of this study, data were processed anonymously. Additionally, the authors declare that all clinical investigation has been conducted according to the principles expressed in the Declaration of Helsinki.

Study design and case definitions

Longitudinal study, Córdoba, 2003–2008. To analyze the molecular evolution and clinical characteristics of CA-MRSA infections in children (≤18 years of age) in Córdoba, all consecutive single patient isolates (n: 99) identified as CA-MRSA according to CDC criteria (see definitions) by a laboratory-based surveillance program of *S. aureus* infections during 2007–2008 from three children's hospitals (CBAH1, CBAH2 and CBAH3) were prospectively included.

These molecular data were compared with those obtained in 2005 [12]. In that year, all *S. aureus* infections were identified by the Clinical Microbiology Laboratory of each hospital (CBAH1, CBAH2 and CBAH3) and the medical records were reviewed for epidemiologic classification (see definitions).

Additionally, 22 CA-MRSA isolates prospectively collected in CBAH1 between 2003 and 2006 following the CDC criteria (see definition) were analysed as well, along with those detected for this study (2007–2008).

Transversal study, Argentina, 2007. To examine the clinical and molecular epidemiology of CA-MRSA and HACO-MRSA infections among children from central, northern and eastern regions of Argentina in 2007, random samples representative of each hospital participating in the prospective surveillance of community onset *S. aureus* infections in children from Argentina (CSACHARG) were analyzed. The clinical features, frequency and outcome of CA-MRSA infections identified in that study have already been published [16]. Briefly, a total of 840 *S. aureus* infections were diagnosed during 2007, 582 of them were of community onset; among them, 135 children with HRFs were excluded from that study (75 infected with HACO-MRSA and 60 with HACO-MSSA). Of the remaining 447 isolates, 281 (62%) were CA-MRSA and 160 CA-MSSA. The following sample was selected for this study: CA-MRSA isolates: 213 of 281 (Buenos Aires city: 101, Buenos Aires province: 11, Corrientes: 22, Chaco: 19 and Santa Fe: 60). HACO-MRSA isolates: 51 of 75 (Buenos Aires city: 25, Buenos Aires province: 5, Corrientes: 5, Chaco: 5 and Santa Fe: 11).

For each case of *S. aureus* isolated from community onset infections from both collections (CBAH1-H3 and CSACHARG), the relevant medical information was examined, including diagnosis, site and clinical details of infection, treatment information, demographic data (age, gender), underlying illnesses (chronic conditions) [8,20] and the presence of the following risk factors for healthcare-associated infections: existence of an invasive device (e.g., vascular catheter, G-tube); any history of MRSA infection or colonization, surgery, hospitalization, dialysis, or residence in a long-term care facility within the 12 months prior to the culture [21–23].

Definitions

Community-associated methicillin resistant *S. aureus* (CA-MRSA) infections were defined as cases from patients without HRFs during the previous year, who acquired the infection outside hospital settings or within 48 h of admission, according to the CDC criteria [22].

Healthcare-associated infections (HA-MRSA) were defined using previously published definitions [21,22], which include: i) the classical nosocomial or hospital-onset infection (HO-MRSA), defined as a those occurring >48 h after hospital admission, not present on admission (no cases of this type were analyzed in this study) and ii) Healthcare-associated community-onset (HACO-MRSA) infections: those occurring in patients with HRFs, having a positive culture within ≤48 h after hospital admission. Hence, Community-onset methicillin resistant *S. aureus* (CO-MRSA) infections include both the CA-MRSA and HACO-MRSA infections.

Invasive infections were defined by one or more of the following conditions: bacteremia, endocarditis, pneumonia, pleural abscess, lymphadenitis, septic arthritis, osteomyelitis, necrotizing fasciitis, pyomyositis or another illness in which *S. aureus* was isolated from normally sterile body fluids [20,21]. Sepsis was defined on the basis of the systemic inflammatory response syndrome criteria [24]. Skin diseases (skin and soft tissue, SSTI) were defined as a primary skin infection such as an abscess, cellulitis, folliculitis or a skin infection spreading to contiguous tissues.

Surgical site infections (SSI) were not considered as skin diseases.

Bacterial isolates and antimicrobial susceptibility

Staphylococcus aureus were identified by standard microbiologic procedures. Antimicrobial susceptibility testing was performed by disk diffusion method [25]. A disc approximation test (D test) was used to detect inducible clindamycin resistance [25]. Screening for reduced susceptibility to vancomycin (VISA and h-VISA) was performed on all CO-MRSA isolates. Vancomycin and teicoplanin minimum inhibitory concentrations (MICs) were determined by agar dilution method [25]. In addition, all MRSA isolates with a MIC of 1 or 2 µg/ml were further screened by 2 additional agar methods: MHA5T-Mueller-Hinton-agar and BHI4V-brain-heart-infusion-agar (5 µg/ml teicoplanin and 4 µg/ml vancomycin, respectively) [6,26,27]. MRSA isolates that were positive in at least one screening test were additionally tested by both, the Etest Macromethod (MET) and Etest glycopeptide-resistance detection strip-GRD E-test strips, (bioMérieux-CD) [6,28]. The strains h-VISA-Mu3 and VISA-Mu50 and the vancomycin-susceptible *S. aureus* strain ATCC 29213 were tested for all methods in parallel as positive and negative controls, respectively.

Molecular typing and detection of genes associated with virulence

In all CO-MRSA isolates, the PFGE of *Sma*I digests of chromosomal DNA were performed and interpreted as previously described [12]. *SmaI* restriction patterns (PFGE) were digitized, presented schematically and analyzed to calculate the Dice coefficient of correlation and to generate a dendrogram by the unweighted-pair group method using average linkage clusterings. Isolates differing by up to six fragments were considered to be subtypes of a given clonal type, and the similarity cut-off was 80%.

All CO-MRSA isolates were screened by PCR for accessory gene regulator (*agr*) type and for 22 specific staphylococcal virulence genes, as described elsewhere [12 and reference therein], comprising sequences specific for enterotoxins: *sea, seb, sec, sed, see, seg, seh, sei, sej, sen, seo, sem* and *sek*; toxic shock syndrome toxin 1(TSST-1): *tst*; exfoliative toxins: *eta* and *etb*; PVL genes: *lukS*-PV-*lukF*-PV; leukocidin: *lukE-lukD* and the class F leukocidin: *lukM*; bacteriocine (*bsa*), adhesins: for collagen (*cna*) and for bone sialoprotein-binding protein (*bbp*). Detection of *arcA* gene, an indicator of the arginine catabolic mobile element (ACME), was analyzed with primers designed in this study, based on the previously determined sequence of strain USA300_FPR3757 (accession NC_007793). The primer sequences are as follows: *arc*A-F 5′-TCT ATT ACT GAG CCA GAA GTA CG-3′and *arc*A-R 5′-CAC GTA ACT TGC TAG AAC GAG TA-3′, whose product has 733 bp expected size. USA300-0114 was used as reference strain for the USA300 clone.

Representative isolates of the most prevalent subtype (defined by PFGE) from all CO-MRSA strains were also characterized by multilocus sequence typing and *spa* typing [29,30].

SCC*mec* typing

The SCC*mec* types (I–VI) were evaluated for all CO-MRSA isolates by multiplex PCR [31] and by allotyping by conventional PCR [32]. SCC*mec* type IV was further sub-typed using published primers [33]. Furthermore, the assignment to the class B *mec* complex was confirmed by PCR with primers specific for ψIS*1272* and *mec*R1 [34]and in order to differentiate the types of SCC*mec* IV and VI, the *ccrAB* typing was completed by PCR detection with primers specific for *ccrAB* allotype 4 [34].

To investigate the presence of SCC*mec* IV(2B&5) [35], all isolates belonging to pulsotype C/ST100 associated with a new variant of SCC*mec* IV (IVNv), which was positive by PCR for J1 specific region of the SCC*mec* subtype IVc and *ccrAB*2 but negative for B *mec* complex [15], were further characterized for the *mecA* downstream vicinity with primers designed based on the sequence previously determined of strain ZH47-(ST100), accession AM292304, (File S1).

The primer sequences are as follows (location relative to the ZH47 sequence given in parentheses): **i)** Tn*4001*-1-F, 5′-GCC AAT CGC TTA ATT GGA GCC G-3′ (18.146 to 18.167) and Tn*4001*-1-R, 5′-ACT TCA TCT TCC CAA GGC TCT GT-3′ (18.854 to 18.832); amplifying the region IS1256L-*aac*(2′)—*aph*(6″) within the Tn*4001*. **ii)** Tn*4001*-2-F, 5′-TGG CCA TCA CGT GTT CTG GG-3′ (21.164 to 21.183) and Tn*4001*-2-R, 5′-TCG GAT GTC TGT CCG AGG ACT-3′ (22.131 to 22.111); amplifying the region between the IS256R (Tn*4001*) and IS1272 from *mec* complex B and **iii)** Tn*4001*-3-F, 5′-ACC AAA CCC GAC AAC TAC AAC TAT-3′ (15.976 to 15.999) and Tn*4001*-3-R, 5′-GTG TCG TAA AGC TGC GCT CA-3′ (17.273 to 17.2554); amplifying the region between the *mec*A locus and IS256L (Tn*4001*). The amplicons with the expected size were end sequenced and compared to the SCC*mec* IV(2B&5) sequence, in the ZH47 strain-(ST100) [35]. All primers used for SCC*mec* IVNv characterization are shown in detail in (File S1).

Statistical analysis

Bacteriologic and patient data were compiled in an electronic database using Access (Microsoft). Data were analyzed with Epi Info version 6.0.4 software (Centers for Disease Control and Prevention, Atlanta, GA). Comparisons between groups were performed with chi-square test or Fisher's exact test, as appropriate. $P<0.05$ was considered statistically significant.

Results

Temporal trends in CA-MRSA infections

During 2007–2008, CA-MRSA accounted for 45% (99 CA-MRSA/221 CA-*S. aureus*) of community-associated *S. aureus* infections in pediatric patients cared for in three children's hospitals of Córdoba, [38% (36/94) in 2007 and 49% (63/127) in 2008]. Hence, these data indicate a significant increase of the annual prevalence of CA-MRSA infections since 2005 [33% (7/21) for a three-month period [12] and 25% (18/71) annually, $P<0.01$ for trend]. Additionally, the overall rate of CA-MRSA infections increased significantly (3.6 fold) accounting for 5.1 to 18.6 cases/100,000 annual visits in 2005 and 2008, respectively, $P<0.0001$ (Figure 1). In contrast, the incidence of CA-MSSA infections only increased 1.1 fold, from 16.2 cases in 2005 to 19.1 cases/100,000 annual visits in 2008. The number of children with invasive CA-MRSA infections in three Córdoba children's hospitals increased significantly from 1.3 in 2005 to 11.1 cases/10,000 admissions in 2008, $P<0.001$.

Similar trends were observed yearly in one of these hospitals (CBAH1) upon analysis of the incidence (CA-MSSA, total CA-MRSA and invasive CA-MRSA infections, Figure 1) from 2003 to 2008.

The characteristics, origin and incidence of CA-MRSA during 2007 in all hospitals are shown in Table 1. Importantly, the rates

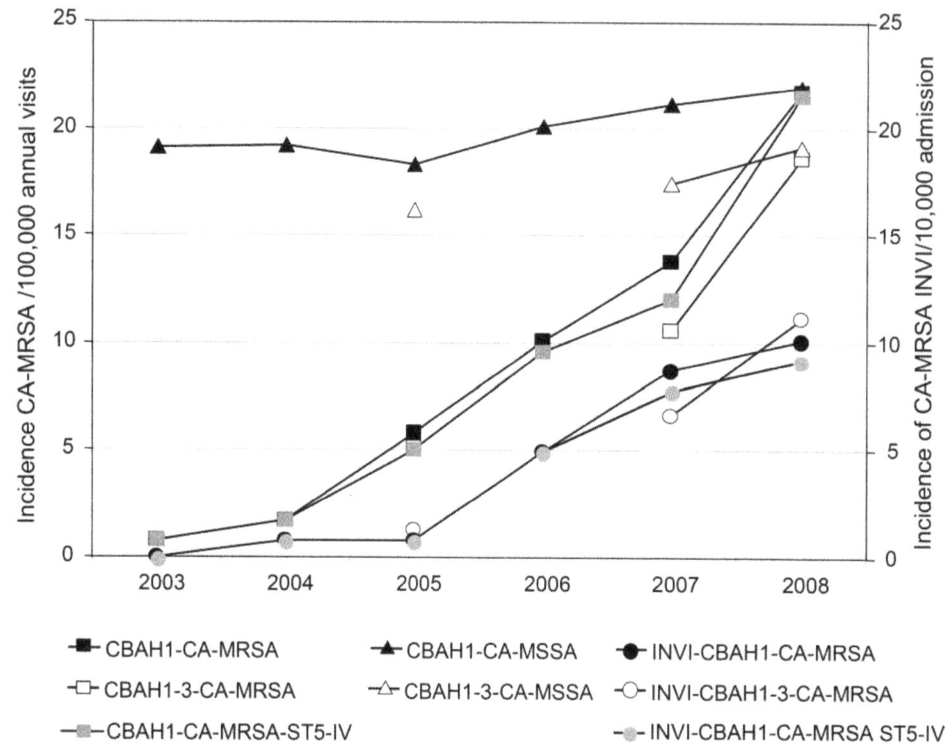

Figure 1. Evolution of community-associated *Staphylococcus aureus* infections from children in Cordoba-Argentina, 2003–2008. Evolution of the rates of all community-associated *Staphylococcus aureus* infections: *i)* methicillin-resistant *S. aureus* (CA-MRSA) infections [total (squares) and invasive-INVI (circles)], and *ii)* total methicillin-susceptible *S. aureus* (CA-MSSA) infections (triangles) in Córdoba children's hospitals, [H1 (CBAH1): 2003–2008: filled figures, and in H1, H2 and H3 (CBAH1-3): 2005 vs 2007–2008: empty figures] *iii)* methicillin-resistant community-associated *Staphylococcus aureus* infections caused by the ST5-IV-PVL$^+$clone [total (gray squares) and invasive (INVI) (gray circles)] in H1 (CBAH1): 2003–2008.

of CA-MRSA infections were highly variable among children from central, eastern and northern regions of Argentina, reaching an overall rate of 14.2 cases/100,000 annual visits (range 6.9–27) in 2007 (Table 1).

Community onset MRSA infections: Demographic and clinical data

The distribution of CA-MRSA infections (Córdoba, 2007–2008 and CSACHARG, 2007) and HACO-MRSA infections (CSA-CHARG, 2007) regarding patient's clinical features, age and sex are shown in Table 2. Although children from Córdoba with CA-MRSA infections were significantly older than children from CSACHARG, both groups were comparable in sex, type and severity of the infections (Table 2).

Similar types of invasive CA-MRSA infections (n: 7) were detected in CBAH1 during 2003–2006: osteomyelitis (n: 2), arthritis (n: 1), pneumonia (n: 1), bacteremia (n: 1), lymphadenitis (n: 1) and necrotizing fasciitis (n: 1).

Among selected children with HACO-MRSA infections (n: 51), multiple risk factors (≥2) were found in 35 (68%). The most common HRFs were: presence of indwelling catheters or percutaneous medical devices (85%) and hospitalization within the previous year (73%). In addition, 70% of the patients had chronic diseases, including immunodeficiencies (human immuno-deficiency virus-HIV/acquired immunodeficiency syndrome-AIDS and malignancies), cardiovascular diseases, chronic pulmonary diseases, chronic renal insufficiency, diabetes, or chronic skin illnesses. These children were more likely to develop invasive infections (65% vs 33%) and presentation with sepsis (27% vs 13%) than children with CA-MRSA infections. Invasive HACO-MRSA cases included mainly lungs and bloodstream infections. In addition, they had significantly lower frequency of SSTI infections (12% vs 67%).

Moreover, 23% of HACO-MRSA isolates were obtained from surgical site infections (Table 2).

The isolates from invasive CA-MRSA infections from CBAH1-H3 and CSACHARG groups (total n: 104) were obtained from blood (74%), other normally sterile body sites including joints (8%), bone (8%), pleural fluid (6%), other body fluids (2%) and other sites (1% each).

Antimicrobial susceptibility profile of community-onset MRSA strains

From all CA-MRSA isolates (n: 312) recovered from the CBAH1-3 and CSACHARG groups during 2007–2008, 20% were resistant to at least one non-β-lactam antibiotic. Resistance to erythromycin (ERY-15%), clindamycin (CLI-14%, 93% of inducible resistance); gentamicin (GEN-8%), rifampin (RIF-2%) and chloramphenicol (CHL-1%) were detected. The HACO-MRSA isolates showed significantly (P>0.001) higher rates of resistance to ERY (45%), CLIN (42%, 23% inducible); GEN (43%) and RIF (14%) than the CA-MRSA isolates. In addition, resistance to ciprofloxacin (22%) and to trimethoprim-sulfameth-oxazole (6%) were only detected among HACO-MRSA isolates. All isolates were susceptible to vancomycin by agar dilution method (MIC90, 1 μg/mL; MIC range, 0.25–2 μg/mL) and teicoplanin (MIC90, 2 μg/mL; MIC range, 0.25–4 μg/mL). From the total 363 CO-MRSA isolates evaluated, only 3 MRSA from children with HRFs (HACO-MRSA infections), were found to be h-VISA.

Table 1. Characteristics, incidence of CA-MRSA infections and location of children's hospitals of northern, eastern and central of Argentina, 2007.

Children's Hospitals	Province	Number of beds	Annual admission	Annual visits[b]	Number of CA-MRSA[a] 2007	Incidence[c]
H1	Córdoba	230	10,375	119,365	16	13.4
H2	Córdoba	75	3,083	123,000	10	8.1
H3	Córdoba	70	1,775	107,000	10	9.3
H4	Santa Fe	96	8,000	220,000	29	13.2
H5	Buenos Aires	274	6,756	202,000	14	6.9
H6	Buenos Aires city surrounding areas	142	7,539	264,938	33	12.5
H7	Santa Fe	178	13,169	175,683	48	27.3
H8	Autonomous city of Buenos Aires	485	18,427	296,452	53	17.9
H9	Autonomous city of Buenos Aires	228	8,917	252,083	42	16.7
H10	Corrientes	152	8,707	181,671	28	15.4
H11	Chaco	78	3,273	214,091	24	11.2

[a]Number of all CA-MRSA isolates detected in the three Cordoba children's hospitals during 2007 and those recovered in each hospital from the surveillance study for community onset *S. aureus* infections in children from Argentina-(CSACHARG) [16].
[b]annual visits: include outpatient facility and emergency service.
[c]Incidence: Number of cases/100,000 annual visits.

Molecular characterization of community-onset MRSA strains: CA-MRSA and HACO-MRSA

The molecular characteristics [sequence type (ST, as defined by MLST), clonal complex (CC), *agr* allotype, PFGE, SCC*mec* and *spaA* types, presence of *pvl* genes and virulence genes profile, along with the drug resistance pattern of the most predominant pulsotypes are shown in Table 3. The distribution of the most predominant genotypes of CO-MRSA isolates involved in invasive and non invasive infections according to the epidemiologic case classification (CA-MRSA and HACO-MRSA) are shown in Table 4. The molecular characterization of the three h-VISA strains demonstrated that they belonged to three different MRSA clones (Table 3).

CA-MRSA clone ST5-IV. PFGE performed on 363 isolates (312 CA-MRSA and 51 HACO-MRSA) revealed a predominant major pulsotype, ("I"; 79%, 285/363 isolates) with a more frequent subtype, I-1 (71%, 202/285). All isolates belonging to the pulsotype "I" were characterized as *agr* 2, ST5, except two isolates belonging to a new single locus variant (SLV) of ST5: ST1524, CC5 (Clonal Complex), *spa*-t311 (91% of isolates) and related (t002, t045; t067; t1094). Most of them were associated with SCC*mec* type IV(2B), 96% with subtype IVa:, 2% with subtype IVc and one isolate was nominated as SCC*mec* type IV non typable (IVNT), since it was positive by PCR for *ccrB2* and *mec* gene complex class B, but negative for J1 regions: a, b, c, d, g and h (Table 3). Two isolates (I18 subtype) were positive only for *ccrC* locus and negative for J1 region of SCC*mec* V and for other SCC*mec* regions analyzed [31] so they were tentatively designated as SCC*mec* related to V (Vr) (Table 3).

The *pvl* genes were not detected in 9% of the "I" pulsotype isolates (26/285) (Table 3 and Figure 2A). There was considerable diversity among the PFGE patterns of these isolates, demonstrating an ongoing evolution: 13 subtypes from 26 PVL$^-$ isolates vs 15 subtypes from 259 PVL$^+$ isolates. Unlike PVL$^+$ isolates, within the PVL$^-$ group, *spa*-t002 (85%) was much more prevalent than *spa*-t311 (4%); and did not have the *sea* gene.

Additionally, all isolates belonging to pulsotype "I" recovered in CBAH1 during 2003–2006 (n: 20) were characterized as ST5, *spa*-t311, associated with SCC*mec*IVa as well as they harbour *pvl* and *sea* genes.

This clone represented 79% of all community-onset MRSA isolates (285/363) in both groups of infections, CA-MRSA (82%, 256/312) and HACO-MRSA (57%, 29/51) (Figure 2 and Table 4). Moreover, this pulsotype predominated among CA-MRSA isolated in CBAH1 during 2003–2006 (91%, 20/22). Longitudinal analysis of CA-MRSA infections at this hospital demonstrated that the significant increase of the incidence of both total CA-MRSA infections and invasive CA-MRSA infections were due to the dissemination of this single pulsotype "I" (ST5-SCC*mec*IV-PVL$^+$) increasing from 1 to 25 cases of CA-MRSA infections between 2003 and 2008 (Figure 1).

On the other hand, both groups, PVL$^+$ and PVL$^-$ variants, produced invasive infections in similar proportions (35%, 90 invasive infections/259 PVL$^+$ MRSA infections vs 35%, 9 invasive infections of 26 pulsotype "I"-PVL$^-$ MRSA infections; $P = 0.96$). Moreover, both groups were comparable regarding sepsis presentation (13%, 33/259 PVL$^+$ vs 12%, 3/26 PVL$^-$; $P = 0.8$).

Southwest Pacific (SWP) clone. The second prevalent clone among total community-onset MRSA isolates (11%, 39/363) was the N pulsotype or Southwest Pacific (SWP) clone. It was characterized as *agr* 3, ST30 (4 isolates as ST196/SLV) belonging to CC30, *spa*-t019 and related t021, t6653 (new *spa* type described for the first time in this study) and *spa*-t975. Most isolates harbored SCC*mec*IVc, (97%) and all of them carried the *pvl* genes. This genetic background accounted for 11.5% (36/312) and 6% (3/51) of CA-MRSA and HACO-MRSA isolates respectively (Table 4). The molecular characteristics of this clone and its distribution in different regions of Argentina during 2007 are shown in Table 4 and Figure 2. In addition, this clone was significantly more frequent in Buenos Aires city and surrounding areas (21%) than in other regions of Argentina (average 8%, range = 7−9, $P = 0.009$, Figure 2B).

Table 2. Demographic and clinical characteristics of children with Community-onset methicillin resistant *S. aureus* infections in central, northern and eastern regions of Argentina.

Characteristics	CA-MRSA CBAH1-H3[a]	CA-MRSA CSACHARG[b]	P[c]	CA-MRSA Total CBAH1-H3[a] and CSACHARG[b]	HACO-MRSA CSACHARG[b]	P[c]
Period	2007–2008	2007			2007	
n(%), [n]	n: 99(%), [n]: 5	n: 213(%), [n]: 25		n: 312(%), [n]: 30	n: 51(%), [n]: 4	
Age, median of years (range)	6.1 (0.24–18)	3.4 (0.08–16)		4.1 (0.08–18)	3.2 (0.08–18)	
Sex (males)[d]	61(61)	128(60)	0.93	189(60)	30(59)	0.88
Type and Severity of Infection[d]						
Skin and soft-tissue (SSTI)						
Abscess and cellulites[e]	72(73)	136(64)	0.11	209(67)	6(12)	<0.001
Necrotizing Fasciitis	1(1)	-		1(0.5)	-	
Surgical Site (SSI)	-	-		-	12(23)	
Musculoskeletal	16(16), [2]	32(15), [11]	0.26	48(15), [13]	6(12), [2]	0.5
Osteomyelitis	11(11), [2]	17(8), [10]		28(9), [12]	5(10), [1]	
Septic arthritis	5(5)	13(6)		18(5.5)	-	
Pyomyositis	-	2(1), [1]		2(0.5), [1]	1(2), [1]	
Respiratory	5(5), [1]	23(11), [7]	0.09	28(9), [8]	9(17), [1]	0.06
Pneumonia	5(5), [1]	11(5), [2]		16(5), [3]	6(12), [1]	
Pleural abscess	-	12(6), [5]		12(4), [5]	3(6)	
Bacteremia	2(2)	15(7)	0.06	17(5.5)	12(23)	<0.001
Endocarditis	1(1), [1]	1(0.5), [5]		2(0.5), [6]	[1]	
Pericarditis	-	1(0.5)		1(0.5)	-	
Deep abscess[f]	[1]	4 (1.5), [1]		4(1), [2]	2(4)	
Lymphadenitis	2(2)	1(0.5)		3(1)	1(2)	
Meningitis	-	[1]		[1]	3(6)	
Invasive Infection[d]	27(27)	77(36)	0.12	104(33)	33(65)	<0.001
Sepsis[d]	11(11)	29(13)	0.38	40(13)	14(27)	0.008

CA-MRSA: Community-associated methicillin resistant *Staphylococcus aureus*, HACO-MRSA: Healthcare-associated community-onset methicillin resistant *Staphylococcus aureus* infections.
[a]CBAH1-H3: Prospective surveillance of CO-*S. aureus* infections in children from three children's hospitals of Córdoba (CBAH1, CBAH2 and CBAH3), 2007 and 2008.
[b]CSACHARG: Prospective surveillance of CO-*S. aureus* infections in children from Argentina, 2007 [16].
[c]*P* values are based on chi-square test or Fisher's exact test, as appropriate, for CA-MRSA,CBAH1-H3 vs. CA-MRSA, CSACHARG and total CA-MRSA vs. HACO-MRSA comparisons by each of categorical variables (males and infection type); $p<0.05$ was considered statistically significant.
[d]Values are number of patients and the percentages are indicated in parentheses. [n]: number of patients with this secondary infection focus (CA-MRSA: 342 infections in 312 patients).
[e]Abscess and cellulites: include 9 cases of impetigo(1 from CBAH1-H3 and 8 cases from CSACHARG).
[f]Deep abscess included: breast (2 cases), psoas (4 cases), liver and renal (1 case each one) abscesses.

Pediatric clone in Argentina: ST100-IVNv. A minor HA-MRSA clone, non-multiresistant to antibiotics, named pulsotype C or D by Sola et al and Corso et al, respectively, clonally related to the Pediatric clone by PFGE analysis [36,37] was also detected. It was characterized as *agr* 2, ST100, belonging to CC5, *spa*-t002, associated with a SCC*mec*IV new variant (SCCmec IVNv), and PVL$^-$ [12,15].

In this study, *Tn*4001 was detected, integrated into the class B *mec* complex upstream of the *mecA* gene (class B2 *mec* gene complex) by means of PCR typing of different regions of SCC*mec*IV in representative isolates of the most frequent subtypes (File S1). Hence, this new variant of SCC*mec*IV, in addition to class B2 *mec* gene complex, also carries type 2 *ccr* gene complex and a J1 region with homology to SCC*mecIVc*, but unlike the SCC*mec*IV(2B&5), it lacks of an SCC with *ccrC* and contains *dcs* gene.

This clone was significantly more frequent among HACO-MRSA infections (10%, 5/51) than among total CA-MRSA infections (2%, 5/312), $P=0.009$, (Table 4).

South American USA300 clone. Four CA-MRSA isolates (one detected in Buenos Aires in 2007 and three in Córdoba during 2007–2008) were clonally related by PFGE to the USA300 MRSA epidemic strain. They belonged to ST8, CC8, *spa*-t008 and to *agr* 1. Three of these isolates were associated with SCC*mec*IVc and one, with subtype IVa. All of them carried the *pvl, bsaA* and *seK* genes. In contrast, all lacked of the *arcA* gene, which is an indicator of the presence of the ACME. The isolate associated with *SCCmec*IVa also carried *sed* and *sej* genes (Figure 2A and Table 3).

Other minor clones. Among CA-MRSA isolates, other minor pulsotypes were also detected accounting cumulatively for only 4% of isolates (n: 10, less than 2% each), (Table 3). Among these, two isolates were characterized as ST188/CC1 and associated with SCC*mec*Vr constituting the first time that this genotype is reported in America [19].

The MRSA strains traditionally associated with nosocomial infections in Argentina [12,15,36,37] only accounted for 37% of the total HACO-MRSA infections (Cordobes/Chilean-pulsotype

Table 3. Characteristics of MRSA clones isolated from children with community onset MRSA infections (CO-MRSA), Argentina.

	Related to Pediatric clone			**Southwest Pacific (SWP) clone**	**South American USA300 clone**	**Cordobes/ Chilean clone**	**Brazilian clone**
Clone	**CA-MRSA clone**		**HA-MRSA clone**				
	n: 285		n: 10	n: 39	n: 4	n: 12	n: 3
Molecular characteristics							
agr allelic group	2		2	3	1	2	1
ST n (%)[a]	ST5: 283 (99); ST1524:2 (1)		ST100: 10 (100)	ST30: 35 (90); ST196: 4 (10)	ST8: 4 (100)	ST5: 12 (100)	ST239: 3 (100)
Clonal complex	5		5	30	8	5	8
SCC*mec* type n (%)[a]	IV(2B): IVa: 275 (96), IVc: 6 (2), IVNT[e]: 1; Vr[f]: 2 (0.7); NT: 1 (0,3)		IVNv: 10 (100)	IV(2B): IVc: 38 (97), IVa: 1 (3)	IV(2B): IVc: 3 (75), IVa: 1 (25)	I	IIIA
PFGE type	I		C	N	USA300	A	B
pvl: n (%)[b]	PVL^+ 259 (91)	PVL^- 26 (9)	PVL^- 10 (100)	PVL^+ 39 (100)	PVL^+ 4 (100)	PVL^- 12 (100)	PVL^- 3 (100)
PFGE Subtype: n (%)[a]	I-1: 202 (71) and 14 minor subtypes	I-2: 7 (2.5) and 12 minor subtypes	C1: 2 (20) and 7 minor subtype	N4: 26 (67) and 3 minor subtypes	USA300, 4 subtypes	A1: 4 (33) and 8 minor subtypes	B15 2 (66) and 1 subtype
RIDOM *spa* type: n (%)[a]	t311: 259 (100)	t002: 22 (85); t311, t045; t067; t1094	t002: 10 (100)	t019: 29 (72); t021: 5 (13); t6653: 4 (10); t975	t008: 4 (100)	t149: 12 (100)	t037: 3 (100)
Virulence genes profile[c]	*sea-egc-lukDE*	*egc-lukDE*	*egc-lukDE*	*egc-lukDE-bbp-cna*	*lukDE-sek-bsa*: 3 (75); *lukDE-sek-sed-sej- bsa*: 1 (25)	*egc-lukDE*	*lukDE-bsa*
Drug resistance non-β-Lactam (%)[d]	ERY(14) CLINi (14) GEN (8) RIF (1) CHL (1) **h-VISA** (1)		GEN (100) ERY (50) CLINi (10); CLINc (30) RIF (30) **h-VISA** (1)	GEN(5) ERY(18) CLINi (18) CHL(3)	GEN(25)	GEN (92) CIP (75) ERY(92) CLIc (92) RIF (17)	GEN (100) CIP (100) ERY (100) CLI (100) RIF(6) CHL (100) SXT (100) **h-VISA** (1)
MINOR CLONES, n: 10							
ST188/CC1, n: 2	PFGE type T1, SCC*mec*Vr, *spa*-t189, *agr* 1, cna^+, PVL^+						
ST917/CC8, n: 4	PFGE type R1, SCC*mec*IVNT, *spa*-t148, *agr* 1, PVL^-						
ST207/CC509, n:3	PFGE type Y1, SCC*mec*IVa, *spa*-t525, *agr* 3, PVL^-						
ST918/Singleton, n:1	PFGE type S1, SCC*mec*IVa, *spa*-t1194, *agr* 3, PVL^-						

agr type, type of accessory gene regulator, ST: Sequence Type, SCC*mec*: Staphylococcal Cassette Chromosome *mec*, PFGE, Pulsed Field Gel Electrophoresis; RIDOM *spa* type: staphylococcal protein A (*spa*) type assigned through the RIDOM databases (http://spaserver.ridom.de).

[a] n (%), total number and % of strains with this molecular characteristic [PFGE subtype (only those more frequent are indicated) or ST or *spa* type or *SCCmec* type]. % is not expressed when only one isolate with this characteristic was detected.

[b] *pvl*, Panton-Valentine leukocidin genes (*lukS-PV-lukF-PV*); indicated as number and % of isolates harboring (PVl^+) or not (PVL^-) *pvl* genes.

[c] virulence genes profile: From all virulence genes analyzed, only those detected are indicated (number and % of positive isolates is expressed when not all isolates harbor this virulence factor).

[d] Drug resistance to non-β-Lactams (%), is indicated as follows: Gentamicin (GEN), Ciprofloxacin (CIP), Erythromycin (ERY), Clindamycin (CLIc and CLIi: constitutive and inducible resistance to macrolides, lincosamide and streptogramine B, respectively), rifampin (RIF), chloramphenicol (CHL), trimethoprim/sulfamethoxazole (SXT) and minocycline (MIN) (%) of strains resistant to these antibiotics within each pulsotype is indicated when more than one isolate was detected. h-VISA (1): means one isolate belonging to this clone with phenotype h-VISA.

[e] IV NT: SCC*mec* type IV non typable.

[f] Vr: SCC*mec* related to V.

Table 4. Genotypes of methicillin resistant *S. aureus* (MRSA) isolates recovered from children with Community-onset infections (invasive and non-invasive) in central, northen and eastern regions of Argentina, by epidemiologic case classification.

	Community onset (CO), N° (%) of cases & N° (%) of INVI isolates in indicated epidemiologic class					
	Total CO	**Community-Associated (CA)**				**Healthcare-associated CO (HACO)**
Genotypes[c]		CBAH1-H3[a] 2008	CBAH1-H3[a] 2007	CSACHARG[b] 2007	Total CA	CSACHARG[b] 2007
I-ST5-IV	285 (79); 99 (72)	57 (90); 14 (82)	29 (80); 7 (70)	170 (80);61 (79)	256 (82);82 (79)	29 (57);17 (51)
N-ST30-IV	39 (11), 11 (8)	3 (5), 2 (12)	3 (8); 1 (10)	30 (14); 7 (9)	36 (11.5); 10(10)	3 (6); 1 (3)
USA300-ST8-IV	4 (1); 3 (2)	2 (3); 1 (6)	1 (3);1 (10)	1 (0.5), 1 (1)	4 (1), 3 (3)	—
C-ST100-IVNv	10 (3); 6 (4)	—	1 (3); —	4 (2); 2 (2.5)	5 (2); 2 (2)	5 (10); 4 (12)
A-ST5-I	12 (3); 10 (7)	—	1 (3); 1 (10)	—	1 (0.5); 1 (1)	11 (21); 9 (27)
B-ST239-IIIA	3 (1); 2 (1.5)	—	—	—	—	3 (6); 2 (6)
OTHERS	10 (2)	1 (2)	1 (3)	8 (3.5)	10 (3)	—
Total	n: 363 & INVI: 137	n: 63 & INVI: 17	n: 36 & INVI: 10	n: 213 & INVI: 77	n: 312 & INVI: 104	n: 51 & INVI: 33

INVI: Invasive infections.
[a]CBAH1-H3: Prospective surveillance of CO-*S. aureus* infections in children from three children's hospitals of Córdoba (CBAH1, CBAH2 and CBAH3) 2007 and 2008.
[b]CSACHARG and: Prospective surveillance of CO-*S. aureus* infections in children from Argentina, 2007 [16].
[c]Genotypes are denoted as: type (by PFGE)-Sequence Type (ST by MLST)-SCC*mec* type.

A-ST5-I-t149, 21%; Pediatric-pulsotype C-ST100-IVNv-t002: 10% and Brazilian-pulsotype B-ST239-IIIA-t037: 6%, Figure 2A and Table 4).

Discussion

Laboratory-based surveillance of community-associated *S. aureus* infections in three children's hospitals in Córdoba-Argentina during 2007–2008 revealed a significant increase of the annual prevalence of CA-MRSA infections since 2005 (49%, 2008 vs 25%, 2005). Moreover, the incidence of CA-MRSA infections among children tripled over that time frame, associated with an 8.5-fold increase in invasive CA-MRSA infections, despite the almost stable overall rate of CA-MSSA infections (1.1 fold increase). A similar pattern with a steady annual increase of CA-MRSA infections and a slight increase of CA-MSSA infections was detected in one (H1) of these hospitals between 2003 and 2008. Hence, we demonstrated that in Córdoba, Argentina, as reported in some regions of United States, particularly in patients with skin and soft-tissue infections, CA-MRSA strains are adding to the burden of CO-*S. aureus* infections, instead of replacing other *S. aureus* strains [8,38].

Unlike in North America, few studies have documented the epidemiology of MRSA infections in the community among Latin-American children [1,12,39]. This study provides the first comprehensive description carried out in Argentina about the evolution of CA-MRSA infections over time (2003–2008) in children from Córdoba.

The types of CA-MRSA infections detected in this study are similar to those described worldwide. Nevertheless, it is important to remark the high proportion of children with invasive CA-MRSA infections in Argentina (33%) compared to previous reports from other countries (1–12%) [20,40]. Regarding HACO-MRSA infections, most children had some type of chronic disease and multiple HRFs, were more susceptible to surgical site and invasive infections as well as sepsis, and had significantly lower frequency of SSTIs compared to children with CA-MRSA infections, in agreement with other studies [4,21,41].

Although variable rates of CA-MRSA infection among children from different regions of Argentina were detected in 2007, one of the most striking finding of our study is that one major CA-MRSA clone (I-ST5-SSC*mec*IV-PVL$^+$) is currently predominanting in both groups: community-associated cases (82%) and healthcare-associated, community-onset cases (57%) in hospitals of northern, eastern and central regions of our country, contrasting with other countries [4].

Therefore, the wide dissemination of this clone over all these regions of Argentina, along with the continued steep rise of its incidence over time in Córdoba, confirm its epidemic nature. Importantly, these results suggest that many children, despite documented contacts with healthcare delivery, are frequently infected with a CA-MRSA clone. This finding, though indirectly, suggests that this clone has entered into the healthcare settings and thus, represents a potentially serious public health challenge for next years, as described elsewhere for other CA-MRSA clones [8–10].

The molecular characteristics shared by the isolates belonging to this major clone corresponded largely to those reported in our previous paper [12], namely, *agr*2, ST5, *spa*-t311 and related ones, *SCCmec*IV(2B) (96% IVa). In addition, most of these isolates carried *pvl* and *sea* genes (91%). Although most of CA-MRSA infections (invasive and non invasive) caused by the "I" clone have been produced by PVL$^+$ isolates, both groups, PVL$^+$ and PVL$^-$, were comparable regarding the proportions of invasive infections and presentation with sepsis. Hence, these results lead to hypothesize that the presence of *pvl* and *sea* genes associated with *spa*-t311 in this lineage would be more related to a possible increase in transmissibility and fitness of this CA-MRSA clone, rather than to its virulence. Further studies are needed to confirm this hypothesis.

Recently, Nübel et al [42], by using single-nucleotide polymorphism analysis, demonstrated that much of the population structure of ST5 is local, with multiple independent introductions of SCC*mec*, producing a regional-specific evolution of particular sublineages. In agreement with that hypothesis, in previous studies we demonstrated the presence of ST5-PVL$^+$ lineages among MSSA strains in our country [12,43]. In this study, 9% of the isolates belonging to I pulsotype were PVL$^-$. Additionally, among the isolates characterized as I9 subtype-*spa*-t311-SCC*mec*IVa, we also found one PVL$^-$ variant and another harboring SCC*mec*IVc

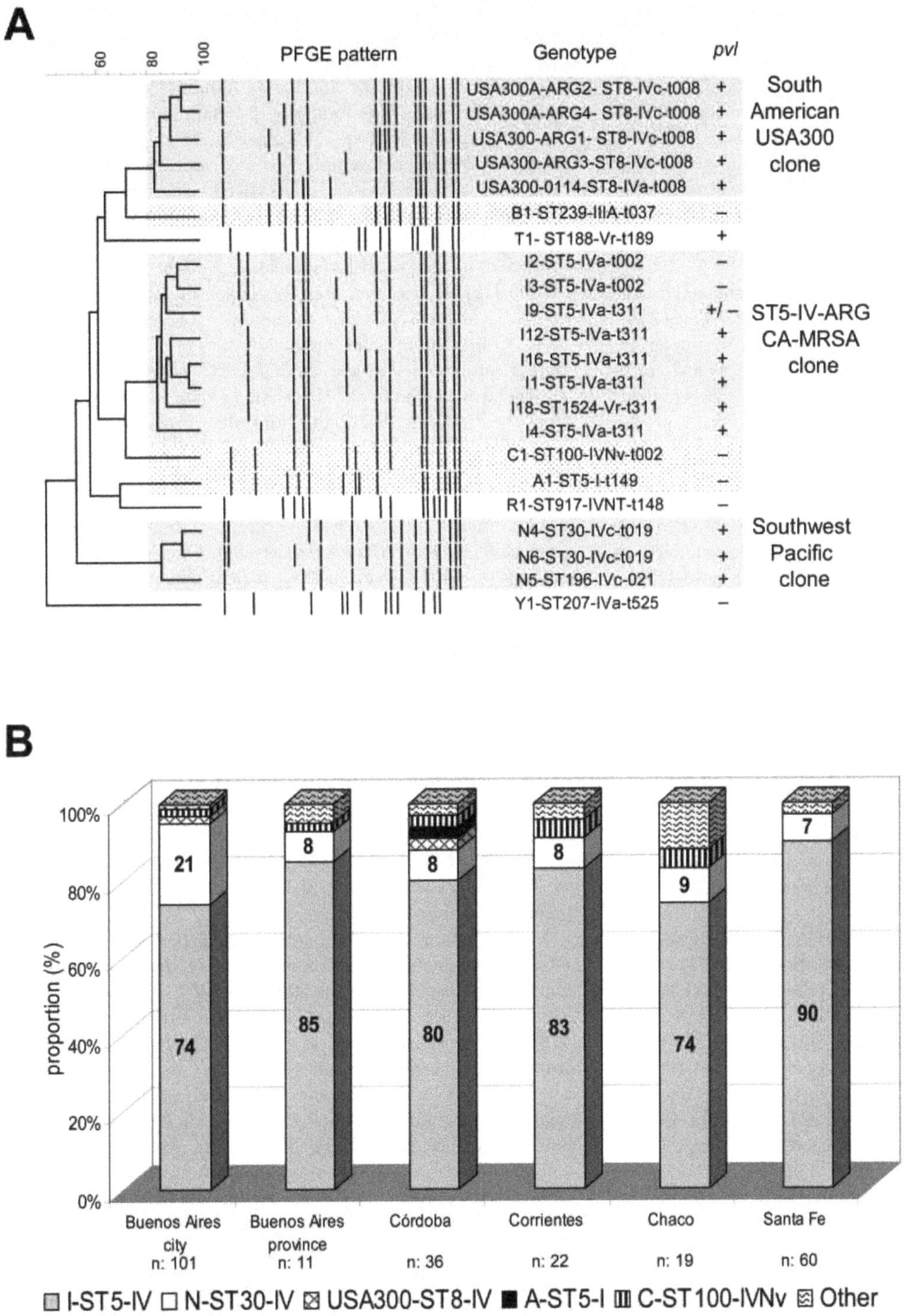

Figure 2. Molecular characteristics and proportion from different regions of Argentina of dominant community methicillin-resistant-*Staphylococcus aureus* clones. A. PFGE pattern analysis for representative isolates belonging to the most prevalent subtypes of community-onset-MRSA clones (CA-MRSA and HA-MRSA) detected in central, eastern and northern regions of Argentina during 2007–2008. The schematic presentation of *SmaI* restriction patterns (middle) and dendrogram (left) by the unweighted-pair group method using average linkage clusterings are shown. Genotypes are denoted as subtype (by PFGE)-ST (by MLST)-SCC*mec* type-*spa* type (right). CA-MRSA clones appear in gray. The presence (+) or absence (−) of *pvl* genes (by PCR) is also indicated for each subtype; strains with and other without *pvl* genes belonging to the same PFGE subtype (I9) are indicated as +/−. The PFGE pattern of USA300-0114 (ST8-IVa-*t008*-ACME+) is shown for comparison purposes. The first (A1-ST5-I-t149-Cordobes/Chilean), second (B1-ST239-IIIA-t037-Brazilian) and third (C1-ST100-IVNv-t002-Pediatric) more frequent HA-MRSA clones in our country, detected among community-onset MRSA infections, are also shown (dotted gray). **B**: Proportion of CA-MRSA clones among representative isolates from different regions of Argentina in 2007.

(Figure 2A). Together, these results support the hypothesis about multiple independent acquisitions of different SCC*mec* types (IVa or IVc or Vr) and virulence genes (*pvl* and *sea*) by a common ST5 MSSA ancestor.

On the other hand, some studies have described the ST5-SCC*mec*IV-PVL$^+$ genotype among CA-MRSA isolates in United States and some countries of Europe and Africa. However in all of them, the isolates had different profiles of virulence genes and/or resistance to antibiotics and so far, its role as dominant genetic background of CA-MRSA over time has not been duplicated outside Argentina [3,44–49].

Accordingly, although this clone is genetically related to the international HA-MRSA "classical" Pediatric clone (ST5-SCC*mec*IV) identified in several countries [50], based on the molecular characterization (CA-MRSA and CA-MSSA) and clinical epidemiology over time, we suggest that this clone is a new epidemic CA-MRSA, probably endowed with increased fitness in this country. Hence, the possibility of being an escaped HA strain should be ruled out.

Conversely, one of the three most predominant HA-MRSA clones in Argentina since 1998 was clonally related to the Pediatric clone by PFGE analysis [36,37] which was characterized as ST100-SCC*mecIV* related to IVc-*spa*-t002-PVL$^-$ [15]. In Córdoba, some community-onset infections were caused by this HA-MRSA clone before the emergence of the new CA-MRSA clone, probably as an "escaped" HA-MRSA strain [12,15]. Accordingly, it was more commonly isolated from HACO-MRSA cases than from CA-MRSA infections (10% vs 2%), as shown herein. The ST100 genotype was also identified in a MRSA isolate from Zurich in 2003 (MRSA-ZH47), associated with the new SCC*mec*IV(2B&5) [35]. In this study, we demonstrated for the first time that the SCC*mec* associated with pulsotype C (Pediatric clone)-ST100 in Argentina is closely related to SCC*mec*IV(2B&5). Therefore, to classify this new variant of SCC*mec*IV, it would be necessary to determine the complete nucleotide sequence, which is currently in progress.

The pandemic Southwest Pacific-(SWP) clone or USA1100 was one of the minor clones found, accounting for 11.5% of CA-MRSA isolates. It was characterized as pulsotype N, ST30, *spa*-t019 and related ones. Most isolates harbored SCC*mec*IVc (97%) all of them carried *pvl* genes and adhesins *cna* and *bbp* genes. Since mid-1990s, this CA-MRSA clone, ST30-IV-PVL$^+$ with different pulsotypes or *spa* types or SCC*mec*IV subtypes has been reported from many regions of the world [1,46]. In Buenos Aires, this clone (ST30-IV) had already been detected as a minor one among CA-MRSA isolates in 2004–2006 [13]. In our study, this clone was significantly more frequent in Buenos Aires city and surrounding areas (21%) than in other regions analyzed, where it accounted for 8% of CA-MRSA isolates in 2007. Although its frequency is still very low, this situation might suggest that this CA-MRSA clone is spreading from Uruguay, where it is highly prevalent at community and hospital settings [11,51].

Recently, the South American USA300 MRSA-(ST8-*SSCmec*IV-*spa*t008-PVL$^+$-ACME$^-$) clone was described as the most predominant (96%) CA-MRSA in northern areas of South America between 2006 and 2008 [14]. An additional important issue of this study was the finding of the first four cases of CA-MRSA infections caused by this highly virulent CA-MRSA clone in the southern cone of Latin America. ACME-negative variants of USA300 also appear to be common in Western Australia and in Spain [52–54], though we were unable to find eventual epidemiological association between Argentinean strains and those from these countries.

Our results confirmed the high prevalence of MRSA infections in the community in Argentinean children, so the characteristics of antimicrobial susceptibility of these strains must be considered for the selection of empiric therapies. Although most CA-MRSA isolates were susceptible to all non-β-lactam antibiotics, inducible resistance to clindamycin (14%), resistance to gentamicin (8%), rifampin (1%) and chloramphenicol (1%) were detected in isolates belonging to ST5-IV-PVL$^+$ CA-MRSA clone (Table 3). It is important to remark that this clone's resistance to antibiotics was only represented by clindamycin, just in 10% of isolates, as described in the previous surveillance performed in Córdoba in2005 [12]. Hence, these results support the ability of the ST5-IV-PVL$^+$ CA-MRSA clone to acquire new resistance determinants. On the other hand, the higher rates of resistance to non-β-lactam antibiotics detected among HACO-MRSA strains were associated with traditional HA-MRSA clones in our country: the Cordobes/Chilean, Brazilian and Pediatric clones. In addition, according to these results, it would be possible to infer that the presence of HRFs should be considered for selection of empirical therapy in children with community-onset MRSA infections.

Importantly, in our study, three strains with h-VISA phenotype from children with HRFs were detected. One of these cases and another one detected in an adult patient without HRFs in 2009 [55] were PVL$^-$ variants of ST5-SCC*mec*-IV CA-MRSA clone. Considering the high proportion of children with invasive CA-MRSA infections caused by this clone, along with the fact that vancomycin is still the centerpiece used for the treatment of this type of CA-MRSA infections [7], this finding constitutes another concern for public health.

Our study was limited by the use of the CDC criteria to identify patients with infections caused by CA-MRSA isolates, which appear to underestimate the burden of diseases produced by these strains. Additionally, evidence from this study, though indirect, indicate that CA-MRSA strains have entered the hospital settings of Argentina and probably the burden of CA-MRSA is even greater than shown here.

In conclusion, we observed a significant increase in the incidence of invasive and non-invasive CA-MRSA infections, in children of Córdoba between 2005 and 2008. This raise could be attributed entirely to the rapid dissemination of an epidemic CA-MRSA clone characterized as I-ST5-*SCCmec*IVa-*spa*-t311-PVL$^+$. Importantly, this highly virulent clone with capacity to express the phenotype h-VISA, predominates in central, northern and eastern regions of Argentina and still more worryingly, it has probably entered the hospital settings. The specific virulence, antibiotic resistance and transmission traits of a CA-MRSA clone distinct from USA300 would need to be identified in order to recognize priority targets for drug and vaccine development. These virulent clones represent a new threat to public health in Argentina and probably worldwide, warranting close monitoring during next years.

Acknowledgments

This article is dedicated to the memory of Hugo Paganini, MD.

We are grateful to Dr. Keiichi Hiramatsu (Department of Bacteriology, Juntendo University, Tokyo, Japan) for providing reference strains Mu3 and Mu50 and to Dr. Alejandra Corso (Instituto Nacional de Enfermedades Infecciosas. *ANLIS.* Dr. C. Malbrán, Buenos Aires – Argentina) for the representative of International Pediatric clone described in Buenos

Aires city hospitals (ARG164). We are grateful to Dario Tosoroni for his excellent technical assistance in the statistic analysis.

The members of Study Group of CA-MRSA in children, Argentina-2007 are:

María P. Della Latta, Lidia Casimir, Claudia Hernández, Andrea Mónaco, José L. Pinheiro, Leonardo Maninno and Claudia Sarkis (*Hospital "Prof. Dr. Juan P. Garrahan", ACBA*), Beatriz Muller Opet, María J. Rial and Norma Schenonne, Catalina De Ricco (*Hospital General de Niños "Dr. Pedro de Elizalde", ACBA*); Gustavo Ezcurra, Estela Ronchi and Celia Bosque (*Hospital de Niños de Santa Fe "Dr. O Alassia", Santa Fe*); Macarena Uranga, María del C. Rodríguez and Fabiana Apriled (*Hospital de Niños de San Justo*, Buenos Aires city surrounding area); Clarisa Aguirre, Viviana García Saito and Claudia Vratnica (*Hospital "Juan Pablo II", Corrientes*); Gabriela Ensinck and Adriana Ernst (*Hospital de Niños "J. Vilela", Rosario-Santa Fe*); Marys Kamiya de Macarrein, Laura Pons and Sandra Morinigo (*Hospital Pediátrico "Dr. A.L. Castelán", Resistencia, Chaco*), Cristina Ciriaci, Victoria Monzani and María del P. López (*Hospital Materno Infantil de Mar del Plata "Don Victorio Tetamanti"* Mar del Plata, Buenos Aires) and members of *S. aureus* Collaborative Study Group in children in Cordoba: Catalina Culasso, Lydia Carvajal and Eduardo Glanstein (*Hospital de Niños de la Santísima Trinidad de Córdoba*), Liliana Gonzalez, Eugenia Tirao (*Hospital Infantil de Córdoba*); Paulo Cortes, Rafael Sanchez Bocco (*Hospital Pediátrico del Niño Jesús, Córdoba*).

We are grateful to all other members members of Cordoba *S. aureus* Collaborative Study Group for their contribution to the surveillance of MRSA infections: Monterisi, Aida and Rocchi, Marta (*Hospital Nacional de Clínicas*); Perlo-Morales, Olga and Aiassa, María S, (*Hospital Córdoba*); Vilaro, Mario and Bongiovanni, María E. (*Hospital Privado de Córdoba*); Mangiaterra, Sandra (*Hospital Italiano de Córdoba*); Diaz, Elda and Lamberghini Ricardo (*Hospital Militar de Córdoba*); Littvik Ana, Lopez Teresa (*Hospital Rawson*); Wolff Lidia and Vercelli B, (*Clínica Privada Velez Sarsfield*); D'Andrea Elena M., Lopez Adriana (*Hospital de Urgencias*); Pino Gladys, Muñoz Veronica (*Hospital San Roque*); Bottiglieri Marina (*Clínica Reina Fabiola*); Gribaudo Germán (*Sanatorio Nosti–Rafaela-Santa Fe*, Decca M Laura (*Clínica del Sud Rio IV-Córdoba*). IK was student of Rotary International's Ambassadorial Scholarships during 2008. CS and JLB are career investigators members of CONICET.

Author Contributions

Conceived and designed the experiments: CS HP JLB. Performed the experiments: CS HP ALE AJM AG IK CC HL JLB. Analyzed the data: CS HP JLB. Contributed reagents/materials/analysis tools: CS HP IK AV JLB. Wrote the paper: CS JLB. Patients' clinical care, collection of clinical and epidemiology data, microbiology diagnostic: Study Group of CA-MRSA in Children, Argentina-2007.

References

1. David MZ, Daum RS (2010) Community-associated methicillin-resistant *Staphylococcus aureus*: epidemiology and clinical consequences of an emerging epidemic. Clin Microbiol Rev 23: 616–87.
2. Deurenberg RH, Stobberingh EE (2009) The molecular evolution of hospital- and community-associated methicillin-resistant *Staphylococcus aureus*. Curr Mol Med 9: 100–15.
3. Deleo FR, Otto M, Kreiswirth BN, Chambers HF (2010) Community-associated meticillin-resistant *Staphylococcus aureus*. Lancet 375: 1557–68.
4. Limbago B, Fosheim GE, Schoonover V, Crane CE, Nadle J, et al. (2009) Characterization of methicillin-resistant *Staphylococcus aureus* isolates collected in 2005 and 2006 from patients with invasive disease: a population-based analysis. J Clin Microbiol 47: 1344–51.
5. Gonzalez BE, Martinez-Aguilar G, Hulten KG, Hammerman WA, Coss-Bu J, et al. (2005) Severe Staphylococcal sepsis in adolescents in the era of community-acquired methicillin-resistant *Staphylococcus aureus*. Pediatrics 115: 642–8.
6. Howden BP, Davies JK, Johnson PD, Stinear TP, Grayson ML (2010) Reduced vancomycin susceptibility in *Staphylococcus aureus*, including vancomycin-intermediate and heterogeneous vancomycin-intermediate strains: resistance mechanisms, laboratory detection, and clinical implications. Clin Microbiol Rev 23: 99–139.
7. Liu C, Bayer A, Cosgrove SE, Daum RS, Fridkin SK, et al. (2011) Clinical practice guidelines by the Infectious Diseases Society of America for the treatment of methicillin-resistant *Staphylococcus aureus* infections in adults and children. Clin Infect Dis 52: e18–55.
8. Gerber JS, Coffin SE, Smathers SA, Zaoutis TE (2009) Trends in the incidence of methicillin-resistant *Staphylococcus aureus* infection in children's hospitals in the United States. Clin Infect Dis 49: 65–71.
9. David MZ, Glikman D, Crawford SE, Peng J, King KJ, et al. (2008) What is community-associated methicillin-resistant *Staphylococcus aureus*? J Infect Dis 197: 1235–43.
10. Maree CL, Daum RS, Boyle-Vavra S, Matayoshi K, Miller LG (2007) Community-associated methicillin-resistant *Staphylococcus aureus* isolates causing healthcare-associated infections. Emerg Infect Dis 13: 236–42.
11. Ma XX, Galiana A, Pedreira W, Mowszowicz M, Christophersen I, et al. (2005) Community-acquired methicillin-resistant *Staphylococcus aureus*, Uruguay. Emerg Infect Dis 11: 973–6.
12. Sola C, Saka HA, Vindel A, Cordoba MRSA Collaborative Study Group, Bocco JL (2008) Emergence and dissemination of a community-associated methicillin-resistant Panton-Valentine leukocidin-positive *Staphylococcus aureus* clone sharing the sequence type 5 lineage with the most prevalent nosocomial clone in the same region of Argentina. J Clin Microbiol 46: 1826–31.
13. Gardella N, von Specht M, Cuirolo A, Rosato A, Gutkind G, et al. (2008) Community-associated methicillin-resistant *Staphylococcus aureus*, eastern Argentina. Diagn Microbiol Infect Dis 62: 343–7.
14. Reyes J, Rincon S, Diaz L, Panesso D, Contreras GA, et al. (2009) Dissemination of methicillin-resistant *Staphylococcus aureus* USA300 sequence type 8 lineage in Latin America. Clin Infect Dis 49: 1861–7.
15. Sola C, Cortes P, Saka HA, Vindel A, Bocco JL (2006) Evolution and molecular characterization of methicillin-resistant *Staphylococcus aureus* epidemic and sporadic clones in Cordoba, Argentina. J Clin Microbiol 44: 192–200.
16. Paganini H, Della Latta MP, Muller Opet B, Ezcurra G, Uranga M, et al. (2008) [Community-acquired methicillin-resistant *Staphylococcus aureus* infections in children: multicenter trial]. Arch Argent Pediatr 106: 397–403.
17. Rodriguez-Noriega E, Seas C, Guzman-Blanco M, Mejia C, Alvarez C, et al. (2010) Evolution of methicillin-resistant *Staphylococcus aureus* clones in Latin America. Int J Infect Dis 14: e560–6.
18. Chua K, Laurent F, Coombs G, Grayson ML, Howden BP (2011) Antimicrobial resistance: Not community-associated methicillin-resistant *Staphylococcus aureus* (CA-MRSA)! A clinician's guide to community MRSA - its evolving antimicrobial resistance and implications for therapy. Clin Infect Dis 52: 99–114.
19. Monecke S, Coombs G, Shore AC, Coleman DC, Akpaka P, et al. (2011) A Field Guide to Pandemic, Epidemic and Sporadic Clones of Methicillin-Resistant *Staphylococcus aureus*. PLoS One 6(4): e17936.
20. Kaplan SL, Hulten KG, Gonzalez BE, Hammerman WA, Lamberth L, et al. (2005) Three-year surveillance of community-acquired *Staphylococcus aureus* infections in children. Clin Infect Dis 40: 1785–91.
21. Klevens RM, Morrison MA, Nadle J, Petit S, Gershman K, et al. (2007) Invasive methicillin-resistant *Staphylococcus aureus* infections in the United States. JAMA 298: 1763–71.
22. Morrison MA, Hageman JC, Klevens RM (2006) Case definition for community-associated methicillin-resistant *Staphylococcus aureus*. J Hosp Infect 62: 241.
23. Klevens RM, Morrison MA, Fridkin SK, Reingold A, Petit S, et al. (2006) Community-associated methicillin-resistant *Staphylococcus aureus* and healthcare risk factors. Emerg Infect Dis 12: 1991–3.
24. Goldstein B, Giroir B, Randolph A (2005) International pediatric sepsis consensus conference: definitions for sepsis and organ dysfunction in pediatrics. Pediatr Crit Care Med 6: 2–8.
25. Clinical and Laboratory Standards Institute. Performance Standards for Antimicrobial Susceptibility Testing Nineteenth Informational Supplement M100-S19. 2009, Wayne, Pennsylvania, USA: CLSI.
26. Wootton M, MacGowan AP, Walsh TR, Howe AR (2007) A multicenter study evaluating the current strategies for isolating *Staphylococcus aureus* strains with reduced susceptibility to glycopeptides. J Clin Microbiol 45: 329–32.
27. Hiramatsu K, Hanaki H, Ino T, Yabuta K, Oguri T, et al. (1997) Methicillin-resistant *Staphylococcus aureus* clinical strain with reduced vancomycin susceptibility. J Antimicrob Chemother 40: 135–6.
28. Satola SW, Farley MM, Anderson KF, Patel JB (2010) Comparison of Detection Methods for Heteroresistant Vancomycin Intermediate *Staphylococcus aureus* (hVISA) using Population Analysis Profile as the Reference Method. J Clin Microbiol 49(1): 177–83.
29. Enright MC, Day NP, Davies CE, Peacock SJ, Spratt BG (2000) Multilocus sequence typing for characterization of methicillin-resistant and methicillin-susceptible clones of *Staphylococcus aureus*. J Clin Microbiol 38: 1008–15.
30. Harmsen D, Claus H, Witte W, Rothganger J, Claus H, et al. (2003) Typing of methicillin-resistant *Staphylococcus aureus* in a university hospital setting by using novel software for spa repeat determination and database management. J Clin Microbiol 41: 5442–8.
31. Milheirico C, Oliveira DC, de Lencastre H (2007) Update to the multiplex PCR strategy for assignment of mec element types in *Staphylococcus aureus*. Antimicrob Agents Chemother 51: 3374–7.

32. Okuma K, Iwakawa K, Turnidge JD, Grubb WB, Bell JM, et al. (2002) Dissemination of new methicillin-resistant *Staphylococcus aureus* clones in the community. J Clin Microbiol 40: 4289–94.
33. Milheirico C, Oliveira DC, de Lencastre H (2007) Multiplex PCR strategy for subtyping the staphylococcal cassette chromosome mec type IV in methicillin-resistant *Staphylococcus aureus*: 'SCCmec IV multiplex'. J Antimicrob Chemother 60: 42–8.
34. Oliveira DC, Milheirico C, de Lencastre H (2006) Redefining a structural variant of staphylococcal cassette chromosome mec, *SCC*mec type VI. Antimicrob Agents Chemother 50: 3457–9.
35. Heusser R, Ender M, Berger-Bachi B, McCallum N (2007) Mosaic staphylococcal cassette chromosome mec containing two recombinase loci and a new mec complex, B2. Antimicrob Agents Chemother 51: 390–3.
36. Corso A, Santos Sanches I, Aires de Sousa M, Rossi A, de Lencastre H (1998) Spread of a methicillin-resistant and multiresistant epidemic clone of *Staphylococcus aureus* in Argentina. Microb Drug Resist 4: 277–88.
37. Sola C, Gribaudo G, Vindel A, Patrito L, Bocco JL (2002) Identification of a novel methicillin-resistant *Staphylococcus aureus* epidemic clone in Cordoba, Argentina, involved in nosocomial infections. J Clin Microbiol 40: 1427–35.
38. Orscheln RC, Hunstad DA, Fritz SA, Loughman JA, Mitchell K, et al. (2009) contribution of genetically restricted, methicillin-susceptible strains to the ongoing epidemic of community-acquired *Staphylococcus aureus* infections. Clin Infect Dis 49: 536–42.
39. Tokumoto MB, Ybarra V, Torreno M, Rodriguez M, Ramirez MS, et al. (2007) Emergence of community-acquired methicillin-resistant *Staphylococcus aureus* (CA-MRSA) paediatric clone among skin and soft-tissue infections in Buenos Aires. Int J Antimicrob Agents 30: 469–71.
40. Niniou I, Vourli S, Lebessi E, Foustoukou M, Vatopoulos A, et al. (2008) Clinical and molecular epidemiology of community-acquired, methicillin-resistant *Staphylococcus aureus* infections in children in central Greece. Eur J Clin Microbiol Infect Dis 27: 831–7.
41. Zaoutis TE, Toltzis P, Chu J, Abrams T, Dul M, et al. (2006) Clinical and molecular epidemiology of community-acquired methicillin-resistant *Staphylococcus aureus* infections among children with risk factors for health care-associated infection: 2001–2003. Pediatr Infect Dis J 25: 343–8.
42. Nubel U, Roumagnac P, Feldkamp M, Song JH, Ko KS, et al. (2008) Frequent emergence and limited geographic dispersal of methicillin-resistant *Staphylococcus aureus*. Proc Natl Acad Sci U S A 105: 14130–5.
43. Sola C, Saka HA, Vindel A, Cordoba S. aureus Collaborative Study Group, Bocco JL (2007) High frequency of Panton-Valentine leukocidin genes in invasive methicillin-susceptible *Staphylococcus aureus* strains and the relationship with methicillin-resistant Staphylococcus aureus in Cordoba, Argentina. Eur J Clin Microbiol Infect Dis 26: 281–286.
44. Breurec S, Zriouil SB, Fall C, Boisier P, Brisse S, et al. (2011) Epidemiology of methicillin-resistant *Staphylococcus aureus* lineages in five major African towns: emergence and spread of atypical clones. Clin Microbiol Infect 17: 160–5.
45. Ellington MJ, Perry C, Ganner M, Warner M, McCormick Smith I, et al. (2009) Clinical and molecular epidemiology of ciprofloxacin-susceptible MRSA encoding PVL in England and Wales. Eur J Clin Microbiol Infect Dis 28: 1113–21.
46. Tristan A, Bes M, Meugnier H, Lina G, Bozdogan B, et al. (2007) Global Distribution of Panton-Valentine Leukocidin-positive Methicillin-resistant *Staphylococcus aureus*, 2006. Emerg Infect Dis 13: 594–600.
47. Bhattacharya D, Carleton H, Tsai CJ, Baron EJ, Perdreau-Remington F (2007) Differences in clinical and molecular characteristics of skin and soft tissue methicillin-resistant *Staphylococcus aureus* isolates between two hospitals in Northern California. J Clin Microbiol 45: 1798–803.
48. Rossney AS, Shore AC, Morgan PM, Fitzgibbon MM, O'connell B, et al. (2007) The Emergence and Importation of Diverse Genotypes of MRSA Harboring the Panton-Valentine Leukocidin Gene *pvl* Reveals that pvl is a Poor Marker for Community-Acquired MRSA in Ireland. J Clin Microbiol 45: 2554–63.
49. Monecke S, Berger-Bachi B, Coombs G, Holmes A, Kay I, et al. (2007) Comparative genomics and DNA array-based genotyping of pandemic *Staphylococcus aureus* strains encoding Panton-Valentine leukocidin. Clin Microbiol Infect 13: 236–49.
50. Dauwalder O, Lina G, Durand G, Bes M, Meugnier H, et al. (2008) Epidemiology of invasive methicillin-resistant *Staphylococcus aureus* clones collected in France in 2006 and 2007. J Clin Microbiol 46: 3454–8.
51. Benoit SR, Estivariz C, Mogdasy C, Pedreira W, Galiana A, et al. (2008) Community Strains of Methicillin-Resistant Staphylococcus aureus as Potential Cause of Healthcare-associated Infections, Uruguay, 2002–2004. Emerg Infect Dis 14: 1216–23.
52. Monecke S, Ehricht R, Slickers P, Tan HL, Coombs G (2009) The molecular epidemiology and evolution of the Panton-Valentine leukocidin-positive, methicillin-resistant *Staphylococcus aureus* strain USA300 in Western Australia. Clin Microbiol Infect 15: 770–6.
53. Blanco R, Tristan A, Ezpeleta G, Larsen AR, Bes M, et al. (2011) Molecular epidemiology of Panton-Valentine leukocidin-positive Staphylococcus aureus in Spain: emergence of the USA300 clone in an autochthonous population. J Clin Microbiol 49: 433–6.
54. Cercenado E, Cuevas O, Marin M, Bouza E, Trincado P, et al. (2008) Community-acquired methicillin-resistant Staphylococcus aureus in Madrid, Spain: transcontinental importation and polyclonal emergence of Panton-Valentine leukocidin-positive isolates. Diagn Microbiol Infect Dis 61: 143–9.
55. Sola C, Lamberghini RO, Ciarlantini M, Egea AL, Gonzalez P, et al. (2011) Heterogeneous vancomycin-intermediate susceptibility in a community-associated methicillin-resistant Staphylococcus aureus epidemic clone, in a case of Infective Endocarditis in Argentina. Ann Clin Microbiol Antimicrob 10(1): 15.

13

Risk Factors Associated with Increased Mortality among HIV Infected Children Initiating Antiretroviral Therapy (ART) in South Africa

Brian C. Zanoni[1,2,3], Thuli Phungula[3], Holly M. Zanoni[3], Holly France[3], Margaret E. Feeney[1,4*]

1 The Ragon Institute of Massachusetts General Hospital, Massachusetts Institute of Technology, and Harvard, Charlestown, Massachusetts, United States of America, 2 Harvard Medical School, Boston, Massachusetts, United States of America, 3 Sinikithemba Clinic and Philani Program, McCord Hospital, Durban, South Africa, 4 Division of Experimental Medicine, University of California San Francisco, San Francisco, California, United States of America

Abstract

Objective: To identify demographic and clinical risk factors associated with mortality after initiation of antiretroviral therapy (ART) in a cohort of human immunodeficiency (HIV) infected children in KwaZulu-Natal, South Africa.

Methods: We performed a retrospective cohort study of 537 children initiating antiretroviral therapy at McCord Hospital in KwaZulu-Natal, South Africa. Data were extracted from electronic medical records and risk factors associated with mortality were assessed using Cox regression analysis.

Results: Overall there were 47 deaths from the cohort of 537 children initiating ART with over 991 child-years of follow-up (median 22 months on ART), yielding a mortality rate of 4.7 deaths per 100 child years on ART. Univariate analysis indicated that mortality was significantly associated with lower weight-for-age Z-score ($p<0.0001$), chronic diarrhea ($p=0.0002$), lower hemoglobin ($p=0.002$), age <3 years ($p=0.003$), and CD4% <10% ($p=0.005$). The final multivariable Cox proportional hazards mortality model found age less than 3 years ($p=0.004$), CD4 <10% ($p=0.01$), chronic diarrhea ($p=0.03$), weight-for-age Z-score (<0.0001) and female gender as a covariate varying with time ($p=0.03$) all significantly associated with mortality.

Conclusion: In addition to recognized risk factors such as young age and advanced immunosuppression, we found female gender to be significantly associated with mortality in this pediatric ART cohort. Future studies are needed to determine whether intrinsic biologic differences or socio-cultural factors place female children with HIV at increased risk of death following initiation of ART.

Editor: Landon Myer, University of Cape Town, South Africa

Funding: This work was generously supported by the Sullivan Family Foundation and the Elizabeth Glaser Pediatric AIDS Foundation (M.E.F.). M.E.F. is the recipient of the Jewelers for Children Elizabeth Glaser Scientist Award. The funders had no role in study design, data collection and analysis, decision to publish, or preparation of the manuscript.

Competing Interests: The authors have declared that no competing interests exist.

* E-mail: margaret.feeney@ucsf.edu

Introduction

Pediatric HIV remains prevalent in sub-Saharan Africa. As of 2009, South Africa alone had more than 280,000 HIV-infected children [1]. Untreated pediatric HIV infection carries a high mortality rate [2,3]. However, access to ART in sub-Saharan Africa has increased dramatically since 2005 [1,4,5,6]. Until recently, few data were available regarding clinical risk factors associated with mortality in children after they initiate ART [7,8,9,10,11]. Recent studies from Southern Africa have consistently found low absolute CD4 and CD4% at the time of ART initiation to be associated with early mortality on ART [5,7,8,11]. Additionally, several studies confirmed that stunting, wasting, anemia, and WHO stage 4 conditions at the time of ART initiation significantly contribute to early pediatric mortality on ART [5,8,10,11].

Although, gender has not previously been associated with mortality in these African cohorts, several studies have documented gender discrepancies in response to HIV infection [12,13,14,15]. Two small studies documented lower HIV RNA in girls compared to boys after initiation of ART [13,14]. However, an additional study found no difference in viral loads between the genders [16].

Expanded knowledge of baseline factors associated with early mortality could improve local guidelines regarding the timing and choice of ART regimen and help target intensity of medical surveillance after ART initiation towards those children at highest risk of early death.

Materials and Methods

Ethics Statement

The protocol was approved by McCord Hospital's Research Ethics Committee and the Partners Human Research Committee. All patients accessing care at McCord Hospital sign a written consent to have their medical information stored on an electronic medical record database that is used for clinical and research purposes.

Study design

We performed a retrospective cohort study using electronic medical records from HIV infected pediatric patients (≤18 years old) who initiated antiretroviral therapy at McCord Hospital's Sinikithemba Clinic in KwaZulu-Natal, South Africa from August 2003 to December 2008. We analyzed clinical and demographic characteristics at the time of initiation of ART therapy as potential predictors of mortality.

Study population and standard of care

McCord Hospital is a semi-private, urban hospital providing care for a mostly Zulu speaking population in Durban, South Africa. Between August 2003 and December 2008, 537 children initiated ART at McCord Hospital's Sinikithemba Clinic. Patients were followed from the time they initiated ART until they died, transferred care to another facility, were lost to follow-up, or until the study end date of May 31, 2009. In this clinical setting, children were diagnosed with tuberculosis based on a combination of available clinical, radiographic, microscopic, and contact information. During the study period, children were initiated on ART when their HIV disease reached World Health Organization (WHO) stage 3 or 4 and/or their CD4 percentage was less than 20% in children younger than 18 months, or less than 15% in children older than 18 months, in accordance with South African National Treatment Guidelines [17]. Based on national guidelines in South Africa, children less than 3 years of age received a Protease Inhibitor (PI)-based first line treatment regimen comprised of lopinavir/ritonavir, stavudine, and lamivudine [17]. Children older than 3 years initiated a Non-Nucleotide Reverse Transcriptase Inhibitor (NNRTI) based treatment regimen comprised of efaverinez, stavudine, and lamivudine [17]. According to local guidelines routine laboratory monitoring includes baseline CD4 and 6 monthly CD4 and viral loads [17]. Throughout the duration of the study period, children taking an efaverinez based regimen who had HIV-TB co-infection did not have any alterations to their treatment while children receiving protease inhibitor based treatment were either changed from lopinavir/ritonavir to ritonavir or received double dosed lopinavir/ritonavir.

Data Collection

We evaluated medical records from all patients who were ≤18 years old when they initiated ART at McCord Hospital's Sinikithemba Clinic from August 2003 to December 2008. TrackCare Software was used to maintain electronic medical records, which were cross referenced with paper charts. Data were entered into a Microsoft Access database, and we then reviewed 10% of all medical records for accuracy. Collected data included age at ART initiation, gender, ART regimen, presence of tuberculosis (TB) and non-TB opportunistic infections, chronic diarrhea (longer than 14 days), baseline laboratory results including absolute and CD4 percentage, and hemoglobin, and baseline weight-for-age Z-scores (calculated for all children less than 10 years of age using the WHO macro for STATA; https://www.who.int/childgrowth/software). Children older than 10 years were assigned a dummy variable for missing weight-for-age z-score so that they could be included in the multivariable model. The presence of chronic diarrhea and opportunistic infections were recorded based on their presence in the electronic medical record as well as review of the hard copy paper records. If these conditions were not documented in the electronic medical record or paper charts they were reported as absent.

Lost to Follow up, Transfers and Deaths. Children were considered lost to follow up if they did not collect treatment for 3 consecutive months. Attempts were made to contact all children who were lost to follow up to determine their status. All lost to follow ups and transfers were censored on the date of their last visit. Otherwise follow-up time was censored at the end of the study period. Death events were defined as all-cause deaths occurring after ART initiation but before the May 31, 2009 end of the study period. Deaths were confirmed by hospital records or family interview. Cause of death was determined by the primary care physician or by verbal autopsy from family members.

Missing Data. In multivariate analysis, only subjects with complete data were analyzed. In univariate analysis subjects were included if they had complete data for the covariate of interest. No data was imputed for this analysis. Since weight-for-age Z-score was systematically missing for children older than 10 years, two variables were included simultaneously in the model for Z-score as a continuous variable and the other as a categorical indicating the absence of Z-score. Including both variable simultaneously allows children >10 years to be included in the multivariable model without imputing values.

Statistical Analysis

Statistical analyses were conducted using SAS statistical software (Release 9.2, Carey, NC). Time to mortality was assessed for subjects from the date of ART initiation to the date of death occurring before May 31, 2009 (end of the study period).

We used Cox proportional hazards regression models to assess associations between demographic and clinical characteristics and mortality. We first determined univariate associations between nine demographic and clinical covariates that, based upon clinical observations and prior studies, were suspected to be potentially important correlates of post-ART mortality. Age was stratified into 2 categories (<3 years and ≥3 years old) to account for the age related difference in ART treatment regimens. We did not assess the association between type of ART regimen (Protease Inhibitor verses Non-Nucleotide Reverse Transcriptor Inhibitor) and mortality in these analyses because the ART regimen was selected based on age, and thus these variables were highly correlated (Pearson correlation coefficient = 0.83). Gender was added in *a priori* to assess age and sex matched controls. Female gender was found to violate the proportional hazard assumption of the Cox model; therefore, was evaluated as a time varying hazard in the final model. We constructed Kaplan-Meier survival curves stratified by age and gender and assessed the difference between the curves using the log rank test. Since CD4 <15% is required for initiation of ART in most children in South Africa [17], the data was highly skewed; therefore, we stratified the CD4 percent variable at <10% and ≥10%. Using the remaining eight variables assessed in univariate analysis, we constructed a multivariable mortality model and used the Score Test criterion in combination with Akaike Information Criterion (AIC) to determine the most parsimonious model [18].

We evaluated the proportional hazards assumptions for the variables in the final multivariable mortality model using the Schoenfeld residuals method. This tests whether the residuals for each variable are uncorrelated (P>0.05) with the ordering of times to death events. We found that the female gender was significantly correlated with death event times (P = 0.02). The other variables were not significantly correlated with death event times. We therefore further evaluated the proportional hazards assumption for the female gender variable by assessing it within

Table 1. Demographic and Clinical Characteristics.

Baseline Characteristics	N Total	Complete Cohort	Males	Females	p-value
N	537		261 (48.6%)	276 (51.4%)	
Age at ART initiation (median; years) [IQR]	537	6.0 [2.4–9.3]	5.95 [2.23–8.75]	6.25 [3.1–9.7]	0.08
<3 years		149 (27.8%)	80 (30.7%)	69 (25%)	0.15
3–18 years		388 (72.2%)	181 (69.3%)	207 (75%)	
CD4 absolute (median; cells/μL)[IQR]	535	226 [70–447]	242 [80–467]	205 [69–438]	0.50
CD4 <10%	524	250 (47.7%)	126 (49.4%)	124 (46.1%)	0.48
Documented OI at baseline	537	138 (25.7%)	63 (24.1%)	75 27.2%)	0.43
Chronic Diarrhea	537	112 (20.9%)	59 (22.6%)	53 (19.2%)	0.34
Hemoglobin (median; g/dl)[IQR]	482	10.0 [8.9–11]	10 [8.8–10.9]	10.1 [8.9–11.1]	0.37
Weight-for-age z-score† (median) [IQR]	403	−1.4 [−2.6–−0.5]	−1.5 [−2.8–−0.6]	−1.3 [−2.4–−0.5]	0.14
TB at initiation of ART	537	228 (42.5%)	107 (41.1%)	121 (43.8%)	0.54
NNRTI treatment*		414 (77.1%)	195 (74.7%)	219 (79.4%)	0.22
Deaths		47 (8.8%)	19 (7.3%)	28 (10.1%)	0.29

*20 children in the <3 year old group were started on NNRTI while all children over 3 years old were initiated on NNRTI based treatment.
†WHO weight-for-age Z-score is only valid for children <10 years old.

the full multivariable Cox proportional hazards regression model as a time-varying covariate with time considered as natural log of time. This time varying covariate was significant ($P = 0.03$) after adjusting for the other covariates within the multivariable model.

Results

Patient Characteristics and Mortality

Demographic and clinical characteristics of the 537 analyzed subjects are described in Table 1. Forty-seven subjects died during the study period, with deaths occurring a median of 60 days after starting ART (range 5 days–2.7 years). The overall mortality in this cohort was low, with only 4.7 deaths per 100 child years on ART. Of the 490 surviving subjects, 18 (3.7%) (10 females, 8 males) were lost to medical follow-up and 72 (14.7%) (41 females, 31 males) subjects were no longer followed because they transferred care to another clinic. Median follow-up for the surviving subjects was 22 months, with follow-up ranging from 14 days to 5.3 years.

Most of these deaths occurred early; 64% (30) occurred within 3 months, and 83% (39) within 6 months of ART initiation. Only 3 children died after 12 months of ART, accounting for 0.56% of the entire cohort with a total follow up time in the study of over 991 child-years. Of the early deaths that occurred before 6 months on ART,28% (11) died of tuberculosis and 18% (7) died of diarrhea, dehydration or malnutrition. Among the children who died between 6 months and one year after initiation of ART, all 5 had plasma HIV RNA levels of <400 copies/ml measured after 6 months on ART. The cause of death was determined to be culture confirmed tuberculosis in 2 children (40%) (both with multiple episodes of tuberculosis treatment), severe malnutrition with chronic diarrhea in 2 children (40%) and unknown in 1 child (20%). Of the 3 children that died after completing one year of ART, 2 (66%) died with high levels of viremia on second-line ART and 1 child died of disseminated tuberculosis.

Table 2. Unadjusted Cox Proportional Hazard Ratios for Mortality after Initiating HIV Treatment.

Demographic and Clinical Variables† n = 537	Hazard Ratio (95% Confidence Interval) 47 death events	P value
Age <3 years	2.42 (1.37–4.30)	0.003
Female gender	1.43 (0.80–2.56)	0.23
Absolute CD4 count (cells/μL)	0.999 (0.998–1.000)	0.05
CD4 <10%	2.49 (1.33–4.66)	0.005
Hemoglobin (gm/dL)	0.76 (0.63–0.90)	0.002
Opportunistic infection not tuberculosis	1.85 (1.03–3.33)	0.04
Tuberculosis at or after initiation of HIV therapy	1.63 (0.92–2.92)	0.10
Chronic diarrhea	3.02 (1.69–5.39)	0.0002
Weight-for-age Z-score	0.53 (0.43, 0.64)	<0.0001

†*Absolute CD4, hemoglobin* and *weight-for-age Z-score* were treated as continuous variables. Reference groups for the binary variables include: *Age <3 years* – reference age 3–18 years; *CD4 <10%* - reference CD4 >10%, *Opportunistic infection* includes children with the presence of candidiasis, Kaposi's sarcoma, Pneumocystis jiroveci pneumonia, cryptococcosis, toxoplasmosis, or cryptosporidiosis, while the reference group did not have any of these opportunistic infections; *Tuberculosis at or after initiation or HIV therapy* – reference was the absence of HIV-tuberculosis co-infection; *chronic diarrhea* – reference children not documented to have chronic diarrhea.

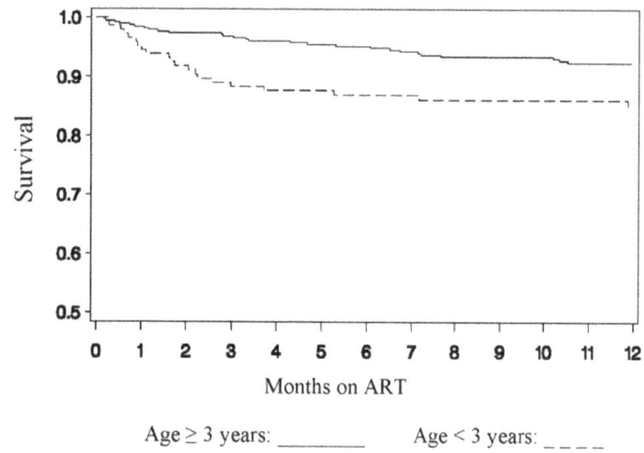

Figure 1. The age-stratified Kaplan-Meier graph of survival after ART initiation.

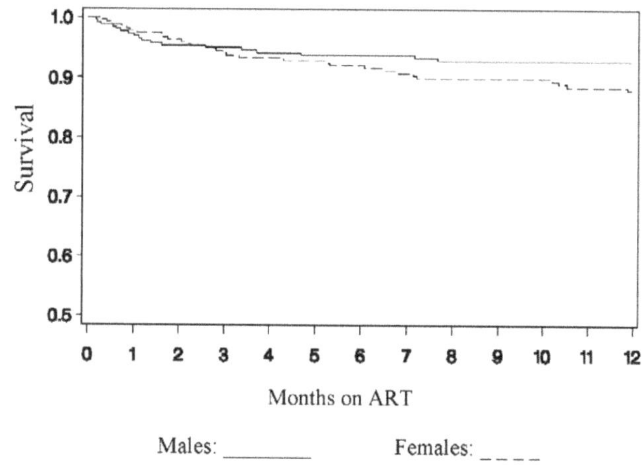

Figure 2. The gender-stratified Kaplan-Meier graph of survival after ART initiation.

Univariate Assessment of Mortality Risk

Univariate associations between demographic and clinical characteristics and mortality are shown in Table 2. Weight-for-age Z-score ($p<0.0001$), chronic diarrhea ($p=0.0002$), lower hemoglobin ($p=0.002$), age <3 years ($p=0.003$), and CD4% <10% ($p=0.005$) were all strongly associated with mortality. The age stratified Kaplan Meier survival curves for time after initiation of ART are shown in Figure 1. Non-TB opportunistic infections ($p=0.04$) and absolute CD4 count ($p=0.05$) were also significantly associated with death.

Multivariable Assessment of Mortality Risk

A multivariable Cox proportional hazards mortality model was developed using the following covariates: weight-for-age Z-score, chronic diarrhea, hemoglobin, CD4%, tuberculosis coinfection, presence of opportunistic infection, age <3 years, and gender. The final model, selected from the best fit model with the lowest AIC using the Score Test [13], is shown in Table 3. In multivariate analysis, age, CD4 <10%, chronic diarrhea, and weight-for-age Z-score were all shown to be strongly and independently predictive of mortality. Interestingly, this analysis also revealed a difference in the survival rate between males and females following initiation of ART. Although female gender was not significantly associated with mortality in univariate analysis, it was significantly associated ($p=0.03$) with mortality when controlling for age, weight-for-age Z-score, chronic diarrhea, and CD4%. The unadjusted Kaplan-Meier graph is illustrated in Figure 2. Female gender was best described as varying linearly with the natural log (ln) of time within the multivariable model.

Table 3. Adjusted Cox Proportional Hazard Ratios for Mortality after Initiating HIV Treatment.

Predictors † n = 524*	Hazard Ratio (95% Confidence Interval) 46 death events	P value
Age <3 years	2.66 (1.37–5.17)	0.004
CD4 <10%	2.39 (1.21–4.71)	0.01
Chronic diarrhea	1.91 (1.05–3.49)	0.03
Weight-to-age Z-score	0.59 (0.47–0.73)	<0.0001
Female*ln time‡	1.79 (1.05–3.49)	0.03

†*Weight-for-age Z-score* and *Female*ln time* were treated as continuous variables. Reference groups for the binary variables include: *Age <3 years* - reference age 3–18 years; *CD4 <10%* - reference CD4 >10%; *chronic diarrhea* - reference children not documented to have chronic diarrhea.
*13 subjects were missing one or more of the model's predictor variables and were not included in the analysis.
‡*Female*ln time* represents the interaction term of female gender and the natural log of time in weeks since ART initiation.

6 Month Viral Response

At six months of ART therapy there were 424 subjects with viral load data available. There was no significant difference ($p=0.56$) in viral suppression rates to <400 copies/ml between males 170/198 (86%) and females 199/226 (88%).

Sensitivity Analysis

In order to determine the impact of lost to follow-up, a sensitivity analysis was performed including the composite endpoint of lost to follow-up and death. This did not significantly change any results in the univarite analysis. In the multivariate analysis only the presence of chronic diarrhea was no longer significant with a p value of 0.12. Age less than three years ($p=0.006$), CD4 <10% ($p=0.016$), weight for age Z-score ($p<0.001$), and female gender ($p=0.007$) all remained significant.

Discussion

The increased availability of ART in sub-Saharan Africa has dramatically improved outcomes for pediatric patients infected with HIV. However, treatment guidelines and algorithms continue to evolve, and there is a pressing need for clinical outcomes data to further refine HIV management strategies for children in resource-limited settings. There is a particularly pressing need for data regarding clinical factors that place these children at increased risk of early mortality despite initiation of ART. Our findings agree with published data from other African cohorts that age <3 years, severely reduced CD4 percent (<10%), chronic diarrhea, and reduced weight-for-age Z-scores are strongly associated with mortality among HIV positive children initiating ART [5,7,8,9,10,11,19,20].

The mortality risk factors identified in this study highlight several areas for potential improvement in pediatric treatment and monitoring algorithms. The increased mortality in younger children and those with low CD4 plus the growing body of evidence of improved outcomes in infant ART initiation argues for the early initiation of ART in HIV positive children [21]. In response, WHO treatment guidelines have recently been altered to recommend expansion of ART to all infants younger than 24 months and all young children with CD4 percentages lower than 25% [22]. Importantly, the vast majority of deaths in our cohort occurred prior to the first set of monitoring labs, which are drawn after six months of therapy per South African guidelines. It would seem prudent to target children with multiple risk factors to receive earlier clinical and laboratory follow-up to ensure an adequate response to therapy. The increased mortality in children with chronic diarrhea and low weight-for-age Z-score at the time of initiation of ART indicates the importance of monitoring nutritional status at the time of ART initiation and argues for earlier ART initiation in these children. Future studies on early aggressive nutritional monitoring and interventions could lead to improved outcomes in children with malnutrition or chronic diarrhea. An unexpected finding from our study was the increased risk of mortality observed among females after controlling for other risk factors. The mortality risk associated with female gender increased progressively with time after initiation of ART therapy. It is unclear whether this disparity is attributable to intrinsic biological differences between the sexes [13,14,23,24,25] or social differences such as delayed presentation for care, differences in parental supervision of boys and girls, or devaluation of the female gender that could place females at a higher risk of mortality after ART initiation in South Africa. Among adults, females tend to have lower viral loads early in HIV-1 infection but progress faster to AIDS for a given viral load than males [15,25,26]. Therefore, it has been suggested that initiating HAART based on CD4 and viral load criteria without accounting for gender differences may disadvantage women [25]. Although pediatric data are limited, two prior studies have suggested gender differences in HIV viral loads among children [13,14], which could provide a biologically plausible basis for our observation of a gender difference in survival on HAART. This finding has not been seen in other HIV mortality analyses of African children [5,7,8,9], most of which utilized smaller cohorts or pooled data from multiple centers. However, a similar increase in mortality was seen among female children in the Women and Infants Transmission Study (WITS), a longitudinal study of HIV-infected children in North America [14]. In addition, the European Collaborative group found more rapid disease progression in HIV infected females less than 4 years old [13]. The published data regarding the impact of gender on survival in HIV-infected adults are significantly confounded by differences in healthcare utilization, as several North American studies have reported lower healthcare utilization and viral suppression rates among women [27,28,29], while several African studies have reported better health utilization and outcomes among HIV positive women on ART [30,31,32,33,34]. However, data from adult studies may not be generalizable to young girls, who are dependent on adult caregivers for accessing clinic services. Therefore, local societal devaluation of female children may place them at unique risk for poor outcomes on ART.

Although tuberculosis co-infection was not significantly associated with mortality in this analysis, this cohort did exhibit a high incidence of tuberculosis infections and TB was a major contributor to deaths. The high incidence of TB may represent over diagnosis and overlap with lymphocytic interstitial pneumonitis [35]. Given the clinical setting many of these were not bacteriologically confirmed cases tuberculosis; however, represented clinical diagnosis based on symptoms, radiography, and contact information. This highlights the pressing need for improved diagnostics for pediatric tuberculosis infections.

One limitation of our study is that it assesses a single cohort of HIV positive children from KwaZulu-Natal, South Africa, and a relatively small number of subjects (8.8%) died during the study period. It is possible that larger studies with increased statistical power may identify other risk factors that significantly predict mortality after initiation of ART in pediatric HIV patients. Given the small number of children lost to follow-up (LTFU), sensitivity analysis using the composite endpoint of LTFU and mortality did not significantly alter the major findings of this study. In addition, this study was located in a semi-private institution which had nominal user fees of R50 (approximately $7 USD) per month which could result in a selection bias toward a wealthier population. In contrast to many sub-Saharan pediatric populations, our cohort generally had access to daily meals and water, as well as medical care at a semi-private clinic, and thus our results may not be generalizable to more impoverished settings.

Further studies are needed to define gender differences in the biological manifestations of HIV infection in boys and girls, and to determine the relationship between gender and survival among children receiving treatment for HIV infection. Our expanding knowledge of the risk factors associated with mortality in HIV infected children on ART can help to further refine HIV treatment guidelines and monitoring practices.

Acknowledgments

The authors would like to thank the dedicated clinical staff at McCord Hospital, especially Janet Giddy, Zinhle Gwala, and Jill Dorse. The authors would also like to thank Roger Davis and Amanda Fox for their guidance and assistance with the statistical analysis for this project.

Author Contributions

Conceived and designed the experiments: BCZ MEF. Performed the experiments: BCZ TP HMZ HF. Analyzed the data: BCZ MEF. Contributed reagents/materials/analysis tools: BCZ MEF. Wrote the paper: BCZ MEF.

References

1. UNAIDS (2009) Aids Epidemic Update. Geneva, Switzerland: Joint United Nations Programme on HIV/AIDS (UNAIDS) and World Health Orginization (WHO).
2. Taha TE, Graham SM, Kumwenda NI, Broadhead RL, Hoover DR, et al. (2000) Morbidity among human immunodeficiency virus-1-infected and -uninfected African children. Pediatrics 106: E77.
3. Prendergast A, Tudor-Williams G, Jeena P, Burchett S, Goulder P (2007) International perspectives, progress, and future challenges of paediatric HIV infection. Lancet 370: 68–80.
4. Bolton-Moore C, Mubiana-Mbewe M, Cantrell RA, Chintu N, Stringer EM, et al. (2007) Clinical outcomes and CD4 cell response in children receiving antiretroviral therapy at primary health care facilities in Zambia. JAMA 298: 1888–1899.
5. Leyenaar JK, Novosad PM, Ferrer KT, Thahane LK, Mohapi EQ, et al. (2010) Early clinical outcomes in children enrolled in human immunodeficiency virus infection care and treatment in lesotho. Pediatr Infect Dis J 29: 340–345.
6. Havens PL, Gibb DM (2007) Increasing antiretroviral drug access for children with HIV infection. Pediatrics 119: 838–845.
7. Kiboneka A, Wangisi J, Nabiryo C, Tembe J, Kusemererwa S, et al. (2008) Clinical and immunological outcomes of a national paediatric cohort receiving combination antiretroviral therapy in Uganda. AIDS 22: 2493–2499.
8. Bong CN, Yu JK, Chiang HC, Huang WL, Hsieh TC, et al. (2007) Risk factors for early mortality in children on adult fixed-dose combination antiretroviral treatment in a central hospital in Malawi. AIDS 21: 1805–1810.
9. Fenner L, Brinkhof MW, Keiser O, Weigel R, Cornell M, et al. (2010) Early mortality and loss to follow-up in HIV-infected children starting antiretroviral therapy in Southern Africa. J Acquir Immune Defic Syndr 54: 524–532.

10. Wamalwa DC, Obimbo EM, Farquhar C, Richardson BA, Mbori-Ngacha DA, et al. (2010) Predictors of mortality in HIV-1 infected children on antiretroviral therapy in Kenya: a prospective cohort. BMC Pediatr 10: 33.
11. Callens SF, Shabani N, Lusiama J, Lelo P, Kitetele F, et al. (2009) Mortality and associated factors after initiation of pediatric antiretroviral treatment in the Democratic Republic of the Congo. Pediatr Infect Dis J 28: 35–40.
12. Sterling TR, Lyles CM, Vlahov D, Astemborski J, Margolick JB, et al. (1999) Sex differences in longitudinal human immunodeficiency virus type 1 RNA levels among seroconverters. The Journal of infectious diseases 180: 666–672.
13. European Collaborative Study (2002) Level and pattern of HIV-1-RNA viral load over age: differences between girls and boys? AIDS 16: 97–104.
14. Foca M, Moye J, Chu C, Matthews Y, Rich K, et al. (2006) Gender differences in lymphocyte populations, plasma HIV RNA levels, and disease progression in a cohort of children born to women infected with HIV. Pediatrics 118: 146–155.
15. Farzadegan H, Hoover DR, Astemborski J, Lyles CM, Margolick JB, et al. (1998) Sex differences in HIV-1 viral load and progression to AIDS. Lancet 352: 1510–1514.
16. Richardson BA, Mbori-Ngacha D, Lavreys L, John-Stewart GC, Nduati R, et al. (2003) Comparison of human immunodeficiency virus type 1 viral loads in Kenyan women, men, and infants during primary and early infection. Journal of virology 77: 7120–7123.
17. South African National Department of Health (2004) National Antiretroviral Treatment Guidelines. In: Health NDo, ed. Johannesberg, South Africa: Minutemann Press.
18. Collett D (2003) Modeling Survival Data in Medical Research. New York: Chapman and Hall.
19. Yotebieng M, Van Rie A, Moultrie H, Cole SR, Adimora A, et al. (2010) Effect on mortality and virological response of delaying antiretroviral therapy initiation in children receiving tuberculosis treatment. AIDS 24: 1341–1349.
20. Reddi A, Leeper SC, Grobler AC, Geddes R, France KH, et al. (2007) Preliminary outcomes of a paediatric highly active antiretroviral therapy cohort from KwaZulu-Natal, South Africa. BMC Pediatr 7: 13.
21. Violari A, Cotton MF, Gibb DM, Babiker AG, Steyn J, et al. (2008) Early antiretroviral therapy and mortality among HIV-infected infants. N Engl J Med 359: 2233–2244.
22. World Health Organization (2010) Antiretroviral Therapy for HIV Infection in Infants and Children: Toward Universal Access. Geneva, Switzerland: World Health Organization.
23. Meier A, Chang JJ, Chan ES, Pollard RB, Sidhu HK, et al. (2009) Sex differences in the Toll-like receptor-mediated response of plasmacytoid dendritic cells to HIV-1. Nat Med 15: 955–959.
24. Sterling TR, Vlahov D, Astemborski J, Hoover DR, Margolick JB, et al. (2001) Initial plasma HIV-1 RNA levels and progression to AIDS in women and men. N Engl J Med 344: 720–725.
25. Sterling TR, Lyles CM, Vlahov D, Astemborski J, Margolick JB, et al. (1999) Sex differences in longitudinal human immunodeficiency virus type 1 RNA levels among seroconverters. J Infect Dis 180: 666–672.
26. Gandhi M, Bacchetti P, Miotti P, Quinn TC, Veronese F, et al. (2002) Does patient sex affect human immunodeficiency virus levels? Clin Infect Dis 35: 313–322.
27. Sohler NL, Li X, Cunningham CO (2009) Gender disparities in HIV health care utilization among the severely disadvantaged: can we determine the reasons? AIDS Patient Care STDS 23: 775–783.
28. Shapiro MF, Morton SC, McCaffrey DF, Senterfitt JW, Fleishman JA, et al. (1999) Variations in the care of HIV-infected adults in the United States: results from the HIV Cost and Services Utilization Study. JAMA 281: 2305–2315.
29. Box TL, Olsen M, Oddone EZ, Keitz SA (2003) Healthcare access and utilization by patients infected with human immunodeficiency virus: does gender matter? J Womens Health (Larchmt) 12: 391–397.
30. Kipp W, Alibhai A, Saunders LD, Senthilselvan A, Kaler A, et al. (2010) Gender differences in antiretroviral treatment outcomes of HIV patients in rural Uganda. AIDS Care 22: 271–278.
31. Braitstein P, Boulle A, Nash D, Brinkhof MW, Dabis F, et al. (2008) Gender and the use of antiretroviral treatment in resource-constrained settings: findings from a multicenter collaboration. J Womens Health (Larchmt) 17: 47–55.
32. Muula AS, Ngulube TJ, Siziya S, Makupe CM, Umar E, et al. (2007) Gender distribution of adult patients on highly active antiretroviral therapy (HAART) in Southern Africa: a systematic review. BMC Public Health 7: 63.
33. Collazos J, Asensi V, Carton JA (2007) Sex differences in the clinical, immunological and virological parameters of HIV-infected patients treated with HAART. AIDS 21: 835–843.
34. Chen SC, Yu JK, Harries AD, Bong CN, Kolola-Dzimadzi R, et al. (2008) Increased mortality of male adults with AIDS related to poor compliance to antiretroviral therapy in Malawi. Trop Med Int Health 13: 513–519.
35. Zanoni BC, Phungula T, Zanoni HM, France H, Feeney ME (2011) Impact of tuberculosis cotreatment on viral suppression rates among HIV-positive children initiating HAART. AIDS 25: 49–55.

14

Close Encounters in a Pediatric Ward: Measuring Face-to-Face Proximity and Mixing Patterns with Wearable Sensors

Lorenzo Isella[1], Mariateresa Romano[2], Alain Barrat[1,3], Ciro Cattuto[1], Vittoria Colizza[1], Wouter Van den Broeck[1], Francesco Gesualdo[2], Elisabetta Pandolfi[2], Lucilla Ravà[2], Caterina Rizzo[4], Alberto Eugenio Tozzi[2]*

1 Complex Networks and Systems Group, Institute for Scientific Interchange (ISI) Foundation, Torino, Italy, **2** Epidemiology Unit, Bambino Gesù Hospital, Rome, Italy, **3** Centre de Physique Théorique de Marseille, CNRS UMR 6207, Marseille, France, **4** National Centre for Epidemiology, Surveillance and Health Promotion, Istituto Superiore di Sanità Rome, Rome, Italy

Abstract

Background: Nosocomial infections place a substantial burden on health care systems and represent one of the major issues in current public health, requiring notable efforts for its prevention. Understanding the dynamics of infection transmission in a hospital setting is essential for tailoring interventions and predicting the spread among individuals. Mathematical models need to be informed with accurate data on contacts among individuals.

Methods and Findings: We used wearable active Radio-Frequency Identification Devices (RFID) to detect face-to-face contacts among individuals with a spatial resolution of about 1.5 meters, and a time resolution of 20 seconds. The study was conducted in a general pediatrics hospital ward, during a one-week period, and included 119 participants, with 51 health care workers, 37 patients, and 31 caregivers. Nearly 16,000 contacts were recorded during the study period, with a median of approximately 20 contacts per participants per day. Overall, 25% of the contacts involved a ward assistant, 23% a nurse, 22% a patient, 22% a caregiver, and 8% a physician. The majority of contacts were of brief duration, but long and frequent contacts especially between patients and caregivers were also found. In the setting under study, caregivers do not represent a significant potential for infection spread to a large number of individuals, as their interactions mainly involve the corresponding patient. Nurses would deserve priority in prevention strategies due to their central role in the potential propagation paths of infections.

Conclusions: Our study shows the feasibility of accurate and reproducible measures of the pattern of contacts in a hospital setting. The obtained results are particularly useful for the study of the spread of respiratory infections, for monitoring critical patterns, and for setting up tailored prevention strategies. Proximity-sensing technology should be considered as a valuable tool for measuring such patterns and evaluating nosocomial prevention strategies in specific settings.

Editor: Benjamin Cowling, University of Hong Kong, Hong Kong

Funding: This work has been partially supported by the Italian Ministry of Health (Grant n. 1M22) to C.R., A.T. and C.C.; by the EC FET-Open project DYNANETS (contract number 233847) to L.I. and V.C.; and by the ERC Ideas grant EpiFor (contract no. ERC-2007-Stg204863) to V.C. The funders had no role in study design, data collection and analysis, decision to publish, or preparation of the manuscript. No additional external funding was received for this study.

Competing Interests: The authors have declared that no competing interests exist.

* E-mail: alberto.tozzi@gmail.com

Introduction

The knowledge of contact patterns among individuals is of paramount importance in the control of infections transmitted from person to person. Patterns of transmission of infections in a given population can be studied using data on contact patterns, knowing the transmission route of the infection, the characteristics of the infectious agent, and the immunity profiles of individuals. The knowledge of patterns of transmission is essential to identify specific mechanisms that favor transmission and thus to set up tailored intervention strategies such as social or physical barriers, targeted immunization, pharmaceutical interventions, and other measures aimed at preventing transmission and controlling the spread of the disease [1–8].

The parameters relevant to contact patterns are mostly obtained from surveys conducted in samples of individuals or can be indirectly estimated from seroprevalence data or from time-use data, and are then extrapolated to the general population [9–15]. Several empirical studies have been recently conducted to determine the pattern of contacts between and within groups in different social settings to model the spread of infectious diseases, most often relying on self-reported methods [10,16]. The study of contacts through interviews and recall of previous encounters has however some limitations, as the data collection is not based on objective measurements and is generally performed on a random day, thus lacking the longitudinal dimension [17]. Most importantly, this approach has a limited applicability to specific settings, such as, e.g., hospitals, that require high-resolution information both at the spatial and temporal level to accurately characterize the interactions among individuals, in an objective way and by means of non-obtrusive methodologies.

The lack of such information has so far limited the guidelines on preventive strategies for the epidemiology of hospital acquired infections mostly to general and qualitative recommendations, that cannot take into account the characteristics of patients, procedures, hospital wards, structures and logistics, and the related heterogeneities across diverse hospital settings [18]. Similarly, while mathematical models have begun to provide insights into many important questions in the epidemiology of nosocomial infections [19], these results mostly focus on qualitative predictions [20], due to the very basic and homogeneous approaches adopted in the description of the population contact structure. On the other hand, fine-grained behavioral information may be used to inform and validate agent-based models of nosocomial infection [21].

To overcome such limitations and address the lack of empirical data relevant to the study of nosocomial infections, we rely on the technology of networked wearable sensors, that provides a novel approach to obtain accurate and tailored estimates of the contact patterns at the individual level in a given community [22–27]. Specifically, we use active Radio-Frequency Identification Devices (RFID) as wearable sensors to measure face-to-face proximity with a high spatial and temporal resolution [24–26]. The deployment of these devices may support the collection of accurate and timely information useful to inform and parameterize models for the study and prediction of the transmission of nosocomial infections, as well as to tailor containment measures for the control of potential outbreaks. To this aim, we present here the results of a study on the measurement and analysis of contact patterns within a pediatric hospital involving patients, caregivers, and health care workers. Our work illustrates the feasibility of contact measures through RFID devices in hospital settings, aimed at providing data-driven knowledge to inform models and prevention strategies.

Methods

Study setting

The study was performed in a general pediatric ward of the Bambino Gesù Hospital in Rome, Italy, a large third level pediatric hospital. The ward under study has 44 beds arranged in 22 rooms with 2 beds each, and mostly admits children with acute diseases who do not require intensive care or surgery. The occupancy rate of the ward is rarely below 95%. The pediatric ward is located in the Department of Pediatrics and is physically separated from other wards and facilities of the Hospital. In a typical workday 10 physicians, 20 nurses, and 6 ward assistants are on duty. Patients admitted into the ward are accompanied by one parent or tutor who spends the night in the same room on a chair. Visitors are allowed to visit the ward during the scheduled visit time of 1 hour in the afternoon. The study was conducted from the 9th to the 16th of November 2009 (weeks 46 and 47), during the incidence peak of the influenza A/H1N1v pandemic in Italy [28].

Data collection infrastructure

Data were obtained and collected through the deployment of an infrastructure consisting of a distributed sensing component, comprising wearable active Radio-Frequency Identification Devices (RFID), and of a data collection and processing component made of RFID readers installed in the ward, a local area network (LAN), and a central computer system for data collection and storage. The deployed RFID devices exchange ultra-low power radio packets in a peer-to-peer fashion. The devices perform a scan of their neighborhood by alternating transmit and receive cycles. During the transmit phase, low-power packets are sent out on a specific radio channel; during the receive phase, the devices listen on the same channel for packets sent by nearby devices. By including the transmitting signal strength in the payload, the receiving device can estimate the degree of proximity of the transmitting device, and this operation can be carried out in a decentralized fashion throughout the sensing network. A more detailed description of the data gathering infrastructure is reported in Refs. [24–26].

The lowest power level used in this deployment was selected to allow packet exchange only between devices within 1–1.5 meters of one another. This setting ensures that when individuals wear the devices on their chest, exchange of radio packets between RFID devices is only possible when they are facing each other, as the human body acts as a RF shield at the carrier frequency used for communication. When a relation of face-to-face proximity is detected, it is relayed from the RFID devices to the RFID readers installed in the hospital ward. The receiving infrastructure only covered the area within the hospital ward under study. The RFID devices are embedded in small hermetically sealed badges to comply with the security regulations of the hospital, and to minimize potential damage arising from their use. Each device has a unique identification number that was used to link the information on the contacts established by the person carrying the device with his/her profile.

Study design

The study was approved by the Ethical Committee of the Bambino Gesù Hospital. Before the study started, health care workers were invited to participate in a meeting where the project was fully explained and its procedure was illustrated in detail. Health care personnel, patients, and their caregivers (defined as tutors, accompanying persons and visitors) were systematically invited to participate in the study. At the time of enrollment, all participants signed an informed consent form, were given an RFID badge, and were asked to wear it at all times within the ward. The RFID tags of a patient and accompanying persons were returned to the study personnel at patient discharge or when moved to another ward. Visitors returned their tag at the end of the visit, whereas health care workers wore RFID tags for the entire duration of the study during working hours. Correct wearing of the RFID tags was monitored daily, and in case of loss or other anomalies the tag was replaced with a new one. The correct operation of devices was also monitored by reviewing the quality of the received signals on a daily basis, and replacing malfunctioning devices. While patients were fully identified to link personal information to pattern of contacts detected by RFID devices, no personal identifiers were used for caregivers or health care workers participating in the study, which were only associated to their professional category. However, the association between a given health care worker and the corresponding RFID tag was fixed throughout the study, i.e., it was possible to track the behavior of the (anonymous) given individual across hospital shifts and across working days. Overall, individuals were distinguished into the following classes or roles for the purpose of the present study: ward assistants (A), who are health care workers in charge of cleaning the ward and distributing the meals, physicians (D), nurses (N), patients (P), and caregivers (C), who comprise tutors and non professional visitors.

Data processing and analysis

We tuned the rate at which low-power packets are emitted and the fraction of time the devices spend listening on the contact channel so that the face-to-face proximity of two individuals wearing the RFID tags can be assessed with a probability in excess of 99% over an interval of 20 seconds. This sets the time scale over which we perform the temporal aggregation of the collected data, allowing for an adequate description of person-to-person interactions that includes brief encounters. Faster timescales are prone to increasing noise and do not result in a higher accuracy of the detection process. We defined that a 'contact' occurs between two individuals during an interval of 20s if and only if the RFID devices worn by the individuals exchanged at least one packet at the lowest power level during that interval. After a contact is established, it is considered ongoing as long as the devices continue to exchange at least one such packet for every subsequent 20s interval. Conversely, a contact is considered broken if a 20s interval elapses with no exchange of low-power packets.

The patterns of close encounters between individuals and the mixing patterns among classes of individuals were analyzed through several indicators. The high spatial and temporal resolution of the infrastructure allows us to monitor the number of contacts that each individual establishes with any other individual, to record the time spent on each such encounter, the cumulative time spent in contact between two individuals, and the frequency of encounters between any two individuals. More in detail, for each pair of individuals i and j we define several possible weights w_{ij}, each corresponding to a different quantity measured on the collected data: the *occurrence of the contact* w^p_{ij}, with $w^p_{ij}=1$ if at least one contact between i and j has been established, and 0 otherwise; the *frequency of the contact* w^n_{ij}, indicating how many times the contact between i and j is observed during the study; the time spent on each such encounter; the *cumulative duration of the contact* w^t_{ij}, indicating the sum of the durations of all contacts established between i and j observed during the study. In addition to the above quantities, that are weights defined for pairs of individuals i and j, it is possible to define corresponding quantities s_i for each individual i, aggregating on all individuals j who had a contact with i, i.e., $s_i = \sum w_{ij}$. In relation to the previously defined weights, one obtains the following quantities: the *number of distinct contacts* s^p_i, indicating the number of distinct individuals with whom i has established at least one contact (i.e., a contact between i and j that occurs $w^n_{ij} > 1$ times is counted only once); the *number of contacts* s^n_i, indicating the overall number of contacts established by individual i, counting repeated contacts with the same individual j as distinct events; the *cumulative time in contact* s^t_i, corresponding to the total sum of the duration of all contacts involving individual i.

In the following, unless otherwise stated, all measures are normalized on a 24-hour (daily) interval, e.g., all cumulative times in contact are divided by the duration of the study expressed in days (8 days). Figure 1 provides an example on how the above quantities are computed for a schematic sequence of contact data, where the individuals i and j belong to two different classes, nurses (N) and patients (P).

Results

Sample characteristics

A total of 195 individuals were invited to participate in the study, and 7 of them (3.6%, 5 health care workers, 1 patient, 1 caregiver) declined participation. A total of 188 individuals were provided with an RFID tag. Before performing the analysis, we reviewed the collected data with specific regard to the quality of signals, and monitored the continuous detection of signals from the devices. In particular, for patients and caregivers classes, we compared the duration of their physical presence at the ward, as obtained from hospital records, with the presence recorded from the RFID infrastructure. We identified and excluded 69 RFIDs belonging to patients or caregivers whose signals were not continuously detected by the receiving infrastructure and were missing for at least 25% of the time they were assigned to the individuals. Given that patients and caregivers spend most of the time at a fixed location in the ward, the above exclusion criterion mainly has the purpose of ensuring good radio coverage of the corresponding rooms. No exclusion was considered in the case of health care workers, as their RFID tags were anonymized and therefore not traceable to their duties; no comparison with paper records was possible, and all signals from those tags were thus retained in the analysis. Results were statistically assessed in terms of their robustness with respect to such filtering procedure and to the chosen 25% threshold, and no strong dependence on the selected subset of individuals was found, as shown in Fig. S1 of the Supplementary Information, which displays unfiltered data.

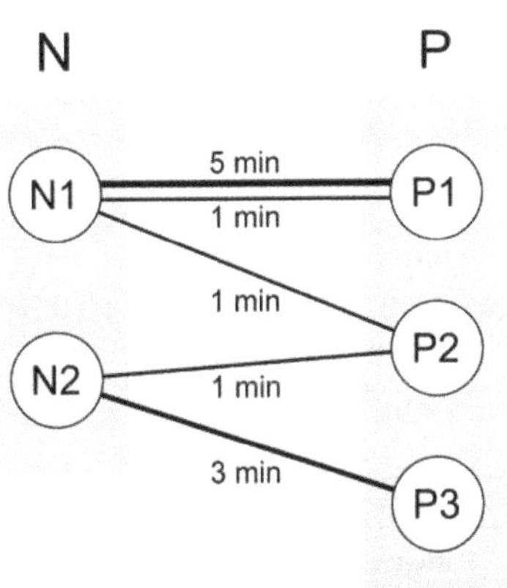

$w^p_{N1,P1} = 1$	$s^p_{N1} = 2$
$w^n_{N1,P1} = 2$	$s^n_{N1} = 3$
$w^t_{N1,P1} = 6$ min	$s^t_{N1} = 7$ min

Figure 1. Schematic representation of detected contacts among 2 nurses (N1, N2) and 3 patients (P1, P2, P3) and corresponding measured quantities. Each individual is represented by a node and a link corresponds to a contact established between two individuals. The width of the link is a measure of the duration of the contact, also indicated explicitly in terms of minutes. Multiple links can occur between two individuals, as highlighted in the pair N1-P1, indicating a contact of frequency larger than 1. The quantities introduced in the Materials and Methods section are calculated for the pair of individuals N1 and P1. The pair established one contact $\left(w^p_{ij}=1\right)$ with frequency equal to two $\left(w^n_{ij}=2\right)$ for a total duration of six minutes $\left(w^t_{ij}=6\text{min}\right)$. By taking into account all interactions, individual N1 has established three contacts $(s^n_i=3)$, two of which were distinct contacts $(s^p_i=2)$, for a total duration of contacts equal to seven minutes $(s^t_i=7\text{min})$.

The analysis therefore included a total of 119 individuals: 10 ward assistants (8.4% of the total number of individuals), 20 physicians (16.8%), 21 nurses (17.6%), 37 patients (31.1%) and 31 caregivers (26.1%). Table 1 reports the characteristics of patients and their discharge diagnoses with regard to airborne infections. Age, length of stay, and the proportion of children with any respiratory infections were similar when comparing the two subsets of patients retained and excluded from the study because of the filtering procedure. We used the median test for comparing age and length of stay, and the chi- square test for the distribution of diagnoses, and the statistical comparison did not yield results signaling any significant difference between the two subsets. Despite the majority of patients was discharged with a diagnosis of a potentially transmissible disease, during the study period no evidence of transmission of nosocomial infection in patients or health care workers was reported according to the routine nosocomial infection surveillance system.

Number, frequency and duration of contacts by category

A total of nearly 16,000 contacts were recorded during the study period, with a median of approximately 20 contacts per participants per day. Table 2 reports the total number of contacts established by individuals for each class, and the median values per participant of the given category. A very large number of contacts involve at least a ward assistant or a nurse. In addition, significant fractions of the overall number of contacts are found to involve at least a patient or a caregiver, representing approximately 22% of the total in both cases. The minimum number of contacts is observed for physicians (8%).

The daily median number of contacts per individual, shown in Figure 2A, is highest among ward assistants, and it is much higher than the values observed for other classes (the second largest value is 45.5 contacts established by an average nurse, compared to 99.5 contacts in the ward assistant case). This pattern is explained by the organization of the staff duties, as ward assistants are requested mainly to clean up, to transport patients, and to distribute food, and they mostly work in pairs. Figure 2B reports the daily median number of distinct contacts s^p that participants of a given class establish with any other participant, showing that health-care workers are involved in interactions with a larger number of distinct individuals, typically 3–5 distinct contacts, whereas patients and caregivers mostly interact with a single person, with high frequency. In addition to the number and the frequency of contacts, the RFID infrastructure enables the accurate measurement of the duration of contacts between individuals, providing a more detailed characterization of proximity events, which is generally hard to achieve by using traditional survey methodologies. Figure 2C shows the cumulative time in contact, s^t, spent by individuals belonging to each of the roles. This quantity is highly heterogeneous, ranging, daily, from a few minutes for physicians up to approximately one hour for ward assistants.

The computed quantities show large heterogeneities among individuals of the same class and across the various days of the study. Figure 3A reports the probability density function $P(s^n)$ (number of events in each bin divided by the bin width) of the number of contacts s^n obtained for each class of participants. The distribution $P(s^n)$ for a given class is defined as the probability that a randomly selected participant of that class has established a total of s^n contacts with any other individual during a given day. Large fluctuations are visible in the number of contacts per individual, varying over 2 or 3 orders of magnitude, and the largest fluctuations are observed in the case of patients and caregivers. Figure 3B reports the probability density functions of the cumulative time in contact, for individuals of each class. The longest durations, up to nearly 4 hours, are observed for contacts that involve at least one patient or one caregiver. The observed broad probability distributions are typical of human-driven systems and have been already observed elsewhere [25,26]. Figure 4 shows boxplots for the distributions of cumulative contact durations w^t between pairs of individuals belonging to given categories. Overall, about 95% of the contacts have a cumulated duration w^t of less than 4 minutes.

Besides characterizing the overall behavior of a given class of participants interacting with any other individual, the collected data allow to further inspect the interaction behavior by focusing on face-to-face proximity between pairs of categories. Figure 5 reports three contact matrices defined on the classes of participants, taking into account the different numbers of individuals in each class [3], and measured using the three quantities defined above: the number of contacts s^n (panel A), the number of distinct contacts s^p (panel B), and the cumulative time in contact s^t (panel C). Panel A shows that the majority of contacts occur within the ward assistant class, followed by nurse-nurse interactions. A number of contacts larger than 10 is also observed for patient-caregiver interactions, considering both the number of contacts that a patient had with any caregiver, and the number of contacts that a caregiver had with any patient. These contacts, however, are characterized by a very high frequency, as signaled by the very small number of distinct contacts reported in panel B for the same two classes, consistent with a strong one-to-one patient-caregiver interaction. A smaller number of distinct contacts is also observed among ward assistants, compared to the median value of 63 contacts, whereas the nurse-nurse interaction remains strong also in terms of number of distinct contacts. The number of contacts (both distinct and non-distinct) among patients is noticeably very low and close to zero. The contact matrix computed in terms of the cumulative time in contact provides yet another characterization of the interaction behavior among classes. Long interactions are observed between

Table 1. Characteristics of patients included and excluded from the analysis.

	Patients excluded from analysis due to poor signal quality	Patients included in the analysis	Total
Number	39	37	76
Age, years; median (range)	3.04 (41 d–17 y)	3.54 (44 d–17 y)	3.38 (41 d–17 y)
Length of stay, days; median (range)	5 (1–36)	7 (1–29)	6 (1–36)
No. of patients with H1N1 infection (%)	7 (17.9%)	12 (32.4%)	19 (25.0%)
No. of patients with acute respiratory infections other than H1N1 (%)	18 (46.1%)	14 (37.8%)	32 (42.1%)

Table 2. Characteristics of the study sample in terms of classes and number of contacts.

Role	No. participants (%)	Total no. daily contacts	No. daily contacts per participant [90% confidence interval] [90% CI]
(A) Ward assistants	10 (8.4%)	991.1	99.5 [38.3–172.8]
(N) Nurses	21 (17.6%)	920.2	45.5 [9.2–83.1]
(C) Caregivers/Accompanying persons/Visitors	31 (26.1%)	910.2	18.1 [3.4–69.4]
(P) Patients	37 (31.1%)	880.6	16.1 [0.5–63.6]
(D) Physicians	20 (16.8%)	325	14.0 [0.4–41.8]

The total number of daily contacts measured per class is the sum of all contacts s^n established by individuals in that class. The number of daily contacts per participant is the median value of the number of contacts s_i^n, with i belonging to the given class.

patients and caregivers, among nurses, and among ward assistants. The time spent in close proximity by a pair of patients or by a pair of visitors is extremely small, and interactions between a health care worker and a non-health care worker are very limited. Fluctuations of these values are reported in Tables S1, S2, and S3 of the Supplementary Information.

Individual level resolution

The results presented so far are broken down into categories of participants and provide an aggregated quantitative estimation of the interaction behavior inter- and intra-classes. Additional information can however be gathered at the individual level, given the high resolution of the infrastructure used for the data collection. A reconstruction of the network of interactions among single individuals can be achieved to inspect in a deeper fashion the aggregated features reported above. Figure 6 shows a set of interaction networks for each pair of classes and within each class, corresponding to the entire monitoring period. In these networks, a node represents an individual, and an edge is drawn between two individuals whenever a face-to-face proximity event involving them was recorded. The networks restricted to physicians, nurses or ward assistants are rather dense, indicating a large diversity of contacts: within a given role, each health care worker interacts with many others. The picture is completely different for patients and caregivers: not only are there very few contacts between caregivers or between patients, but, as expected, the patient-caregiver contacts are very specific. Each patient has contacts with essentially one caregiver, and vice-versa, which corresponds to the fact that each patient was accompanied by one caregiver, confirming at the individual level the results previously observed at the class level. Contacts among caregivers and among patients are barely observed.

Discussion

Mathematical and computational models play an increasingly important role in the assessment and control of epidemics. In addition to studies focusing on the general population, models are also used to study the spread of infectious diseases in specific settings, such as, e.g., hospitals. Nosocomial infections represent a major public health issue with high morbidity and mortality and high costs associated with prolonged treatments, which deserve urgent and efficacious prevention strategies. The sources and transmission paths of nosocomial infections are indeed often unknown and unrecognized. The application of epidemic models to hospitals is therefore crucial to provide valuable insights on the routes of infection propagation and to identify tailored measures for prevention and control of hospital acquired infections. Models need to be informed with the pattern of interactions among individuals along which the transmission of infection can occur, however only simple homogeneous assumptions have been considered so far. Our

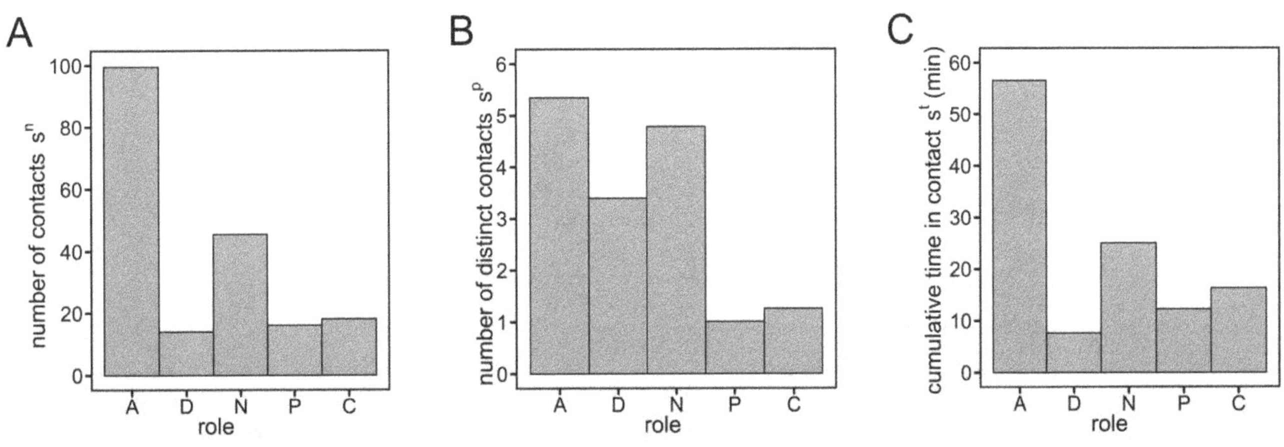

Figure 2. Contact number and duration per role (A: ward assistants; D: Doctor; N: Nurse; P: Patients; C: Caregiver). The plots show the median values per participant in each class of: the number of contacts s^n (panel A), the number of distinct contacts s^p (panel B), the cumulative time in contact s^t (panel C). All quantities for a given class are computed on the contacts established by participants in that class with any other participant. Data are normalized to a 24-hour interval.

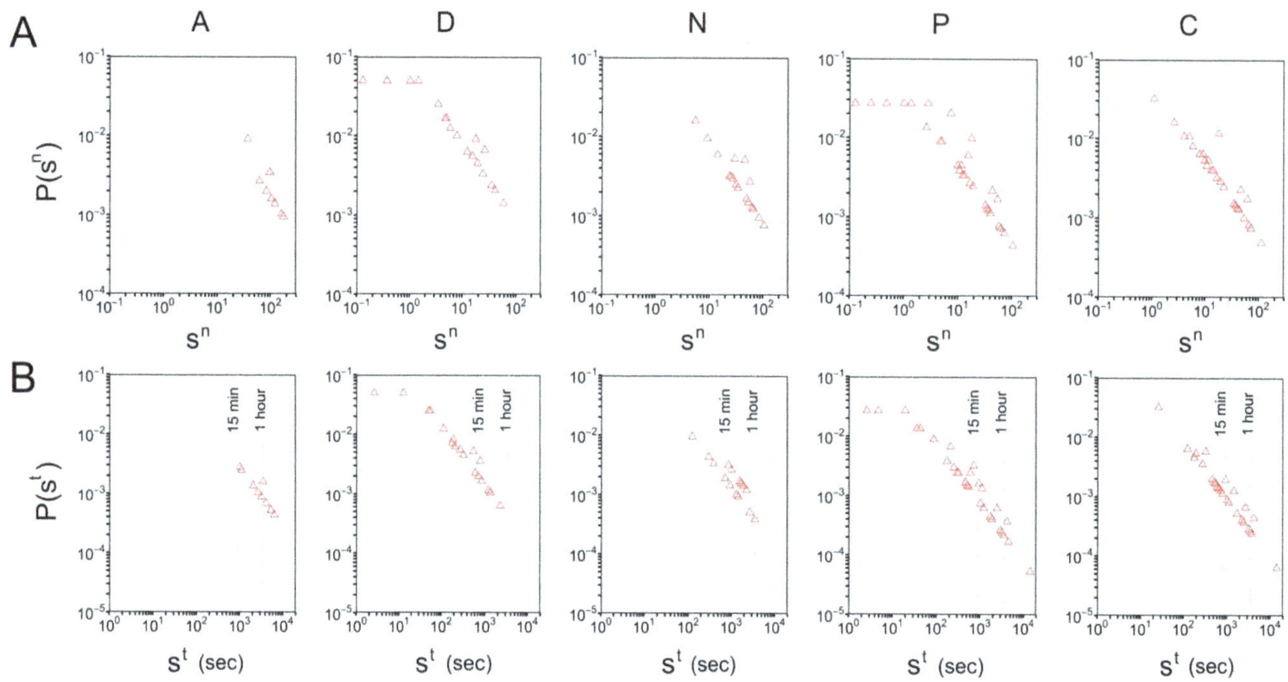

Figure 3. Probability density functions of the number of contacts per individual, s^n (panel A), and of the cumulative time in contact s^t (panel B). Each plot corresponds to a given class and considers the contacts that an individual in that class established with any other individual. Contact duration is expressed in seconds and is normalized to a 24-hour interval.

study provides for the first time direct measures of the number and duration of close contacts by different role and at the individual level in a hospital setting. By taking advantage of the RFID technology, our results account for important heterogeneities in the hospital population and in the interactions among patients, health care workers, and visitors, that enable an accurate parameterization of models for infectious disease spread on the close-contact route.

Our main finding is the very limited interaction that we observed between pairs of patients or between pairs of caregivers, and between health care workers and caregivers. This is empirically found both in the number of contact events, taking into account both distinct and repeated events, and in the duration of such contacts. This result has immediate practical implications for the development of prevention measures for respiratory infections within the hospital, which represent the most frequent

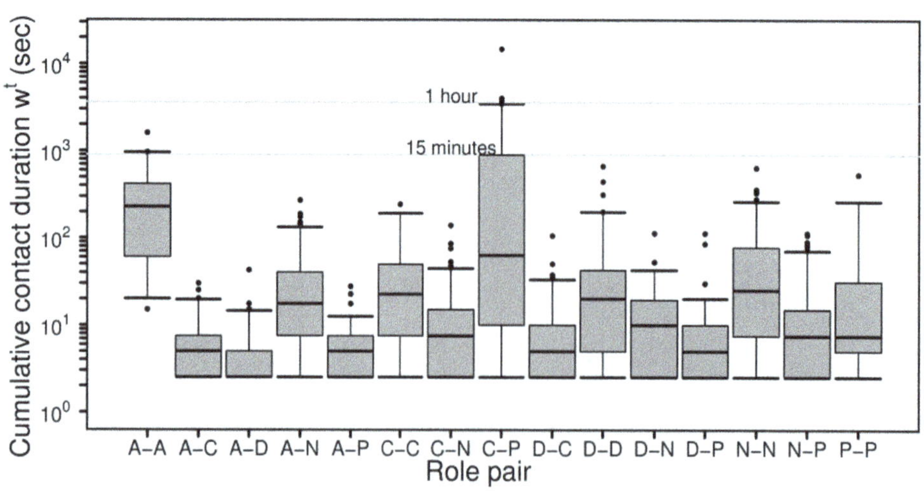

Figure 4. Boxplots for the distributions of cumulative contact durations w^t between individuals belonging to given role pairs (horizontal axis), given the occurrence of a contact. Here we only consider non-zero values of w^t, and contact durations are expressed in seconds and are normalized to a 24-hour interval. On normalizing, the experimental resolution of 20 seconds yields the lowest value of 2.5 seconds visible in the figure. As usual, the bottom and top of the boxes correspond to the 25th and 75th percentiles, and the horizontal segment indicates the median. The ends of the whiskers correspond to the 5th and 95th percentiles. The dots are outliers located outside the 90% confidence interval, i.e., events falling below the 5th percentile or above the 95th percentile.

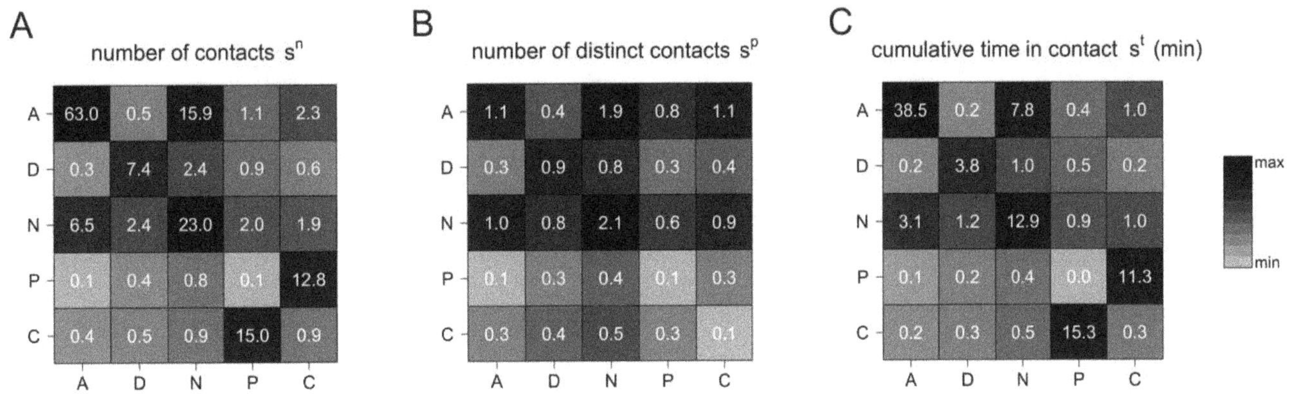

Figure 5. Contact matrices defined on the classes of individuals. Matrices are displayed for the number of contacts s^n (panel A), the number of distinct contacts s^p (panel B), and the cumulative time in contact s^t (panel C). The matrix entry for classes X (row) and Y (column) is the median value of the node strengths for individuals of class X, computed on the contacts they had with individuals of class Y; the asymmetry of the matrices depends on the different numbers of individuals populating each class [3]. Individuals of class X that did not have contacts with individuals of class Y count as nodes with zero strength, i.e., they affect the median value for the corresponding matrix entry. To increase the readability of the figure, matrix entries are grayscale-coded according to the median values, with the lightest and darkest shade of gray respectively corresponding to the minimum and maximum value for each matrix. Contact durations are expressed in minutes and normalized to a 24-hour interval.

nosocomial infections [29,30]. Current guidelines [18] identify the caregiver class as the priority group that control strategies should target [31], given that they may carry asymptomatic or mild community acquired respiratory illnesses and then spread the infection within the hospital to susceptible patients and staff. While caregivers may represent a source of the infection, our results show that their pattern of interaction is very stable and mostly spent in contact with the corresponding patient, thus not favoring the spread of a potential infection to a large number of individuals in the ward. This observation can inform models aimed at testing different prevention recommendations, exploring control resources focused mainly on the caregiver-patient interaction as opposed to resources focused on all possible interactions that a caregiver may have in the ward.

Another major insight concerns patients. Our results show that in addition to intense and continuative interactions with the caregivers, patients are contacted most frequently and with the longest duration by nurses, among all health care categories. Nurses were also found to have a pattern of frequent and long contacts among each other. Thus, in our setting, where a high proportion of patients had a diagnosis of respiratory infection, the intensive professional contact of nurses with patients and among themselves may result in a higher risk for airborne infections among nurses. These observations highlight the crucial importance of prioritizing nurses in local infection control interventions, and confirm the findings of a recent study where data on contacts were collected through a questionnaire [32]. On the other hand, the pattern of contacts between physicians and patients showed a small number of contacts of short duration suggesting a less important role of this health care category in infection transmission. It is worth to mention that, although our study was conducted during the peak of influenza A/H1N1v activity in Italy, no case of influenza transmission was observed among the individuals included in the study. This observation is in line with a strict application of H1N1 containment guidelines in the hospital setting established by the Italian Ministry of Health [33].

We have studied the statistics associated with the collected data and we found a large degree of heterogeneity in the number of contacts and in the duration of contacts across classes. Large fluctuations up to 2 or 3 orders of magnitude are observed in the number of contacts established by an individual in a given class with any other individual, and similar results are observed in the duration of contacts. These fluctuations are however reduced when considering specific class-class interactions, highlighting the presence of well-defined interaction behaviors that are class-specific. Large variations are observed in the patient-caregiver interaction, providing additional empirical evidence for the importance of focusing control efforts on such interactions as they may lead to large variations in a potential outbreak.

Though observed in the hospital context, the large variability observed in the contact number and contact duration is consistent with empirical data collected in other settings. As an example, the same RFID technology was applied to investigate contact patterns in scientific conferences [24,26] showing also in this case a strong heterogeneity of the contact durations between individuals – most contacts were very short in this setting, but contacts of very different durations were observed, including very long ones. This similarity points to the presence of common statistical signatures in the way people interact, that go beyond the constraints and behavioral patterns imposed by the specific context.

Our study allows to define risks of transmission between classes of individuals by calculating matrices of contacts of class-class type along the three quantities describing a contact event that we considered – the number of contacts, the number of distinct contacts, the overall duration of contacts. These contact matrices represent the input ingredients for the parameterization of mathematical and computational models of nosocomial infections, going beyond simple homogeneous assumptions and simple structuring of the population into two classes – patients and health care workers – as in previous studies [20,34]. This work complements similar efforts that focus on the community level [9,10], though our data collection method ensures a higher objectivity of the measure of contact events, and a higher resolution both in time and in space. By taking full advantage of this resolution, RFID technology can be used to inform increasingly complex models that require a finer classification of contacts by personal characteristics [35,36]. Differently from survey methodologies, our method affords data collection and behavior characterization at the individual level, and thus may be used to inform agent-based modeling approaches. This could provide additional insights and uncover unexpected behaviors induced by the fluctuations observed even within the class-class structuring of the population.

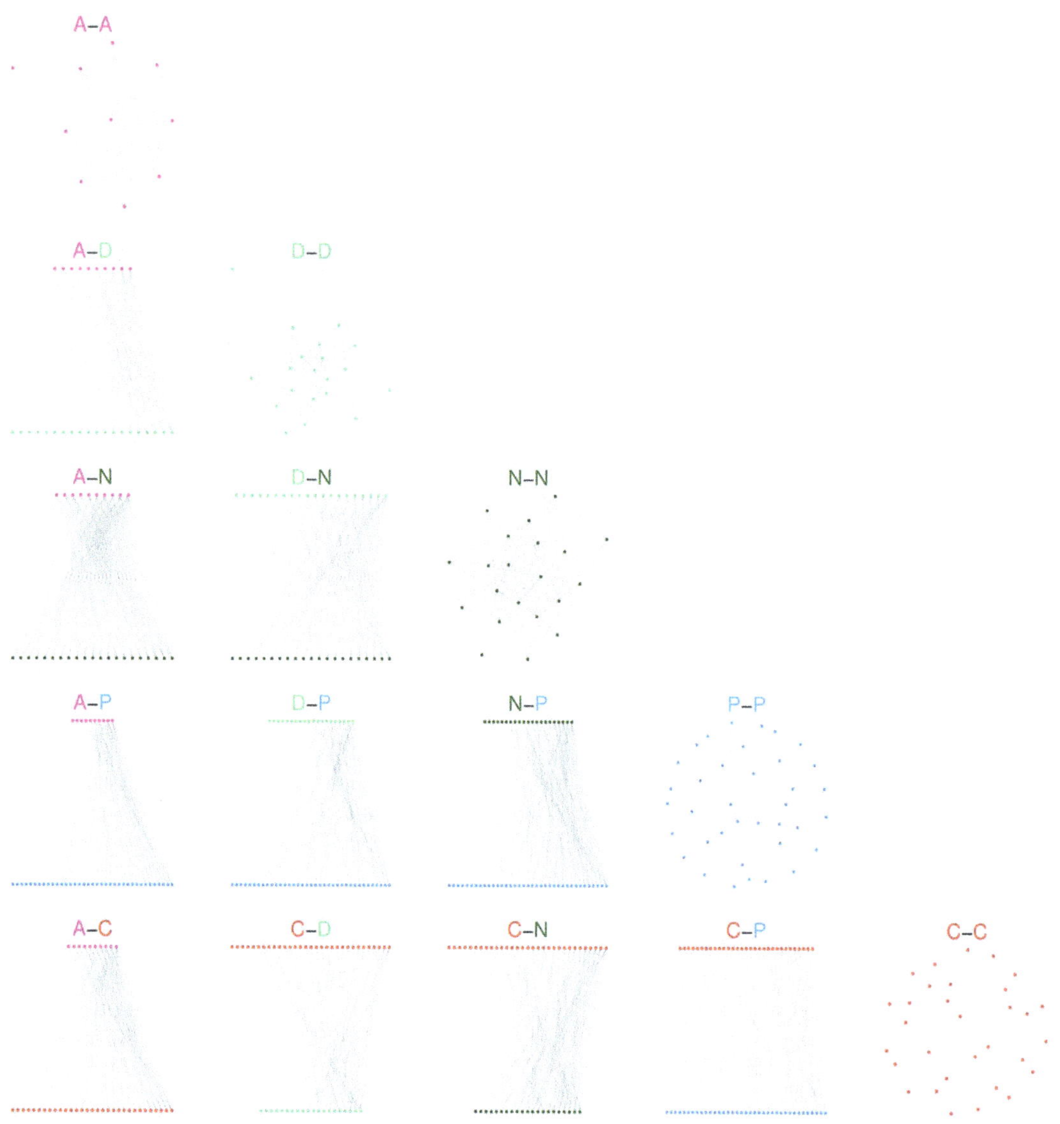

Figure 6. Cumulative contact networks of individuals, for all pairs of classes and within each class. Nodes represent unique individuals, and edges between nodes represent a cumulative face-to-face time over the whole monitoring period. In the off-diagonal layouts, nodes are positioned from left to right in increasing order of number of edges.

However, in order to obtain reliable and statistically significant results from numerical simulations, longer and more extensive deployments should be considered to better characterize expected behaviors and the associated fluctuations. Although this study was carried out over a period of one week, it was conducted in a period when strict rules for infection control were applied because of the threat of cross infection with the 2009 A/H1N1 pandemic influenza virus. We do not believe that the conduction of the study itself has changed the behavior of health care workers, but longer deployments would in this respect be needed to assess the stability of the results over time.

A strength of the present study is the high participation rate of individuals in our experiment. We did not encounter major opposition in the acceptance of the experimental procedure by health care workers, patients, or caregivers, and only a very limited fraction of them (3.6%) declined participation. Once enrolled in the study, most participants regularly wore the RFID devices according to the instructions, thus contributing to the collection of high quality data. These observations suggest that if appropriate protocols are provided, and privacy protection is ensured, measures of contacts through RFID devices are easily replicable, and it is conceivable to aim at fully covering entire wards or hospitals. In this respect, such an approach would constitute a major improvement in the collection of high quality data, if compared to available studies based on interviews where the participation rate was much lower and where logistics and resources limited the length and coverage of the survey [9,30].

Our method presents limitations as well. First of all, given that the RFID tags exchange radio-frequency signals, the collected data can only provide information on the proximity of two badges (and therefore of the persons carrying the badges), but no information on the possible occurrence of a physical contact between the two persons is available. Our measures can thus be used for properly estimating the transmission parameters of respiratory infections but they are less informative for infections transmitted by direct contact. Note however that physical contact can only occur between persons who are already in spatial proximity. Therefore, it would be very interesting to study the fraction of close encounters that result in a physical contact, as this may help to identify useful parameters for modeling infections transmitted through physical contact. In the future, the use of sensors that can directly resolve physical contact may be explored. Another possible limitation is the fact that settings with no wireless connections involve additional complexity in the implementation of the measurements and in the definition of procedures, as limited by the available communication infrastructure. However, upcoming new technology that will allow operating the RFID sensing layer in a fully distributed fashion with on-board storage on the devices, will have minimal requirement on the host infrastructure and is expected to provide increasingly larger opportunities for deployment of wearable sensing systems for the measurement of contacts patterns. This new technology would be also very important to run similar data collection campaigns that cover full hospitals, to assess whether logistic and behavioral characteristics and procedures that are ward-specific are reflected in the observed contact patterns. Finally, a comparative study between different hospitals may provide valuable insights into how structural organization and procedural management may impact the contact patterns among individuals, and therefore the potential epidemic spreading within the hospital. This would also allow us to assess the specificity of the results obtained in the present study. On the other hand, human behavior has been shown in many studies to exhibit important regularities, and a certain number of characteristics of our results can be expected to hold across different wards or hospitals: for example the broad distributions of Fig. 3, or the overall structure of the interaction networks, with the strong specificity of patient-caregiver contacts contrasted to the HCW interactions.

Our study represents, to our knowledge, the first example of unsupervised data collection of face-to-face contacts in a hospital setting by means of wearable radio frequency devices. The obtained results provide significant advances in our knowledge of the mixing patterns taking place in a hospital ward, and allow for a fine structuring of the population into classes of individuals based on their role, along with the evaluation of the corresponding contact matrices. The resulting analysis may help to identify specific interactions at increased risk of transmission, and to explore a variety of possible interventions by means of numerical simulations obtained with modeling approaches informed by measured contact matrices. Outbreak investigations conducted concurrently with proximity sensing by wearable devices may further augment the knowledge we have on the routes of transmission and thus help in reducing the burden of nosocomial infection.

Supporting Information

Figure S1 Contact matrices for classes of individuals, with no filtering of RFID badges. The matrices are computed in the same way as those of Figure 5, but no filtering procedure is applied and the data for all RFID badges are retained. Matrices are displayed for the number of contacts s^n (panel A), the number of distinct contacts s^p (panel B), and the cumulative time in contact s^t (panel C). Matrix entries are grayscale-coded according to the median values, with the lightest and darkest shade of gray respectively corresponding to the minimum and maximum value for each matrix. Contact durations are expressed in minutes and normalized to a 24-hour interval. Comparison with Figure 5 shows the robustness of the data with respect to the filtering procedure.

Table S1 Median number of contacts measured by different roles (D: Physician; N: Nurse; A: Ward assistant; P: Patient; E: Visitor) together with 5th and 95th percentiles (brackets).

Table S2 Median number of distinct contacts measured by different roles (D: Physician; N: Nurse; A: Ward assistant; P: Patient; E: Visitor) together with 5th and 95th percentiles (brackets).

Table S3 Median cumulative duration (in minutes) of contacts measured by different roles (D: Physician; N: Nurse; A: Ward assistant; P: Patient; E: Visitor) together with 5th and 95th percentiles (brackets).

Acknowledgments

We warmly thank Bitmanufaktur and the OpenBeacon project. We also thank the health care workers who participated in the study and helped at the Bambino Gesù Hospital, the Head of the Department of Pediatrics, Prof. A.G. Ugazio, the personnel from the Information System Department, their Head, Eng. Giulio Siccardi, and the families of participating patients.

Author Contributions

Conceived and designed the experiments: AET CC AB CR VC. Performed the experiments: MR FG EP LR CC WVdB. Analyzed the data: LI CC AB VC AET. Contributed reagents/materials/analysis tools: CC WVdB. Wrote the manuscript: AET CC CR LI VC AB.

References

1. Anderson R, May R (1991) Infectious Diseases of Humans: Dynamics and Control. Oxford: Oxford University Press.
2. Diekmann O, Heesterbeek JAP (2000) Mathematical Epidemiology of Infectious Diseases: Model Building, Analysis and Interpretation. New York: Wiley series in mathematical and computational biology.
3. Glass RJ, Glass LM, Beyeler WE, Min HJ (2006) Targeted social distancing design for pandemic influenza. Emerg Infect Dis 12: 1671–1681.
4. Germann TC, Kadau K, Longini IM Jr., Macken CA (2006) Mitigation strategies for pandemic influenza in the United States. Proc Natl Acad Sci USA 103: 5935–5940.
5. Ferguson NM, Cummings DA, Fraser C, Cajka JC, Cooley PC, et al. (2006) Strategies for mitigating an influenza pandemic. Nature 442: 448–452.
6. Perisic A, Bauch CT (2009) Social contact networks and disease eradicability under voluntary vaccination. PLoS Comput Biol 5: e1000280.
7. Longini IM Jr., Halloran ME (2005) Strategy for distribution of influenza vaccine to high-risk groups and children. Am J Epidemiol 161: 303–306.
8. Longini IM Jr., Halloran ME, Nizam A, Yang Y (2004) Containing pandemic influenza with antiviral agents. Am J Epidemiol 159: 623–633.
9. Wallinga J, Teunis P, Kretzschmar M (2006) Using data on social contacts to estimate age-specific transmission parameters for respiratory-spread infectious agents. Am J Epidemiol 164: 936–944.
10. Mossong J, Hens N, Jit M, Beutels P, Auranen K, et al. (2008) Social contacts and mixing patterns relevant to the spread of infectious diseases. PLoS Med 25(5): e74.
11. Edmunds WJ, Kafatos G, Wallinga J, Mossong JR (2006) Mixing patterns and the spread of close-contact infectious diseases. Emerg Themes Epidemiol 3: 10.
12. Beutels P, Shkedy Z, Aerts M, Van Damme P (2006) Social mixing patterns for transmission models of close contact infections: exploring self-evaluation and diary-based data collection through a web-based interface. Epidemiol Infect 134: 1158–66.
13. Kretzschmar M, Mikolajczyk RT (2009) Contact profiles in eight European countries and implications for modelling the spread of airborne infectious diseases. PloS One 4: e5931.
14. Del Valle SY, Hyman JM, Hethcote HW, Eubank SG (2007) Mixing patterns between age groups in social networks. Soc Networks 29: 539–554.

15. Zagheni E, Billari FC, Manfredi P, Melegaro A, Mossong J, et al. (2008) Using Time-use Data to Parameterize Models for the Spread of Close-contact Infectious Diseases. Am J Epidemiol 168: 1082–1090.
16. Mikolajczyk RT, Akmatov MK, Rastin S, Kretzschmar M (2008) Social contacts of school children and the transmission of respiratory-spread pathogens. Epidemiol Infect 136: 813–822.
17. Ogunjimi B, Hens N, Goeyvaerts N, Aerts M, Van Damme P, et al. (2009) Using empirical social contact data to model person to person infectious disease transmission: an illustration for varicella. Math Biosci 218: 80–7.
18. WHO (2002) Guidelines on prevention and control of hospital associated infections WHO/CDS/CSR/EPH/2002.12.
19. Grundmann H, Hellriegel B (2006) Mathematical modelling: a tool for hospital infection control. Lancet Infect Dis 6: 39–45.
20. Cooper BS, Medley GF, Scott GM (1999) Preliminary analysis of the transmission dynamics of nosocomial infections: stochastic and management effects. J Hosp Infect 43: 131–147.
21. Temime L, Opatowski L, Pannet Y, Brun-Buisson C, Boëlle PY, et al. (2009) Peripatetic health-care workers as potential superspreaders. Proc Natl Acad Sci USA 106: 18420–18425.
22. Pentland A (2008) Honest signals: how they shape our world. MIT Press.
23. Olguin O, Gloor D, Pentland PA (2009) Wearable sensors for pervasive healthcare management. 3rd International Conference on Pervasive Computing Technologies for Healthcare, London.
24. The SocioPatterns project. Available: http://www.sociopatterns.org/. Accessed 2010 Sep 6.
25. Alani H, Szomsor M, Cattuto C, Van den Broeck W, Correndo G, et al. (2009) Live Social Semantics. Proceedings of the 8th International Semantic Web Conference (ISWC2009). LNCS 5823: 698–714.
26. Cattuto C, Van den Broeck W, Barrat A, Colizza V, Pinton J, et al. (2010) Dynamics of person-to-person interactions from distributed RFID sensor networks. PLoS ONE 5: e11596.
27. Kazandjieva M, Lee JW, Salathé M, Feldman MW, Jones JH, et al. (2010) Experiences in Measuring a Human Contact Network for Epidemiology Research. ACM Workshop on Hot Topics in Embedded Networked Sensors (HotEmNets) .
28. National Center for Epidemiology, Surveillance and Health Promotion, Istituto Superiore di Sanità. Flunews Italy, 2009. Available: http://www.epicentro.iss.it/focus/h1n1/pdf/flunews/FluNews_46.pdf. Accessed 2010 Sep 6.
29. Muller MP, McGeer A (2006) Febrile respiratory illness in the intensive care unit setting: an infection control perspective. Curr Opin Crit Care 12: 37–42.
30. Brankston G, Gitterman L, Hirji Z, Lemieux C, Gardam M (2007) Transmission of influenza A in human beings. Lancet Infect Dis 7: 257–265.
31. Cavalcante SS, Mota E, Silva LR, Teixeira LF, Cavalcante LB (2006) Risk factors for developing nosocomial infections among pediatric patients. Pediatr Infect Dis J 25: 438–445.
32. Bernard H, Fischer R, Mikolajczyk RT, Kretzschmar M, Wildner M (2009) Nurses' contacts and potential for infectious disease transmission. Emerg Infect Dis 15: 1438–44.
33. Italian Health Ministry. Nuova influenza A(H1N1) - Recommendations, 21 May 2009. Available: http://www.nuovainfluenza.salute.gov.it/nuovainfluenza/archivioOrdinanzeCircolariNuovaInfluenza.jsp. Accessed 2010 Sep 6.
34. Donker T, Wallinga J, Grundmann H (2010) Patient referral patterns and the spread of hospital-acquired infections through national health care networks. PLoS Comput Biol 6: e1000715.
35. Halloran ME (2006) Invited commentary: Challenges of using contact data to understand acute respiratory disease transmission. Am J Epidemiol 164: 945–6.
36. Read JM, Eames KT, Edmunds WJ (2008) Dynamic social networks and the implications for the spread of infectious disease. J R Soc Interface 5: 1001–7.

15

Ulcerogenic *Helicobacter pylori* Strains Isolated from Children: A Contribution to Get Insight into the Virulence of the Bacteria

Inês Vitoriano[1], Kathy D. Saraiva-Pava[1], Alexandra Rocha-Gonçalves[2], Andrea Santos[3], Ana I. Lopes[4], Mónica Oleastro[3], Mónica Roxo-Rosa[1]*

1 Faculdade de Engenharia, Universidade Católica Portuguesa, Rio de Mouro, Portugal, **2** Chymiotechnon, Departamento de Química, Universidade de Coimbra, Coimbra, Portugal, **3** Departamento de Doenças Infecciosas, Instituto Nacional Saúde Dr. Ricardo Jorge, Lisboa, Portugal, **4** Departamento de Pediatria, Hospital Universitário de Santa Maria/Faculdade de Medicina de Lisboa, Lisboa, Portugal

Abstract

Infection with *Helicobacter pylori* is the major cause for the development of peptic ulcer disease (PUD). In children, with no other etiology for the disease, this rare event occurs shortly after infection. In these young patients, habits of smoking, diet, consumption of alcohol and non-steroid anti-inflammatory drugs and stress, in addition to the genetic susceptibility of the patient, represent a minor influence. Accordingly, the virulence of the implicated *H. pylori* strain should play a crucial role in the development of PUD. Corroborating this, our *in vitro* infection assays comparing a pool of five *H. pylori* strains isolated from children with PUD to a pool of five other pediatric clinical isolates associated with non-ulcer dyspepsia (NUD) showed the greater ability of PUD strains to induce a marked decrease in the viability of gastric cells and to cause severe damage in the cells cytoskeleton as well as an impairment in the production/secretion of mucins. To uncover virulence features, we compared the proteome of these two groups of *H. pylori* strains. Two-dimensional gel electrophoresis followed by mass-spectrometry allowed us to detect 27 differentially expressed proteins between them. In addition to the presence of genes encoding well established virulence factors, namely *cagA*, *vacAs*1, *oipA* "on" status, *homB* and *jhp562* genes, the pediatric ulcerogenic strains shared a proteome profile characterized by changes in the abundance of: motility-associated proteins, accounting for higher motility; antioxidant proteins, which may confer increased resistance to inflammation; and enzymes involved in key steps in the metabolism of glucose, amino acids and urea, which may be advantageous to face fluctuations of nutrients. In conclusion, the enhanced virulence of the pediatric ulcerogenic *H. pylori* strains may result from a synergy between their natural ability to better adapt to the hostile human stomach and the expression of the established virulence factors.

Editor: Yoshio Yamaoka, Veterans Affairs Medical Center (111D), United States of America

Funding: This work was supported by PPCDT/SAL-IMI/57297/2004 research grant from the Fundação para a Ciência e a Tecnologia (FCT), Portugal. I. Vitoriano and K.D. Saraiva-Pava are the recipients of doctoral fellowships (SFRH/BD/38634/2007, FCT and SFRH/BD/72849/2011, respectively). The funders had no role in study design, data collection and analysis, decision to publish, or preparation of the manuscript.

Competing Interests: The authors have declared that no competing interests exist.

* E-mail: roxorosa@hotmail.com

Introduction

Helicobacter pylori is a spiral-shaped, microaerophilic, gram-negative bacterium that inhabits the human stomach. Depending on the socioeconomic status of the country, the prevalence of infection varies from 40 to over 80% of the population, with higher rates for developing countries [1]. Infection is usually acquired during childhood and always elicits an acute immune response which, in the absence of effective treatment, persists throughout the patient's life, resulting in chronic gastritis. Although this condition may be asymptomatic, some patients develop dyspeptic symptoms, *i.e.*, the so-called non-ulcer dyspepsia (NUD) [2]. In about 15% of infected patients, gastritis may progress further to severe gastric diseases, namely peptic ulcer disease (PUD) and gastric cancer (GC) [1,3].

PUD is a multifactorial disease which leads to considerable patient morbidity and mortality [4]. It is considered to be a disease of adulthood being its progression highly dependent on environmental factors, such as the use of non-steroid anti-inflammatory drugs (NSAID), alcohol consumption, diet, smoking and stress. Some viral infections (*e.g.* cytomegalovirus and herpes simplex infections), Crohn's disease and syndromes where an increase in acid secretion occurs (*e.g.*, Zollinger-Ellison syndrome), may also contribute to the onset of PUD [4]. However, a long-term infection with *H. pylori* is considered as the major causative factor for PUD. This is easily demonstrated by the high number of patients infected with *H. pylori* among those who are affected by PUD, and by the fact that, with the successful eradication of the bacteria, non-NSAID-related PUD is healed and rarely recurs [2,4]. PUD can be subdivided into duodenal ulcer (DU) and gastric ulcer (GU) diseases which are considered divergent. DU is basically a duodenal acid injury that results from acid hypersecretion due to infection of the antrum by *H. pylori* [2]. In contrast, GU is usually associated with acid hyposecretion that results from the gastric atrophy caused by a proximal spread of the infection, and hence, of inflammation [2]. Supporting differences in the pathogenesis of these two clinical outcomes, the prevalence of *H. pylori* infection is higher than 95% in DU cases and around 60% to 80% in GU [5,6].

The development of PUD in *H. pylori* infected children is a very rare event and usually occurs soon after infection. In Portugal, for example, only about 2% of the estimated 40% of the Portuguese infected children suffer from this disease [7]. Besides genetic susceptibility [8], the aforementioned environmental factors should have a minor influence on the pathogenesis of PUD in infected children. Therefore, we believe that the virulence factors of the implicated strain must play a crucial role in the onset of PUD in children [2]. We have reported some data on genetic studies of clinical isolates which show the association of some bacterial genes with the development of PUD in infected children [9–12]. Indeed, in addition to the most well known virulence factors, namely the *cytotoxin-associated gene A* (*cagA*) gene, the "on" genotype (*i.e.*, functional) of the *outer inflammatory protein A* (*oipA*) gene, the s1/m1 allele of the *vacuolating cytotoxin gene* (*vacA*), and the *A2* allele of the *blood group antigen binding adhesin* (*BabA*) gene [1,3], we found that *homB* and *jhp562* genes are closely associated with PUD in children and may be useful in determining the clinical outcome of infection [9–12]. HomB protein is an antigenic outer membrane protein which was shown to be involved in the host inflammatory response, inducing the secretion of interleukin-8 (IL8), and in the adhesion of *H. pylori* to gastric epithelial cells [9,10]. The *jhp562* gene encodes a glycosyltransferase involved in the synthesis of lipopolysaccharide and may also be implicated in the regulation of Lewis antigen expression [12]. The presence of the triple genotype *cagA*, *jhp562* and *homB* in *H. pylori* strains provides a good discriminatory basis to distinguish PUD and NUD outcomes in infected children [12].

Motivated by these findings, we further characterized five *H. pylori* strains, isolated from Portuguese children with PUD, all positive for *cagA*, *jhp562* and *homB* genes. Their virulence profile was first compared to that of five other clinical isolates collected from children with NUD, by co-culture assays with the NCI-N87 cell line (American Type Culture Collection (ATCC) CRL 5822). We report here the differences that we found in the impact of these two groups of *H. pylori* strains on the viability, phenotype and cytoskeleton organization of the NCI-N87 cells. Moreover, in order to understand the molecular mechanisms that underlie their more pathogenic phenotype, we compared the proteomes of the ulcerogenic *H. pylori* strains with those of the NUD strains.

Results

Ten *H. pylori* strains isolated from Portuguese pediatric patients, five suffering from NUD (mean age 10.2 years, range 7 to 14) and five other affected by PUD (mean age 11.8 years, range 10 to 15, having no other etiology for the disease), were carefully selected to be genetically homogeneous within the respective group (Table 1). The difference between the mean ages of these two groups was not statistically significant. According to their previously reported genotype [12], all PUD strains were positive for some important virulence factors associated with PUD in children. These include *cagA*, *vacA* s1 (*i.e.*, the toxic allele), *oipA* "on", *homB* and *jhp562* (with the exception of strain 1846/05) genes (Table 1). In contrast, all of the NUD strains were *cagA*, *homB* and *jhp562* negative and carried the *oipA* "off" status and the *vacA* s2 (*i.e.*, the non-toxic allele) gene (Table 1).

Co-culture assays

To clarify whether the virulence of the strains was the determining factor for the development of PUD in children from whom they were collected, we compared their impact on human gastric epithelial cells with that of NUD strains, by *in vitro* infection experiments. These experiments were carried out using the NCI-N87 cell line, known for its unique differentiation status as it is able to form coherent monolayers, expressing the correct cellular distribution of both *E*-cadherin and ZO-1 junction proteins [13]. Confluent NCI-N87 cells monolayers were thus incubated in parallel with two different pools of *H. pylori* strains, one including the five PUD associated strains, and another including the five NUD strains, both at a multiplicity of infection (MOI) of 100. Under our experimental co-culture conditions, the viability of NCI-N87 cells was clearly reduced over time with both pools of *H. pylori* strains (Figure 1). However, this effect was more pronounced in the first hours following infection with the pool of PUD-associated strains. Indeed, cell viability was significantly lower ($p<0.05$) in NCI-N87 cells infected with PUD-*H. pylori* strains at

Table 1. Characterization of the *H. pylori* strains included in the study and of the patients from whom each of them was isolated.

H. pylori						Patient		
Strain	***cagA***	***vacA***	***oipA***	***homB***	***jhp562***	**Histologic Analysis**	**Age**	**Gender**
173/00	–	s2	off	–	–	NUD	14	M
207/99	–	s2	off	–	–	NUD	7	F
228/99	–	s2	off	–	–	NUD	8	M
655/99	–	s2	off	–	–	NUD	11	M
1786/05	–	s2	off	–	–	NUD	11	M
499/02	+	s1	on	+	+	GU	11	M
1089/03	+	s1	on	+	+	DU	10	M
1152/04	+	s1	on	+	+	DU	10	M
1198/04	+	s1	on	+	+	DU	15	M
1846/05	+	s1	on	+	–	DU	13	M

All strains are indicated by their collection number. All patients were from Portugal. In columns *cagA*, *homB* and *jhp562*: + indicates strain containing the gene; – indicates strain lacking the gene. *vacA* column: s1 indicates strains containing the toxic allele of the gene; and s2, strain containing the non-toxic allele of the gene. *oipA* column: on indicates strains containing the functional allele of the gene; and off, strains containing the non-functional allele of the gene. NUD - non-ulcer dyspepsia; DU – duodenal ulcer; GU – gastric ulcer. M - Masculine; F - Feminine.

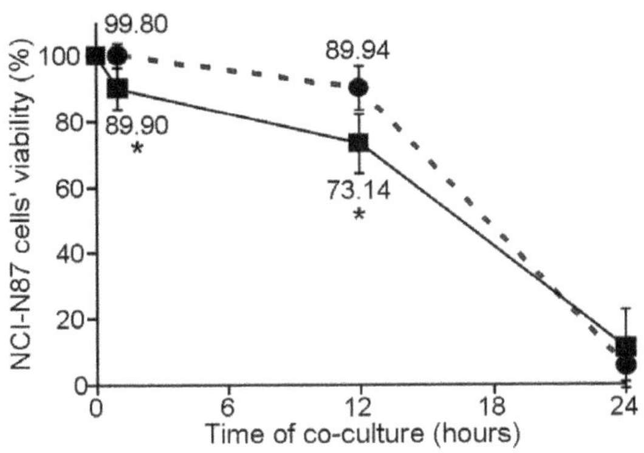

Figure 1. Impact of the two isogenic groups of pediatric *H. pylori* strains on NCI-N87 cells viability. The viability of NCI-N87 cells was assessed by the trypan blue exclusion assay after 1, 12 and 24 h of co-culture with a pool of five pediatric PUD-associated strains (■ in full line) and a pool of five pediatric NUD-associated strains (● in dashed line). For normalization, the value of 100% corresponds to the viability of non-infected NCI-N87 cells. * indicates values that were determined as significantly different ($p<0.05$) between the viability of cells infected with PUD strains and that of cells infected with NUD-strains at the same time-point of co-culture. Symbols and error bars are means ± SD of the values at each point for 3 observations.

1 h (89.90%±6.23) and 12 h post-infection (73.14%±8.96), compared to cells infected with NUD strains (99.80%±3.52 and 89.94%±6.70, respectively) (Figure 1). At 24 h post-infection, the viability of the epithelial cells was very low in both cases, 5.40%±4.51 and 10.78%±11.91, for cells infected with NUD and PUD strains, respectively (Figure 1). However, the morphological analysis of the remaining cells (Figure 2) showed dramatic differences in the impact of each pool of *H. pylori* strains. Indeed, light microscopy observations revealed much more pronounced cell damage in NCI-N87 cells infected with the pool of PUD-*H. pylori* strains (Figures 2A, 2B and 2C). Moreover, the pool of PUD strains caused the total destabilization of the NCI-N87 cells' microtubule network, as demonstrated by the immunocytochemical assays (Figures 2F), which seemed almost unchanged in cells infected with NUD-*H. pylori* strains (Figure 2E). In addition, epithelial cells infected with the PUD-*H. pylori* strains showed a drastic reduction in the cytoplasmic Periodic Acid Schiff (PAS) reactivity (Figure 2G, 2H and 2I), which was supported by the destruction of the cell membrane observed with hematoxylin and PAS double staining (Figure 2J, 2L and 2M). We also observed that the nuclear envelope of the NCI-N87 cells infected with the *H. pylori* strains associated with PUD was undisrupted, despite having a very irregular appearance, suggesting cell death by necrosis (Figure 2I and 2M). In contrast, NCI-N87 cells co-cultured with the NUD-associated *H. pylori* strains showed an accumulation of extracellular vesicles positive for PAS (dark arrow in Figure 2L) suggesting the expected exocytosis of intracellular mucus-containing vesicles, also observed in the non-infected control (data not shown). After 24 h of co-culture, NUD strains maintained their bacillary shape and were adherent to the epithelial cell surface (Figure 2H and 2L), however, PUD strains acquired a coccoidal shape (Figure 2I and 2M) which was already observed at 12 h post infection (data not shown).

H. pylori proteome profile

Total soluble protein extracts from each of the 10 *H. pylori* strains were resolved by 2-dimensional gel electrophoresis (2DE), first in a non-linear pH range of 3–11 and then in a 7–16% (w/v) SDS-PAGE. After Coomassie Brilliant Blue (CBB) staining, the digitalized images of the gels were analyzed using the ImageMaster™ 2D Platinum software. Protein spots were automatically detected and manually corrected and the best resolved 2DE-gel, that of NUD-associated *H. pylori* strain 655/99, was used as the reference map during computer assisted analysis. After automatic matching, followed by a manual correction, gels were separated into two classes, NUD and PUD, according to the pathology with which the strain was associated. Gel-to-gel matching was confirmed by MS identification of matched spots from different 2DE gels. The 2DE maps obtained for each group of strains were found to be highly reproducible and consistent (Figure 3). No statistically difference was observed for the number of detected spots (on average 485±77 *vs.* 443±43 in NUD and PUD 2DE gels, respectively) between these two classes.

Comparative proteomic analysis

In order to search for a protein signature for pediatric *H. pylori* PUD-associated strains, a computer-assisted analysis was performed by statistical evaluation of changes in the % Vol, *i.e.*, the normalized volume, for each protein spot within the two disease-associated classes of 2DE gels. As a result, irrelevant variations between images were eliminated. From this analysis, we observed that the proteome of the *H. pylori* strain 499/02, the unique strain associated with GU, was not fully consistent with the proteome of the other four strains included in the group of PUD related strains isolated from children with DU. Therefore, from this point onward the strain 499/02 was analyzed separately. Table 2 lists the identification by peptide mass fingerprinting (PMF) analysis and/or by comparison with 2DE databases [14] of 26 protein spots detected as being differentially expressed: 24 of them were statistical significant ($p<0.05$) between the NUD and DU classes of strains; and one spot detected at a different position within the 2DE-gels.

These include 15 proteins which were highly abundant in DU-associated *H. pylori* strains (solid arrows in Figure 3; upward arrows in Table 2), when compared to NUD strains: flagellar hook protein (FlgE, spot 2) and flagellin A (FlaA, spot 3), both components of the bacteria's flagella; the heat shock protein B (HspB, spot 4), a homolog of Hsp60 involved in protein folding; both beta and alpha subunits of urease (UreB, spot 5, and UreA, spot 20), which catalyzes the hydrolysis of urea into ammonia and CO_2; phosphoglycerate kinase (Pgk, spot 12), 3-dehydroquinate dehydratase (AroQ, spot 22) and flavodoxin A (FldA, spot 25), involved in bacteria metabolic cycles; putative aldo-keto reductase (spot 15), a protein of the cell detoxification system; an isoform of UPF0174 protein HP_1588 (spot 17), a protein whose function is unknown; the non-heme iron-containing ferritin (Pfr, spot 23), involved in iron metabolism; the virulence factor neutrophil activating protein (NapA, spot 26); and the HPG27_1480 protein (spot 27), homologous to the HP1542 protein which has a putative function in cell shape [15]. Interestingly, a thirteenth protein, the hypothetical protein HPAG1_1081 (spot 13), was detected exclusively in the DU- associated *H. pylori* strains. This protein is a homolog of HP1143, another protein with a putative function in cell shape [16]. Further experiments are needed to clarify whether the expression of this protein is unique to the DU strains, or it also occurs in NUD and GU strains but at levels below our detection threshold. As previously shown, only the PUD-*H. pylori* strains were *cagA* positive and this was confirmed by the total absence of CagA protein in the 2DE maps of the NUD-strains. This protein corresponds to spot 1 in the PUD-2DE maps (Figure 3; Table 2).

Amongst the group of differentially expressed proteins, we found the following 11 protein spots to be less abundant in DU-

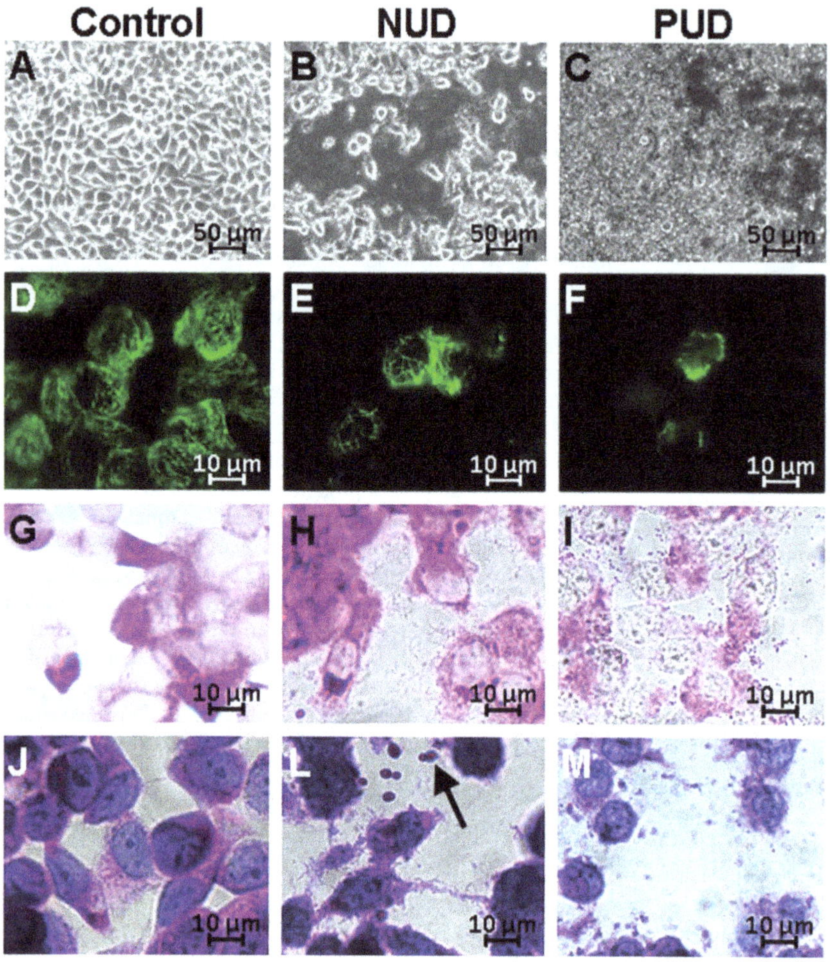

Figure 2. Impact of the two isogenic groups of pediatric *H. pylori* strains on the NCI-N87 cells morphology. NCI-N87 cells grown to 80–90% confluence were co-cultured for 24 h with the pool of five isogenic NUD-associated *H. pylori* strains (NUD) and in parallel with the pool of five isogenic PUD strains (PUD). The control corresponds to non-infected NCI-N87 cells. A), B), and C) light microscopy observations. D), E), and F) immunodetection of the microtubule network (green) (1:1000 α-tubulin antibody plus a FITC conjugated secondary antibody). G), H), and I) PAS staining alone, and in J), L), and M) in conjugation with hematoxylin. Dark arrow indicates extracellular vesicles that reacted with PAS.

associated *H. pylori* strains (dotted arrows in Figure 3; downward arrows in Table 2), when compared with NUD strains: hydantoin utilization protein A (HyuA, spot 6), aspartate ammonia-lyase (AspA, spot 11), succinyl-CoA-transferase (SCOT) subunits A and B (ScoA and ScoB, spots 19 and 21, respectively), pyruvate flavodoxin oxidoreductase, gamma subunit (Porγ, spot 24), proteins involved in bacteria metabolic cycles; ribosomal protein S1 (RpsA, spot 8) and cysteinyl-tRNA synthetase (CysS, spot 10), proteins involved in protein biosynthesis; catalase (KatA, spot 9), involved in the cell detoxification system; HELPY_0944 (spot 16), homologous to HP0958, which is a protein with a putative function in cell motility; and another isoform of UPF0174 protein HP_1588 (spot 18), a protein whose function is unknown. Spot 7, which we were unable to identify, was only detected in NUD strains, with the exception of the *H. pylori* strain 228/99. As before, we cannot say that the expression of this protein is completely absent in DU strains, rather that its expression levels were below our detection threshold.

Besides differences in protein expression between these two groups of strains, we detected a difference in the position of the protein spot 14 within the 2DE-gel (Figure 3) that was identified as being elongation factor Ts (EF-Ts) (Table 2). Indeed, in the 2DE-maps of the DU strains, this protein spot was shifted to the right relative to its position in the NUD 2DE-maps (Figure 3).

Interestingly, we found differences in the abundance of some of these protein spots in GU-associated *H. pylori* strain 499/02, when compared to that of the DU strains (Figure 3; Table 2). Showing the same tendency of that observed in DU strains compared to NUD strains, we found FlgE (spot 2), FlaA (spot 3), Pgk (spot 12) and aroQ (spot 22). Showing the opposite tendency of that observed for DU strains compared to NUD strains, and with abundance levels similar to those observed in the latter group of strains, we found UreB (spot 5), HPAG1_1081 (spot 13), putative aldo-keto reductase (spot 15), one isoform of the HP_1588 (spot 17), and UreA (spot 20). CagA (spot 1) was less abundant in the GU strain (Table 2). All of the other protein spots followed the same pattern of expression observed for the *H. pylori* strains associated with DU (Table 2).

Although the MOWSE score in the MS identification did not reach statistical significance ($p>0.05$) for the CagA (spot 1), CysS (spot 10), AspA (spot 11), ScoA (spot 19), Pfr (spot 23) and HPG27_1480 (spot 27) protein spots, we are confident in our

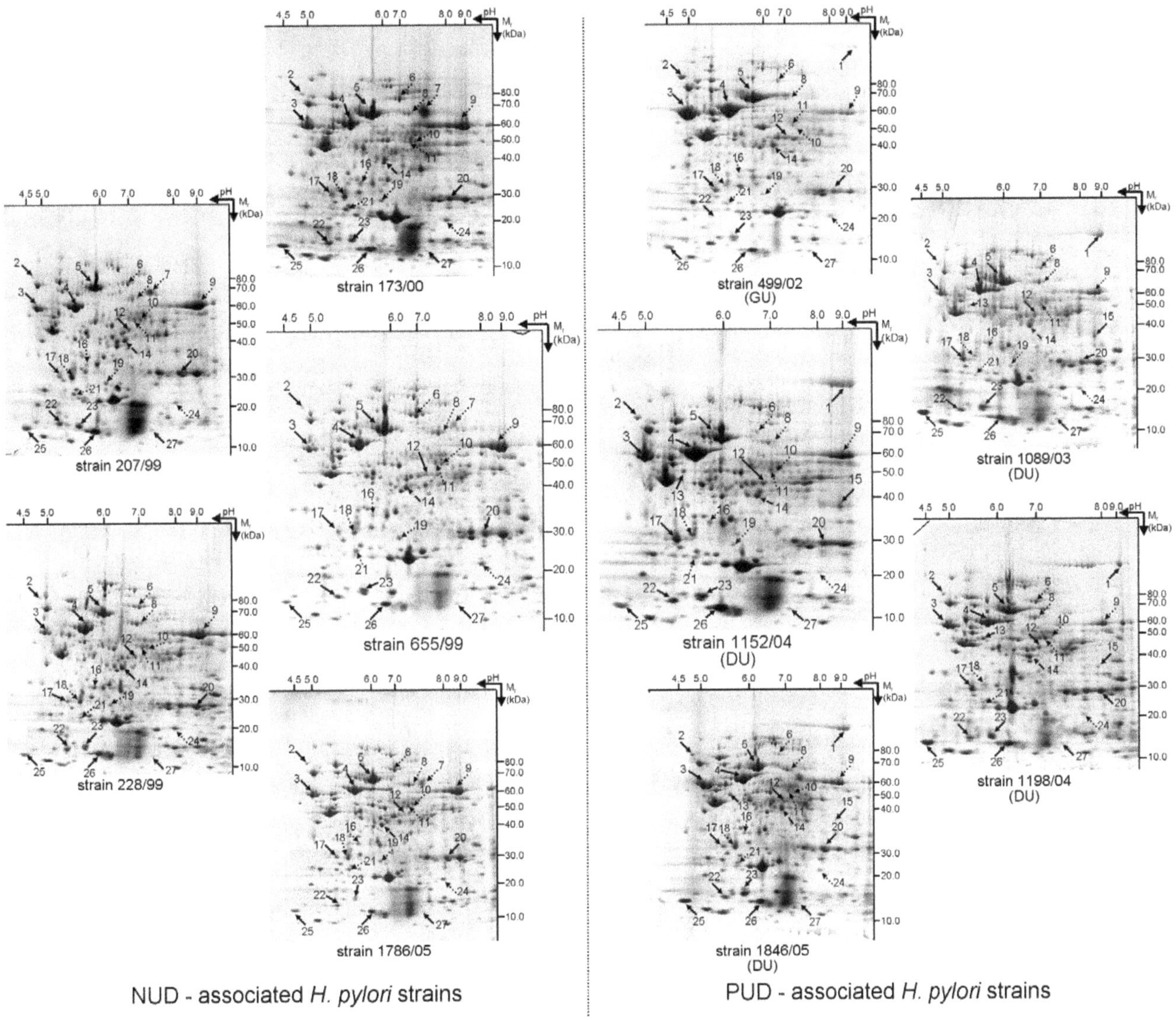

Figure 3. Profile of the soluble proteome of the 10 studied pediatric *H. pylori* strains. These include five strains associated with NUD (173/00, 207/99, 228/99, 655/99 and 1786/05), four from patients affected by DU (1089/03, 1152/04, 1198/04 and 1846/05) and a strain associated with GU (499/02). Proteins from the total biomass recovered from a 24 h grown plate were separated by 2DE, *i.e.*, first in a non-linear pH 3–11 and than in a 7–16% (w/v) SDS-PAGE. After CBB-staining, gels were analyzed using ImageMaster^{TM} 2-D Platinum software. Black arrow indicates spots that were more abundant in PUD (DU+GU) strains when compared to NUD strains; Dotted arrow indicates spots that were less abundant in PUD (DU+GU) strains when compared to NUD strains; Dashed arrow indicates the spot that was shifted right in DU strains when compared to NUD strains. Spot numbers indicated in the 2DE maps are the same as used in Table 2.

results because the same identification was obtained for equivalent spots from different 2DE gels and it also matched with the identification in the 2DE *H. pylori* database [14].

Motility assay

As there were proteins related somehow to bacteria motility included in the group of proteins which were expressed differentially between NUD and PUD strains, we further evaluated whether this was translated into differences in motility. Accordingly, the pools of five NUD strains and of five PUD strains under study were inoculated in an agar motility medium and, at 5, 7 and 11 days the diameter of the growth halo was measured (Figure 4). In agreement with the higher abundance of FlgE (spot 2), FlaA (spot 3) in PUD strains (both in DU and GU strains), the *H. pylori* strains associated with PUD in children showed bigger growth halos (Figure 4), indicating that they have higher motility than the strains associated with NUD. These experiments were carried out twice, leading to consistent results.

Discussion

The development of PUD in children is a rare consequence of infection by *H. pylori*. Environmental factors should have a minor influence on its pathogenesis since pediatric PUD develops soon after infection. Its dependence on the genetic susceptibility of these children is still poorly understood. The expression of sialyl-Lewis (x) antigens in gastric epithelial cells in association with *H. pylori*-dependent DU in pediatrics was recently reported. However, in contrast to the aberrant expression found in adults patients, the gastric mucosa of these children presents a normal pattern of

Table 2. Identification of proteins found to be differentially expressed in *H. pylori* strains from PUD patients (n = 5) compared to NUD patients (n = 5).

					Theoretical						% Vol					
Spot no.	Protein	Cellular function	ORF	Swiss-Prot/ NCBI no.	Mw (kDa)	pI	MOWSE score		Peptides matched	Sequence coverage (%)	Average NUD ± S.D	Average DU ± S.D	Variation (DU/ NUD)	*p value*		Variation (GU/DU)
1	CagA, Cytotoxin associated protein A	Induces abnormal proliferation; tight junctions disruption; cytoskeleton rearrangements	HP0547	gi|307135439	131	8.9	82	*	10/16	7	absent	1.558±0.487	↑	5.265E-08	*	↓
2	FlgE, Flagellar hook protein	Component of bacteria flagellum basal body	HP0870	Q9ZKY0	76	5.0	71	*	12/35	17	0.077±0.036	0.136±0.055	↑	2.099E-02	*	↑
3	FlaA, Flagellin A	Major component of bacteria flagellum	HP0601	P0A0S2	53	6.0	121	*	14/37	14	2.130±0.794	3.063±0.941	↑	4.706E-02	*	↑
4	HspB, Chaperone and heat shock protein	Protein folding/ stress response	HP0010	B6JPA7	58	5.4	93	*	18/55	26	5.021±0.556	5.856±0.533	↑	7.801E-03	*	-
5	UreB, Urease beta subunit	Urea metabolism	P14917	P69996	62	5.6	Comparison to 2DE database				8.815±1.310	10.477±1.455	↑	3.551E-02	*	↓
6	HyuA, Hydantoin utilization protein A	Arginine and proline metabolism	HP0695	gi|108563105	79	6.4	105	*	24/100	20	0.503±0.128	0.204±0.110	↓	4.079E-04	*	-
7	Unknown	—	—	—	—	—	—				1.094±0.702	absent	↓	2.706E-04	*	-
8	RpsA, 30S Ribosomal protein s1	Translation process	HP0399	P56008	63	6.3	Comparison to 2DE database				0.126±0.029	0.085±0.022	↓	1.141E-02	*	-
9	KatA, Catalase	Detoxification	HP0875	P77872	59	8.7	161	*	21/48	37	4.833±0.962	2.669±0.621	↓	1.292E-04	*	-
10	CysS, Cysteinyl-tRNA synthetase	Translation process	HP0886	B5Z7P5	53	6.0	28		4/23	8	0.152±0.091	0.027±0.024	↓	2.615E-03	*	-
11	AspA, Aspartate ammonia-lyase	Catalyzes the deamination of aspartate originating fumarate	HP0649	gi|207108618	35	8.5	58		5/23	10	0.396±0.097	0.252±0.089	↓	9.261E-03	*	-
12	Pgk, Phosphoglycerate kinase	Glucose metabolism	HP1345	gi|261838924	44	6.3	86	*	10/33	27	0.213±0.064	0.303±0.069	↑	2.525E-02	*	↑
13	HPAG1_1081, Hypothetical protein	Putative function in cell shape	HP1143	gi|108563506	51	5.5	77	*	11/23	15	absent	0.200±0.072	↑	3.577E-07	*	absent
14	EF-Ts, Elongation factor Ts	Translation process	HP1555	B6JP47	40	6.2	76	*	7/13	16	0.606±0.101	0.613±0.185	↔	9.206E-01		normal position
15	Putative aldo-keto reductase	Catalyze the reduction of aldehydes and ketones to the corresponding alcohol product	HP1193	gi|254779741	37	6.7	86	*	8/18	22	0.015±0.040	0.147±0.224	↑	7.418E-03	*	↓
16	HELPY_0944, Hypothetical protein	Motility	HP0958	gi|254779556	30	5.6	99	*	13/46	41	0.231±0.080	0.165±0.026	↓	8.453E-02		-
17	HP_1588, UPF0174 protein	Unknown	HP1588	O26107	29	5.5	85	*	8/17	15	0.322±0.123	0.563±0.373	↑	2.293E-03	*	↓

Table 2. Cont.

					Theoretical						% Vol					
Spot no.	Protein	Cellular function	ORF	Swiss-Prot/ NCBI no.	Mw (kDa)	pI	MOWSE score		Peptides matched	Sequence coverage (%)	Average NUD ± S.D	Average DU ± S.D	Variation (DU/ NUD)	*p value*		Variation (GU/DU)
18	HP_1588, UPF0174 protein	Unknown	HP1588	O26107	29	5.5	90	*	10/30	28	0.853±0.192	0.399±0.167	↓	5.076E-04	*	-
19	ScoA, Succinyl-CoA-transferase subunit A	Citric acid cycle	HP0691	P56006	26	5.8	41		3/7	11	0.199±0.051	0.052±0.053	↓	3.739E-05	*	-
20	UreA, Urease subunit alpha	Urea metabolism	HP0073	Q9ZMZ4	27	8.5	145	*	12/26	43	0.798±0.078	1.082±0.214	↑	3.314E-03	*	↓
21	ScoB, Succinyl-CoA-transferase subunit B	Citric acid cycle	HP0692	gi|208434607	22	5.4	104	*	10/33	33	0.242±0.066	0.149±0.061	↓	1.070E-02	*	-
22	AroQ, 3-dehydroquinate dehydratase	Aromatic aminoacid biosynthesis	HP1038	B6JKY5	19	5.1	77	*	8/36	35	0.520±0.108	0.622±0.077	↑	5.503E-02		↑
23	Pfr, Ferritin	Iron storage protein	HP0653	Q9ZLI1	19	5.4	40		4/23	23	0.728±0.295	1.185±0.193	↑	4.285E-03	*	-
24	Porγ, Pyruvate flavodoxin oxidoreductase, gamma subunit	Decarboxylation of pyruvate in acetyl-CoA	HP1108	gi|15645722	21	8.5	88	*	10/33	36	0.313±0.086	0.141±0.033	↓	1.133E-04	*	-
25	FldA, Flavodoxin	Electron transport process	HP1161	O25776	17	4.5	73	*	5/14	42	0.657±0.277	1.259±0.430	↑	6.800E-03	*	-
26	NapA, Neutrophil activating protein A	Protects DNA from oxidative damage; activates neutrophils, mast cells and monocytes	HP0243	gi|7188724	17	5.7	103	*	16/100	79	1.350±0.567	1.933±0.360	↑	2.996E-02	*	-
27	HPG27_1480	Putative function in cell shape	HP1542	gi|208435422	11	5.6	48		3/13	35	0.065±0.016	0.088±0.007	↑	4.953E-03	*	-

"Comparison to 2DE databases" indicates spots for which identification was done by finding the corresponding spot on the standard *H. pylori* 2DE gel from the database [14]. All of the others were identified by PMF analysis. For each spot the average of the % Vol ± S.D. is indicated. In the Variation (DU/NUD) column: ↑, proteins for which the average of the % Vol of spots on DU 2DE maps was higher than that on NUD 2DE maps; ↓, proteins for which the average of the % Vol of spots on DU 2DE maps was lower than that on NUD 2DE maps; ↔, proteins that were shifted right in the DU 2DE-maps regarding their position on the NUD 2DE-maps. In the Variation (GU/NUD) column: ↑, proteins for which the average of the % Vol of spots on GU 2-DE maps was higher than that on the DU 2DE maps; ↓, proteins for which the average of the % Vol of spots on GU 2DE maps was lower than that on DU 2DE maps; =, proteins showing the same pattern of expression observed for the *H. pylori* strains associated with DU. Asterisks indicate statistical significant results ($p<0.05$). [1]Indicates the identified ORF in the 26695 reference strain.

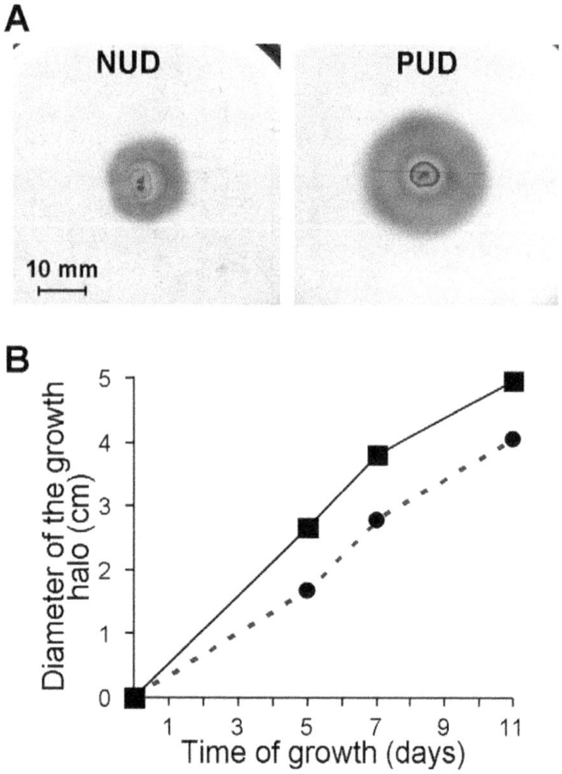

Figure 4. Motility of the two isogenic groups of pediatric *H. pylori* strains in study. The five strains of each class, recovered from 24 h grown plates, were pooled together, inoculated on semi-solid BHI broth −5% FBS medium plates and incubated for 11 days at 37°C under microaerophilic conditions. A) The growth halo observed at day 5 for the pool of PUD and of NUD strains. B) Variation of the diameter of the growth halo along the time (■ in full line refers to PUD strains and ● in dashed line refers to NUD strains). Symbols are means of the values at each point for 2 observations.

expression and glycosylation of MUC6 or MUC2 [8]. Moreover, the susceptibility associated to male gender has been described and the hypothesis that female hormones, before the onset of the menopause, somehow protect against the development of PUD has been raised [17,18]. In agreement, we have recently reported that pediatric PUD is significantly more frequent in boys than in girls (63.6% *vs* 36.4%, $p<0.025$) when analyzing a large cohort of 1,115 Portuguese children [19]. Notwithstanding, the involvement of more pathogenic strains is surely a key factor in pediatric *H. pylori*-dependent PUD, as was clearly demonstrated by our previous reported data [9]. In order [10–12] to better characterize the virulence of such strains, we studied a group of five *H. pylori* strains isogenic for important virulence factors associated with pediatric PUD, namely *cagA*, *vacA* s1 allele, *oipA* "on", *homB* and *jhp562* (with the exception of the strain 1846/05) genes (Table 1). These were compared to another group of five strains, isolated from Portuguese children presenting NUD, all negative for those virulence factors (Table 1).

In agreement with the more pathogenic behavior of PUD *H. pylori* strains, our co-culture assays showed that, indeed, the five PUD-associated strains, when pooled together, caused a more pronounced reduction in the viability of NCI-N87 cells than the pool of five NUD-associated strains (Figure 1). In contrast to NCI-N87 cells in co-culture with NUD strains, the remaining epithelial cells after 24 h of co-culture with PUD strains presented a dramatic destabilization of the microtubule network (Figure 2F) and a decrease in the cytoplasmic reactivity to PAS (Figure 2I), suggesting lower amounts of mucins . These results are consistent with the decreased levels of mucins observed in gastric biopsies of infected adult patients with PUD and in cell lines in co-culture with *H. pylori* strains positive for both *cagA* and *vacAs1* genes [20,21]. Double staining with PAS and hematoxylin showed that *H. pylori* PUD strains induce the destruction of the cytoplasmic membrane of some host cells, leading them to release their cytoplasmic content (Figure 2M). This is similar to necrosis, a required step in the PUD pathogenesis process. Probably due to changes in environmental conditions caused by massive cell death, PUD strains acquired a coccoidal form (Figures 2I and 2M). This phenotype was already observed at 12 h of co-culture.

Taking advantage of our pediatric strains, we decided to evaluate the proteome of each of the 10 Portuguese *H. pylori* strains. Their proteome profiles were consistent (Figure 3) and comparable with proteome profiles in databases [14]. Moreover, 27 proteins were found to be differentially expressed between PUD and NUD strains (Table 2). It should be stressed that these differences in protein expression profile are intrinsic to the bacteria and were not induced by the environment. In fact, despite having experienced completely different environmental conditions *in vivo*, in this study they were grown under the same controlled conditions which did not fully resemble their natural niche. An important observation was noted for the group of PUD-associated strains: the strain 499/02 presented unique features which required special attention given that it was isolated from a child with GU and the other four were associated with DU. Although these diseases share important molecular mechanisms in their pathogenesis, they are characterized by different patterns of colonization, gastritis and gastric acid secretion [2]. Our results suggest that the ability to induce one of these situations is reflected in the proteome of the implicated *H. pylori* strains and should be investigated further. Thus, the strain 499/02 was considered separately in the subsequent analysis. Figure 5 resumes the following discussion of the differentially expressed proteins grouped according to their known function. We were not able to identify spot 7 but its role should be important role as it was absent from the proteome of all PUD strains.

Motility

For efficient colonization of the gastric niche, *H. pylori* depends on its ability to swim [22]. The results of the five pediatric strains associated with PUD (Figure 4) show higher levels of FlgE (spot 2) and FlaA (spot 3) compared to NUD strains, justifying their enhanced motility. We must stress that spot 3 may result from the overlap of FlaA and FlaB (flagellin B), another component of the *H. pylori* flagellum filament, both having equal p*I* and similar molecular weight (53 and 54 kDa, respectively). If that is the case, our results reflect a change in the abundance of both FlaA and FlaB.The abundance of HELPY_0944 protein (spot 16) was decreased in the five PUD strains compared to the NUD strains. Despite its homology with the protein HP0958 (*H. pylori* strain 26695), these results point to a different cellular function for these two proteins. Contrary to our data on the expression of FlgE, FlaA (and FlaB) and HELPY_0944 proteins, *HP0958* mutants result in non-flagellated strains, showing a total abrogation of *flgE* and *flaB* transcription [23,24] and very low levels of FlaA [25]. In fact, HP0958 protein is known to induce the transcription of *flgE* and *flgB* through stabilization of the RNA polymerase sigma factor RpoN [23,24] and the synthesis of FlaA in an RpoN-independent manner [25].

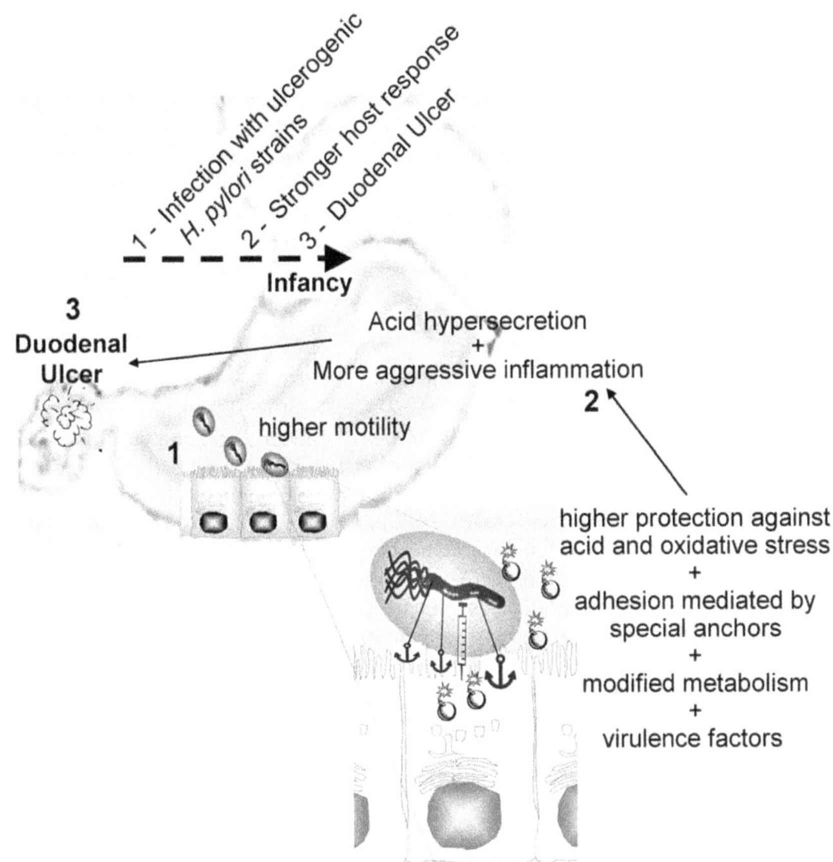

Figure 5. Schematic diagram of the DU development in children upon *H. pylori* infection. The virulence of the pediatric PUD-associated *H. pylori* strains results from a synergy between their natural ability to better adapt to the hostile human stomach and their virulence factors. Adaptation is ensured by: higher motility (↑ FlaA, ↑ FlgE, ↓ HELP_0944, ↑ HPAG1_1081, and ↑ HPG27_1480), higher ability to survive under low pH conditions (↑ UreA and B and ↑ putative aldo-keto reductase), better antioxidant defenses against inflammation (↑ Pfr, ↑ NapA and ↓ KatA), modified metabolism (↓ HyuA, ↓ AspA, ↑ Pgk, ↓ ScoA and B, ↑ AroQ, ↓ Porγ, ↑ FldA, ↓ RpsA and ↓ CysS), adhesion (indicated by a anchor) mediated by "on" OipA and HomB. Virulence factors (indicated by a bomb): cagA and VacAs1. 1 – Infection; 2 – Host response (acid hypersecretion and inflammation); 3 – duodenal acid injury (Duodenal Ulcer, indicated by an explosion symbol). Dotted arrow - Time line.

Besides its polar flagella, *H. pylori*'s spiral morphology is a requirement for its motility. In line with this, HPAG1_1081 (spot 13) was exclusively detected in DU-*H. pylori* strains. HPAG1_1081 is a homolog of HP1143, a coiled-coil protein with a predicted intermediate filament-like function [26], thus contributing to the morphology maintenance [16]. HPG27_1480 protein (spot 27), another protein found more abundantly in all PUD strains, is homolog to HP1542, a protein involved in spiral shape maintenance [15].

Antioxidant system

For a sustained infection of the inflamed gastric mucosa, characterized by the presence of large amounts of reactive oxygen species (ROS), *H. pylori* depends on the concerted activity of several proteins for its antioxidant defense [27]. Here we report higher levels of Pfr (spot 23) and NapA (spot 26) proteins and lower levels of KatA (spot 9) for the PUD strains.

Pfr is an essential protein for *H. pylori* which serves as a storage of iron in a bioavailable form [28]. Thus, besides protecting the bacterium against oxidative stress caused by the iron-mediated Fenton reaction in the presence of excessive amounts of this ion, Pfr also guarantees the necessary amount of iron for the normal metabolism of the cell under iron-limited conditions [29]. Like Pfr, NapA is capable of sequestering iron under oxidative stress conditions and these two share a protective role of the bacterial DNA [30]. NapA is, however, better known for its role in mediating the adhesion of *H. pylori* to host mucins and its ability to recruit neutrophils and monocytes to the infected gastric mucosa, inducing the secretion of chemokines [31]. According to the literature, abnormally high levels of NapA are expressed in mutant strains lacking KatA. Instrumental in catalyzing the decomposition of H_2O_2 into H_2O and O_2 [27], this enzyme has been described as being essential to the survival of *H. pylori* in a sustained long-term inflammation [27]. We therefore propose that the NUD strains analyzed in this study are prepared to resist in a long-term but less aggressive inflammation. However, the five pediatric strains associated with PUD are able to survive an acute inflammation that results in the early development of PUD.

Two isoforms of HP1588 protein (spots 17 and 18) were also differentially expressed between PUD and NUD strains. The exact function of this protein is not known although some studies indicate a potential role in stress resistance, as it is over-expressed under acidic [32] or iron starvation conditions [33].

Acid Resistance

Urease is a key enzyme in the colonization and persistence of *H. pylori*, playing a central role in the bacteria resistance to gastric acidity by catalyzing the hydrolysis of urea into ammonia and

CO_2. Ammonia is, however, cytotoxic to the host cells, causing their necrosis. This multimeric protein of approximately 1100 kDa is composed of twelve small subunits, UreA (27 kDa), and twelve large subunits, UreB (62 kDa) [34]. In agreement with our previous findings [35], urease (UreA plus UreB) was one of the most abundant proteins in the proteome of all of the *H. pylori* strains in the current study. However, the strains collected from children with DU had higher levels of both UreA and UreB, than either the NUD or the GU strains. Higher levels of HspB (spot 4), a protein which functions as an extracellular chaperonin for urease [36] among other key roles, were observed in all PUD strains.

According to the literature, excessive urease activity under neutral conditions is lethal to the bacteria [34]. Considering that no difference was detected neither in the growth rate nor in the urease activity among these pediatric strains at pH 7 (results not shown), we hypothesize that the highest amount of urease produced by the DU strains does not reflect a higher activity *per se*. Instead, urease activity must be acid–dependent and thus, once in their natural niche, DU strains are better protected against a sudden drop in pH and/or in Ni^{2+} concentration which explains their ability to survive under abnormally acidic conditions [34]. Moreover, since urease has also been proposed to play a role in adherence to gastric mucins [37], again in a acid dependent manner [38], higher levels of urease may facilitate the processes of colonization and infection, contributing to the ulcerogenic phenotype of DU strains.

Lastly the putative aldo-keto reductase (spot 15) was also found to be more abundant in DU strains. It was described as an essential enzyme for growth at acidic pH [39], and is involved in the removal of toxic aldehydes and ketones of the cell. Again, the abundance of this protein in the proteome of the GU-associated strain 499/02 was equivalent to that in NUD strains, further corroborating the idea that only the DU-associated pediatric *H. pylori* strains are prepared to face a hyper-acidic environment.

Metabolism

Among the proteins expressed differentially between NUD and PUD strains, there were 10 proteins involved in the metabolism of the bacterium.

A lower abundance of HyuA (spot 6), the enzyme responsible for the conversion of N-methyl hydantoin to N-carbamoyl sarcosine, was observed in all PUD-associated *H. pylori* strains. Not much is known about the role of this protein in *H. pylori* but this was described as a key step in the metabolism of creatine in other bacteria [40], a final pathway in the urea cycle and amino acid metabolism. Whether this may favor the endogenous production of urea we do not know and it should be investigated. In line with our findings, other authors have indicated HyuA as a biomarker for GC, since positive antibodies against it were found in sera from patients suffering with GC but not with PUD [41,42]. Interestingly, AspA (spot 11), the enzyme that by catalyzing the deamination of Asp to fumarate ensures the aneuplerotic replenishment of the latter in Krebs cycle [43,44], was in low abundance in all PUD strains compared with NUD strains. Asp and fumarate link the Krebs cycle to the urea cycle [45], therefore, we may suppose that in the former group of strains, Asp is primarily involved in the urea cycle with the concomitant production of urea. However, as *H. pylori* uses amino acids as a primary source of carbon, nitrogen and energy, with Asp being one of the eight most consumed amino acids [46], we cannot rule out that in PUD strains, Asp is used in the biosynthesis of Asp-derived amino acids. Indeed, the metabolism of amino acids was recently connected to virulence, colonization and stress resistance of *H. pylori* [46]. In *H. pylori*, the Krebs cycle is characterized by the absence of succinate dehydrogenase [44]. Although controversial, the SCOT complex which catalyzes the conversion of succinyl-CoA to succinate in an acetoacetate-dependent manner was proposed to substitute the missing enzyme [47]. Here *H. pylori* strains isolated from children with PUD presented lower levels of both subunits of the SCOT-complex, ScoA and ScoB (spots 19 and 21, respectively) which suggests a down-regulation of its catalytic activity.

Since *H. pylori* is a microaerophilic organism, the initiation of the Krebs cycle, *i.e.* the oxidative descarboxylation of pyruvate is catalyzed by an oxygen sensitive enzyme, pyruvate flavodoxin oxidoreductase (POR), instead of the aerobic pyruvate dehydrogenase or the strictly anaerobic pyruvate-formate lyase. Although its stoichiometry is unknown, POR is composed of four subunits, all essential for the *in vitro* viability of *H. pylori*. These are encoded by the *porCDAB* operon [48]. In this reaction, the FldA protein is the electron acceptor [43,44,49], a low potential one, which in turn is re-oxidized by the flavodoxin-quinone reductase (FqrB), generating NADPH. *In vitro* experiments have shown that POR is the rate limiting enzyme in this pathway [50]. The reverse reaction of this POR-FldA-FqrB-NADP reductase complex is believed to be important in the fixation of CO_2, which is essential for replenishing pyruvate consumed by gluconeogenesis [50]. Interestingly, we found significantly lower levels of one isoform of the PORγ subunit (spot 24), encoded by the *porC* gene, in the pediatric PUD-associated *H. pylori* strains compared to the NUD strains. As far as we known, the role of PORγ subunit and its isoforms in the POR complex is still unclear. However, because of the observed higher levels of FldA (spot 25), we interpret our findings as PUD strains having a more functional POR. In this case, we would expect a higher production of NADPH and acetyl-CoA in PUD strains. Further experiments are needed to clarify this. Moreover, the Pgk protein (spot 12), a glycolytic/gluconeogenic enzyme which catalyzes the reversible conversion of 1,3-biphosphoglycerate into 3-phosphoglycerate [44], was found to be more abundant in the DU-associated strains and even more abundant in the GU related *H. pylori* strain.

Chorismate, a precursor of aromatic amino acids, is formed from phosphoenol pyruvate and erythrose 4-phosphate by means of seven enzymes [44]. AroQ (spot 22), an enzyme that catalyzes the conversion of 3-dehydroquinate into 3-dehydroshikimate which is a key step in chorismate synthesis, showed an augmented expression in DU-associated *H. pylori* strains and, again, an even higher expression in the GU strain. This is suggestive of an enhancement in aromatic amino acid biosynthesis in DU strains compared to NUD strains and even more pronounced in the GU strain over all of the other [51].

In *H. pylori*, amino acids in excess of those needed for protein synthesis cannot be stored and are catabolised. Our data point out that this ability is potentiated in the pediatric PUD-*H. pylori* strains. In fact, lower levels of both RpsA (spot 8), one of the 21 ribosomal proteins of the small 30S subunit [44], and aminoacyl-tRNA synthetase CysS (spot 10) were observed for these strains when compared to NUD strains. These data suggest a down-regulation of translation in general saving amino acids for degradation. If that is the case, the aforementioned higher levels of HspB registered for PUD strains would also play an important role in avoiding protein misfolding. The elongation factor EF-Ts (spot 14), also involved in translation, showed a shift in 2DE gels of DU strains, suggesting a post-translational modification which may influence its activity. In fully agreement with these results, two studies reported that under stress, nutritional or low pH conditions, the stringent response of *H. pylori* included the down-regulation of ribosomal genes and of aminoacyl-tRNAs and, in contrast, the enhancement of amino acid biosynthesis [44,52]. The beauty of the data presented here is that are not induced by stress conditions but, as mentioned above, are intrinsic to PUD strains, making them much more adapted and, therefore, virulent.

Virulence factors

As already mentioned, all of the *H. pylori* strains associated with PUD in children that we have analyzed carried the genes of some well known virulence factors (Table 1) from which we could only detect the expression of *cagA*. CagA (spot 1 in our 2DE gels) which is known to induce abnormal proliferation, disruption of tight junctions, cytoskeleton rearrangements and IL-8 secretion in the host cells [53], was less abundant in the GU strain when compared to the other four DU associated strains.

It was important to disclose whether the special features of the proteome profile of the PUD-*H. pylori* strains of this study were linked to their *cagA/vacA*s1 positive genotype. For that, we checked the abundance of the aforementioned 26 proteins in the proteome of ten other Portuguese *H. pylori* strains isolated from children and adult patients with NUD and from adults patients with PUD and GC (five *cagA/vacA*s1 positive and five others negative for these virulence factors), all currently under study in our lab. Of those proteins, only HspB and Pfr showed a pattern of abundance in the comparison between *cagA* positive and negative strains (data not shown) similar to that presented when comparing pediatric PUD and NUD strains (data from this study). This supports our hypothesis that the pediatric *H. pylori* strains associated with PUD present a specific protein signature which provides them a natural ability of adaptation to the human stomach. This profile combined with the expression of virulence factors (*cagA*, *vacA*s1, *oipA* "on" status, *homB* and *jhp562*) appears to be responsible for their enhanced virulence. Asian isolates which present marked differences in their genetic background compared to European strains, namely being nearly all positive for *cagA*, are an interesting group to study in the future.

Conclusion

The data that we report here clearly show that the pediatric ulcerogenic *H. pylori* strains in our study share a particular proteome profile that, in addition to the well established virulence factors, provides them with higher motility. They also highlight for the strains' better antioxidant defenses and metabolism favoring the biosynthesis of aromatic amino acids, perhaps to be used as source of energy. Additionally, DU strains are apparently better fitted than all the other studied strains to survive under low pH conditions, which may justify their survival following acid hypersecretion which is characteristic of this disease. We believe that the virulence of pediatric ulcerogenic strains is strongly dependent on the synergy of their well established virulence factors and their better adaptation to the natural niche. Despite the relevance of these data, further research is required to determine their biological meaning under stressful conditions (acidic, oxidative and nutrient limited conditions). Moreover, host susceptibility should be evaluated in order to clarify its role in the pathogenesis of pediatric DU. Finally, it will be important to characterize all of the differences in the proteome profile of DU- and GU-associated *H. pylori* strains, to better understand the divergence of these diseases.

Methods

Bacteria and cell growth conditions

A total of 10 *H. pylori* strains isolated from children attending the pediatric gastroenterology units in the Lisbon area (Portugal) for upper diagnostic gastrointestinal symptoms were analyzed. These included five patients presenting NUD and five others with PUD (one GU and four DU) (Table 1). None of the children had received anti-*H. pylori* antibiotic or anti-secretory therapy prior to endoscopy. All of the children suffering from PUD had no other etiology for the disease. These strains belong to the collection of bacterial strains of the Department of Infectious Diseases of the National Institute of Health Dr. Ricardo Jorge, in Lisbon, Portugal. Bacteria were grown in *H. pylori* selective medium (Biogerm, Maia, Portugal) at 37°C in a microaerobic environment (Anoxomat®, MART Microbiology BV, Drachten, The Netherlands) for 24 h. For motility and co-culture assays, a pool of the five NUD strains and a pool of the five PUD strains were prepared by mixing biomasses recovered from 24 h grow plates of each strain (equal amount of each strain).

For co-culture assays, the NCI-N87 (ATCC CRL 5822) cell line was grown at 37°C with 5% CO_2 and 99% humidity in Dulbecco's modified Eagle's medium (DMEM/F12) (Invitrogen, Life Technologies, Carlsbad, CA, USA) supplemented with 10% (v/v) of heat inactivated (56°C for 30 min) fetal bovine serum (FBS) (Invitrogen).

Co-culture assays

A pool of the five NUD-associated strains and a pool of the five PUD-associated strains were prepared in NCI-N87 cell growth medium, and diluted to a final concentration of 1×10^8 CFU/mL. NCI-N87 cells grown on 8-well chamber slides (Nalge Nunc, Roskilde, Denmark) for immunocytochemistry assays or on 24 multi-well plates (Nalge Nunc) for cellular viability determination, until 80 to 90% confluence were rinsed twice with phosphate-buffered saline (PBS) (Invitrogen) and fresh growth medium was added. Bacterial pools were then added at a MOI of 100 and the plates were maintained under NCI-N87 cell growth conditions. Non-infected NCI-N87 cells were used as a control. At 1, 12 and 24 h post-infection, cells were analyzed by light microscopy and stained using PAS (Sigma-Aldrich Co., St. Louis, MO, USA) and hematoxylin (Sigma-Aldrich). Cell viability was determined using the classical trypan blue exclusion test (Sigma-Aldrich).

Immunocytochemistry analysis

After co-culture with the pools of *H. pylori* strains, NCI-N87 cells were rinsed twice with cold PBS and fixed for 30 min at 4°C in a 4% (v/v) formaldehyde (Sigma-Aldrich) and 3.7% (w/v) sucrose (Merck, Darmstadt, Germany) solution, in PBS. After two washes with PBS, cells were permeabilized for 15 min with 0.2% (v/v) Triton X-100 (Sigma-Aldrich) in PBS at room temperature (RT), washed three times more with PBS and blocked with 1% (w/v) bovine serum albumin (BSA) in PBS for 30 min at RT, prior to incubation for 2 h at 37°C with the anti-α-tubulin (clone DM1A) (Sigma-Aldrich) monoclonal antibody (diluted 1:1000 in 0.5% (w/v) BSA in PBS). Cells were then washed three times with PBS and incubated for 1 h at 37°C with the fluorescein isothiocyanate (FITC)-conjugated anti-mouse IgG (Sigma-Aldrich) diluted 1:100 and washed three times again. Cell slides were mounted in Vectashield (Vector Laboratories, Burlingame, CA, USA) and their immunofluorescence was observed and recorded on an Axiovert 40CFL fluorescence microscope (Carl Zeiss, Jena, Germany) equipped with an Axiocam MRc5 (Carl Zeiss) camera. Images were processed with the software AxioVision Rel. 4.6.3 (Carl Zeiss).

2DE

Bacterial total protein extracts and their separation by 2DE was performed as previously described [35]. Briefly, 800–1000 μg of protein in 450 µL re-hydration buffer were loaded onto 18 cm Immobiline DryStrips (GE Healthcare, Uppsala, Sweden) with a non-linear wide range pH gradient (pH 3–11). After active gel strip re-hydration, IEF was run on an Ettan IPGphor 3 unit (GE Healthcare) for a total of 100 kVh during which the voltage was gradually increased up to 5,000 V for a total of 66 h. For SDS-PAGE, the second dimension analysis, the proteins on the gel strips were equilibrated by soaking the strip in equilibration buffer for 15 min at RT and then for another 15 min in blocking buffer. Strips were finally applied onto 7–16% (w/v) gradient polyacrylamide gels and run overnight at 1 W/gel (Ettan DALT*six* System, GE Healthcare). Protein visualization was carried out by CBB staining (Sigma Aldrich).

2DE map analysis

CBB-stained 2DE gels were scanned in the ImageScanner (GE Healthcare) operated by the software LabScan 5 (GE Healthcare) in transparency mode with a red color filter. Scanning was carried out at 300 dpi and 16 bit grayscale. Images were analyzed using the ImageMaster^{TM} 2D Platinum software (GE Healthcare) as before [35], taking into account the standardized relative intensity volume of spots (or % Vol, *i.e.* the volume of each spot over the volume of all spots in the gel). Differences in protein abundance among strains were statistically assessed. To assure result reproducibility, all samples were subjected to 2DE twice, making a total of 20 analyzed 2DE gels.

Sample preparation and mass spectrometry analysis

The selected differentially expressed proteins were identified by PMF using an Autoflex III MALDI-TOF/TOF mass spectrometer (Bruker Daltonics, Bremen, Germany), as previously reported, with some minor modifications [35]. Protein spots were excised from the CBB-stained 2DE gels and enzymatically digested in-gel with proteomics grade porcine trypsin (Sigma-Aldrich). Trypsin-digested peptides were loaded in a disposable ready-to-use MALDI target prespotted with α-cyano-4-hydroxycinnaminic acid (Prespotted AnchorChip PAC 384/96, Bruker Daltonics) and were assayed with the mass spectrometer in the positive ion mode. Spectra acquired with the FlexControl (Compass software, version 1.2, Bruker Daltonics) in reflection mode, were processed by using FlexAnalysis (Compass software, version 1.2, Bruker Daltonics). Monoisotopic peptide masses were used to search protein databases (*H. pylori* NCBI nr. 2011.03.04, 13254464 sequences; or Swissprot databases nr. 2010.10, 521016 sequences) using MASCOT software (version 2.3.01, Matrix Science, London, UK). A mass accuracy of 50–100 ppm and 1 missed cleavage were allowed in the searches. In the absence of matches, the mass window was extended up to 200 ppm. Cysteine carbamidomethylation was considered as a fixed modification and protein *N*-terminal acetylation, oxidation of methionine and pyroglutamic-acid on N-terminal glutamic acid were allowed as variable modifications. Proteins with significant MOWSE scores ($p<0.05$) are reported. In a few special cases, MS identification based on MOWSE scores with no statistical significance were also reported and discussed since the same identification was obtained for the equivalent spot from different 2DE gels and because it matched the identification in the 2DE *H. pylori* database.

Motility assays

5 µl of each pool of *H. pylori* prepared as mention above, were inoculated with a sterile pipette tip into motility agar plates, consisting of brain-heart infusion (BHI) medium (Oxoid, Hampshire, UK) supplemented with 5% (v/v) of heat-inactivated (56°C for 30 min) FBS, *H. pylori* selective supplement (10 mg/L of vancomycin, 5 mg/L of trimethoprim, 5 mg/L of cefsulodin and 5 mg/L of amphotericin B) (Oxoid) and 0.35% (w/v) agar. Motility was scored by measuring the bacterial halo diameter at 5, 7 and 11 days of incubation of the plates under microaerobic conditions (Campygen CN0025, Oxoid), at 37°C. Differences in motility of the two pools of strains, tested in three independent experiments, were statistically assessed.

Statistics

Whenever necessary, differences were tested by Student's *t* test, being considered as statistically significant when $p<0.05$. Results are expressed as averages ± standard deviations (SD) of *n* observations.

Acknowledgments

The authors thank Professor Filipa Vale (Faculdade de Engenharia, Universidade Católica Portuguesa) for the scientific revision of the manuscript and Lindsay Mégraud for the careful revision of the English.

Author Contributions

Conceived and designed the experiments: MO MRR. Performed the experiments: IV KDSP ARG AS MO. Analyzed the data: IV AIL MO MRR. Contributed reagents/materials/analysis tools: AIL MO MRR. Wrote the paper: IV MO MRR.

References

1. Konturek PC, Konturek SJ, Brzozowski T (2009) Helicobacter pylori infection in gastric cancerogenesis. J Physiol Pharmacol 60: 3–21.
2. Lai LH, Sung JJ (2007) Helicobacter pylori and benign upper digestive disease. Best Pract Res Clin Gastroenterol 21: 261–279.
3. Atherton JC (2006) The pathogenesis of Helicobacter pylori-induced gastro-duodenal diseases. Annu Rev Pathol 1: 63–96.
4. Malfertheiner P, Chan FK, McColl KE (2009) Peptic ulcer disease. Lancet 374: 1449–1461.
5. Walsh JH, Peterson WL (1995) The treatment of Helicobacter pylori infection in the management of peptic ulcer disease. N Engl J Med 333: 984–991.
6. Kalach N, Bontems P, Koletzko S, Mourad-Baars P, Shcherbakov P, et al. (2010) Frequency and risk factors of gastric and duodenal ulcers or erosions in children: a prospective 1-month European multicenter study. Eur J Gastroenterol Hepatol 22: 1174–1181.
7. Oleastro M, Pelerito A, Nogueira P, Benoliel J, Santos A, et al. (2011) Prevalence and incidence of *Helicobacter pylori* infection in a healthy pediatric population in the Lisbon area. Helicobacter 16: 363–372.
8. Linden S, Semino-Mora C, Liu H, Rick J, Dubois A (2010) Role of mucin Lewis status in resistance to Helicobacter pylori infection in pediatric patients. Helicobacter 15: 251–258.
9. Oleastro M, Cordeiro R, Yamaoka Y, Queiroz D, Megraud F, et al. (2009) Disease association with two Helicobacter pylori duplicate outer membrane protein genes, homB and homA. Gut Pathog 1: 12.
10. Oleastro M, Cordeiro R, Ferrand J, Nunes B, Lehours P, et al. (2008) Evaluation of the clinical significance of homB, a novel candidate marker of Helicobacter pylori strains associated with peptic ulcer disease. J Infect Dis 198: 1379–1387.
11. Oleastro M, Monteiro L, Lehours P, Megraud F, Menard A (2006) Identification of markers for Helicobacter pylori strains isolated from children with peptic ulcer disease by suppressive subtractive hybridization. Infect Immun 74: 4064–4074.
12. Oleastro M, Santos A, Cordeiro R, Nunes B, Megraud F, et al. (2010) Clinical relevance and diversity of two homologous genes encoding glycosyltransferases in Helicobacter pylori. J Clin Microbiol 48: 2885–2891.
13. Basque JR, Chenard M, Chailler P, Menard D (2001) Gastric cancer cell lines as models to study human digestive functions. J Cell Biochem 81: 241–251.
14. Max Planck Institute for Infection Biology website. Available: http://web.mpiib-berlin.mpg.de. Accessed 2011 March 15.
15. Sycuro LK, Pincus Z, Gutierrez KD, Biboy J, Stern CA, et al. (2010) Peptidoglycan crosslinking relaxation promotes Helicobacter pylori's helical shape and stomach colonization. Cell 141: 822–833.

16. Waidner B, Specht M, Dempwolff F, Haeberer K, Schaetzle S, et al. (2009) A novel system of cytoskeletal elements in the human pathogen Helicobacter pylori. PLoS Pathog 5: e1000669.
17. Andreica V, Dumitrascu D, Sasca N, Toganel E, Suciu A, et al. (1990) Helicobacter-like organisms in gastroduodenal diseases. Gastroenterol Clin Biol 14: 437–441.
18. Schubert TT, Bologna SD, Nensey Y, Schubert AB, Mascha EJ, et al. (1993) Ulcer risk factors: interactions between Helicobacter pylori infection, nonsteroidal use, and age. Am J Med 94: 413–418.
19. Oleastro M, Cabral J, Ramalho PM, Lemos PS, Paixao E, et al. (2011) Primary antibiotic resistance of Helicobacter pylori strains isolated from Portuguese children: a prospective multicentre study over a 10 year period. J Antimicrob Chemother 66: 2308–2311.
20. Byrd JC, Bresalier RS (2000) Alterations in gastric mucin synthesis by Helicobacter pylori. World J Gastroenterol 6: 475–482.
21. Byrd JC, Yunker CK, Xu QS, Sternberg LR, Bresalier RS (2000) Inhibition of gastric mucin synthesis by Helicobacter pylori. Gastroenterology 118: 1072–1079.
22. Ottemann KM, Lowenthal AC (2002) Helicobacter pylori uses motility for initial colonization and to attain robust infection. Infect Immun 70: 1984–1990.
23. Pereira L, Hoover TR (2005) Stable accumulation of sigma54 in Helicobacter pylori requires the novel protein HP0958. J Bacteriol 187: 4463–4469.
24. Ryan KA, Karim N, Worku M, Moore SA, Penn CW, et al. (2005) HP0958 is an essential motility gene in Helicobacter pylori. FEMS Microbiol Lett 248: 47–55.
25. Douillard FP, Ryan KA, Caly DL, Hinds J, Witney AA, et al. (2008) Posttranscriptional regulation of flagellin synthesis in Helicobacter pylori by the RpoN chaperone HP0958. J Bacteriol 190: 7975–7984.
26. Ausmees N, Kuhn JR, Jacobs-Wagner C (2003) The bacterial cytoskeleton: an intermediate filament-like function in cell shape. Cell 115: 705–713.
27. Wang G, Alamuri P, Maier RJ (2006) The diverse antioxidant systems of Helicobacter pylori. Mol Microbiol 61: 847–860.
28. Waidner B, Greiner S, Odenbreit S, Kavermann H, Velayudhan J, et al. (2002) Essential role of ferritin Pfr in Helicobacter pylori iron metabolism and gastric colonization. Infect Immun 70: 3923–3929.
29. Kelly DJ (2001) The physiology and metabolism of Campylobacter jejuni and Helicobacter pylori. Symp Ser Soc Appl Microbiol. pp 16S–24S.
30. Wang G, Hong Y, Olczak A, Maier SE, Maier RJ (2006) Dual Roles of Helicobacter pylori NapA in inducing and combating oxidative stress. Infect Immun 74: 6839–6846.
31. D'Elios MM, Montecucco C, de Bernard M (2007) VacA and HP-NAP, Ying and Yang of Helicobacter pylori-associated gastric inflammation. Clin Chim Acta 381: 32–38.
32. Ang S, Lee CZ, Peck K, Sindici M, Matrubutham U, et al. (2001) Acid-induced gene expression in Helicobacter pylori: study in genomic scale by microarray. Infect Immun 69: 1679–1686.
33. Merrell DS, Thompson LJ, Kim CC, Mitchell H, Tompkins LS, et al. (2003) Growth phase-dependent response of Helicobacter pylori to iron starvation. Infect Immun 71: 6510–6525.
34. Stingl K, De Reuse H (2005) Staying alive overdosed: how does Helicobacter pylori control urease activity? Int J Med Microbiol 295: 307–315.
35. Vitoriano I, Rocha-Goncalves A, Carvalho T, Oleastro M, Calado CR, et al. (2011) Antigenic Diversity Among Portuguese Clinical Isolates of Helicobacter pylori. Helicobacter 16: 153–168.
36. Pyndiah S, Lasserre JP, Menard A, Claverol S, Prouzet-Mauleon V, et al. (2007) Two-dimensional blue native/SDS gel electrophoresis of multiprotein complexes from Helicobacter pylori. Mol Cell Proteomics 6: 193–206.
37. Loke MF, Lui SY, Ng BL, Gong M, Ho B (2007) Antiadhesive property of microalgal polysaccharide extract on the binding of Helicobacter pylori to gastric mucin. FEMS Immunol Med Microbiol 50: 231–238.
38. Icatlo FC, Goshima H, Kimura N, Kodama Y (2000) Acid-dependent adherence of Helicobacter pylori urease to diverse polysaccharides. Gastroenterology 119: 358–367.
39. Cornally D, Mee B, MacDonaill C, Tipton KF, Kelleher D, et al. (2008) Aldo-keto reductase from Helicobacter pylori–role in adaptation to growth at acid pH. FEBS J 275: 3041–3050.
40. Wyss M, Kaddurah-Daouk R (2000) Creatine and creatinine metabolism. Physiol Rev 80: 1107–1213.
41. Gao L, Michel A, Weck MN, Arndt V, Pawlita M, et al. (2009) Helicobacter pylori infection and gastric cancer risk: evaluation of 15 H. pylori proteins determined by novel multiplex serology. Cancer Res 69: 6164–6170.
42. Krah A, Miehlke S, Pleissner KP, Zimny-Arndt U, Kirsch C, et al. (2004) Identification of candidate antigens for serologic detection of Helicobacter pylori-infected patients with gastric carcinoma. Int J Cancer 108: 456–463.
43. Doig P, de Jonge BL, Alm RA, Brown ED, Uria-Nickelsen M, et al. (1999) Helicobacter pylori physiology predicted from genomic comparison of two strains. Microbiol Mol Biol Rev 63: 675–707.
44. Marais A, Mendz GL, Hazell SL, Megraud F (1999) Metabolism and genetics of Helicobacter pylori: the genome era. Microbiol Mol Biol Rev 63: 642–674.
45. Mendz GL, Hazell SL (1996) The urea cycle of Helicobacter pylori. Microbiology 142(Pt 10): 2959–2967.
46. Leduc D, Gallaud J, Stingl K, De Reuse H (2010) Coupled amino acid deamidase-transport systems essential for Helicobacter pylori colonization. Infect Immun 78: 2782–2792.
47. Corthesy-Theulaz IE, Bergonzelli GE, Henry H, Bachmann D, Schorderet DF, et al. (1997) Cloning and characterization of Helicobacter pylori succinyl CoA:acetoacetate CoA-transferase, a novel prokaryotic member of the CoA-transferase family. J Biol Chem 272: 25659–25667.
48. Chalker AF, Minehart HW, Hughes NJ, Koretke KK, Lonetto MA, et al. (2001) Systematic identification of selective essential genes in Helicobacter pylori by genome prioritization and allelic replacement mutagenesis. J Bacteriol 183: 1259–1268.
49. Hughes NJ, Chalk PA, Clayton CL, Kelly DJ (1995) Identification of carboxylation enzymes and characterization of a novel four-subunit pyruvate:-flavodoxin oxidoreductase from Helicobacter pylori. J Bacteriol 177: 3953–3959.
50. St Maurice M, Cremades N, Croxen MA, Sisson G, Sancho J, et al. (2007) Flavodoxin:quinone reductase (FqrB): a redox partner of pyruvate:ferredoxin oxidoreductase that reversibly couples pyruvate oxidation to NADPH production in Helicobacter pylori and Campylobacter jejuni. J Bacteriol 189: 4764–4773.
51. Bottomley JR, Clayton CL, Chalk PA, Kleanthous C (1996) Cloning, sequencing, expression, purification and preliminary characterization of a type II dehydroquinase from Helicobacter pylori. Biochem J 319(Pt 2): 559–565.
52. Mouery K, Rader BA, Gaynor EC, Guillemin K (2006) The stringent response is required for Helicobacter pylori survival of stationary phase, exposure to acid, and aerobic shock. J Bacteriol 188: 5494–5500.
53. Kusters JG, van Vliet AH, Kuipers EJ (2006) Pathogenesis of Helicobacter pylori infection. Clin Microbiol Rev 19: 449–490.

Viral Etiologies of Acute Respiratory Infections among Hospitalized Vietnamese Children in Ho Chi Minh City, 2004–2008

Anh Ha Lien Do[1]*, H. Rogier van Doorn[1,2], My Ngoc Nghiem[4], Juliet E. Bryant[1,2], Thanh Hang thi Hoang[1], Quang Ha Do[1], Tan Le Van[1], Tan Thanh Tran[1], Bridget Wills[1,2], Vinh Chau van Nguyen[4], Minh Hien Vo[4], Cong Khanh Vo[4], Minh Dung Nguyen[4], Jeremy Farrar[1,2], Tinh Hien Tran[4], Menno D. de Jong[1,2,3]

1 Oxford University Clinical Research Unit, Wellcome Trust Major Overseas Program, Ho Chi Minh City, Vietnam, **2** Nuffield Department of Clinical Medicine, University of Oxford, Oxford, United Kingdom, **3** Department of Medical Microbiology, Academic Medical Center, University of Amsterdam, Amsterdam, The Netherlands, **4** Hospital for Tropical Diseases, Ho Chi Minh City, Vietnam

Abstract

Background: The dominant viral etiologies responsible for acute respiratory infections (ARIs) are poorly understood, particularly among hospitalized children in resource-limited tropical countries where morbidity and mortality caused by ARIs are highest. Improved etiological insight is needed to improve clinical management and prevention.

Objectives: We conducted a three-year prospective descriptive study of severe respiratory illness among children from 2 months to 13 years of age within the largest referral hospital for infectious diseases in southern Vietnam.

Methods: Molecular detection for 15 viral species and subtypes was performed on three types of respiratory specimens (nose, throat swabs and nasopharyngeal aspirates) using a multiplex RT-PCR kit (Seeplex™ RV detection, Seegene) and additional monoplex real-time RT-PCRs.

Results: A total of 309 children were enrolled from November 2004 to January 2008. Viruses were identified in 72% (222/309) of cases, including respiratory syncytial virus (24%), influenza virus A and B (17%), human bocavirus (16%), enterovirus (9%), human coronavirus (8%), human metapneumovirus (7%), parainfluenza virus 1–3 (6%), adenovirus (5%), and human rhinovirus A (4%). Co-infections with multiple viruses were detected in 20% (62/309) of patients. When combined, diagnostic yields in nose and throat swabs were similar to nasopharyngeal aspirates.

Conclusion: Similar to other parts in the world, RSV and influenza were the predominant viral pathogens detected in Vietnamese hospitalized children. Combined nasal and throat swabs are the specimens of choice for sensitive molecular detection of a broad panel of viral agents. Further research is required to better understand the clinical significance of single versus multiple viral coinfections and to address the role of bacterial (co-)infections involved in severe respiratory illness.

Editor: Dong-Yan Jin, University of Hong Kong, Hong Kong

Funding: This study was funded by the Wellcome Trust of Great-Britain. The funders had no role in study design, data collection and analysis, decision to publish, or preparation of the manuscript.

Competing Interests: The authors have declared that no competing interests exist.

* E-mail: hadla@oucru.org

Introduction

Acute respiratory illnesses (ARIs) are a leading cause of infectious disease-related morbidity, hospitalization, and mortality among children worldwide, particularly in developing countries and in young children (age < 5 years) [1]. Regardless of geographic location, the most common etiologic agents of ARIs in children are viruses [2]. The most frequently implicated viruses among hospitalized children are respiratory syncytial virus (RSV), human metapneumovirus (hMPV), influenza A and B viruses (InfV A and InfV B), parainfluenza viruses (PIV1-2-3) and adenoviruses (AdV) [3]. Other commonly implicated causes are human rhinoviruses (hRV), human coronaviruses (hCoV), enteroviruses (EnV) and human bocavirus (HBoV) [4,5,6,7,8].

The development of molecular methods such as conventional or real-time reverse transcriptase polymerase (RT-PCR) has facilitated rapid and sensitive simultaneous diagnostic detection of the variety of viruses causing respiratory tract infection [9]. However, limited resources and laboratory capacity precludes the routine use of molecular diagnostics in tropical lower-income countries such as Vietnam. As a consequence, insight into the aetiology of ARIs is lowest in regions of the world where morbidity and mortality are highest. Better understanding of the full spectrum of respiratory viruses causing ARIs in hospitalized patients in these settings is essential for improving preventive and therapeutic strategies and prioritizing diagnostic efforts.

Here we performed a 3-year prospective descriptive study to report on viral aetiologies, clinical features and epidemiological patterns of ARIs in hospitalized Vietnamese children using established commercially available and in-house nucleic acid amplification techniques. In addition, we used these techniques to evaluate which clinical specimen had the highest yield for ARI diagnostics by comparing nasopharyngeal aspirates and individual or combined throat and nasal swabs.

Methods

Study design

Patients were enrolled from November 2004 to January 2008 from the Paediatric Intensive Care Unit (PICU) and the Paediatric Respiratory Ward (PRW) at the Hospital for Tropical Diseases (HTD) in Ho Chi Minh City, the largest referral hospital for infectious diseases in southern Vietnam. Children were eligible for inclusion if less than 15 years of age and if admitted for an ARI or ARI-related condition (respiratory distress, pneumonia, bronchiolitis, croup) with an onset of illness less than 5 days before hospitalization. Excluded were patients who were discharged from a hospital in the previous 4 days, newborns who never left the hospital, patients with uncomplicated upper respiratory illness (e.g. rhinitis, sinusitis, otitis media), or patients with proven or suspected non-infectious respiratory symptoms (e.g asthma). Demographic, socio-economic, and clinical data were documented in case report forms (CRFs). Three types of respiratory specimens (nasal swabs, throat swabs, and nasopharyngeal aspirates) were collected on admission by trained personnel using standard operating procedures, and were placed in viral transport medium [10]. Specimens were kept at 4°C for a maximum of 24 h and then aliquotted and stored at −80°C until further processing.

Ethics

The study was approved by the Scientific and Ethical Committee of the Hospital for Tropical Diseases and the Oxford University Tropical Research Ethical Committee.

Written informed consent was obtained from parents or legal guardians of children enrolled in the study.

Diagnostic testing

For specimens collected between November 2004 to June 2007, RNA was extracted from 100 μl of each respiratory specimen using an inhouse GuSCN based extraction protocol [11] or Qiagen Viral RNA mini kits, according to the instructions of the manufacturer (Qiagen, Hilden, Germany). Since July 2007, an automated commercial GuSCN-based method was used, according the instructions of the manufacturer (Easy MAG 2.0, bioMérieux, Marcy l'Étoile, France). For each individual patient, all three respiratory specimens were extracted simultaneously. An internal RNA-virus control (equine arteritis virus (EAV)) was added to each sample prior to extraction at a standard concentration yielding a Ct value of 30 to 35 cycles in real-time RT-PCR. RNA was reversely transcribed using Superscript III reverse transcriptase (Invitrogen, Carlsbad, USA) and random hexamers (Roche, Mannheim, Germany). Each 20 μl reaction mixture contained 5 μl extracted RNA, 4 μl 1 of 5X RT-buffer, 0.5 mM of each dNTP (Roche), 2 ng random hexamer, 10 mM DTT (Invitrogen), 1 UI of RNAse inhibitor and 2 UI RT Superscript III. The cDNA synthesis was performed using an Eppendorf Master thermocycler gradient system (Perkin-Elmer Corporation, Foster City, USA) under the following conditions: 10 min at 25°C, 60 min at 50°C and 15 min at 75°C.

Detection of 12 respiratory viral pathogens, including influenza A (InfV A), influenza B (InfV B), RSV types A and B (RSV A, RSV B), hCoV (229E, OC43), hMPV, PIV types 1, 2 and 3 (PIV1, 2, 3), hRV A and AdV, was performed using a commercially available, internally controlled multiplex RT-PCR (Seeplex™ RV Detection kit, Seegene, Inc., Seoul, Korea) according to the manufacturer's instructions[12]. In addition, three previously described monoplex real-time PCRs were performed for detection of HBoV [7], enteroviruses (EnV) [13] and hCoV NL63[14] (**Table 1**).

Data analysis

A positive case was defined as the presence of any viral pathogen detected in any specimen type of a given patient. A patient was considered to have a single viral infection if only one pathogen was detected in one or more of the tested specimens. In case more than one viral pathogen detected, patients were considered to have viral co-infections. Severe disease was defined as being admitted to PICU. Fast breathing was classified according to WHO standards [15], i.e, ≥ 60 per minute in a child aged < 2 months, ≥ 50 per minute in a child aged 2 to 11 months and ≥ 40 per minute in a child aged ≥12 months.

We used a consensus standard to assess sensitivity: a patient was considered a true-positive (TP) for a given virus if any specimen type or testing method yielded a positive result. Thus, the specificity of each specimen type for any given virus was by definition 100%. Sensitivity per sample and virus was assessed using the following definitions: true negatives (TN), defined as the number of patients negative in all three specimens and false negatives (FN), defined as a negative sample while an alternative specimen from the same patient tested positive for a given virus. For the comparison of independent groups, we used the Mann-Whitney U test for continuous data and the Fisher exact test for categorical data. The Wilcoxon signed-rank test was used for pairwise comparisons of matched pairs of Ct values of the three types specimens from monoplex real-time RT-PCRs for HBoV, enteroviruses and hCoV NL63. Sensitivities of the different specimen types were compared using McNemar's test. All statistical tests were conducted at the two-tailed 5% significance level. Analyses were performed with R 2.9.1 (R Foundation for Statistical Computing, Vienna, Austria) and Intercooled Stata 9.2 (College Station, TX, USA).

Table 1. Primers and probes used in monoplex real-time RT-PCRs to detect HBoV, enterovirus and hCoV-NL63.

Virus name	Gene target	Primers/ probes name	Nucleotide sequence
hBoV[7]	NP-1	Boca-F	5′-GGAAGAGACACTGGCAGACAA-3′
		Boca-R	5′-GGGTGTTCCTGATGATATGAGC-3′
		Boca probe	FAM-5′-CTGCGGCTCCTGCTCCTGTGAT-3′-TAMRA
EnV[13]	5′_NC	Entero-F	5′-CCCTGAATGCGGCTAAT-3′
		Entero-R	5′- ATTGTCACCATAAGCAGCC-3′
		Entero-probe	FAM-5′-CGGAACCGACTACTTT-GGGT-3′-TAMRA
hCoV NL63[14]	Spike gene	NL63-F	5′ -GCGTGTTCCTACCAGAGAGGA-3′
		NL63-R	5′-GCTGTGGAAAACCTTTGGCA- 3′
		NL63-probe	FAM-5′-ATGTTATTCAGTGCTTTGG-TCCTCGTGAT-3′-TAMRA

Results

Study population

A total of 309 patients were enrolled in the study between November 2004 and January 2008. Ages ranged from 2 months to 13 years, and 181 (59%) patients were less than 2 years old. 79 (26%) of 309 patients were admitted to the PICU. Demographic and clinical characteristics of the PICU and PRW cohorts are shown in **Table 2**. At admission, most patients had fever, cough, runny nose, and fast breathing (154/309; 51%). Twenty percent (61/309) had indrawings, 33% (101/309) had wheezing, 31% (95/309) had crepitations, and 2% (6/309) had stridor. Patients with clinical symptoms suggestive of severe pneumonia [16], i.e fast breathing with cyanosis, indrawings or stridor, were all admitted to PICU. Oxygen support was required in 49% (39/79) of PICU patients, only one case required mechanical ventilation. Compared to PRW admitted patients, a significant higher number of PICU patients were hospitalized for more than 7 days (**Table 2**). In addition, they were more likely to have been exposed to cooking smoke and more often had other family members who were sick at home. A history of previous hospitalizations for respiratory illness was observed more frequently in patients admitted to PRW (**Table 2**).

Diagnoses at admission were based on clinical and laboratory information and Xray interpretation; physicians were unaware of diagnostic results for respiratory viruses during data collection, except for two suspected H5N1 cases as these were diagnosed for public health purposes by specific PCR. Nearly half of cases (46%, 142/309) were diagnosed as ARI at admission, followed by bronchiolitis in 34%, broncho-pneumonia in 16%, pneumonia in 3% and laryngitis or laryngotracheitis in 1% (4/309). Broncho-pneumonia was more frequently diagnosed among PICU than PRW patients (**Table 2**).

The median duration of hospitalisation was 6 days, and 25% of patients were hospitalized for more than 7 days. Discharge information was available for 295 of 309 cases: 93% of patients fully recovered; 1% (4/295) had an incomplete recovery at the time of discharge; 5% (15/295) went home without permission of ward doctors; and 2 patients (1%) died. One fatal case was diagnosed with influenza A (H5N1)-associated viral pneumonia and died on day of admission. The second fatal case was negative for all viruses tested, and was diagnosed with severe pneumonia with shock syndrome of unknown aetiology. Diagnosis of bacterial pathogens was not systematically performed. However, 98% of patients received antibiotic treatment during admission. The two suspect cases of Influenza A/H5N1 infection received oseltamivir treatment.

Viral etiologies, age distribution, seasonality and severity

One or multiple viral pathogens were detected in respiratory specimens of 222 of 309 (72%) patients. RSV was most frequently detected (24%, 73/309), followed by influenza viruses (17%, 51/309), HBoV (16%, 50/309) and enteroviruses (9%, 28/309) (**Table 3**). Single infections accounted for 52% (160/309) of cases. Infections with multiple viruses were found in 20% (62/309): dual infections were identified in 18% of cases (55/309), triple infections in 2% (6/309), while in one case 4 different viruses were detected.

RSV and influenza viruses were the leading causes of single infections, followed by hBoV and hMPV. Human bocavirus was most frequently involved in co-infections (n = 27), followed by RSV, influenza viruses (both n = 21), hCoV-NL63 (n = 16) and enteroviruses (n = 15). Among RSV cases, co-infection with hBoV was most frequent (8/21), followed by influenza viruses (7/21) and hCoV (5/21). For influenza cases, co-infection with hCoV was most frequent (8/21), followed by RSV (7/21) and HBoV (6/21). 16/21 additional viruses were also detected among hCoV-NL63 infection cases.

RSV was the most common virus detected in children less than 5 years whereas influenza virus was most prevalent virus among children over 5 (**Table 4**). Wheezing was significantly more frequent among RSV-positive cases (32/72 (44%)) than among RSV-negative cases (69/233 (30%); p = 0.02), as were crepitations (36/72 (50%) vs. 59/175 (25%); p = 0.001). Among HBoV-infected children, throat viral loads were higher in patients with wheezing symptoms than in those without, as indicated by lower Ct values in the former (p = 0.03).

Except for RSV, influenza and HBoV, no significant associations were observed between viral etiologies and age distributions, signs or symptoms, clinical diagnosis, or duration of hospital stay (**Table 2** and **Table 5**). Similarly, there were no apparent differences in clinical characteristics or severity between single and multiple infections, nor between virus-positive and virus-negative cases. However, among virus -positive patients, we found that PICU patients were significantly younger than respiratory ward patients (Mann-Whitney's test p = 0.001).

RSV infection showed seasonal variation with peaks during the rainy season from May to October. Seasonality of hMPV infection was also apparent during the rainy season. Influenza cases occurred throughout the year (**Figure 1**). The numbers of remaining viral aetiologies were insufficient to detect seasonal patterns.

Optimal specimen for viral diagnosis

Virus was detected in a total of 226 respiratory specimens from 222 patients. 117 (40%) patients tested positive in all three specimens collected, 33 (11%) were positive only in nasal swabs, 29 (10%) only in throat swabs, and 46 (16%) only in NPA specimens. The diagnostic yield of the three specimen types are shown in **Table 6**. Overall, diagnostic yield from NPAs was superior although pair-wise differences were not significant. However, separate analyses of specific viruses demonstrated significantly superior yield of NPA specimens for influenza viruses (p = 0.05 and p = 0.006 for NPA versus nasal swab and throat swab, respectively). For enteroviruses, throat swabs were superior (p = 0.01 and p = 0.02 for throat swab versus nasal swab and NPA, respectively). In addition, Ct values of enteroviruses from throat swabs were significantly lower, indicating higher viral loads, compared to nasal swabs (median Ct value of throat swab was 30.8 (IQR 28.2–33.7) versus median Ct value of nasal swab 34.6 (IQR 33–37.1), p = 0.003).

We evaluated our dataset to examine the diagnostic yield from a combination of the results of nasal and throat swabs (NTS) relative to NPA (**Table 6**). Our analysis indicated that testing of combined NTS should yield comparable sensitivities to NPAs for detection of all respiratory viruses of our panel, and is likely to significantly improve the detection of enteroviruses (McNemar's test p = 0.001).

Discussion

Here we report the viral etiologies of ARIs in 309 hospitalized children in southern Vietnam enrolled during a period of more than three years (11/2004-1/2008). Seventy-two percent of patients were diagnosed with single virus infections and 20% were co-infected with multiple respiratory viruses. Overall, RSV was the most frequently detected virus, and accounted for 24% of infections in children less than 5 years old. Influenza (17%) was the

Table 2. Demographic and clinical characteristics of study cohort.

	PICU		PRW	
	N	Value(%)	N	Value(%)
Demographic				
Median age in months (IQR)	78	15.5 (10–25)	230	24 (17–36)
Infant (<12months)	78	30 (38.0)	230	26 (11)
Male	79	44 (56)	223	128 (57)
Mean birth weight (kg) (IQR)	74	3.2 (2.9–3.4)	171	3.1 (2.8–3.4)
Median number of family members (IQR)	78	5 (4–7)	222	5 (4–6)
Exposed to cooking smoke [1]	79	**69 (87)**	230	**45 (20)**
Living with smokers	79	60 (76)	230	165 (81)
Medical story and clinical characteristics				
Previous hospitalization with respiratory diseases [2]	76	**27 (36)**	226	**120 (53)**
Other family members sick at home [3]	78	**20 (26)**	226	**30 (13)**
Median (IQR) onset of illness [4]	79	**4 (3–5)**	229	**3 (3–4)**
Fast breathing [5]	77	**55 (71)**	224	**102 (46)**
Cyanosis	79	4 (5.)	228	0 (0)
Indrawings	79	61 (77)	228	0 (0)
Stridor	78	5 (6)	227	1 (0)
Wheezing [6]	79	**65 (82)**	226	**36 (16)**
Crepitations [7]	79	**55 (70)**	227	**40 (18)**
Fever (>37.5°C) **Fever ≥ 38.5°C** [8]	79	77 (97) **25 (32)**	229	229 (100) **159 (69)**
Rash	79	1 (1)	227	17 (7)
Cough	79	77 (97)	229	226 (99)
Runny noses	76	49 (61)	228	220 (96)
Oxygen	79	39 (49)	229	0 (0)
Diagnosis at admission				
Bronchiolitis	79	24 (30)	230	81 (35)
Broncho-pneumonia [9]	79	**42 (53)**	230	**6 (3)**
Pneumonia	79	10 (13)	230	0 (0)
Laryngitis	79	3 (4)	230	1 (0)
ARIs	79	0 (0)	230	142 (62)
Median of duration of hospitalization (IQR) **Duration of hospitalization >7 days** [10]	78	7 (6–9) **34 (44)**	218	6 (4–7) **44(20)**
Median of number of white cells in blood (K/mm^3) (IQR)	79	14.2 (10.0–19.5)	223	11.1 (7.9–15.0)
Clinical outcomes				
Fully recovery (%)	78	69 (88)	217	205 (94)
Death	78	2 (3)	217	0 (0)
Viral pathogen				
Virus positive (%)	79	58 (73.4)	230	164 (71.3)
Single infection (%)	79	43 (54.4)	230	117 (50.9)
Co-infection (%)	79	15 (19.0)	230	47 (20.4)
Single RSV infection (%)	79	14 (17.7)	230	38 (16.5)
Single Influenza virus infection (%)	79	5 (6.3)	230	25 (10.9)
Single HBoV infection (%)	79	6 (7.6)	230	17 (7.4)
Single hMPV infection (%)	79	4 (5.1)	230	12 (5.2)
Single EnV infection (%)	79	2 (2.5)	230	11 (4.8)
Single hRV A infection (%)	79	4 (5.1)	230	1 (0.4)

Table 2. Cont.

PICU, Pediatric Intensive Care Unit; PRW, Pediatric Respiratory Ward. Values in bold and underline indicate statistical significance ($p < 0.05$).
[1]p value Fisher's exact = 0.001.
[2]p value Fisher's exact = 0.008.
[3]p value Fisher's exact = 0.01.
[4]p value Mann-Whitney'test = 0.003.
[5, 6, 7]Fast breathing, wheezing and crepitations (p value Fisher's exact = 0.001).
[8]p value Fisher's exact = 0.001.
[9]p value Fisher's exact = 0.001.
[10]p value of Fisher's test = 0.001.

second most common virus detected, while the recently discovered hBoV, hMPV and hCoV-NL63 were detected in 16%, 7%, and 7% of cases, respectively. Enteroviruses were found in 9% of cases, supporting studies from both Europe [6], [17] and southeast Asia [18] which also detected enteroviruses in a large fraction of children with respiratory infections.

Our findings are consistent with other reports from Asia and elsewhere indicating that RSV and influenza are dominant causes of severe respiratory tract infections in children [19,20,21,22]. However, the clinical significance of co-infections and the relative ranking of the other respiratory viruses in our panel remain unclear. A recent study of ARI in Nha Trang (Central Vietnam) reported almost identical prevalence rates for RSV and influenza A but found a lower percentage of co-infections (11% versus 20% in our study) and different prevalence rates for rhinovirus (28% versus 4% in our patients) and bocavirus (5% verus 16% in our patients) [23,24]. These differences likely reflect differences in study design and testing protocols: Yoshida *et al.* included a large number of ambulatory outpatients whereas our study focused exclusively on hospitalized cases; their diagnostic testing was based on nasal swab alone; their PCR for rhinovirus was able to detect rhinovirus types A, B and C whereas ours detected only rhinovirus A and B; and their panel of viruses did *not* include either enteroviruses or hCoV NL63.

We found that RSV and hMPV cases were detected mainly during the rainy season from May to October, supporting previous observations from tropical or subtropical regions [23,24]. In contrast, influenza seems to occur throughout the year with no discernable peak incidences.

Our results confirm and extend previous observations regarding the importance of RSV in children under 5 [23,24], and the clinical association between wheezing and RSV infection [25] [26,27]. Increasing evidence suggests that RSV infections may be related to asthma phenotypes, with progressive disappearance of

Table 3. Viral etiologies identified.

	Single infection			Co- infection			Total positive cases
Viral causes	**PICU**	**PRW**	**Subtotal n (%)**	**PICU**	**PRW**	**Subtotal n (%)**	**n (%)**
RSV	14	38	52 (17)	6	15	21 (7%)	73 (24)
RSV A	7	23	30 (10)	3	9	12 (4)	42 (14)
RSV B	7	15	22 (7)	3	6	9 (3)	31 (10)
Influenza	5	25	30 (10)	5	16	21 (7)	51 (17)
InfV A	2	15	17 (6)	2	8	10 (3)	27 (9)
InfV B	3	10	13 (4)	3	8	11 (4)	24 (8)
HBoV	6	17	23 (7)	6	21	27 (9)	50 (16)
EnV	2	11	13 (4)	3	12	15 (5)	28 (9)
hMPV	4	12	16 (5)	1	4	5 (2)	21 (7)
Parainfluenza virus	4	7	11 (3)	2	6	8 (3)	19 (7)
PIV-1	1	3	4 (1)	1	3	4 (1)	8 (3)
PIV-2	1	0	1 (0)	0	2	2 (1)	3 (1)
PIV-3	2	4	6 (2)	1	1	2 (1)	8 (3)
Coronavirus	4	3	7 (2)	5	12	17 (5)	24 (8)
hCoV-NL63	3	2	5 (2)	5	11	16 (5)	21 (7)
hCoV-229E	1	0	1 (0)	0	0	0 (0)	1 (0)
hCoV-OC43	0	1	1 (0)	0	1	1 (0)	2 (1)
AdV	0	3	3 (1)	3	9	12 (4)	15 (5)
hRV A	4	1	5 (2)	1	5	6 (2)	11 (4)
Total	43	117	160 (52)	32	100	62 (20)	222 (72)

Case numbers reflect combined results from all three specimen types. All percentages were calculated as the fraction of the total study population (N = 309).

Table 4. Age group distribution of viral etiologies.

Virus detected	Age groups <1 year (N = 56)		1-5 years (N = 239)		>5 years (N = 13)	
	n	%	n	%	n	%
RSV A& B	12	21%	60	25%	1	8%
InfV A&B	6	11%	41	17%	4	31%
HBoV	12	21%	36	15%	1	8%
EnV	5	9%	23	10%	0	0%
hMPV	0	0%	20	8%	1	8%
PIV (1-3)	8	14%	11	5%	0	0%
hCoV	5	9%	16	7%	3	23%
AdV	1	2%	14	6%	0	0%
hRV A	2	4%	9	4%	0	0%
Single infections	28	50%	126	53%	5	38%
Co-infections	10	18%	50	21%	2	15%
Positives cases	38	68%	176	74%	7	54%

Percentages were calculated based on the fraction of study population within each age group. (Note, age data was not available for one case.)

this effect with increasing age [28]. As such, our findings emphasize the importance of screening for RSV in paediatric cases of asthma. Our results also confirm observations of Allander *et al* suggesting an association between HBoV levels and symptoms of wheezing [7], indicating that information about viral load may be important for better understanding of disease pathogenesis.

We found significant associations between disease severity and a history of exposure to household cooking smoke. Indoor pollution due to biomass fuels (wood, crop residues and animal dung) or coal burning is a known risk factor for ARI mortality and morbidity in developing countries[29,30]. Disease severity was also associated with longer delays between onset of illness and presentation to

Table 5. Summary of associations between clinical characteristics and viral single/co-infection or viral positive cases and viral negative cases.

Characteristic	Single infection (n = 160)	Co-infection (n = 62)	Virus positive (n = 222)	Virus negative (n = 87)
Age[a]	21 (14–36)	24 (14–35)	22 (14–35)	24 (14–36)
Fever (%)	99 (61.9)	35 (56.5)	134 (60.4)	50 (57.5)
Fast breathing[b] (%)	84 (52.5)	28 (45.2)	112 (50.5)	45 (51.7)
Cyanosis (%)	3 (1.9)	0 (0)	3 (1.4)	1 (1.1)
Oxygen (%)	22 (13.8)	5 (8.1)	27 (12.2)	12 (13.8)
Indrawing (%)	34 (21.3)	9 (14.5)	43 (19.4)	18 (20.7)
Stridor (%)	2 (1.3)	2 (3.2)	4 (1.8)	2 (2.30
Wheeze (%)	58 (36.3)	18 (29.0)	76 (34.2)	25 (28.70
Crepitations (%)	58 (36.3)	13 (21.0)	71 (32.0)	24 (27.6)
Bronchiolitis (%)	59 (36.9)	16 (25.8)	75 (33.8)	30 (34.5)
Broncho-pneumonia (%)	32 (20.0)	9 (14.5)	41 (18.5)	7 (8.0)
Pneumonia (%)	3 (1.9)	2 (3.2)	5 (2.3)	5 (5.7)
Laryngitis (%)	1 (0.6)	2 (3.2)	3 (1.40	1 (1.0)
ARIs (%)	65 (40.6)	33 (53.2)	98 (44.1)	44 (50.6)
Hospital duration[c]	7 (5–8)	6 (4–8)	6 (5–8)	6 (5–8)
Duration > 7 days [d] (%)	40 (25.0)	15 (24.2)	55 (24.8)	23 (26.4)

Percentages were calculated based on the fraction of patients having a specific symptom within each group.
[a]Median (IQR) of age of each group.
[b]fast breathing was defined according to the standard WHO [15].
[c]Median (IQR) of duration of hospitalization (days).
[d]Number and percentage of patients having duration of hospitalization lasted longer than 7 days.

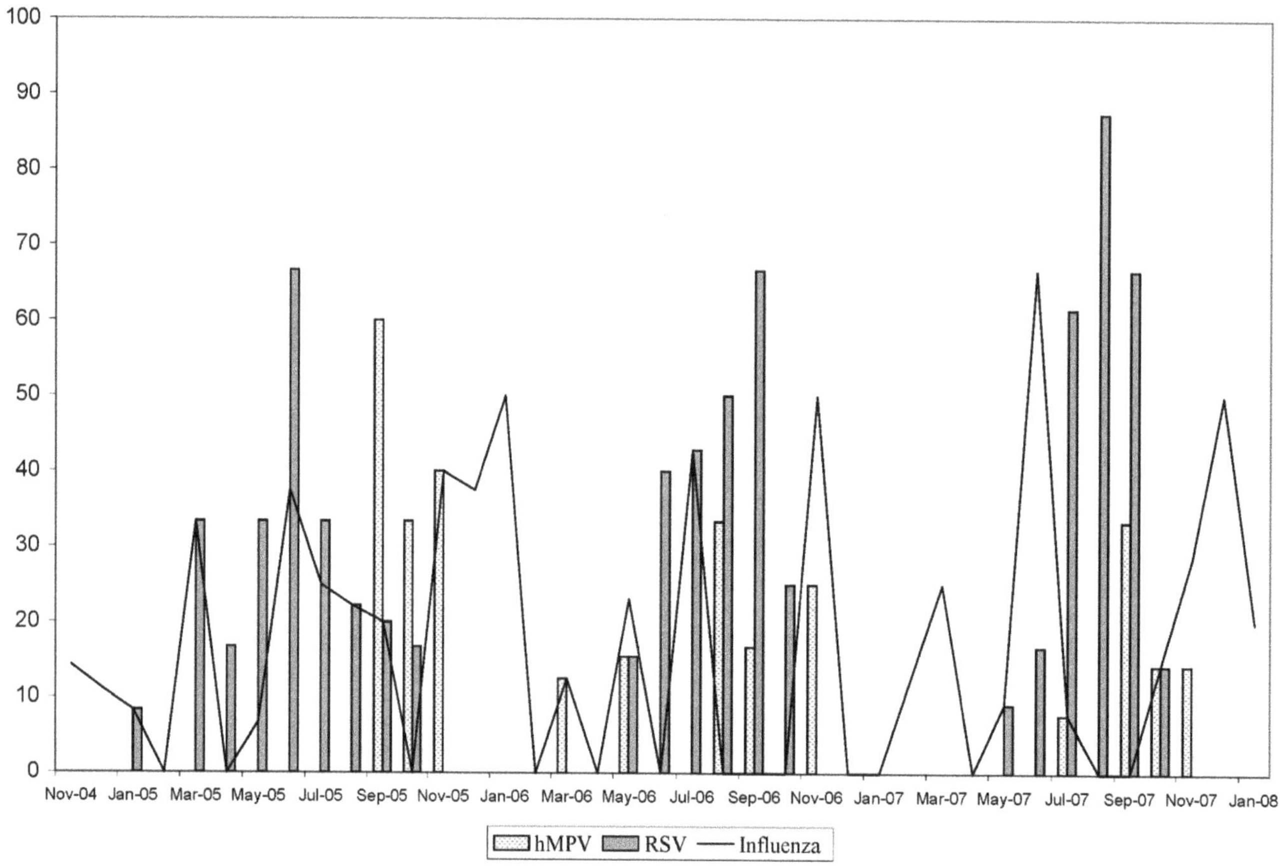

Figure 1. Proportion of RSV and hMPV positive cases recruited each month from November 2004 to January 2008. Time in months is displayed on the X-axis and the percentage of positive cases of each virus among all cases recruited in that month on the y-axis.

Table 6. Diagnostic sensitivity and efficacy of respiratory specimens and combined nasal-throat (NT) swabs by viral etiology.

Virus detected	Total positive cases (N)	Nasal swabs		Throat swabs		NPA		NT swabs	
		Sensitivity % (n)	95%CI	Sensitivity % (n)	95%CI	Sensitivity % (n)	95%CI	Sensitivity % (n)	95%CI
Any virus*	222	75(166)	69–81	73(161)	67–78	78(173)	73–83	79(176)	73–84
RSV	73	84(61)	75–92	81(59)	72–90	90(66)	84–97	93(68)	85-98
InfV	51	**53**[i](27)	39–67	**45**[ii](23)	31–59	**75**[i,ii](38)	63–87	73(37)	58-84
HBoV	50	65(32)	51–78	52(26)	38–66	65(32)	52–79	78(39)	64-89
EnV	28	**50**[iii](14)	32–69	**85** [iii,iv](23)	72–99	**48**[iv, v](13)	29–67	**93**[v](26)	77-99
hMPV	21	67(14)	47–87	71(15)	52–91	71(15)	52–91	81(17)	58-95
PIV	19	74(14)	49–91	44(8)	22–67	72(13)	52–93	79(15)	54-94
AdV	15	73(11)	51–96	87(13)	70 -100	73(11)	51–96	100(15)	78-1
hRV A	11	64(7)	35–92	73(8)	46–99	91(10)	74–100	82(9)	48-98
hCoV	24	58(14)	39–78	58(14)	39–78	50(12)	30 -70	83(20)	63-95
Picornavirus[#]	36	58(21)	41–75	83(30)	67–91	64(23)	46–79	92(33)	78-98

Underlined and bold numbers indicate significant differences in paired values by McNemar's test:
[i]between nasal swabs and NPA ($p = 0.05$);
[ii]between NPA and throat swabs ($p = 0.006$);
[iii]between nasal swabs and throat swabs ($p = 0.01$);
[iv]between throat swabs and NPA ($p = 0.02$);
[v]between NT swabs and NPA ($= 0.001$).
*refers to the total number of positive cases, defined as the detection of any viral pathogen in any specimen per patient.
[#]refers to cases in whose samples enterovirus or human rhinovirus A was detected.

hospital. Delays in presentation are typical of health seeking behavior in lower income households of developing countries [31]. Our patient survey questionnaire did not include explicit questions regarding household income, however our findings clearly indicate the need for further research on the socio-economic risk factors associated with ARI.

Numerous previous studies have investigated optimal sampling methods for diagnosis of respiratory viruses by culture, immunofluorescence, or molecular techniques [32,33,34,35,36,37]. Regardless of the diagnostic approach, NPA specimens typically exhibit increased sensitivity (15-31%) relative to nasal swabs or throat swabs. However, the differential increase appears less marked for molecular based methods [32]. Indeed, results of the present study indicate that, although NPAs yielded the highest overall yield of virus detection (78%, 173/222), the differential improvement over nasal or throat swabs was marginal and not statistically significant across all viruses (**Table 6**). Nevertheless, NPAs were significantly superior to nasal or throat swabs for detection of influenza viruses ($p \leq 0.05$), whereas throat swabs were superior for enteroviruses ($p \leq 0.05$). Combining the results of nasal and throat swabs rendered comparable sensitivities to NPAs for detection of all respiratory viruses of our panel and increased sensitivity for enteroviruses. As nasal and throat swabs are easier to obtain and less distressing for patients, these samples are preferred in our setting.

There were several limitations to our study. Firstly, we focused only on viral aetiologies since these are common causes of ARI and understudied in this region. However, this prevented the possibility of addressing key questions about bacterial pathogens and the possible role of viral and bacterial co-infections. As nearly all children in our study received antibiotic treatment, and issues involving judicious use of antibiotics and resistance development is becoming increasingly important in Vietnam, inclusion of bacterial pathogens in future studies will be essential. Second, our testing algorithm did not include measles virus. We suspect there may have been undiagnosed measles cases within our cohort, since 6/18 cases who presented with rash on admission were negative for all viruses tested; furthermore, national surveillance data indicates that Vietnam experienced a rise in measles cases in 2005–2006 [38]. Lastly, our sample size was limited and insufficient to allow more refined observations regarding differences in age distributions, clinical characteristics, or determinants of severity between specific viral species. The principle reasons for limited enrollment were a) resource constraints and feasibility (overburdening of doctors and nurses in wards where admission of 2 to 3 patients per bed is common practice), and b) limited familiarity with clinical research among patients and parents in this setting and thus additional challenges to obtaining consent. In total, during the 3-year study period, only 4.1% of all admitted ARI patients at the respiratory ward (40 beds) were enrolled in the

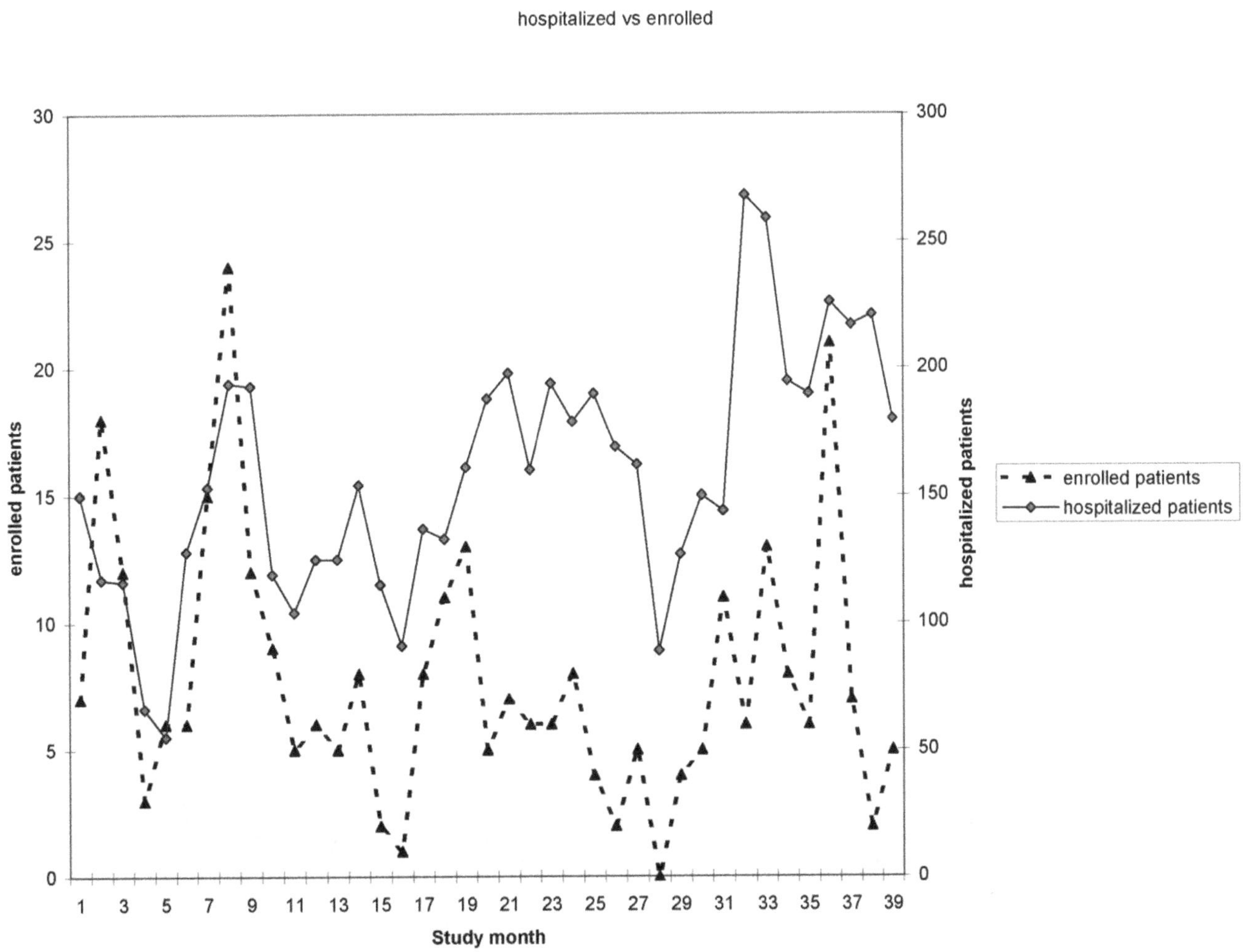

Figure 2. Number of cases enrolled and total numbers of ARI children hospitalized in HTD, November 2004 to January 2008.

study, and 14.2% of ARI patients admitted to the PICU (15 beds). While the sample size of enrolled patients relative to the total number of admitted patients was small, the proportion remained stable throughout the study period and the number of enrolled patients followed a similar pattern as the number of admitted patients over time (**Figure 2**). For these reason, we believe that our study population nevertheless provided a reasonable representation of the overall ARI patient population in Ho Chi Minh City at the time.

In conclusion, our study contributes critical baseline epidemiological data on ARI in Vietnam, and highlights the importance of RSV and influenza as dominant viral etiologies of severe pediatric ARI. Our findings indicate that combined nasal-throat swabs are the specimens of choice for sensitive molecular detection of a broad panel of viral agents. Pneumonia remains a leading cause of death among children less than 5 years old in developing countries, and continues to be a salient public health problem in Vietnam. Enhancing existing surveillance systems to better understand disease burden of respiratory pathogens is one step forward to development of therapeutic and prevention strategies.

Acknowledgments

The study would not have been possible without the excellent support from all clinicians from the Paediatric Intensive Care Unit and from the Paediatric Respiratory Ward of the Hospital for Tropical Diseases. Special thanks to Marcel Wolbers, Hoang thi Thanh Hang for statistical advice and to Tran Thuy Ngan, Duong thi Tam, Le thi Tam Uyen from the Molecular Diagnostic Group of the Virology Department of OUCRU for help with the work.

Author Contributions

Conceived and designed the experiments: MDJ THT JF BW. Performed the experiments: MNN. Analyzed the data: AHLD THtHJB HRvD MDJ. Contributed reagents/materials/analysis tools: AHLD QHD TLV TTT VCvN MHV CKV MDN. Wrote the paper: AHLD JB HRvD MDJ.

References

1. Williams BG, Gouws E, Boschi-Pinto C, Bryce J, Dye C (2002) Estimates of world-wide distribution of child deaths from acute respiratory infections. Lancet Infect Dis 2: 25–32.
2. Cilla G, Onate E, Perez-Yarza EG, Montes M, Vicente D, et al. (2008) Viruses in community-acquired pneumonia in children aged less than 3 years old: High rate of viral coinfection. J Med Virol 80: 1843–1849.
3. Yeolekar LR, Damle RG, Kamat AN, Khude MR, Simha V, et al. (2008) Respiratory viruses in acute respiratory tract infections in Western India. Indian J Pediatr 75: 341–345.
4. Sloots TP, Whiley DM, Lambert SB, Nissen MD (2008) Emerging respiratory agents: new viruses for old diseases? J Clin Virol 42: 233–243.
5. Papadopoulos NG (2004) Do rhinoviruses cause pneumonia in children? Paediatr Respir Rev 5(Suppl A): S191–195.
6. Jacques J, Moret H, Minette D, Leveque N, Jovenin N, et al. (2008) Epidemiological, molecular, and clinical features of enterovirus respiratory infections in French children between 1999 and 2005. J Clin Microbiol 46: 206–213.
7. Allander T, Jartti T, Gupta S, Niesters HG, Lehtinen P, et al. (2007) Human bocavirus and acute wheezing in children. Clin Infect Dis 44: 904–910.
8. Weiss SR, Navas-Martin S (2005) Coronavirus pathogenesis and the emerging pathogen severe acute respiratory syndrome coronavirus. Microbiol Mol Biol Rev 69: 635–664.
9. Henrickson KJ (2004) Advances in the laboratory diagnosis of viral respiratory disease. Pediatr Infect Dis J 23: S6–10.
10. WHO (2006) Collecting, preserving and shipping specimens for the diagnosis of avian influenza A(H5N1) virus infection.
11. Boom R, Sol CJ, Salimans MM, Jansen CL, Wertheim-van Dillen PM, et al. (1990) Rapid and simple method for purification of nucleic acids. J Clin Microbiol 28: 495–503.
12. Kim SR, Ki CS, Lee NY (2009) Rapid detection and identification of 12 respiratory viruses using a dual priming oligonucleotide system-based multiplex PCR assay. J Virol Methods 156: 111–116.
13. Beld M, Minnaar R, Weel J, Sol C, Damen M, et al. (2004) Highly sensitive assay for detection of enterovirus in clinical specimens by reverse transcription-PCR with an armored RNA internal control. J Clin Microbiol 42: 3059–3064.
14. Pyrc K, Bosch BJ, Berkhout B, Jebbink MF, Dijkman R, et al. (2006) Inhibition of human coronavirus NL63 infection at early stages of the replication cycle. Antimicrob Agents Chemother 50: 2000–2008.
15. Peter F, Wrigh FTC (2000) Generic protocol to examine the incidence of lower respiratory infection due to respiratory syncytial virus in children less than five years of age.
16. WHO U Model IMCI Handbook: Integrated Management of Childood illness. Geneva, Switzerland: Division of Child and Adolescent Health and Development, World Health Organisation; 2005: WHO/FCH/CAH/0012.
17. Tapparel C, Junier T, Gerlach D, Van-Belle S, Turin L, et al. (2009) New respiratory enterovirus and recombinant rhinoviruses among circulating picornaviruses. Emerg Infect Dis 15: 719–726.
18. Vongphrachanh P, Simmerman JM, Phonekeo D, Pansayavong V, Sisouk T, et al. (2010) An early report from newly established laboratory-based influenza surveillance in Lao PDR. Influenza Other Respi Viruses 4: 47–52.
19. Mathisen M, Strand TA, Sharma BN, Chandyo RK, Valentiner-Branth P, et al. (2010) Clinical presentation and severity of viral community-acquired pneumonia in young Nepalese children. Pediatr Infect Dis J 29: e1–6.
20. Kim YK, Nyambat B, Hong YS, Lee CG, Lee JW, et al. (2008) Burden of viral respiratory disease hospitalizations among children in a community of Seoul, Republic of Korea, 1995–2005. Scand J Infect Dis 40: 946–953.
21. Izurieta HS, Thompson WW, Kramarz P, Shay DK, Davis RL, et al. (2000) Influenza and the rates of hospitalization for respiratory disease among infants and young children. N Engl J Med 342: 232–239.
22. Weber MW, Milligan P, Sanneh M, Awemoyi A, Dakour R, et al. (2002) An epidemiological study of RSV infection in the Gambia. Bull World Health Organ 80: 562–568.
23. Yoshida LM, Suzuki M, Yamamoto T, Nguyen HA, Nguyen CD, et al. Viral pathogens associated with acute respiratory infections in central vietnamese children. Pediatr Infect Dis J 29: 75–77.
24. Weber MW, Mulholland EK, Greenwood BM (1998) Respiratory syncytial virus infection in tropical and developing countries. Trop Med Int Health 3: 268–280.
25. Durani Y, Friedman MJ, Attia MW (2008) Clinical predictors of respiratory syncytial virus infection in children. Pediatr Int 50: 352–355.
26. Djelantik IG, Gessner BD, Soewignjo S, Steinhoff M, Sutanto A, et al. (2003) Incidence and clinical features of hospitalization because of respiratory syncytial virus lower respiratory illness among children less than two years of age in a rural Asian setting. Pediatr Infect Dis J 22: 150–157.
27. Loscertales MP, Roca A, Ventura PJ, Abacassamo F, Dos Santos F, et al. (2002) Epidemiology and clinical presentation of respiratory syncytial virus infection in a rural area of southern Mozambique. Pediatr Infect Dis J 21: 148–155.
28. Perez-Yarza EG, Moreno A, Lazaro P, Mejias A, Ramilo O (2007) The association between respiratory syncytial virus infection and the development of childhood asthma: a systematic review of the literature. Pediatr Infect Dis J 26: 733–739.
29. Dherani M, Pope D, Mascarenhas M, Smith KR, Weber M, et al. (2008) Indoor air pollution from unprocessed solid fuel use and pneumonia risk in children aged under five years: a systematic review and meta-analysis. Bull World Health Organ 86: 390–398C.
30. Smith KR, Samet JM, Romieu I, Bruce N (2000) Indoor air pollution in developing countries and acute lower respiratory infections in children. Thorax 55: 518–532.
31. Okiro EA, Ngama M, Bett A, Cane PA, Medley GF, et al. (2008) Factors associated with increased risk of progression to respiratory syncytial virus-associated pneumonia in young Kenyan children. Trop Med Int Health 13: 914–926.
32. Lambert SB, Whiley DM, O'Neill NT, Andrews EC, Canavan FM, et al. (2008) Comparing nose-throat swabs and nasopharyngeal aspirates collected from children with symptoms for respiratory virus identification using real-time polymerase chain reaction. Pediatrics 122: e615–620.
33. Macfarlane P, Denham J, Assous J, Hughes C (2005) RSV testing in bronchiolitis: which nasal sampling method is best? Arch Dis Child 90: 634–635.
34. Heikkinen T, Salmi AA, Ruuskanen O (2001) Comparative study of nasopharyngeal aspirate and nasal swab specimens for detection of influenza. Bmj 322: 138.
35. Heikkinen T, Marttila J, Salmi AA, Ruuskanen O (2002) Nasal swab versus nasopharyngeal aspirate for isolation of respiratory viruses. J Clin Microbiol 40: 4337–4339.
36. Stensballe LG, Trautner S, Kofoed PE, Nante E, Hedegaard K, et al. (2002) Comparison of nasopharyngeal aspirate and nasal swab specimens for detection of respiratory syncytial virus in different settings in a developing country. Trop Med Int Health 7: 317–321.
37. Covalciuc KA, Webb KH, Carlson CA (1999) Comparison of four clinical specimen types for detection of influenza A and B viruses by optical immunoassay (FLU OIA test) and cell culture methods. J Clin Microbiol 37: 3971–3974.
38. WHO website. Available: http://www.who.int/immunization_monitoring/en/globalsummary/timeseries/TSincidenceByCountry.cfm?C=VNM.Accessed 2011 March 1.

17

Estimating the Burden of Malaria in Senegal: Bayesian Zero-Inflated Binomial Geostatistical Modeling of the MIS 2008 Data

Federica Giardina[1,2], Laura Gosoniu[1,2], Lassana Konate[3], Mame Birame Diouf[4], Robert Perry[5], Oumar Gaye[6], Ousmane Faye[3], Penelope Vounatsou[1,2]*

1 Department of Epidemiology and Public Health, Swiss Tropical and Public Health Institute, Basel, Switzerland, 2 University of Basel, Basel, Switzerland, 3 Faculté des Sciences et Techniques, UCAD Dakar, Sénégal, 4 National Malaria Control Programme, Dakar, Sénégal, 5 Center for Global Health, Centers for Disease Control and Prevention, Atlanta, Georgia, United States of America, 6 Faculté de Médecine, Pharmacie et Odontologie, UCAD Dakar, Sénégal

Abstract

The Research Center for Human Development in Dakar (CRDH) with the technical assistance of ICF Macro and the National Malaria Control Programme (NMCP) conducted in 2008/2009 the Senegal Malaria Indicator Survey (SMIS), the first nationally representative household survey collecting parasitological data and malaria-related indicators. In this paper, we present spatially explicit parasitaemia risk estimates and number of infected children below 5 years. Geostatistical Zero-Inflated Binomial models (ZIB) were developed to take into account the large number of zero-prevalence survey locations (70%) in the data. Bayesian variable selection methods were incorporated within a geostatistical framework in order to choose the best set of environmental and climatic covariates associated with the parasitaemia risk. Model validation confirmed that the ZIB model had a better predictive ability than the standard Binomial analogue. Markov chain Monte Carlo (MCMC) methods were used for inference. Several insecticide treated nets (ITN) coverage indicators were calculated to assess the effectiveness of interventions. After adjusting for climatic and socio-economic factors, the presence of at least one ITN per every two household members and living in urban areas reduced the odds of parasitaemia by 86% and 81% respectively. Posterior estimates of the ORs related to the wealth index show a decreasing trend with the quintiles. Infection odds appear to be increasing with age. The population-adjusted prevalence ranges from 0.12% in Thillé-Boubacar to 13.1% in Dabo. Tambacounda has the highest population-adjusted predicted prevalence (8.08%) whereas the region with the highest estimated number of infected children under the age of 5 years is Kolda (13940). The contemporary map and estimates of malaria burden identify the priority areas for future control interventions and provide baseline information for monitoring and evaluation. Zero-Inflated formulations are more appropriate in modeling sparse geostatistical survey data, expected to arise more frequently as malaria research is focused on elimination.

Editor: Roly D. Gosling, London School of Hygiene and Tropical Medicine, United Kingdom

Funding: This investigation was conducted as part of the Swiss-South Africa Joint Research Project No. IZLSZ3 122926. The authors also thank the Bill and Melinda Gates Foundation (Project No. OPP1032350) for financial contribution. The funders had no role in study design, data collection and analysis, decision to publish, or preparation of the manuscript.

Competing Interests: The authors have declared that no competing interests exist.

* E-mail: penelope.vounatsou@unibas.ch

Introduction

More than two hundred million cases of malaria were estimated worldwide in 2008 and the majority (85%) was in African countries. Malaria accounted for 850 thousand deaths in the same year, 89% of which occurred in Africa. Over 85% of deaths were in children under five years of age [1]. Senegal is one of the 45 countries in Africa where malaria is endemic and represents the leading cause of morbidity and hospital mortality [2]. The main parasite transmitted by anopheline mosquitoes is *Plasmodium falciparum* and transmission occurs seasonally in the entire country, from June to November. Rapid diagnostic tests (RDTs) have been provided free of charge since 2007. Two years later, almost 86% of suspected malarial fever cases were screened with an RDT [3]. Malaria incidence in children under five decreased from 400 000 suspected cases in 2006 to 30 000 confirmed cases in 2009 [4]. Routine surveillance provides some evidence that the number of malaria inpatient cases and deaths during the same period are decreasing. However, these estimates must be interpreted with caution since they are affected by poor reporting, introduction of RDTs as well as changes in case definition [1]. Furthermore, the lack of nationally representative surveys makes these estimates unreliable. Almost all malaria surveys in Senegal were carried out in five parts of the country: Dakar and its suburbs, specific areas around the Senegal River, Fatick region and Niakhar province. Few studies have been conducted in the rest of the country, particularly in the regions of Tambacounda and Casamance.

The Senegal Malaria Indicator Survey (SMIS) is the second nationally representative household survey focusing on malaria-related indicators and the first that collected parasitological data. The survey was supported by the National Malaria Control Program (NMCP) and carried out between November 2008 and January 2009 by the Research Center for Human Development in Dakar (CRDH) with the technical assistance of ICF Macro and funding from the President's Malaria Initiative (PMI). Malaria control interventions have been implemented in the country recently. The SMIS collected information on interventions such as ownership and use of insecticide treated nets (ITNs) or long lasting impregnated nets (LLINs) as well as intermittent preventive treatment for pregnant women (IPTp). ITN coverage, measured by ownership of at least one mosquito net per household, reached 82% in 2010 [4]. In 2006, Artemisin-based combination therapies (ACTs) were introduced and they were made freely available in 2010. However, indoor residual spraying (IRS) has not been implemented as a routine intervention in the country. During the SMIS only three districts had introduced IRS as a mean of malaria control and therefore no related information was collected in the survey. The number of districts using IRS increased to six in 2010.

A national contemporary map of malaria distribution is an essential tool in order to prioritize control interventions in areas with higher burden and to achieve a better resource allocation and health management. Several maps presenting the distribution of malaria risk in Senegal have been generated over the last few years as part of mapping efforts covering larger areas. A West Africa malaria risk map [5] was obtained using Bayesian geostatistical models on entomological inoculation rate estimates produced by applying the Garki transmission model [6] on historical survey data from the MARA database [7]. An updated malaria risk map for West Africa was estimated using geostatistical models on MARA survey data considering a different effect of environmental factors on malaria depending on the ecological zones [8]. A Senegal malaria risk map was also embedded in a worldwide map based on historical survey data and geostatistical models [9]. All these efforts made use of old and heterogeneous survey data, collected over different seasons, diagnostic tools and overlapping age groups across locations.

Common exposures such as environmental or climatic conditions as well as socio-economic status influence the transmission of malaria similarly in neighboring regions introducing spatial correlation. Geostatistical models including location-specific random effects were employed to model spatial correlation as a function of the distance between sampled locations. The data consisted of a large number of locations with zero prevalence; therefore the commonly used Binomial distribution may underestimate the zero-prevalence probability. Zero-Inflated Binomial (ZIB) models provide a flexible way to address this problem [10]. ZIB models for prevalence data have not been applied before in the context of geostatistical modelling of infectious disease data. To our knowledge, the only application is in the modeling of sparse malaria entomological data [11]. Zero-Inflated Poisson/

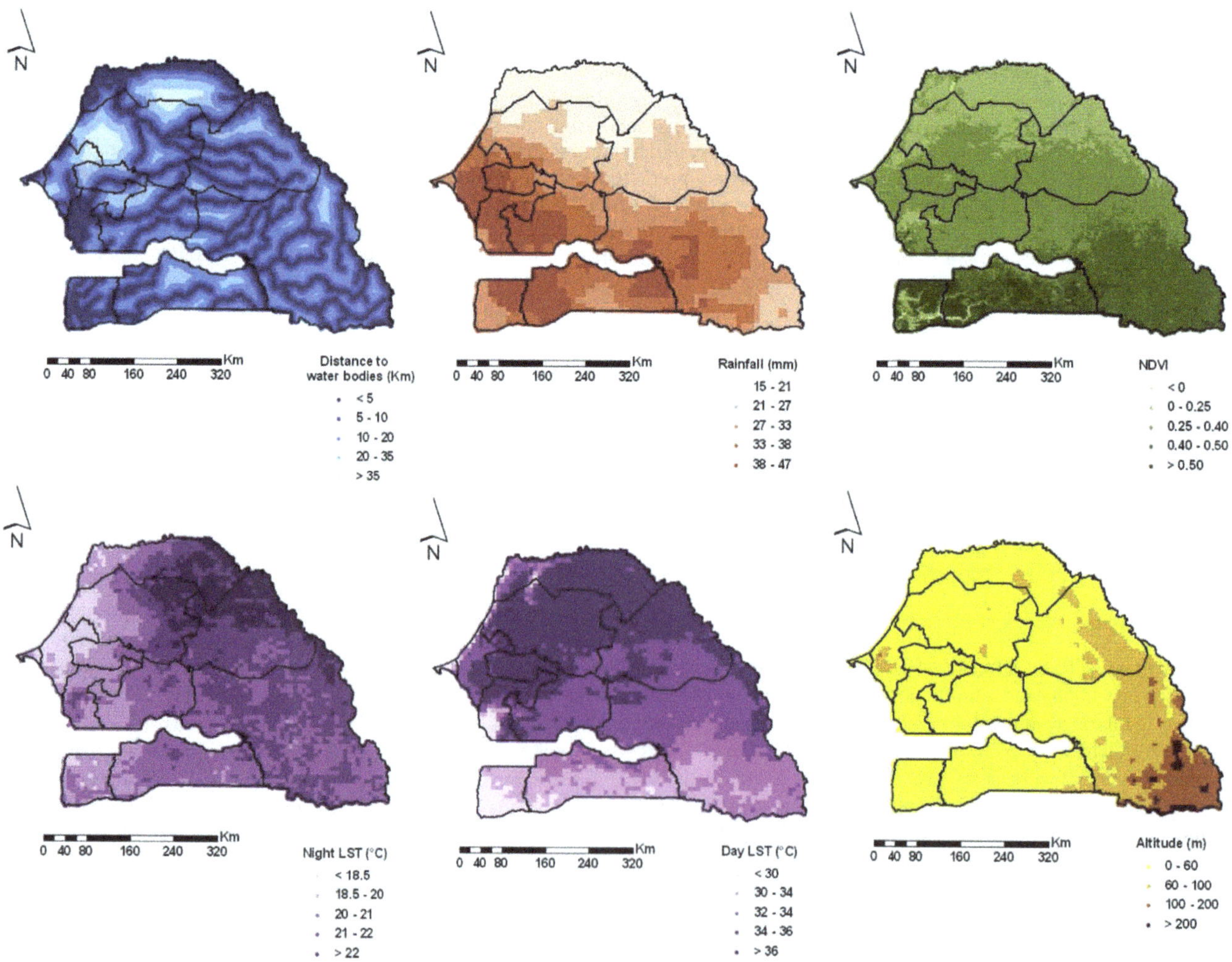

Figure 1. Environmental and climatic factors. Distance to water bodies, Rainfall, NDVI (Normalized Differenced Vegetation Index), Night and Day LST (Land Surface Temperature) and altitude at 4 km^2 resolution in Senegal. Regional boundaries are overlaid.

Negative Binomial models have been formulated for geostatistical count data (i.e. mapping isopod nest burrows [12] and child HIV/TB mortality [13]), however applications are rather limited.

In this paper, we provide spatially explicit burden estimates of malaria in Senegal using the SMIS data and Bayesian geostatistical Zero-Inflated Binomial models based on variable selection methods for spatial data.

Materials and Methods

Country Profile

Senegal is located in Western Africa, facing the North Atlantic Ocean between Guinea-Bissau and Mauritania. Its borders run south of the Casamance River and along the Senegal River respectively. The Gambia penetrates more than 320 km into the country, from the Atlantic coast to the centre along the Gambia River which bisects Senegal's territory. Northern Senegal is characterized by a Sahelian ecological zone with semiarid grasslands and acacia savannas. Malaria is unstable hypoendemic and immunity is acquired later in life. A Sudano-Sahelian zone in the centre of the country is dominated by a flat wooded savanna with very few prominent topographical features. Malaria is endemic in this area and immunity is acquired around the age of ten. The southern part of Senegal is occupied by a Sudano-Guinean ecological zone, with annual rainfall exceeding 800 mm. Malaria is hyperendemic and immunity is acquired in the first five years of life. The urban malaria burden is concentrated in the cities of Dakar, Rufisque, Kaolack and Saint-Louis where the anopheles vector density is very low. The high transmission season in Senegal occurs mainly between July and October. However, in the Senegal River delta area, there are two annual peaks of the disease caused by river flooding: one in the rainy and the other in the dry season.

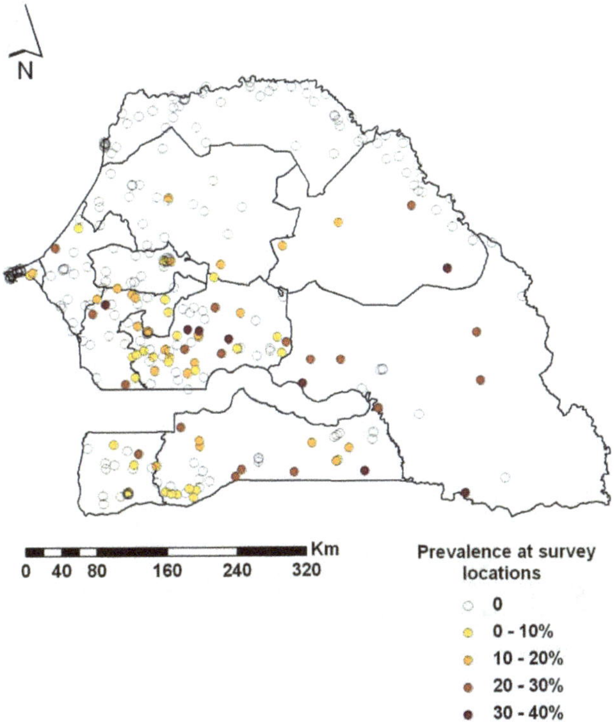

Figure 2. Prevalence at survey locations. Prevalence reported in the 317 locations of the SMIS 2008. Regional boundaries are overlaid.

Ethical statement

Participation in the survey was voluntary and written informed consent was obtained in the local language before questionnaire administration and blood collection for parasitaemia and anemia testing. Individuals were told about the general purpose of the survey, possible risks and benefits of the survey and those presenting malaria parasites and/or anaemia were treated. The survey protocol was submitted to and approved by the Ethical Review Committee at the National Malaria Control Program and the Institutional Review Board (IRB) of Macro International.

Malaria Data (SMIS 2008–2009)

A nationally representative random sample of 320 clusters and 9600 households was selected through a stratified two-stage sampling procedure. The clusters were the census units (CU) used by the National Agency for Statistics and Demography (ANSD) in the census carried out in 2002 (Recensement Général de la Population et de l'Habitat, RGPH-2002). However, in the three regions of Kaolack, Kolda and Saint-Louis, the health districts served as sampling clusters. At the first sampling stage, 320 clusters were drawn with probability proportional to the number of households in each cluster. The sampling procedure was stratified by the area type (urban/rural) of the clusters: 67.5% of the selected ones were in rural areas and 32.5% in urban areas. At the second sampling stage 30 households were selected randomly from each cluster. Rural areas are slightly overrepresented due to over-sampling in the three regions of Kaolack, Kolda and Saint-Louis. Geographical information is available at cluster level. As part of the final sampling, one every third village was randomly selected and every child between 6 and 59 months of age was tested for parasitaemia. Two tests were performed, RDT and blood smear test [14]. This study is based on the results of microscopic examination since thick blood smear test is considered as the gold standard [15].

Malaria predictors

Three sets of malaria predictors were considered in the study, namely environmental/climatic proxies, socio-economic factors and malaria intervention measures. The environmental/climatic variables were extracted from remote sensing sources. Decadal rainfall data were downloaded via the Africa Data Dissemination Service (ADDS). Weekly day/night land surface temperature (LST) and biweekly normalized difference vegetation index (NDVI) data were obtained from Moderate Resolution Imaging Spectroradiometer (MODIS). Permanent rivers and lakes were extracted from Health Mapper. The shortest Euclidean distance between the centroid of each pixel and the closest water body was calculated in ArcGIS version 9.1 (ESRI; Redlands, CA, USA).

Table 1. Posterior model probabilities obtained using Gibbs Variable Selection (First stage).

Model	Environmental Variables	Binomial	ZIB
1.	Night LST, NDVI	2.46%	2.52%
2.	Night LST, NDVI, Area type	72.21%	74.28%
3.	Night LST, Rainfall, NDVI, Area type	12.13%	13.23%
4.	Others	13.2%	9.97%

In the model with the highest posterior probability (72.21% with Binomial model and 74.28% with ZIB), Night LST, NDVI and Area type were included as covariates. This model was selected and used to predict the malaria risk.

Altitude data were obtained from an interpolated digital elevation model (DEM) developed by the U.S. Geological Survey - Earth Resources Observation and Science (USGS EROS) Data Center. The geographical distributions of the environmental factors are displayed in Figure 1. Data on the rural extents in Senegal are provided by the Global Rural-Urban Mapping Project (GRUMP). According to the UN definition for Senegal, agglomerations with more than 10 000 inhabitants were considered as urban [16]. The above data were available at 1 km^2 spatial resolution, with the exception of rainfall which has a resolution of 8 km^2.

Socioeconomic disparities were measured by a wealth index, included in the SMIS data and calculated by a weighted sum of household assets. The weights were estimated through principal components analysis [17]. ITN related information in the SMIS was used to calculate the following ITN coverage indicators ([18] and [19]): i) a binary variable reporting whether the child has a bed net for sleeping; ii) the proportion of children under the age of 5 years reported to have slept under an ITN the night before the survey visit; iii) the total number of nets per household (irrespective of the number of household members); iv) a binary indicator representing the availability of at least one ITN per every two household members and v) at least one ITN per every two children under the age of 5 years in the household. Human population data estimates for the year 2010 were obtained from the Gridded Population of the World version 3 (GPWv3) database at 1 km^2 spatial resolution. These data were used to convert spatially explicit parasitaemia risk estimates into number of infected children under the age of 5 years. The total number of children under 5 years of age was obtained from the International Data Base of the U.S. Census Bureau, Population Division for the year 2010.

Bayesian geostatistical modeling

Let Y_i and N_i be the number of infected with malaria parasites and the number of screened children under the age of 5 years at location s_i (i.e. cluster centroid) respectively. Y_i is typically assumed to arise from a Binomial distribution, $Y_i \sim Bin(N_i,p_i)$ where p_i indicates the probability of parasitaemia at s_i. However, in the presence of excessive number of zeros, a Binomial model may be inadequate to estimate the zero-prevalence probability and to identify relevant covariates related to the outcome. To take into account the sparsity of the data, a Zero-Inflated Binomial (ZIB) model $Y_i \tilde{} ZIB(N_i,p_i,\theta_i)$ was fitted and compared to the standard Binomial analogue. A ZIB model assumes two sources of zeros: θ_i% (mixing probabilities) of the zeros are structural, not random and the remaining $(1-\theta_i)$% arise with a frequency defined by a Binomial distribution, see equation (1)

$$Y_i|p_i,\theta_i \sim \begin{cases} 0 & \text{with probability } \theta_i \\ Bin(N_i,p_i) & \text{with probability } 1-\theta_i \end{cases} \quad (1)$$

In the above formulation, p_i does not have a direct interpretation of parasitaemia risk since it is influenced by the proportion of structural zeros.

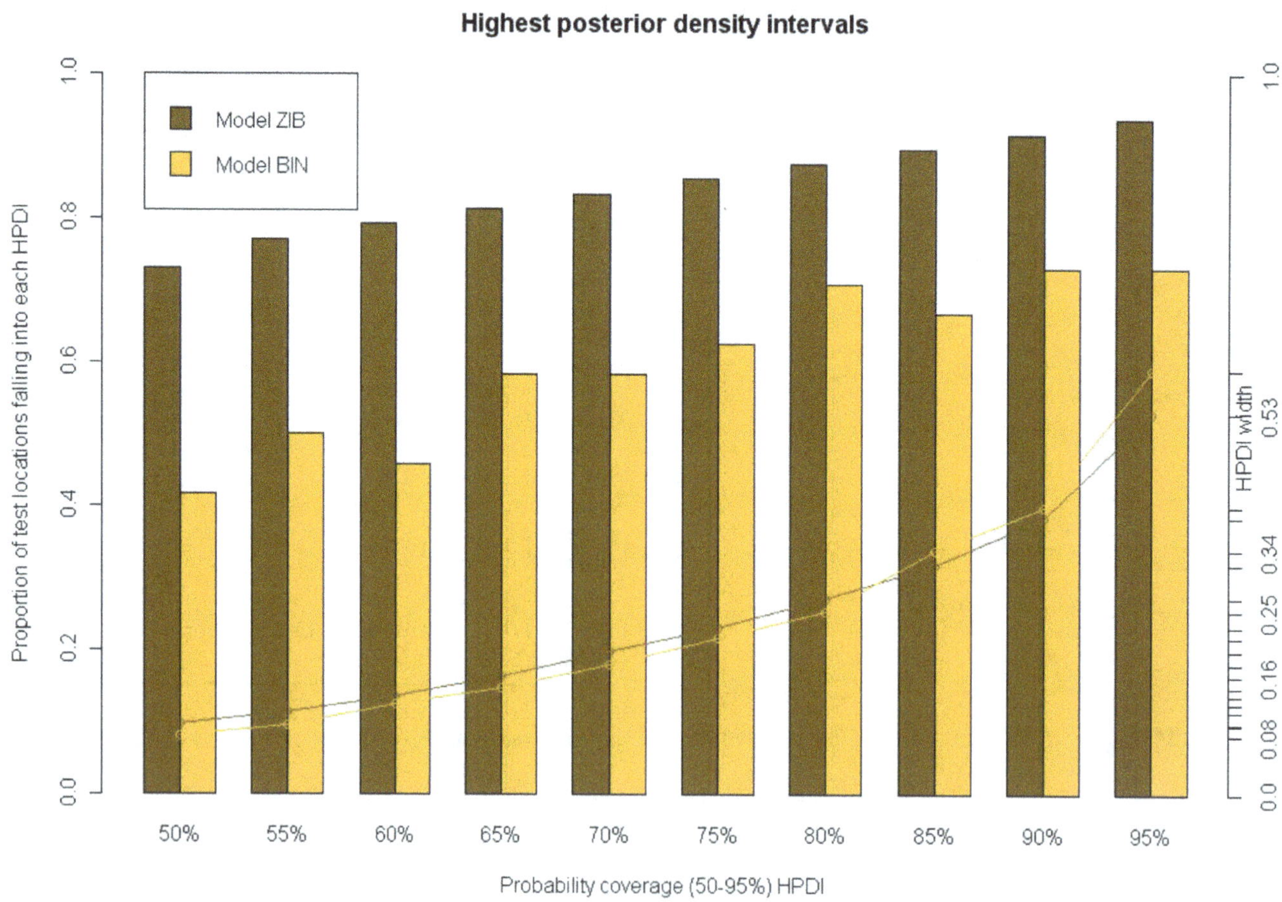

Figure 3. Model comparison and validation. Percentage of test locations with malaria prevalence falling in the highest posterior density intervals (HPDI) predicted from Binomial and Zero-Inflated Binomial models (bars). Lines indicate the corresponding HPDI length.

The relation between p_i and the vector of k associated predictors $X_i=(X_{i1},X_{i2},...,X_{ik})^T$ observed at location s_i is modeled via the equation $logit(p_i)=X_i\boldsymbol{\beta}+\omega_i+\phi_i$, where $\boldsymbol{\beta}_i=(\beta_1,\beta_2,...,\beta_k)$ is the regression coefficient vector, ω_i and ϕ_i are location-dependent random effects. Spatial dependence is introduced by assuming that the random effects $\boldsymbol{\phi}=(\phi_1,\phi_2,...,\phi_n)$ are distributed according to a MVN distribution with mean 0 and covariance matrix $\boldsymbol{\Sigma}$ where each element σ_{jl} is defined by an exponential parametric function of the distance d_{jl} between two locations s_j and s_l, i.e. $\sigma_{jl}=\sigma_\phi^2\exp(-\rho d_{jl})$. The parameter σ_ϕ^2 represents the spatial variation and ρ is the parameter controlling the rate of correlation decay with increasing distance. In the case of exponential correlation function, $3/\rho$ can be used to calculate the distance above which spatial correlation is negligible, known as range. Any remaining non-spatial variation is estimated by the random effects ω_i, assumed independent and normally distributed with mean 0 and variance σ_ω^2.

Bayesian variable selection approaches were employed using the above geostatistical models to choose the best set of predictors. In particular, three variable selection methods, namely Gibbs variable selection (GVS) by Dellaportas et al. [20], Stochastic Search Variable Selection (SSVS) by George and McCulloch [21] and the variable selection sampler of Kuo and Mallick (KM) [22] were compared. The best set of covariates was indicated by the model with the highest posterior probability. Details of the geostatistical variable selection methods are given in the Appendix.

The model includes over 330 parameters. To enable model fit and prediction a Bayesian formulation and MCMC estimation was adopted. To complete model specification, prior distributions were assigned to the parameters. An inverse-gamma prior was assumed for the variance and a gamma distribution for the spatial decay parameter ρ. The priors for the regression coefficients were non-informative Gaussian distributions with mean 0 and variance 100. Covariates were standardized in order to acquire better correlation properties and reduce MCMC computational time [23].

Bayesian kriging was employed to predict the parasitaemia risk at unsampled locations and produce a parasitaemia risk map at high spatial resolution [24]. A regular grid of 4 km^2 resolution covering the whole country was created, resulting in around 60 000 pixels. Predictions were based on a geostatistical model using only environmental/climatic factors since data on malaria interventions or socio-economic status are not available at high resolution scale for the whole country. Therefore, a two stage geostatistical variable selection approach was applied. In the first stage, only climatic predictors were included to identify the best prediction model. In the second stage, geostatistical variable selection was carried out to select among the five ITN coverage indicators defined above. The models were adjusted for age, wealth index and the climatic predictors determined during the first stage.

The predictive model was validated on a test subset of the data. In particular, a randomly selected sample of 269 locations (85% of the data locations) was used as a training set for model fit. The predictive performance of the model was assessed by calculating the proportion of observed prevalence data at the remaining 15% of (test) locations, correctly estimated within Highest Posterior Density Intervals (HPDI) of probability coverage ranging from 50 to 100% [25]. The above validation procedure was also used to compare the ZIB model with its Binomial analogue. The number of malaria infected children under five years of age was estimated at pixel level by multiplying the geostatistical model-based risk estimates with the total number of children under the age of 5 years provided by the International Data Base of the U.S. Census Bureau, Population Division for the year 2010. The previous values were added to calculate the total infected children under the age of 5 years at district level. Subsequently, dividing by the number of children under the age of 5 years living in the district, population-adjusted estimates of parasitaemia risk were obtained.

Fortran 95 (Compaq Visual Fortran Professional 6.6.0) and standard numerical variables (NAG, The Numerical Algorithms Group Ltd.) were used to implement the MCMC code. Open-BUGS [26] was also employed in the model fit.

Results

A total of 4138 children between 6 and 59 months of age from 320 clusters were tested for parasitaemia with both RDT and blood smear test. The overall observed malaria prevalence was 6.74%. The number of children under the age of 5 years tested with both Rapid Diagnostic Test and blood smear test was 3960. Almost 12.05% of the children under the age of 5 years tested with RDT were found positives. The percentage of children under the age of 5 years that were positives to both tests was 5.44%. Due to the observed discordance between the diagnostic tools, the standard microscopy test was considered in the analysis [15].

A large number of survey locations (around 70%) had zero prevalence. No children under the age of 5 years were tested in two clusters of Saint-Louis region and one cluster in Kaolack, thus reducing the actual number of GPS coordinates to 317. Figure 2 shows that the lowest malaria prevalence in the country was recorded in Saint-Louis (0%), followed by the regions of Dakar (1.72%) and Louga (1.43%).

Posterior model probabilities obtained from MCMC runs of 100 000 iterations using the GVS are presented in Table 1. Similar results were obtained with the other two variable selection methods, SSVS and KM. As shown in the table, the set of

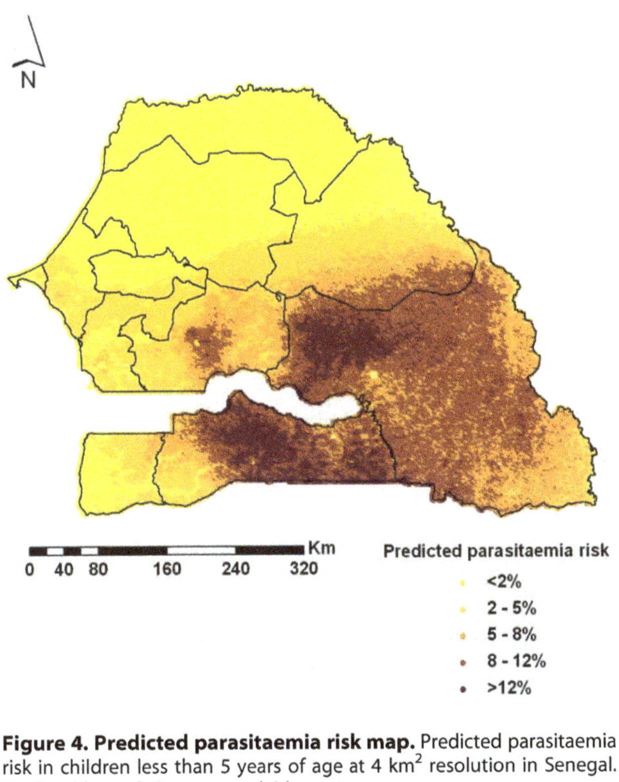

Figure 4. Predicted parasitaemia risk map. Predicted parasitaemia risk in children less than 5 years of age at 4 km^2 resolution in Senegal. Regional boundaries are overlaid.

covariates that defined the Binomial as well as the ZIB geostatistical models with the highest posterior probabilities consisted of night LST, NDVI and area type (urban/rural). The predictive performance of the selected models is shown in Figure 3. The proportion of test locations falling into the 50–95% HPDIs was constantly higher under the ZIB model. Furthermore, the latter model estimated narrower HPDIs. Based on the above results, the ZIB was adopted to predict the parasitaemia risk at high spatial resolution and to assess the effects of interventions on the infection risk.

Geostatistical ZIB model parameter estimates are given in Table 2. Model I includes only climatic covariates. The posterior estimate of the OR indicates a positive association between NDVI, night LST and parasitaemia, however the corresponding 95% credible intervals include one. Living in urban areas reduces the parasitaemia odds by 81% (95% BCI: 55%–93%). Raw data summaries estimate a parasitaemia prevalence of 1.3% in urban compared to the 8.47% in rural areas. The range parameter suggests that spatial correlation is present up to a distance of 2.4° which is equivalent to 265 km (1° = 111.12 km). The spatial variance ($\sigma_{\phi}^2=2.49$) was around 5 times higher than the non-spatial one ($\sigma_{\omega}^2=0.52$) indicating high geographical variation. Model based predictions, obtained through Bayesian kriging over a grid of around 60 000 pixels of 2 km×2 km spatial resolution are depicted in Figure 4. The plotted values correspond to the medians of the pixel-specific posterior predictive distributions. Low values of parasitaemia prevalence are concentrated in the northern Senegal, particularly in the region of Saint-Louis, Louga and Matam. Malaria risk increases in some areas of central Senegal and reaches the highest values in the southern Kolda and eastern Tambacounda where the predicted risk was 10.66% and 9.45%, respectively. Another high-risk area is located in the centre of Kaolak region with an estimated prevalence of 5.6%.

Table 2. Association of parasitaemia risk with environmental/climatic factors, socio-economic status and malaria interventions resulting from raw data summaries and geostatistical Zero-Inflated Binomial models.

Variable	Raw Data	Geostatistical model I[a]		Geostatistical model II[b]	
	Prevalence	OR	95% BCI[c]	OR	95% BCI[c]
Night LST		1.16	(0.66, 1.86)	0.83	(0.53, 1.26)
NDVI		1.48	(0.88, 2.48)	0.91	(0.61, 1.83)
Area type					
Rural	8.47%	1		1	
Urban	1.30%	0.19	(0.07,0.45)	0.43	(0.16, 1.06)
Wealth Index[d]					
Most poor	13.75%			1	
Very poor	6.51%			0.77	(0.57, 1.03)
Poor	1.51%			0.22	(0.08, 0.51)
Less poor	0.96%			0.12	(0.05, 0.41)
Least poor	0.65%			0.09	(0.01, 0.26)
Age					
0–1	3%			1	
1–2	4.54%			1.20	(0.70, 2.43)
2–3	8.07%			2.93	(1.62, 5.33)
3–4	7.95%			2.96	(1.66,5.74)
4–5	8.11%			2.77	(1.44, 5.21)
ITNs[e]					
<1	6.84%			1	
≥1	1.41%			0.14	(0.03, 0.7)
Spatial parameters		**Posterior median**	**95% BCI[c]**	**Posterior median**	**95% BCI[c]**
σ_{ω}^2		2.49	(1.07, 6.41)	3.04	(2.22, 4.02)
σ_{ω}^2		0.52	(0.25,1.03)	0.35	(0.15,0.73)
Range[f]		2.40	(1.11, 2.98)	1.689	(0.003,2.93)
Mixing probabilities					
θ		0.29	(0.19,0.39)	0.35	(0.24,0.46)

[a]Model I includes only environmental/climatic factors.
[b]Model II includes ITN coverage, children's age and wealth index.
[c]Bayesian Credible intervals.
[d]Household wealth index.
[e]Number of available ITNs per every two household members.
[f]The range parameter (degrees), defined as $3/\rho$ indicates the distance above which the spatial correlation becomes negligible.

The predicted number of malaria infected children under the age of 5 years is displayed in Figure 5 and the estimates of population-adjusted prevalence obtained at the smallest administrative level (*arrondissement*) are summarized in Table 3. Kriging enabled the estimation of parasitaemia prevalence in areas where no survey locations were selected by the sampling procedure. For instance, the population-adjusted prevalence is 0.61% in the *arrondissement* of Barkedji, Louga region and 9.54% in Keniaba, Tambacounda region. The total number of infected children under the age of 5 years in the country below the age of five was estimated to be around 48 thousand. The map of the estimated number of children under the age of 5 years infected with malaria and the predicted parasitaemia prevalence show very different patterns, because of the population density, higher in the urban regions of Dakar and Saint-Louis.

Geostatistical variable selection among the five different ITN coverage indicators (Table 4) showed that having at least one available ITN per every two household members was most related with the parasitaemia risk after adjusting for climatic/environmental factors, age and wealth index. The posterior probability of the model was around 34% indicating that the model was chosen 34% of the times among the $2^5 = 32$ possible models including all combinations of the five coverage indicators. Estimates of the posterior distribution of the parameters are given in Table 2 (Model II). Living in a household with at least one ITN per every two members was found to have a protective effect on parasitaemia, reducing the odds by 86% (95% BCI: 30%–97%). This result was also seen in the raw data summaries as shown by the second column of Table 2. The observed parasitaemia risk in the two categories, i.e. "less than one ITN" and "at least one ITN" per every two members was 6.84% and 1.41% respectively. Posterior estimates of the ORs related to the wealth index show a decreasing trend with the quintiles. The second quintile (very poor) had an OR of 0.77 (95% BCI: 0.57–1.03) whereas the last one (least poor) was 0.09, (95% BCI: 0.01–0.26). A similar pattern was presented in the prevalence calculated from the raw data. The highest (13.75%) and lowest (0.65%) infection risk were observed in the most and least poor group, respectively. Infection odds appear to be increasing with age. For instance, the OR is 1.2 (95% BCI: 0.70–2.43) in children 1–2 years old and 2.77, (95% BCI: 1.44–5.21) in children 4–5 years old. Observed parasitaemia prevalence was the lowest in infants (3%) reaching 8.11% in children 4–5 years old.

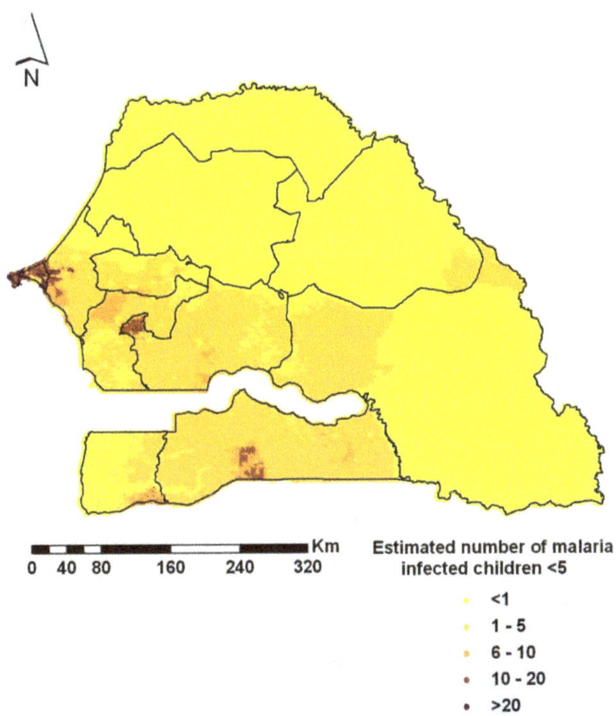

Figure 5. Estimated number of malaria infected children <5 years. The smooth map depicts the estimated number of malaria infected children less than 5 years of age at 4 km^2 resolution in Senegal. Regional boundaries are overlaid.

Discussion

This study estimated the number of infected children under the age of 5 years at different geographical scales in Senegal and produced the first parasitaemia risk map in the country using contemporary data collected under the nationally representative malaria survey of 2008/2009. Geostatistical Zero-Inflated Binomial models were developed and Bayesian variable selection methods for spatially correlated data were employed to build a predictive model and assess the effectiveness of the ITN intervention adjusting for climatic and socio-economic confounders.

A large number of zeros was observed when modeling the number of infected children under the age of 5 years, probably due to the fact that the survey was carried out at the beginning of the dry season, when transmission starts to decrease. To address the issue of sparsity a ZIB model was derived. Model validation revealed that the ZIB model had higher predictive ability than the Binomial analogue suggesting that, when a large number of zeros occurs in the data, a ZIB model should be considered. Since malaria research is focused on elimination and eradication of the disease, it is expected that forthcoming surveys will include a large number of locations with zero prevalence and the ZIB models would provide a suitable alternative to the standard Binomial ones for geostatistical modeling.

Geostatistical variable selection is an important topic in malaria mapping. The predictive ability of a model depends on the covariates included in the multivariate regression setting. Modeling approaches in malaria mapping treat selection of predictors separately than the geostatistical model fit. Variable selection is often based on regression models that ignore spatial correlation, leading to wrong estimates of covariates effects and their significance. Geostatistical variable selection not only identifies the best set of predictors but builds parsimonious models with the best predictive ability [27]. In addition, it can be used to avoid overfitting due to the inclusion of unnecessary predictors or random effects. In this work, we have employed three Bayesian variable selection methods within a geostatistical model formulation. The climatic model with the highest posterior probability selected by the three methods included the following combination of covariates: night LST, NDVI and area type. Altitude in Senegal presents very little variation throughout the country therefore it was not considered as a potential predictor of malaria transmission in the variable selection procedure.

As mentioned above, maps showing the distribution of malaria risk in Senegal can be found in [5], [8] and [9] as part of efforts in mapping malaria risk at regional and continental level using historical data. Nevertheless, compilations of historical data obtained from surveys, heterogeneous in the age groups involved and the seasons considered, require methods for standardizing risk estimates into a common scale for mapping purposes. Different statistical methods have been employed; the work by Gemperli

Table 3. Estimates of infected children less than 5 years old per *arrondissernent.*

Region	Department	*Arrondissement*	OP[a]	EIC[b]	PEP[c]	Region	Department	*Arrondissement*	OP[a]	EIC[b]	PEP[c]
Dakar	Dakar	Parcelles Assainies	0%	360	0.20%	Louga	Louga	Keur Monar Sarr	2.27%	72	0.31%
Dakar	Guédiawaye	Guédiawaye	0%	112	0.17%	Louga	Louga	Sakal	0%	48	0.13%
Dakar	Pikine	Niayes	0%	356	0.21%	Matam	Matam	Agnam-Civol	0%	376	1.56%
Dakar	Rufisque	Diamnadio	12.5%	272	1.16%	Matam	Matam	Ogo	3.09%	1044	4.07%
Dakar	Rufisque	Rufisque-Bargny	4.35%	72	0.27%	Matam	Ranérou	Ranérou	4.65%	1464	4.29%
Diourbel	Bambey	Baba-Garage	0%	176	0.87%	Matam	Kanel	Sinthiou Bamambé	25%	532	5.08%
Diourbel	Bambey	Lambaye	0%	236	1.17%	Saint-Louis	Dagana	Ross-Béthio	0%	120	0.28%
Diourbel	Diourbel	Ndindy	0%	516	1.41%	Saint-Louis	Podor	Gamadji Sarré	0%	72	0.30%
Diourbel	Diourbel	Ndoulo	0%	384	0.93%	Saint-Louis	Podor	Thillé-Boubacar	0%	80	0.12%
Diourbel	Mbacké	Taif	15.38%	436	1.96%	Saint-Louis	Dagana	Mbane	0%	48	0.28%
Diourbel	Mbacké	Ndame	1.52%	356	0.44%	Tambacounda	Bakel	Moudéry	27.08%	2436	7.49%
Fatick	Fatick	Diakhao	14.29%	420	2.94%	Tambacounda	Bakel	Kéniaba	—	384	9.54%
Fatick	Fatick	Niakhar	8.11%	636	2.75%	Tambacounda	Bakel	Kidira	0%	204	7.13%
Fatick	Fatick	Tattaguine	7.55%	840	2.99%	Tambacounda	Kédougou	Bandafassi	—	244	8.24%
Fatick	Foundiougne	Djilor	7.14%	128	1.94%	Tambacounda	Kédougou	Salémata	—	172	6.89%
Fatick	Foundiougne	Colobane	6.98%	676	2.21%	Tambacounda	Kédougou	Saraya	37.04%	208	6.35%
Fatick	Gossas	Ouadiour	5.17%	540	2.98%	Tambacounda	Tambacounda	Koumpentoum	36.84%	3464	10.49%
Kaolack	Kaffrine	Maka Yop	6.91%	2240	5.53%	Tambacounda	Tambacounda	Koussanar	17.31%	800	4.12%
Kaolack	Kaffrine	Malem Hoddar	11.87%	1740	6.15%	Tambacounda	Tambacounda	Makacoulibantang	0%	1884	10.14%
Kaolack	Kaolack	Sibassor	15.79%	1208	5.07%	Tambacounda	Tambacounda	Missirah	6.67%	424	5.71%
Kaolack	Kaolack	Ndiédieng	5.1%	452	3.01%	Thiès	Mbour	Ndaganiao	—	224	2.47%
Kaolack	Kaolack	Koumbal	4%	884	1.41%	Thiès	Mbour	Sèsséne	5.08%	540	2.62%
Kaolack	Nioro du Rip	Paoscoto	3.77%	1264	3.48%	Thiès	Mbour	Sindia	0%	684	1.84%
						Thiès	Thiès	Keur Moussa	0%	1312	1.31%
Kaolack	Kaffrine	Birkelane	8.2%	656	3.54%	Thiès	Thiès	Thiénaba	—	120	1.12%
Kolda	Kolda	Dabo	39.18%	3212	13.1%	Thiès	Tivaouane	Méouane	1.59%	360	1.09%
Kolda	Kolda	Médina Yoro Foula	27.17%	3240	8.59%	Thiès	Tivaouane	Médina Dakar	0%	156	0.99%
Kolda	Sédhiou	Bounkiling	19.23%	1632	6.84%	Thiès	Tivaouane	Niakhène	0%	288	0.92%
Kolda	Sédhiou	Diendé	3.49%	1280	3.62%	Thiès	Tivaouane	Pambal	27.78%	136	1.71%
Kolda	Sédhiou	Djibabouya	5.56%	460	5.23%	Ziguinchor	Bignona	Sindian	6.25%	408	3.52%
Kolda	Vélingara	Bonconto	5.45%	2644	8.98%	Ziguinchor	Bignona	Tendouck	0%	208	2.19%
Kolda	Vélingara	Kounkané	9.76%	1472	10.47%	Ziguinchor	Bignona	Tenghory	3.33%	196	1.44%
Louga	Kébémer	Ndande	0%	92	0.33%	Ziguinchor	Oussouye	Loudia-Ouoloff	0%	32	1.17%
Louga	Linguère	Barkedji	—	64	0.61%	Ziguinchor	Ziguinchor	Niaguis	—	24	1.37%
Louga	Linguère	Dodji	4.92%	348	1.50%	Ziguinchor	Ziguinchor	Niassia	1.25%	348	0.78%
Louga	Linguère	Yang Yang	0%	68	0.52%	Ziguinchor	Bignona	Diouloulou	6.25%	120	1.72%

[a]Observed Prevalence.
[b]Estimated number of infected children under 5 years of age.
[c]Population-adjusted estimated prevalence.
Data based on the old administrative division (Decret n° 2002-166).

Table 4. Posterior model probabilities obtained using Gibbs Variable Selection (Second stage).

Model	ITN coverage indicators	Posterior Probabilities
1.	None	25.20%
2.	Ownership of 1 ITN per 2 household members	34.00%
3.	Child has ITN for sleeping, ownership of 1 ITN per 2 household members, n. of ITNs per household	7.80%
4.	Others	33.0%

The model with the highest posterior probability (34%) includes "Ownership of 1 ITN per 2 household members" as the selected ITN coverage indicator.

and colleagues [5], for instance, made use of the Garki transmission model to take into account the heterogeneity in the surveys. The model developed by Pull and Grab [28] was instead employed by the MAP project [9], standardizing age-groups to produce a world map of Plasmodium falciparum malaria endemicity. The parasitaemia risk map presented in this paper, has been estimated from a contemporary survey and shows similar patterns to the one obtained from previous efforts [5], especially in the Southern and Eastern part of Senegal, at the border with Mali where the risk is higher. However, Gemperli et al. [5] predicted a lower risk in the Central part of the country and higher in the urban areas of Dakar and Saint-Louis, as well as throughout the Sahelian region. In terms of absolute values, those results are uniformly higher than the current ones, due to the fact that the SMIS was carried out at the beginning of the low transmission season. The predicted pattern of malaria produced by the more recent work by Gosoniu et al. [8] is more consistent with the map we generated, however the absolute values are still far from our estimates. The map of Senegal from the MAP project [9] does not show any relevant variations or geographical differences in the intensity of malaria risk throughout the country. For logistic reasons the survey took place at the start of the dry season, thus projections from our model are likely to underestimate the burden during the highest transmission season.

Furthermore, the differences between observed and population adjusted risk estimates are mainly due to low prevalence observed in highly populated areas. The urban area of Dakar, for example, is the most populated one, and the majority of surveys were carried out in that area although the parasitaemia risk is very low.

Geostatistical variable selection enabled the assessment of the effect on parastaemia risk of different ITN coverage indicators after taking into account climatic factors and socio-economic disparities. Recent work by [18] and [19] proposed a number of ITN coverage measures related to the ownership and use of nets at individual or household level. Five indicators have been assessed in the study and only one suggested a reduction in malaria risk with increasing coverage. This may explain the lack of relation between ITN coverage and malaria risk in similar analyses of MIS data. The Senegal data revealed that the presence of at least one ITN per every two household members reduced the odds of parasitaemia by 86%. In a recent analysis in Tanzania [29], ownership of at least one ITN was the only indicator assessed, showing no protective effect. On the other hand, the analysis of Zambia MIS 2005 [30] measured ITN coverage by the ownership of at least one bednet per household and found a preventive effect on malaria risk. Gosoniu et al. [31] reported a reduction in risk for areas having at least 0.2 ITNs per person, a measure similar to the one presented in this paper. Different indicators of ITN coverage were considered in a spatial analysis of the Liberia MIS data [27], however none of them was associated with a reduction in the infection risk.

The model does not include some known risk factors for malaria such as maternal education, proximity to health services as this information was not readily available from the MIS data. It is however interesting to collect this data and include them in future MIS analyses aiming to assess ITN effects on parasitaemia.

This study found that the malaria risk in children less than five years old increases with age. Infants had the lowest risk. The risk rises especially after the age of two and levels off in older children. Similar results were observed in other low endemic settings.

All the results presented in the paper are based on the estimation of parasitaemia prevalence using the blood smear test. Malaria prevalence estimated using the RTDs was almost twice as high as the one based on the microscopy results. This confirms earlier findings suggesting that RDTs might present a large number of false positives when used in field conditions probably due to high temperatures during storage and transport as well as poor training on RDTs use.

In the model formulation, a linear relation between the parasitaemia odds and the environmental covariates was assumed. Geostatistical variable selection could be used to determine the best functional form that describes the above relation. Furthermore, a stationary geostatistical model was fitted assuming that spatial correlation depends only on the distance between locations irrespective of the locations themselves. This assumption may not be true when there are unobserved factors, such as health system performance, that vary across the country. The relation between climatic predictors and malaria may differ as well among the ecological zones.

Future control interventions can be planned and implemented by decision-makers according to the priority of the areas. A better resource allocation and health management can be achieved by monitoring the impact of prevention and control activities. The produced map and estimates generated in this study can be considered as baseline for comparisons with future national surveys to evaluate the effectiveness and progress of on-going intervention programmes as well as the changes of the parasitaemia risk over space and time.

Author Contributions

Analyzed the data: FG PV. Wrote the paper: FG LG PV. Gave intellectual content and critically reviewed manuscript: LK RP OF MDB OG.

References

1. World Health Organization (2009) World Malaria Report. Available: http://whqlibdoc.who.int/publications/2009/9789241563901_eng.pdf. Accessed 2012 Feb 5.
2. World Health Organization (2008) World Health Report. Available: http://www.searo.who.int/LinkFiles/Reports_whr08_en.pdf. Accessed 2012 Feb 5.
3. Thiam S, Thior M, Faye B, Ndiop M, Diouf ML, et al. (2011) Major Reduction in Anti-Malarial Drug Consumption in Senegal after Nation-Wide Introduction of Malaria Rapid Diagnostic Tests. PLoS ONE 6(4): e18419.
4. Roll Back Malaria Progress & Impact Series: Focus on Senegal. Available: http://www.rollbackmalaria.org/ProgressImpactSeries/report4.html. Accessed 2012 Feb 5.
5. Gemperli A, Sogoba N, Fondjo E, Mabaso M, Bagayoko M, et al. (2006) Mapping malaria transmission in West and Central Africa. Tropical Medicine and International Health 11: 1032–1046.
6. Dietz K, Molineaux L, Thomas A (1974) A malaria model tested in the African savannah. Bull World Health Organ 50: 347–57.
7. MARA/ARMA (1998) Towards an atlas of malaria risk in Africa. First technical report of the MARA/ARMA collaboration. Durban, South Africa.
8. Gosoniu L, Vounatsou P, Sogoba N, Maire N, Smith T (2009) Mapping malaria risk in West Africa using a Bayesian nonparametric non-stationary model. Computational Statistics & Data Analysis 53: 3358–3371.
9. Hay SI, Guerra CA, Gething PW, Patil AP, Tatem AJ, et al. (2009) A world malaria map: Plasmodium falciparum endemicity in 2007. PLoS Medicine 6(3): e48.
10. Hall DB (2000) Zero-inflated Poisson and Binomial regression with random effects: a case study. Biometrics 56: 1030–1039.
11. Amek N, Bayoh N, Hamel M, Lindblade KA, Gimnig J, et al. (2011) Spatio-temporal modeling of sparse geostatistical malaria sporozoite rate data using a zero inflated Binomial model. Journal of Spatial and Spatio-Temporal Epidemiology 2: 283–290.
12. Agarwal DK, Gelfand AE, Cintron-Pousty S (2002) Zero-Inflated models with application to spatial count data. Environmental and Ecological statistics 9: 341–355.

13. Musenge E, Vounatsou P, Kahn K (2011) Space-time confounding adjusted determinants of child HIV/TB mortality for large zero-inflated data in rural South Africa. Journal of Spatial and Spatio-Temporal Epidemiology 2: 205–217.
14. Ndiaye S, Ayad M (2009) Enquéte Nationale sur le Paludisme au Sénégal 2008–2009. Calverton, Maryland, USA: Centre de Recherche pour le Développement Humain (Sénégal) et ICF Macro.
15. Wongsrichanalai C, Barcus MJ, Muth S, Sutamihardja A, Wernsdorfer WH (2007) A review of malaria diagnostic tools: microscopy and rapid diagnostic test (RDT). Am J Trop Med Hyg 77: 119–127.
16. Collection and dissemination of data from the *Demographic Yearbook*. UN statistics division website. Available: http://unstats.un.org/unsd/demographic/sconcerns/densurb/Defintion_of%20Urban.pdf. Accessed 2012 Feb 5.
17. Rutstein SO, Johnson K (2004) The DHS Wealth Index. DHS Comparative Reports No. 6. Calverton, Maryland: ORC Macro.
18. Thwing JI, Perry R, Townes DA, Diouf MB, Ndiaye S, et al. (2011) Success of Senegal's first nationwide distribution of long-lasting insecticide-treated nets to children under five-contribution toward universal coverage. Malaria Journal 10: 86.
19. Kilian A, Wijayanandana N, Ssekitoleeko J (2010) Review of delivery strategies for insecticide treated mosquito nets – are we ready for the next phase of malaria control efforts? Available: http://www.malariaconsortium.org/userfiles/file/Malaria%20resources/Review%20of%20delivery%20strategies%20for%20ITNs.pdf.
20. Dellaportas P, Forster JJ, Ntzoufras I (2002) On Bayesian Model and Variable Selection Using MCMC. Statistics and Computing 12: 27–36.
21. George EI, McCulloch RE (1993) Variable Selection via Gibbs Sampling. Journal of the American Statistical Association 88: 881–889.
22. Kuo L, Mallick B (1998) Variable Selection for Regression Models. Sankhya B 60: 65–81.
23. Gelfand AE, Sahu SK, Carlin B (1995) Efficient parametrisations for normal linear mixed models. Biometrika 82: 479–488.
24. Diggle PJ, Tawn JA (1998) Model-based geostatistics. Appl Stats 47: 299–350.
25. Gosoniu L, Vounatsou P, Sogoba N, Smith T (2006) Bayesian modelling of geostatistical malaria risk data. Geospatial Health 1: 127–139.
26. Lunn D, Spiegelhalter D, Thomas A, Best N (2009) The BUGS project: Evolution, critique, and future directions, Statistics in Medicine 28: 3049–3067.
27. Gosoniu L, Vounatsou P (2011) Geostatistical variable selection in malaria risk mapping: an application to the Liberia Malaria Indicator Survey data. Parasites and Vectors. Submitted.
28. Pull JH, Grab B (1974) A simple epidemiological model for evaluating the malaria inoculation rate and the risk of infection in infants. Bull World Health Organ 51: 507–516.
29. Gosoniu L, Msengwa A, Lengeler C, Vounatsou P (2011) Spatially explicit burden estimates of malaria in United Republic of Tanzania: Bayesian geostatistical modeling of the Tanzania HIV/AIDS and Malaria Indicator Survey data. PLoS OneIn press.
30. Riedel N, Vounatsou P, Miller JM, Gosoniu L, Chizema-Kawesha E, et al. (2010) Geographical patterns and predictors of malaria risk in Zambia: Bayesian geostatistical modelling of the 2006 Zambia national malaria indicator survey (ZMIS). Malaria Journal 9: 37.
31. Gosoniu L, Veta AM, Vounatsou P (2010) Bayesian Geostatistical Modeling of Malaria Indicator Survey Data in Angola. PLoS ONE 5(3): e9322.
32. O'Hara RB, Sillanpää MJ (2009) A review of Bayesian variable selection methods: what, how and which. Bayesian analysis 4: 85–118.

18

Pediatric Acute Q Fever Mimics Other Common Childhood Illnesses

Ingeborg Y. Bart[1], Yvonne Schabos[1], Roeland W. N. M. van Hout[2], Alexander C. A. P. Leenders[3], Esther de Vries[1]*

1 Department of Pediatrics, Jeroen Bosch Hospital's-Hertogenbosch, The Netherlands, 2 Department of Linguistics, Radboud University, Nijmegen, The Netherlands, 3 Department of Medical Microbiology, Jeroen Bosch Hospital's-Hertogenbosch, The Netherlands

Abstract

Knowledge of Q fever has increased over the last decades, but research has mainly focused on adults. Data in children are scarce, and current knowledge is mostly based on case reports. The aim of this study was to determine predictors for acute Q fever in children in the general population. We retrospectively studied all children tested for *Coxiella burnetii* by serology and/or PCR upon request of their general practitioner in the regional laboratory for Medical Microbiology of the Jeroen Bosch during the Q fever outbreak in the Netherlands between 2007 and 2011. A total of 1061 patients was analyzed. Influenza-like illness and respiratory tract infection were the most common presentations of acute Q fever, mimicking other common childhood illnesses. None of the reported symptoms was significantly related to a positive test outcome and therefore presenting signs or symptoms have no predictive value in diagnosing Q-fever in children. Only diagnostic tests are reliable. As the infection generally follows a mild and uncomplicated course, we question if the difficulty of recognizing pediatric Q fever is a problem worth solving.

Editor: Ravi Jhaveri, University of North Carolina School of Medicine, United States of America

Funding: The authors have no funding or support to report.

Competing Interests: The authors have declared that no competing interests exist.

* E-mail: e.d.vries@jbz.nl

Introduction

Between 2007 and 2011, the Netherlands was confronted with the largest human Q fever outbreak ever reported; in 2009, 2,354 Q fever cases were reported to the public health authorities [1]. The outbreak was concentrated in the northeastern part of the province of Noord-Brabant (*figure 1*). During the epidemic, the Regional Laboratory for Medical Microbiology and Infection Prevention of the Jeroen Bosch Hospital was the major provider of *C. burnetii* diagnostics for this region.

Q fever usually presents as a self-limiting febrile disease [2]. It may also manifest with a variety of non-specific symptoms that are commonly encountered in other illnesses [2], or remain asymptomatic [1,3]. Knowledge of Q fever has increased over the last decades, but research has mainly focused on adults. Data in children are scarce; current knowledge is mostly based on case reports [4–17] and small case series [3,18–22]. Fever and pneumonia are most frequently reported in these cases, followed by central nervous system infection and myocarditis. A bias towards more severe cases seems to be likely in the available literature. As a result, selecting the right children for Q fever diagnostics in everyday practice is difficult.

We aimed to determine predictors for a positive Q fever test in children in the general population. With these predictors, the risk profile can be analyzed and used to decide whether or not tests for *C. burnetii* infection are warranted in a particular child.

In the Netherlands, the primary care system is the key entry for health care. Therefore, we studied a case series of children who visited their general practitioner during the Q fever outbreak with complaints that prompted their physician to test for *C. burnetii* infection.

Methods

Study population

We analyzed all data from children (0–18 years) that were tested upon request of their general practitioner for *C. burnetii* by serology and/or PCR in the regional laboratory for Medical Microbiology and Infection Prevention of the Jeroen Bosch Hospital during the Q fever outbreak from September 2007 until June 2010. The study area and period coincided with a high incidence of Q fever [23].

Data collection

In July 2011, all general practitioners who had ordered Q fever tests in pediatric patients were asked to answer a written multiple-choice questionnaire about the child's reported symptoms at the time of sampling. Data were derived from their electronic medical records (EMR), after informed consent from the parents and – if applicable – children was obtained. The items *unexplained fever, lower respiratory tract infection, skin rash, vomiting - diarrhea and/or abdominal pain* and *other* could be chosen. In addition, age, gender and the outcome(s) of the test(s) were noted.

Laboratory diagnosis of acute Q-fever

Laboratory diagnosis of acute Q-fever depends on the duration of symptoms. The first 2 to 3 weeks after the onset of disease, no antibodies are formed and diagnosis can only be made based on a

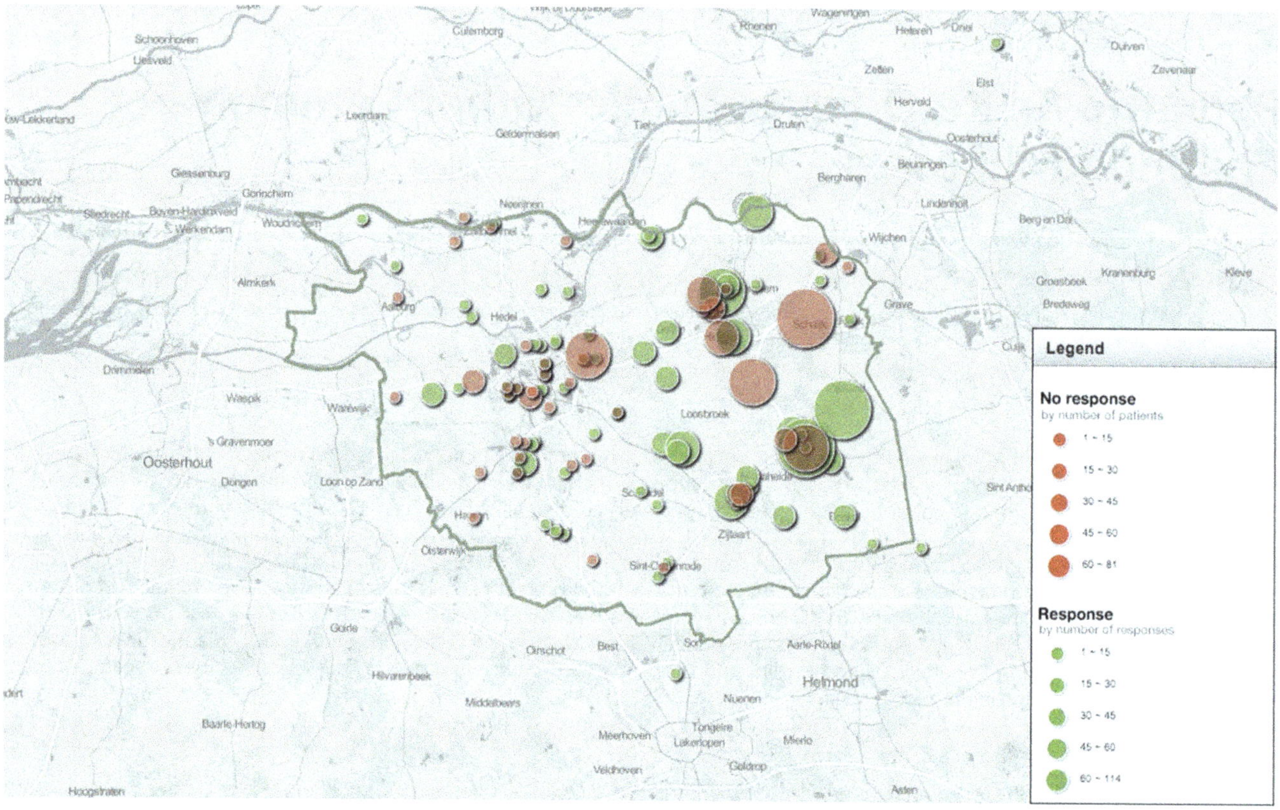

Figure 1. Geographical distribution and number of responders and non-responders to the questionnaire. Dark green line: Jeroen Bosch Hospital laboratory encachment area. Responders and non-responders: see legend within the image.

positive polymerase chain reaction (PCR) [24]. After this, IgM phase I/II antibodies are the first to be detected followed shortly by IgG phase II. IgG phase I antibodies are the last to be formed, sometimes even weeks to months after the onset of infection. Therefore, anti-phase II antibodies predominate during acute Q-fever, while anti-phase I antibodies are more likely to be elevated in chronic Q-fever cases [25,26].

All sera in this study were analyzed in the Regional Laboratory of Medical Microbiology and Infection Prevention at the Jeroen Bosch Hospital, 's-Hertogenbosch, The Netherlands. During the outbreak, a diagnostic screening strategy was implemented to cope with the large number of samples. This strategy combined an enzyme-linked immunoassay (ELISA) IgM phase II (Serion Immundiagnostica, Wurzburg Germany) or an in house PCR test, depending on the time after onset of symptoms, with confirmation and follow-up by an indirect immunofluorescence assay (IFA) (Focus Diagnostics, Cypress, CA, USA) [24,25]. IFA is considered the reference method [26].

Statistical analysis

All possible predictors were investigated by using the Fisher exact test or a t test. We used a binomial test to investigate the differences between the general practitioners in their success of predicting seropositive outcomes (using SPSS). A regression analysis with two successful predictors using mixed models with a binomial outcome, the general practitioners constituting a random factor (using the package lme4 in R) was also performed.

Results

Study population

All 2088 patients for whom tests were ordered by general practitioners were included in the study. A total of 1061 questionnaires were returned (50.8%). In 40 patients, the general practitioners could not retrieve the presenting symptoms from their EMR; these cases were excluded from further analysis.

Patient characteristics

There were no differences in the distribution of age, gender and test outcome between the responder and the non-responder group (*table 1*). The geographical distribution of the general practitioners who did or did not respond to our questionnaire was similar, and equally distributed in the area of the outbreak (*figure 1*).

Table 1. Patient characteristics.

	Responder group	Non-responder group
Patients (number)	1021	1027
Mean age (years)	11,69	11,52
Male gender (percent)	47,4	46,0
Acute Q-fever present (percent)	4,8	4,3
General practitioners (number)	141	99

Of the 1021 children analyzed, 484 were boys, of which 28 were diagnosed with acute Q fever, and 537 were girls, of which 21 were diagnosed with acute Q fever. No significant relation between gender and a positive test result was found (chi square [1, N = 1021] = 1.958, p = 0.162). The age of the children ranged between 0.28 and 17.98 years (M 11.7; SD 4.7); the number of children tested increased with increasing age (*figure 2*).

Children with a positive test were older (positive test M 13.9 years, SD 3.6; negative test M 11.6 years, SD 4.7; no homogeneity of variance, Levene's test, F = 13.104, p = 0.000; Welch t test (57) = 4.337, p = 0.000). This is not merely caused by more tests being performed in older children; the proportion of diagnosed infections is also significantly related to age (r = 0.108, N = 1021, p = 0.001).

Reported symptoms

The original answers to the multiple-choice question are shown in table 2. Most patients presented with more than one symptom (mean 1.8 symptoms per patient). The top 5 reported symptoms in confirmed acute Q-fever cases were fatigue (n = 22), lower respiratory tract infection (n = 13), cough (n = 13), headache (n = 9), and fever (n = 8). *Other* was the multiple-choice item that was most often reported. When the item *unexplained fever* had been chosen, often other symptoms had been added to *other* in writing that could explain the fever, however. In those cases, we reclassified *unexplained fever* to *respiratory tract infection*, *gastro-intestinal tract infection* or *influenza-like infection* as appropriate. The remarks written under the item *other* were grouped as follows (*table 3*): *upper respiratory tract infection* (i.e. cough, aching throat, pharyngitis, tonsillitis, sinusitis, rhinitis, ear pain, cervical lymphadenopathy); *lower respiratory tract infection* (i.e. symptoms described as under *upper respiratory tract infection* but combined with either tachypnea or dyspnea); *undetermined respiratory tract infection* (i.e. single presenting symptoms such as dyspnea or tachypnea); *influenza-like infection* (i.e. 2 or more of: fever, headache, nausea, malaise, myalgia, arthralgia or upper respiratory tract infection with one or more of the above mentioned symptoms excluding fever); *malaise* (i.e. bad thrive, malaise, faint, or tiredness); *Q fever in the direct vicinity of the patient* (i.e. visited a farm with known Q fever, family member or close contact with Q fever).

49 children (4.8%) in the response group were diagnosed with acute Q fever at the time of laboratory testing, but none of the reported presenting symptoms was significantly related to a positive test outcome. No symptoms were significantly related to a negative test outcome either. None of the Fisher exact tests applied to the group of modified symptoms in Table 3 returned a significant outcome (the lowest p value, 0.310, was far above the alpha level of 0.05). None of the modified reported symptoms had a relationship with the presence of acute Q fever; in other words,

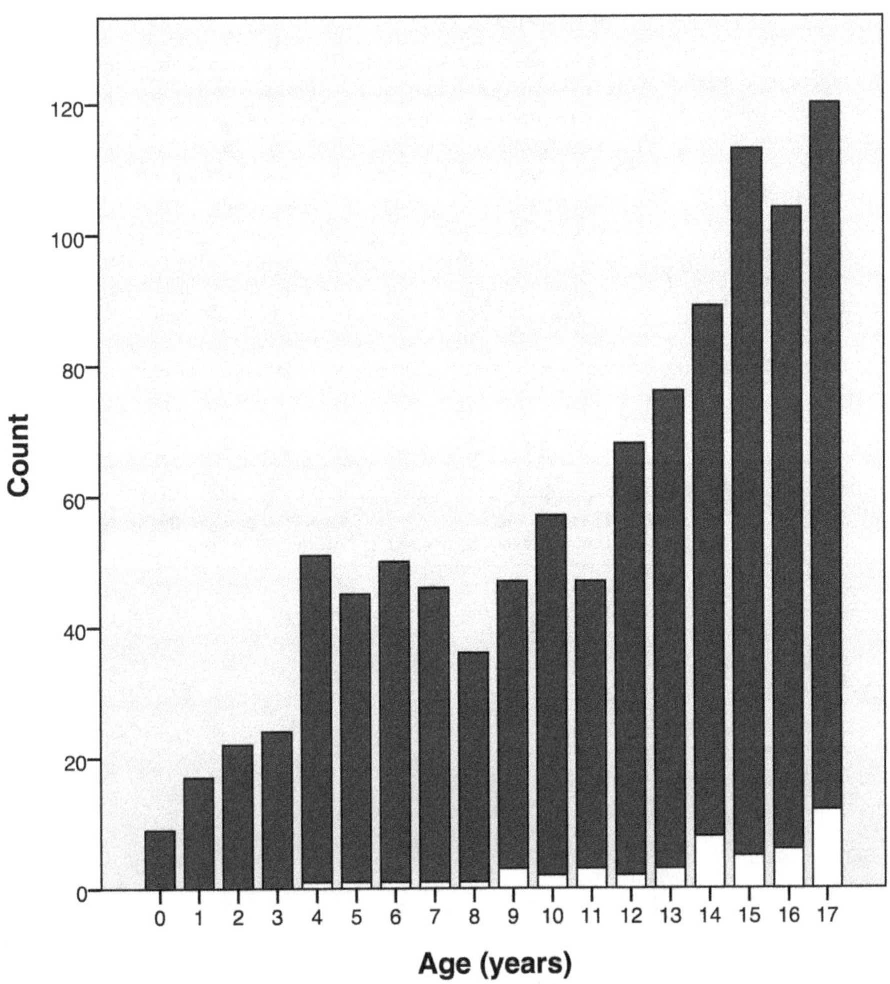

Figure 2. Number of requested tests and test outcome divided per age. White bar: acute Q fever. Dark grey bar: no acute Q fever.

Table 2. Reported items in the original multiple-choice questionnaire.

Items	Reported (number)
Unexplained fever	193
Lower respiratory tract infection	263
Skin rash	5
Vomiting, diarrhea, and/or abdominal pain	122
Other	1310
Total	1893

no predictors for positivity could be identified among the reported presenting symptoms.

Two patients had no disease manifestations but were tested because of Q fever in their direct vicinity. This number is too small for statistical analysis of its predictive value.

General practitioner characteristics

The distance between the epicenter of the epidemic and the practice of the general practitioner ranged between 0.25 and 38.45 kilometers (M = 18.73, SD = 8.27). The number of tests per general practitioner was correlated to the distance of the practice to the epicenter, but the correlation coefficient was moderate ($r = -0.283$, $N = 140$, $p = 0.001$). There were also several general practitioners close to the epicenter who did not request many tests, and some having their practice much further away who did.

There is a significant correlation between distance and positive diagnosis ($r = -0.072$, $N = 1021$, $p = 0.\ 021$). The overall probability of a positive outcome was fairly low for all general practitioners: 4.8% (49 positive outcomes on 1021 tests), but that does not exclude differences in performance between them. Five of the 140 practitioners performed beyond the average level (one-directional binomial test, criterion being a p value of 0.048), a number that is within the range of more extreme performances to be expected purely on the basis of probability. An important observation is that all five practitioners had their practice located near the epicenter.

A regression model to predict acute Q fever

In order to identify factors that needed to be included to predict the probability of a positive test, we applied regression analysis, with general practitioners as a random effect (generalized linear mixed model analysis; lme4, package R). The null model in the analysis contains no effects, only including general practitioners as a random effect. The Akaikes Information Criterion (AIC) of this model was 388.86. Further analyses clarified that both the age of the children and distance from the epicenter play a significant role in predicting a positive test outcome. Testing several models of how to apply these variables, the best implementation (lowest AIC) was a squared value for age (in years) and a categorical distance parameter, distinguishing between a distance of 15 kilometers or less from the epicenter and a distance of more than 15 kilometers. The resulting model has an AIC of 375.19, a clear improvement compared to the null model. Both variables were significant (age squared, $z = 3.087$, $p = 0.002$; distance, two groups, $z = -2.492$, $p = 0.013$). Including these two variables had the effect that no individual practitioners performed significantly better any longer in their test outcome prediction (their normalized random intercept values were all between -1 and 1).

Discussion

Our study shows that it is difficult to accurately identify acute Q fever in children based on signs and symptoms alone. They appear to have no predictive power. Clinicians have to rely on diagnostic tests to confirm or reject the diagnosis. On one hand, this can lead to large numbers of children being tested during an epidemic, with large numbers of negative test results, posing a great burden on the available laboratory facilities. On the other hand, Q fever may be easily missed outside an epidemic. Consistent with earlier reports, respiratory tract infection and influenza-like illness were the most frequently reported presentation in acute Q fever [1,3,18]. These clinical presentations are most often caused by other pathogens in children. Given the frequent mild and self-limiting course of

Table 3. Modified groups of reported symptoms.

Modified groups	Reported cases in the group without acute Q fever (%) (n = 972)	Reported cases in the acute Q fever group (%) (n = 49)
Lower respiratory tract infection	249 (25,6)	12 (24,5)
Upper respiratory tract infection	183 (18,8)	10 (20,4)
Undetermined respiratory tract infection	25 (2,6)	2 (4,1)
Unexplained fever	94 (9,7)	2 (4,1)
Skin rash	5 (0,5)	0
Vomiting, diarrhea, abdominal pain or gastroenteritis-like symptoms	93 (9,6)	4 (8,2)
Influenza-like symptoms	220 (22,6)	12 (24,5)
Malaise	126 (13,0)	8 (16,3)
Q-fever in the direct vicinity of the patient	51 (5,2)	4[1](8,2)
Other[2]	59 (6,1)	2 (4,1)
Total	1105	56

[1]As single 'symptom' in 2 patients.
[2]*Other* contains: patient's request, profuse sweating, myalgia/arthralgia, headache, dizziness, palpitations, sleeping difficulty and weight loss; total number of symptoms in the non-acute Q fever group is 62, three cases having two symptoms.
For explanation of the modification see text.

illness, investigations to define the causative organism are generally not undertaken. It is doubtful whether this is an important clinical problem, since our data also indicate that Q fever is generally mild and uncomplicated in children: there were no children who were diagnosed with chronic Q-fever during our study, and no serious acute illness requiring hospital admission was reported.

Two variables turned out to be predictive of a positive test result: the distance to the epicenter of the epidemic, and the age of the tested child. The best prediction was a squared value for age (years) and a two-valued distance parameter (living <15 or >15 kilometers from the epicenter). Once these predictors were taken into account in the data analysis, no differences were found between the general practitioners in their test outcome performance. None of them was able to increase their efficacy in making a correct clinical diagnosis based on signs and symptoms alone.

An increased incidence of acute Q fever with increasing age has been reported before, and has been explained by increased exposure to *C. burnetii* when children get older, similar to the increased risk of acute Q fever with occupational exposure in adults [18,27]. The recent Dutch epidemic originated from goat farms, and residency or performing recreational activities in the neighborhood of these farms were determined to be important risk factors for infection, probably due to a combination of wind and dry weather [28]. It is not very likely that this kind of exposure increases with increasing age. It has also been suggested that young children are presented less to a general practitioner, as they often remain asymptomatic during an acute Q fever infection [29]. However, even after correcting for this effect, the percentage of positive test outcomes was still correlated to increasing age in our study, which renders this explanation unlikely.

A relationship between the risk of infection and the distance from the infectious source has been reported before. In a recent Dutch study on 96 adults in 2008, residency within 2 km from the source farm greatly increased the risk for infection, whereas residency at a distance of 5 km or more from the source farm seemed protective [30]. The epicenter in our study comprised of multiple affected dairy goat farms distributed over a larger area, and we estimated the distances from the epicenter based on the location of the general practitioner, which makes distance a less precise parameter in our study. Nevertheless, we found a sharp boundary in relation to infection as well, indicating that distance is a direct and determining factor in an acute Q fever epidemic.

Our study poses several limitations. Firstly, we used passive surveillance to determine the predictors of acute pediatric Q fever, creating the possibility of selection bias.

Performing a prospective cohort study would have eliminated this factor because the decision to test for Q fever would no longer depend on the individual general practitioner. Unfortunately, this is so labor intensive and expensive to perform that it is not feasible. The national Q fever epidemic gave us the opportunity to obtain as reliable data as possible. Secondly, our study only included the patients tested by their general practitioner, it is possible that severely sick children are not represented in our data because they were directly referred to the hospital, and primarily tested there. Maltezou et al. reported a low hospitalization rate in pediatric acute Q fever, however, which suggests that such 'direct referrals' are rare [3]. Also, only one pediatric patient was primarily diagnosed with acute Q fever in the Jeroen Bosch Hospital during the study period (encachment area in relation to the epidemic: see figure 1). The patient presented with an influenza-like illness and the course of illness was uncomplicated.

To our knowledge, our study presents the largest specific case series of acute Q-fever in children. We conclude that pediatric acute Q fever mimics other common respiratory and/or influenza-like illnesses, and is clinically difficult to distinguish from other pathogens. Fortunately, pediatric Q fever generally follows a mild and uncomplicated course. We therefore question if the difficulty of recognizing pediatric Q fever is an important problem that is worth solving.

Author Contributions

Conceived and designed the experiments: EV IB. Performed the experiments: IB YS AL. Analyzed the data: EV IB YS RvH. Contributed reagents/materials/analysis tools: AL. Wrote the paper: EV IB YS RvH AL. Designing figures: IB YS.

References

1. Terheggen U, Leggat PA (2007) Clinical manifestations of Q fever in adults and children. Travel Med Infect Dis 5: 159–164. doi:10.1016/j.tmaid.2006.06.001.
2. Raoult D, Marrie T, Mege J (2005) Natural history and pathophysiology of Q fever. Lancet Infect Dis 5: 219–226. doi:10.1016/S1473-3099(05)70052-9.
3. Maltezou HC, Raoult D (2002) Q fever in children. Lancet Infect Dis 2: 686–691.
4. Cohn A, Prebble J, Robson J, Nourse C (2012) Q fever as a cause of recurrent soft-tissue nodules and abscesses in a child. Pediatr Infect Dis J 31: 525–527. doi:10.1097/INF.0b013e3182468f0e.
5. Baquero-Artigao F, del Castillo F, Tellez A (2002) Acute Q fever pericarditis followed by chronic hepatitis in a two-year-old girl. Pediatr Infect Dis J 21: 705–707.
6. Boele van Hensbroek M, de Vries E, Dolan G, Schneeberger P (2000) Rash and petechiae as presenting signs of Q fever. Pediatr Infect Dis J 19: 358.
7. Drancourt M, Raoult D, Xeridat B, Milandre L, Nesri M, et al. (1991) Q fever meningoencephalitis in five patients. Eur J Epidemiol 7: 134–138.
8. Hervás JA, la Fuente de MA, García F, Reynés J, de Carlos JC, et al. (2000) *Coxiella burnetii* myopericarditis and rhabdomyolysis in a child. Pediatr Infect Dis J 19: 1104–1106.
9. Kuroiwa Y, Oyanagi R, Fuse S, Mori T, Ueno H, et al. (2007) Persistent hepatitis and repeated wheezing in an infant. Q fever. Pediatr Infect Dis J 26: 763–768–9. doi:10.1097/INF.0b013e3180f60bfe.
10. Maltezou HC, Kallergi C, Kavazarakis E, Stabouli S, Kafetzis DA (2001) Hemolytic-uremic syndrome associated with Coxiella burnetii infection. Pediatr Infect Dis J 20: 811–813.
11. Ravid S, Shahar E, Genizi J, Schahor Y, Kassis I (2008) Acute Q fever in children presenting with encephalitis. Pediatr Neurol 38: 44–46. doi:10.1016/j.pediatrneurol.2007.09.004.
12. Nourse C, Allworth A, Jones A, Horvath R, McCormack J, et al. (2004) Three cases of Q fever osteomyelitis in children and a review of the literature. Clin Infect Dis 39: e61–e66. doi:10.1086/424014.
13. Téllez A, Sanz Moreno J, Valkova D, Domingo C, Anda P, et al. (1998) Q fever in pregnancy: case report after a 2-year follow-up. J Infect 37: 79–81.
14. Neth OW, Falcon D, Peromingo E, Soledad Camacho M, Rodríguez-Gallego C, et al. (2011) Successful management of chronic multifocal Q fever Osteomyelitis with adjuvant interferon-gamma therapy. Pediatr Infect Dis J 30: 810–812. doi:10.1097/INF.0b013e31821487f5.
15. Tasher D, Stein M, Raucher-Sternfeld A, Somekh E (2012) Coxiella burnetii infection of a bovine jugular vein conduit in a child. Pediatr Cardiol 33: 831–833. doi:10.1007/s00246-012-0215-x.
16. Ohgimi C, Tanaka R, Oh-ishi T (2009) [A case report of acute Q fever showing Kawasaki disease-like symptoms in a 9-year-old girl]. Kansenshōgaku Zasshi 83: 245–250.
17. Ariga T, Nagaoka H, Miyanoshita A, Kusunoki Y, Watanabe T, et al. (2000) Coxiella burnetii lymphadenitis: a possible fever focus in acute Q fever. Pediatr Int 42: 711–714.
18. Maltezou HC, Constantopoulou I, Kallergi C, Vlahou V, Georgakopoulos D, et al. (2004) Q fever in children in Greece. Am J Trop Med Hyg 70: 540–544.
19. Richardus JH, Schaap GJ, Donkers A, Dumas AM, Huisman J (1984) [Q fever in the Netherlands; a description of 33 case reports observed between 1979 and 1983]. Ned Tijdschr Geneeskd 128: 2253–2258.
20. Ruiz-Contreras J, González Montero R, Ramos Amador JT, Giancaspro Corradi E, Scarpellini Vera A (1993) Q fever in children. Am J Dis Child 147: 300–302.
21. Richardus JH, Dumas AM, Huisman J, Schaap GJ (1985) Q fever in infancy: a review of 18 cases. Pediatr Infect Dis 4: 369–373.
22. Barralet JH, Parker NR (2004) Q fever in children: an emerging public health issue in Queensland. Med J Aust 180: 596–597.
23. Schimmer B, Morroy G, Dijkstra F, Schneeberger PM, Weers-Pothoff G, et al. (2008) Large ongoing Q fever outbreak in the south of The Netherlands, 2008. Euro Surveill 13.

24. Meekelenkamp JCE, Schneeberger PM, Wever PC, Leenders ACAP (2012) Comparison of ELISA and indirect immunofluorescent antibody assay detecting Coxiella burnetii IgM phase II for the diagnosis of acute Q fever. Eur J Clin Microbiol Infect Dis 31: 1267–1270. doi:10.1007/s10096-011-1438-0.
25. Wegdam-Blans MCA, Nabuurs-Franssen MN, Horrevorts AM, Peeters MF, Schneeberger PM, et al. (2010) [Laboratory diagnosis of acute Q fever]. Ned Tijdschr Geneeskd 154: A2388.
26. Fournier PE, Marrie TJ, Raoult D (1998) Diagnosis of Q fever. J Clin Microbiol 36: 1823–1834.
27. Georgiev M, Afonso A, Neubauer H, Needham H, Thiery R, Rodolakis A, et al. (2013) Q fever in humans and farm animals in four European countries, 1982 to 2010. Euro Surveill 18.
28. Schimmer B, Lenferink A, Schneeberger P, Aangenend H, Vellema P, et al. (2012) Seroprevalence and risk factors for Coxiella burnetii (Q fever) seropositivity in dairy goat farmers' households in The Netherlands, 2009–2010. PLoS ONE 7: e42364. doi:10.1371/journal.pone.0042364.
29. Parker N, Robson J, Bell M (2010) A serosurvey of Coxiella burnetii infection in children and young adults in South West Queensland. Australian and New Zealand Journal of Public Health 34: 79–82. doi:10.1111/j.1753-6405.2010.00478.x.
30. Barbara Schimmer RTSMWLZA de BPMSTVPVWVDH (2010) The use of a geographic information system to identify a dairy goat farm as the most likely source of an urban Q-fever outbreak. BMC Infectious Diseases 10: 69. doi:10.1186/1471-2334-10-69.

19

Increases in Pediatric Antiretroviral Treatment, South Africa 2005–2010

Sandeep D. Patel[1], Elysia Larson[2], Thobile Mbengashe[3], Heidi O'Bra[4], J. W. Brown[5], Thurma M. Golman[4], Jeffrey D. Klausner[4]*

1 U. S. Indian Health Services, Belcourt, North Dakota, United States of America, **2** American Schools of Public Health at U.S. Centers for Disease Control and Prevention, Pretoria, South Africa, **3** National Department of Health, Pretoria, South Africa, **4** Division of Global HIV/AIDS, U.S. Centers for Disease Control and Prevention, Pretoria, South Africa, **5** U.S. Agency for International Development, Pretoria, South Africa

Abstract

Background: In South Africa in 2010, about 340,000 children under the age of 15 were infected with HIV. We describe the increase in the treatment of South African pediatric HIV-infected patients assisted by the President's Emergency Plan for AIDS Relief (PEPFAR) from 2004 to 2010.

Methods: We reviewed routine program data from PEPFAR-funded implementing partners among persons receiving antiretroviral treatment age 15 years old and less. Data quality was assessed during the reporting period by program officials through routine analysis of trends and logic checks. Based on UNAIDS estimated mortality rates of untreated HIV-infected children, we calculated the number of deaths averted and life-years gained in children under five receiving PEPFAR-assisted antiretroviral treatment.

Results: From October 2004 through September 2010, the number of children newly initiated on antiretroviral treatment in PEPFAR-assisted programs increased from 154 to 2,641 per month resulting in an increase from 2,412 children on antiretroviral treatment in September 2005 to 79,416 children in September 2010. Of those children who initiated antiretroviral treatment before September 2009, 0–4 year olds were 1.4 (95% CI: 1.3–1.5) times as likely to transfer out of the program or die as 5–14 year olds; males were 1.3 (95% CI: 1.0–1.7) times as likely to stop treatment as females. Approximately 27,548 years of life were added to children under-five years old from PEPFAR-assisted antiretroviral treatment.

Conclusions: Pediatric antiretroviral treatment in South Africa has increased substantially. However, additional case-finding and a further acceleration in the implementation of pediatric care and treatment services is required to meet the current treatment need.

Editor: Ann M. Moormann, University of Massachusetts Medical School, United States of America

Funding: This work was completed without any external funding.

Competing Interests: The authors have declared that no competing interests exist.

* E-mail: JDKlausner@mednet.ucla.edu

Introduction

South Africa has the world's greatest burden of Human Immunodeficiency Virus (HIV) infection with an estimated 5.7 million persons infected with HIV in 2010, including 340,000 children under the age of 15 years [1,2]. South Africa's under five mortality rate increased substantially from 1996–2001 [3]. Most of those deaths are caused by conditions that are either preventable or treatable, such as Acquired Immune Deficiency Syndrome (AIDS) (35%), neonatal causes (30%) and pneumonia and diarrhea (17%) [4]. The South African Government (SAG) launched a national strategy to address the HIV epidemic in children and adults in 2003 [5]. The SAG Guidelines for the Management of HIV in Children at that time (in 2004) outlined criteria for commencing antiretroviral therapy (ART) as CD4 percentage <20% in a child under 18 months old and CD4 percentage <15% in a child over 18 months old [6]. In April 2010 those criteria were expanded to include ART for all HIV-infected infants, children 1–5 years old with CD4 T-cell counts <750 cells/mm^3 and 5–15 years olds with CD4 T-cell counts <350 cells/mm^3.

In 2004 the United States President's Emergency Plan for AIDS Relief (PEPFAR) began assisting the SAG to establish and scale up HIV prevention, care and treatment programs in private, non-government and government-supported clinics through partnerships with various implementing organizations [7]. PEPFAR assists the delivery of antiretroviral treatment (ART) through a range of services depending on the resource needs of the facility. Assistance may include the renovation of facilities, hiring of clinical staff, training and mentoring of clinicians, technical expertise, laboratory services, supply chain strengthening, the provision and distribution of drugs, quality assurance, and monitoring and evaluation activities. Approximately 90% of PEPFAR assistance goes toward government facilities with the remaining 10% reaching private facilities. The South African National Department of Health is responsible for policy development and implementation including determination of the eligibility criteria for treatment initiation. Over the period 2004–2010 the National Department of Health took increasing responsibility for procurement of prophylactic and antiretroviral drugs, reimbursement for the laboratory costs, and supply of the professional workforce.

In 2005, of the approximately 93,000 children in need of ART, less than 12,000 (13%) were receiving treatment [2,8]. In 2010, 183,000 South African children were estimated to require ART [2]. The SAG set targets to initiate 38,000 new children on ART between April 2010 and March 2011, and have 150,134 children on ART by March 2011 [9].

Using routine program data, we describe increases in pediatric HIV/AIDS treatment and select outcomes in PEPFAR-assisted programs in South Africa from 2004 through 2010.

Patients and Methods

We reviewed routine quarterly HIV care and treatment program output data submitted by PEPFAR-funded implementing partners, primarily local and international non-governmental organizations who are responsible for the delivery of high-quality HIV care and treatment programs. Those partners submit quarterly data through an open-source web-based platform. Partners reported by healthcare facility the following measures: the number of patients initiating (newly initiated and those transferred in) ART, currently receiving ART, and the cumulative number not receiving ART by age group. Those not receiving ART were defined as those who were seen at a clinic but did not meet eligibility criteria for ART; or had been on ART and categorized as discontinued due to lost-to-follow-up, transferred out, stopped, died or unknown reasons. Data were reviewed for face-validity, trends and logical errors for each submitting partner each quarter by program officials during the reporting period. We could only access data from pediatric HIV programs that were partially or fully supported by PEPFAR. Therefore, we did not include pediatric HIV-infected patients who were cared for by private practitioners or SAG programs not associated with PEPFAR. To assess the reach of the PEPFAR program, we obtained the number of children on ART nationwide from the National Department of Health ART monitoring and evaluation system (a paper-based monthly reporting system) [8].

We completed a retrospective analysis of measures for persons less than 15 years old who ever received ART in PEPFAR-assisted programs in South Africa between October 1, 2004 and September 30, 2010. Detailed data on attrition were only available from April 1, 2008 through September 30, 2009. Using Microsoft Excel® and SAS® version 9.1 (SAS Institute Inc., Cary, NC), data were analyzed at the end of each of the United States Government fiscal year (October 1-September 30). We calculated monthly averages by dividing the total number for a period by the number of months in that period. We calculated prevalence ratios (PR) and 95% confidence intervals (CI) by age group and continuation on antiretroviral therapy. We estimated the number of years of life added due to treatment of HIV-infected 0–4 year olds, up to 30 years of age. To do that, we used the number of children currently on ART at the end of our study period. Mortality estimates for children on ART and children not on ART were derived from UNAIDS/UNICEF recommendations and other published reviews included in Spectrum Software version 4.351 [10]. We used those estimates to calculate the combined number of years the children would have lived if they were not provided with ART and subtracted it from the number of years those children were expected to live now that they are on ART. To simplify the model the mortality estimates for children not on ART assume only perinatal infection. The mortality estimates account for varying mortality risk in each year of life. We also calculated the number of deaths averted in the first five years of life for the 0–4 year olds currently on PEPFAR-assisted ART at the end of the study period by subtracting the number of deaths estimated for children on ART from those not on ART using mortality estimates from Spectrum [10].

In accordance with United States regulations and international guidelines, the Centers for Disease Control and Prevention and the South African Government determined the review of programmatic data and subsequent analyses to be a non-research activity.

Results

The number of children ever initiated on PEPFAR-assisted ART increased from 2,412 children in September 2005 to 79,416 children in September 2010, a 32-fold increase (Figure 1). The rapid increase of ART within PEPFAR-assisted programs contributed substantially to expanding coverage from the estimated 12.5% of HIV-infected children in need of ART in 2005 to over 54% in September 2010. As part of the national effort, PEPFAR-assisted programs contributed to 20% of children receiving ART in 2005 and to over 75% of those receiving treatment in September 2009 (Figure 2).

The number of children in PEPFAR-assisted programs newly initiating ART per month increased 16-fold from 154 new children per month in 2005 to 2,641 new children per month in 2010 (Figure 3). From March to June 2010, 9,107 children were newly initiated on ART by PEPFAR-assisted programs contributing to 24% of the March 2011 SAG target.

Of the 74,549 children started on ART, 66,870 (89.7%) were retained on ART by the end of September 2009. The attrition of 7,679 children from ART in PEPFAR-assisted program between April 2008 and September 2009 can be attributed to multiple causes: of the 74,549 children who ever initiated ART, 0.3% had stopped treatment (0.28% of 0–4 year olds compared to 0.34% of 5–14 year olds (PR = 0.83, CI 0.63–1.09)), 4.0% had transferred care (5.0% of 0–4 year olds compared to 3.5% of 5–14 year olds (PR = 1.41, CI 1.32–1.52)), 1.3% had died (1.6% of 0–4 year olds compared to 1.2% of 5–14 year olds (PR = 1.32, CI 1.17–1.50)), and 4.6% were lost to follow-up (4.8% of 0–4 year olds compared to 4.6% of 5–14 year olds (PR = 1.05, CI 0.98–1.12)), (Figure 4). Males were 1.35 times as likely as females to stop treatment (CI 1.04–1.74).

Just over one-third of the 79,416 HIV-infected children on PEPFAR-assisted ART in South Africa is younger than five years old. After removing an additional 8.9% for children who were lost-to-follow-up, transferred, or stopped treatment, a total of 23,875 children remain for analysis. Those children would live for a total of 59,830 years without treatment and 87,378 years with treatment. This suggests that ART has added 27,548 years of life for children under five who were receiving ART in September 2010. Alternatively, in the first five years of life it is estimated that 13,875 of these children would die without treatment as opposed to 8,046 on treatment, suggesting that in the first five years of life, ART averted 5,829 deaths.

Discussion

The provision of ART to children in South Africa has greatly increased in the past six years through the South African

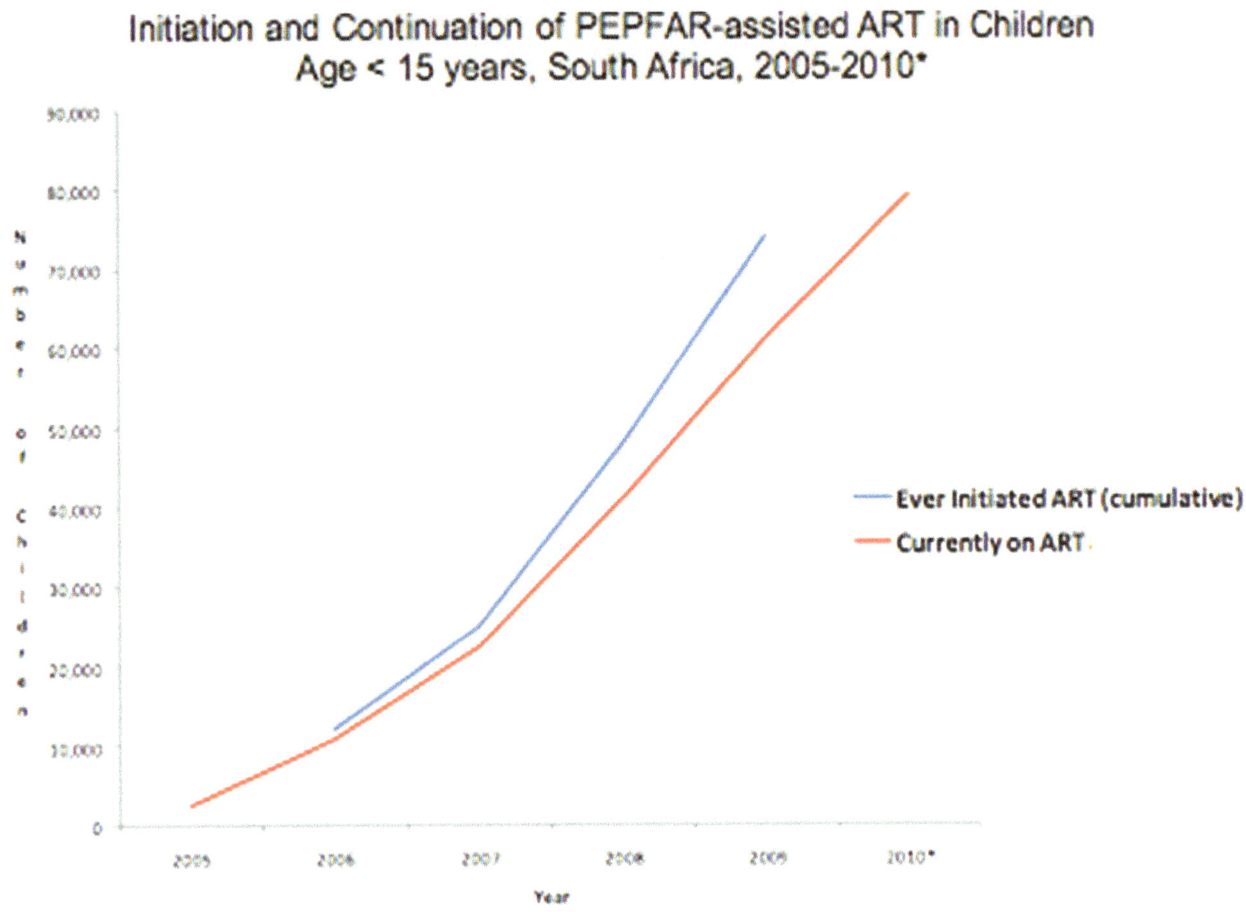

*Data are for the U.S. fiscal year from October 1-September 30, 2005-2010.

Figure 1. Initiation and Continuation of PEPFAR-assisted Antiretroviral Treatment (ART) in Children, South Africa, 2005–2010.

government's treatment programs and with the assistance of PEPFAR. The 79,416 children currently receiving PEPFAR-assisted ART in September 2010 contribute to over 50% of the March 2011 SAG target of 150,134 children receiving ART. In April 2010, the SAG updated the criteria for ART initiation to: all HIV-infected infants <1 year old, 1–5years olds with CD4 T cell counts <750 cells/mm^3 and 5–15 year olds with CD4 T cell counts <350 cells/mm^3 to help prevent high mortality in untreated children [11,12]. As those guidelines are put into effect, the number of children receiving ART should further increase substantially [13].

Pediatric treatment services are largely centralized (based at district hospitals) at present. In 2006, only 6% of children received ART in community (or primary) health centers in the most populated province, Gauteng [14]. However, it has been shown that provision of ART at the primary healthcare clinic level can result in increased number of patients receiving therapy without compromising quality of care [15]. In April 2010, the SAG prioritized Nurse Initiated and Managed Antiretroviral Treatment (NIMART) to decentralize adult services. The addition of pediatric care and treatment components to the NIMART program could further increase the number of children provided with ART.

Similar to other studies in which an administrative database was used, our study had some limitations. Programmatic measures change frequently, undergo inconsistent quality assurance, and are subject to over- and under-reporting. Due to programmatic changes in data collection procedures, data related to pediatric mortality and treatment drop-out were available for only six of the 24 quarters in the study period, and therefore, might not be generalizable. Additionally, the comparisons of outcomes between children age less than 5 years of age and greater than 5 years of age must be interpreted with caution since those on treatment age greater than 5 years of age have a survival bias. The characteristics of survivors might be different than non-survivors. Regardless, the main findings are likely valid and are consistent with past studies that also showed that loss to follow-up in this population secondary to transfer of care to other treatment providers is an issue, thus necessitating additional efforts to understand why 0–4 year olds are more likely to transfer care or die [21]. Other measures, such as the age of ART initiation, provider type, regimen type and duration, serial CD4 T-cell counts, plasma HIV viral load, hospitalization and mortality, should be routinely collected among the pediatric population in order to discern any differences in clinical outcomes at the national level.

The proportion of children continuing on treatment (89.7%) was better than that of the adult population (77%) in PEPFAR-assisted programs in South Africa for a similar period [16] and on the higher end of other reports on children from sub-Saharan Africa [17–19]. Because cumulative attrition data were reported

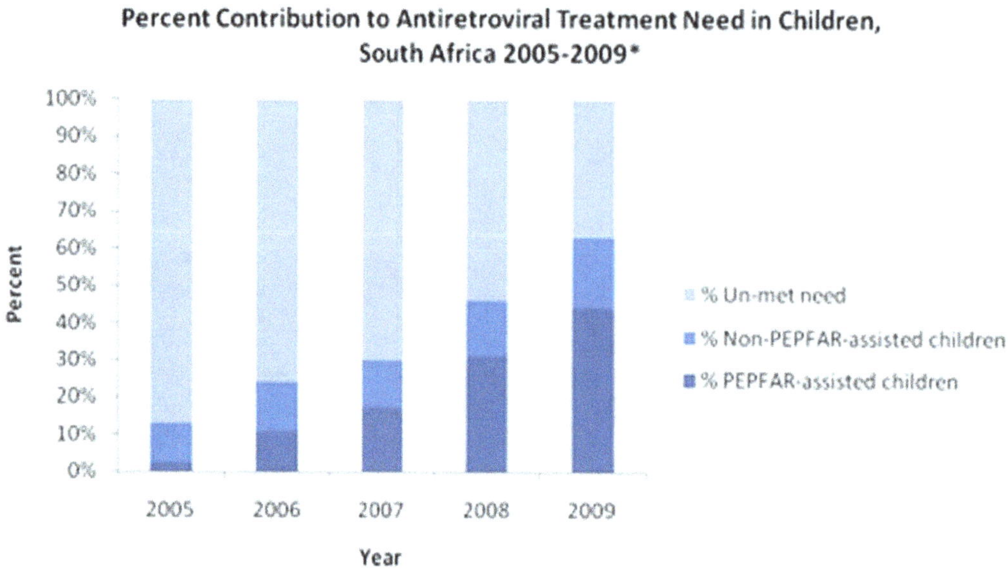

*Annual data are from September each year for PEPFAR-assisted sites and December each year for non-PEPFAR-assisted sites; unmet need was calculated as total need [2] minus the met need

Figure 2. Percent Contribution to Antiretroviral Treatment (ART) Need in Children by PEPFAR Assistance, South Africa 2005–2009.

each quarter, there may have been some misclassification of program outcomes due to reporting error. We were limited by the available data in determining factors that might influence retention. Detailed patient data such as, clinical stage of illness, socioeconomic status, migration status and health of primary caregiver along with facility characteristics such as, the size of the facility, ratio of staff-to-patients, urban versus rural setting, transport costs, and average distance from patient's homes were not available. Further evaluation is needed to understand how those characteristics might contribute to difference in continuation on ART in children.

While the overall reported discontinuation of PEPFAR-assisted treatment was relatively low, the most frequent reason (4.6%) was lost to follow-up, followed by transferred care (4.0%). Current

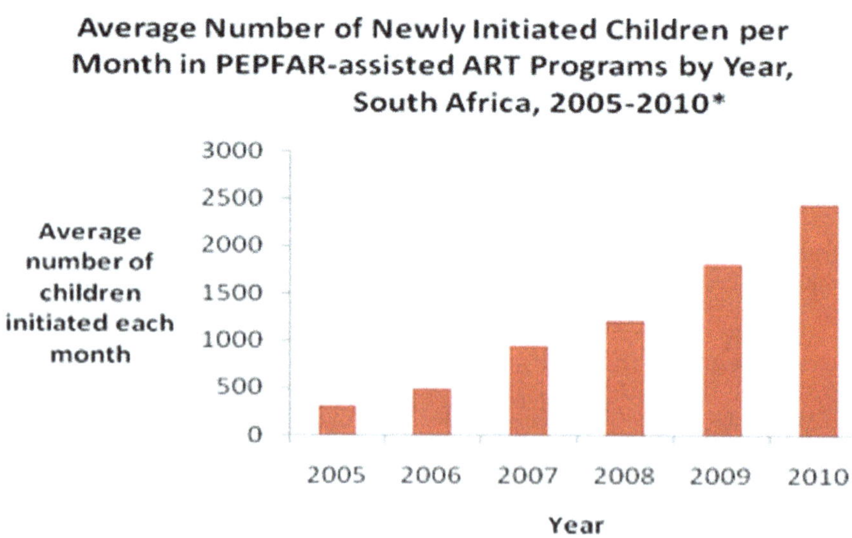

*Data are for the U.S. fiscal year, from October 1-September 30.

Figure 3. Average Number of Newly Initiated Children per Month in PEPFAR-assisted Antiretroviral Therapy (ART) Programs by year, South Africa, 2005–2010.

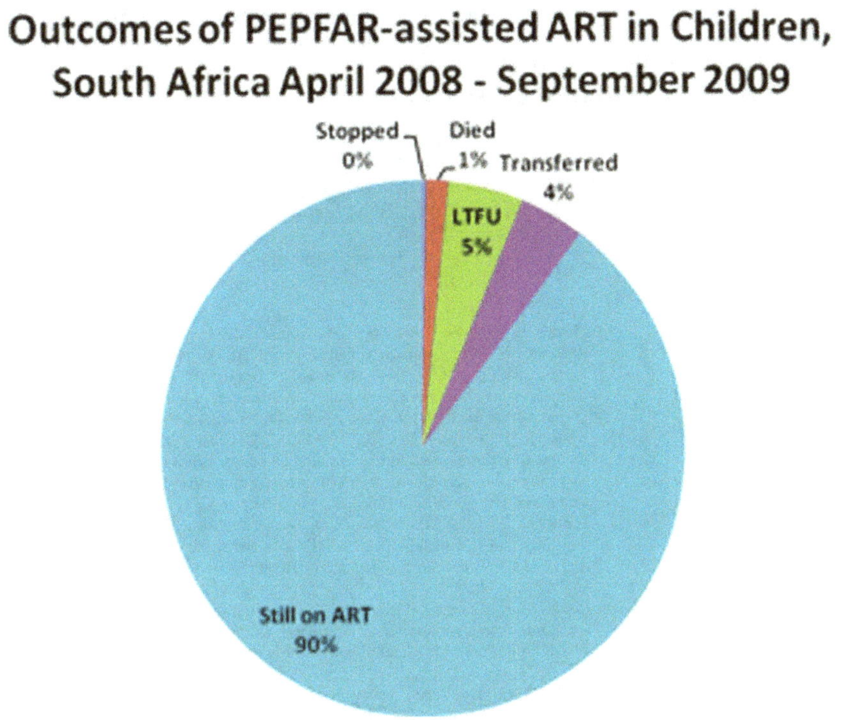

Figure 4. Outcomes of PEPFAR-assisted Antiretroviral Therapy (ART) in Children, South Africa 2008–2009. *Lost to Follow-up (LTFU).

patient monitoring systems for HIV care and treatment in South Africa are unevenly distributed across clinical sites and do not allow for the tracking of individuals at the provincial or national level [20]. A national system utilizing a unique patient identifier could greatly facilitate the care of patients and the monitoring of patient outcomes. However, the system must be designed to ensure patient confidentiality. Furthermore, patient outcomes can be improved by supporting current efforts to initiate an HIV case reporting system.

When estimating number of years of life added for children under five, we only took into account ART administration. Our estimate is conservative in that we did not take into account the impact of pre-ART care interventions, such as nutritional programs and opportunistic infection prophylaxis, which may also lead to reduced mortality [21–22]. However, our assumptions did include perinatal transmission for those children not receiving treatment, which is the worst-case scenario and may overestimate mortality. As interventions to prevent mother to child transmission improve, there will be fewer perinatal infections. We also assumed that children on ART began early in life, which may overestimate the number of life-years added by treatment. South African vital statistics demonstrate a trend in declining all-cause mortality in children under five beginning in 2006, after a steady and dramatic increase in mortality from 2001–2006, further supporting the link between ART and reduced mortality [3,23].

Initiatives to prevent and treat HIV infection are underway in South Africa; however, HIV/AIDS cannot be looked at in isolation without addressing other factors contributing to the increased infant/child mortality, such as infant and child feeding practices and respiratory diseases. The functional separation of services such as Prevention of Mother to Child Transmission programs, immunizations, management of childhood illnesses, and diagnosis of HIV infection leads to decreased continuity of care for children and missed opportunities for intervention resulting in increased morbidity and mortality. Integration of services and increased involvement of community health workers could enhance the probability of achieving national goals [14]. Community health workers help HIV infected patients initiate care at earlier stages and they improve patient retention, especially in rural settings [15]. Also, programs to improve family planning and maternal health are necessary for long-term success with children as the prevalence of HIV infection in child-bearing women is 29% [24] and it is clear that disability and loss of mothers (due to morbidity or mortality) affects the overall welfare of the child.

From 2005–2010, the SAG with assistance from PEPFAR increased ART for children. This collaboration added approximately 27,549 years of life for under-five children currently receiving ART. While that is a major medical achievement, significant challenges lay ahead in terms of reaching the national targets and providing life-long care and treatment. Specific needs to address are: lack of a central system for case reporting, reliable distribution of antiviral and other life-saving drugs to all clinics, decentralization of ART initiation and administration, integrated care, and strengthening the capacity of community-based services. At present, the management of HIV infection necessitates lifelong regular clinical care. Capacitating the South African public medical system and providing care and treatment for HIV-infected children will require increased local community involvement, advocacy, financial investment and political will.

Acknowledgments

The findings and conclusions in this report are those of the authors and do not necessarily represent the official views of the Centers for Disease Control and Prevention.

We'd like to recognize the outstanding contributions of PEPFAR-funded implementing partners, non-government organizations, faith-based organizations, and local and foreign universities who have made the delivery of quality HIV pediatric care and treatment services possible. In addition South African Government officials and advocacy organizations have made important contributions to the provision of lifesaving care and treatment in South Africa. We would also like to thank Jenny K. Cohen for her help with final revisions of this manuscript.

The findings were presented in part at the 5th Annual South African AIDS Conference, Durban, South Africa, June 7–10 and published as abstract for the conference: Patel SD, Larson E, O'Bra H, Brown JW, Goldman TM, and Klausner JD. Scale-up of President's Emergency Plan for AIDS Relief-supported pediatric ART in South Africa, 2005–2010. 5th South African AIDS Conference, June 7–10, 2011, Durban, South Africa.

Author Contributions

Conceived and designed the experiments: SDP EL HO JWB JDK. Performed the experiments: SDP EL JDK. Analyzed the data: SDP EL HO JWB, JDK. Contributed reagents/materials/analysis tools: TM TMG. Wrote the paper: SDP EL JDK. Editing, expert opinion, and insight into statistical modeling: TM, TG.

References

1. Shisana O, Simbayi LC, Rehle T, Zungu NP, Zuma K, et al. (2008) *South African National HIV Prevalence, Incidence, Behaviour and Communication Survey, 2008*: The health of our children. Cape Town: HSRC Press.
2. Mid-year population estimates (2010) Statistics South Africa, Statistical release P0302. Available: http://www.statssa.gov.za/publications/P0302/P03022010.pdf. Accessed 2011 June 27.
3. Nannan N, Dorrington RE, Laubscher R, Zinyakatira N, Prinsloo M, et al. (2012) Under-5 mortality statistics in South Africa: Shedding some light on the trends and causes 1997–2007. Cape Town: South African Medical Research Council.
4. Bradshaw D, Chopra M, Kerber K, Lawn JE, Bamford L, et al. (2008) South Africa Every Death Counts Writing Group. Every death counts: use of mortality audit data for decision making to save the lives of mothers, babies, and children in South Africa. Lancet. 2008; 371: 1294–304.
5. Department of Health. *Operational Plan for Comprehensive HIV and AIDS Care, Management and Treatment for South Africa*. Pretoria, South Africa: Department of Health; 2003. Available: http://www.info.gov.za/otherdocs/2003/aidsplan/index.html. Accessed 2010 Dec 3.
6. *Guidelines for the Management of HIV in Children*. 2004. Department of Health. Republic of South Africa.
7. *The President's Emergency Plan for AIDS Relief; FY 2008 South Africa partners*. Available: http://www.pepfar.gov/partners/2008/128082.htm. Accessed 2011 Jun 27.
8. Day C, Gray A. (2010) Health and related indicators. In: *South African Health Review 2010*. Fonn S, Padarath A (editors). Durban: Health Systems. Available: http://www.hst.org.za/publications/876. Accessed 2011 Jun 27.
9. *HIV & AIDS and STI Strategic Plan for South Africa: 2007–2011*. South African National AIDS Council, Pretoria 0001, South Africa.
10. Stover J, Johnson P, Hallett T, Marson M, BecquetR, et al. (2010) The Spectrum projection package: improvements in estimating incidence by age and sex, mother-to-child transmission, HIV progression in children and double orphans. Sex Transm Infect 86:ii16-ii21.
11. *Guidelines for the Management of HIV in Children*. 2010–2nd edition. Department of Health. Republic of South Africa.
12. Violari A, Paed FC, Cotton MF, Gibb DM, Babiker AG, et al. (2008) Early antiretroviral therapy and mortality among HIV-infected infants. New England Journal of Medicine 2008;359(21): 2233–2244.
13. Lack of treatment of South Africa's infants with HIV. Lancet 2010; 13: 1618.
14. Meyers T, Moultrie H, Naidoo K, Cotton M, Eley B, et al. (2007) Challenges to Pediatric HIV Care and Treatment in South Africa *J Infect Dis* 196: S474–81.
15. Bedelu M, Ford N, Hilderbrand K, Reuter H (2007) Implementing Antiretroviral Therapy in Rural Communities: The Lusikisiki Model of Decentralized HIV/AIDS Care *J Infect Dis*; 196: S464–8.
16. Klausner JD, Serenata C, O'Bra H, Mattson CL, Brown JW, et al. (2011) Scale-up and Continuation of Antiretroviral Therapy in PEPFAR and South African government-supported Treatment Programs, South Africa, 2005–2009. J Acquir Immune Defic Syndr 56: 292–295.
17. Fenner L, Brinkhof MWG, Keiser O, Weigel R, Cornell M, et al. (2010) Early mortality and loss to follow-up in HIV-infected children starting antiretroviral therapy in Southern Africa. Journal of Acquired Immune Deficeincy Syndrom 54(5): 524–532.
18. Davies M-A, Keiser O, Technau K, Eley B, Rabie H, et al. (2009) Outcomes of the South African national antiretroviral treatment programme for children: The IeDEA Southern Africa Collaboration. South African Medical Journal 99: 730–737.
19. Davies M-A, Egger M, Keiser O, Boulle A (2009) Paediatric antiretroviral treatment programmes in sub-Saharan Africa: a review of published clinical studies. African Journal of AIDS Research 8(3): 329–338.
20. Cornell M, Grimsrud A, Fairall L, Fox MP, van CutsemG, et al. (2010) Temporal changes in programme outcomes among adult patients initiating antiretroviral therapy across South Africa, 2002–2007. AIDS. 24: 2263–70.
21. Sutcliffe CG, van Dijk JH, Bolton C, Persaud D, Moss WJ (2008) Effectiveness of antiretroviral therapy among HIV-infected children in sub-Saharan Africa. Lancet Infect Dis. Aug;8(8): 477–89.
22. Mermin J, Lule J, Ekwaru JP, Malamba S, Downing R, et al. (2004) Effect of co-trimoxazole prophylaxis on morbidity, mortality, CD4-cell count, and viral load in HIV infection in rural Uganda. Lancet 364: 1428–34.
23. Mortality and causes of death in South Africa, 2008: Findings from death notification. Statistics South Africa, Statistical release P0309.3. 2010. Available: http://www.statssa.gov.za/publications/P03093/P030932009.pdf. Accessed 2011 Jun 27.
24. *The National HIV and Syphilis Antenatal Prevalence Survey South Africa 2007*, National Department of Health, South Africa 2008. Available: http://www.unaids.org/es/dataanalysis/epidemiology/countryestimationreports/file,29278,es.pdf. Accessed 2011 Jun 27.

20

Detection of Bocavirus in Children Suffering from Acute Respiratory Tract Infections in Saudi Arabia

Ahmed S. Abdel-Moneim[1,2]*, Mahmoud M. Kamel[1,3], Abdullhamid S. Al-Ghamdi[1], Mater I. R. Al-Malky[4]

1 College of Medicine, Taif University, Al-Taif, Saudi-Arabia, **2** Department of Virology, Faculty of Veterinary Medicine, Beni-Suef University, Beni-Suef, Egypt, **3** Department of Clinical Pathology, National Cancer Institute, Cairo University, Cairo, Egypt, **4** Pediatric Hospital, Al-Taif, Saudi Arabia

Abstract

Human bocavirus (HBoV) was recently discovered in children with respiratory distress and/or diarrhea. To our knowledge, no previous study has reported the existence of bocavirus in Saudi Arabia. Swabs samples from 80 children with respiratory tract infections were examined for the presence of HBoV. Real-time polymerase chain reaction was used as a sensitive method to detect the HBoV. Direct gene sequencing was used to determine the genotype of the detected virus isolates. HBoV was detected in 22.5% of the examined patients. The NP1 partial gene sequence from all patients showed that the circulated strains were related to HBoV-1 genotype. Most of HBoV infected patients showed evidence of mixed coinfection with other viral pathogens. The current study clearly demonstrated that genetically conserved HBoV1 circulates in Saudi Arabia. Interestingly, most of the HBoV1 infected cases were associated with high rates of co-infections with other viruses.

Editor: Jianming Qiu, University of Kansas Medical Center, United States of America

Funding: This study was supported by a research grant (Project No. 1652-433-1) through the Research Support of Taif University, Saudi Arabia. The funders had no role in study design, data collection and analysis, decision to publish, or preparation of the manuscript.

Competing Interests: The authors have declared that no competing interests exist.

* E-mail: asa@bsu.edu.eg

Introduction

Bocavirus is a single-stranded DNA virus belonging to the family *Parvoviridae*, subfamily *Parvovirinae*, genus *Bocavirus*. Bocaviruses are unique among parvoviruses because they contain a third ORF between the non-structural and structural coding regions [1–2]. The genus bocavirus includes viruses that infect bovine, canine, feline, porcine and some simian species as well as sea lions [3–8]. Human bocavirus (HBoV) was first found in children with acute respiratory tract infections in 2005 [1]. It was then detected in children with respiratory tract infections in addition to gastroenteritis worldwide [9–12]. The virus exists in four different serotypes HBoV1-4 [1–2,13–14]. Although HBoV 1 and 2 were reported in respiratory samples, all the 4 genotypes of HBoV have been identified in children with acute gastroenteritis.

HBoV has been reported in various countries, indicating its worldwide endemic nature. The virus has been identified in Europe [15–17], America [18–19], Asia [9,20], Australia [21–22], Africa [23], and the Middle East [24]. The prevalence of HBoV ranges between 1.5 to 19.3% [18,25]. Primary infection with HBoV seems to occur early in life and children between the ages of 6–24 months seem to be mostly affected [9–10], but older children can also be infected. Newborn children may become protected by maternally derived antibodies [9]. HBoV infections are rarely found in adults [26–27]. Lindner et al. detected anti-HBoV antibodies in 94% of healthy blood donors >19 years of age [28].

HBoV detection has been mostly performed on nasopharyngeal aspirates and swabs and relies mostly on classical [10,18,19,21,22,26] and real-time PCR [10,23,29]. Real-time PCR possesses many advantages over conventional PCR, as it offers greater sensitivity, specificity, and reduced expenditure of time.

The current study aims to screen the epidemiological status and molecular phylogeny of HBoV isolates prevailing in pediatric patients with respiratory infection in Saudi Arabia.

Results and Discussion

The current study investigated the prevalence of HBoV in patients suffering from respiratory tract infections in Saudi Arabia. The presence of the major viral causes of the respiratory distress in HBoV positive cases was also screened. HBoV was detected in 18/80 of the examined patients (22.5%) with ages ranging from 2 months to 10 years, (Table 1–2). Clinical findings for HBoV-positive patients were indistinguishable from those for patients with other respiratory viruses. Previously, HBoV has been detected in samples from patients aged between 5 months and 2 years [1,29]. Ma et al, speculated that the antibody against HBoV derived from the mother might protect children under 5 months of age from HBoV infection [9], however, we detected HBoV in two cases below 5 months: in a 2-month-old and 4-month-old child (Table 1–2) that may indicate the possibility of HBoV infection in very young children.

The rate of HBoV in respiratory tract infections has been reported to be 1.5 to 19.3% [18,25]. Real-time PCR was used in the current study to screen HBoV due to its high diagnostic sensitivity that could be responsible for the higher rate of HBoV infection in Saudi Arabia than the widely accepted upper limit of infection rates worldwide. Meanwhile, a recent study showed 21.5% prevalence among children [30].

Table 1. Demographic and clinical data of children suffered from respiratory distress in the current study.

Variable	Value [N = 80]	HBoV infected [N = 18]
Age	2 mo- 10 yr	
0–4 Mo	11	2
5–8 Mo	6	1
9–12 Mo	1	1
1–2 yr	27	8
>2–3 yr	8	4
>3–4 yr	4	0
>4–5 yr	6	1
>5–7 yr	4	0
>7–10 yr	4	1
Sex		
Male	39	8
Female	41	10
Clinical symptoms		
Fever	80	18
Nasal discharge	80	18
Watery	70	16
Purulent	10	2
Asthma	16	2
LRTI[a]	41	15
URTI[b]	39	3
Diarrhea	20	3
Nervous manifestations	2	0
Rash	6	0

[a]Lower respiratory tract infection.
[b]Upper respiratory tract infection.

Table 2. Common respiratory viruses among HBoV infected children.

Sample No	Age	Sex	RSV	PIV-1	PIV-3	IAV	Adenovirus
1	2 Mo	Female	+	−	−	−	−
2	10 Mo	Male	−	−	−	−	−
3	8 Mo	Male	−	−	−	+	−
4	18 Mo	Male	+	−	−	+	−
5	19 Mo	Male	+	−	−	−	−
6	36 Mo	Female	+	−	+	+	−
7	12 Mo	Female	+	−	−	+	+
8	36 Mo	Male	+	−	−	−	−
9	17 Mo	Female	+	−	−	+	+
10	13 Mo	Female	+	−	−	+	+
11	5 yr	Female	+	−	−	+	+
12	4 Mo	Female	+	−	−	+	+
13	20 Mo	Male	+	−	−	+	−
14	20 Mo	Male	−	−	−	+	−
15	24 Mo	Female	−	−	−	+	+
16	10 yr	Female	−	−	−	+	−
17	30 Mo	Female	+	−	−	−	−
18	32 Mo	Male	+	−	−	−	−

The evidence of HBoV as the main initiator of the disease in the infected cases is still uncertain because of its high co-infection rate with other pathogens, and it remains unclear whether HBoV is the sole etiologic agent or just a concomitant virus bystander. In previous studies, none of the nasal swabs obtained from healthy children yielded a positive HBoV test. This suggests that HBoV is not a frequent commensal virus inhabiting the respiratory tract [16,19]. HBoV infections are frequently present in concomitant with other viruses and often occur in more than 50% of the tested samples [31]. In the current study, only one case was found to be infected only by HBoV as a single virus entity while most of isolates (17/18) showed coinfection with other viral pathogens. The most frequently detected co-pathogens were RSV (13/18; 72.2%), IAV (12/18 cases, 66.66%), respiratory adenovirus (6/18 cases, 33.33%) while only 1/18 (5.5%) case was coinfected with PIV-3 and none was coninfected with PIV-1 (Table 2). It is assumed that the rate and frequency of coinfections may be higher if more viruses were screened. Consistent with other studies [1,16], the prevalence rate of bocavirus was higher in children under 2 years of age (Table 1).

Partial NP-1 gene sequence of the eighteen detected HBoV strains were obtained in our study. Multisequence analysis showed complete identity (100%) between each other, and phylogenetic analysis demonstrated that they belonged to HBoV1 (data not shown). Blast analysis revealed complete homology to the published sequence of HBoV1. Furthermore, the phylogenetic analysis results of three selected sequences showed that the Saudi HBoV1 strains obtained from respiratory samples belonged to group I human bocaviruses (Fig. 1).

To the best of our knowledge, this is the first report of HBoV1 in Saudi Arabia. Continuous surveillance and genome sequence analysis are needed to obtain more information on the genotypic variation and molecular evolution of HBoV in the country.

Materials and Methods

Ethics Statement

The study protocol was approved by the medical ethics review board of the College of Medicine, Taif University and by the pediatric hospital ethics committee in accordance with the guidelines for the protection of human subjects. Informed written consents from the next of kin of the participants involved in the study were taken.

Sample Collection and Processing

Nasopharyngeal swabs from 80 children suffered from moderate to severe lower respiratory tract infections were collected from January to May 2012 from the Governmental Pediatric Hospital-Al-Taif, Saudi Arabia. The children's age ranged from two months to ten years of age. Clinical manifestations and case histories were recorded. Individual swabs were kept in 1 ml sterile saline containing gentamycin sulphate. Swabs were routinely processed and kept at −80°C until further analysis.

Nucleic Acid Extraction

Viral nucleic acid was extracted from 200 μl of individual samples using DNA/RNA extraction Kit (Koma Bioteck Inc., Seoul, Korea), according to the manufacturer's instructions.

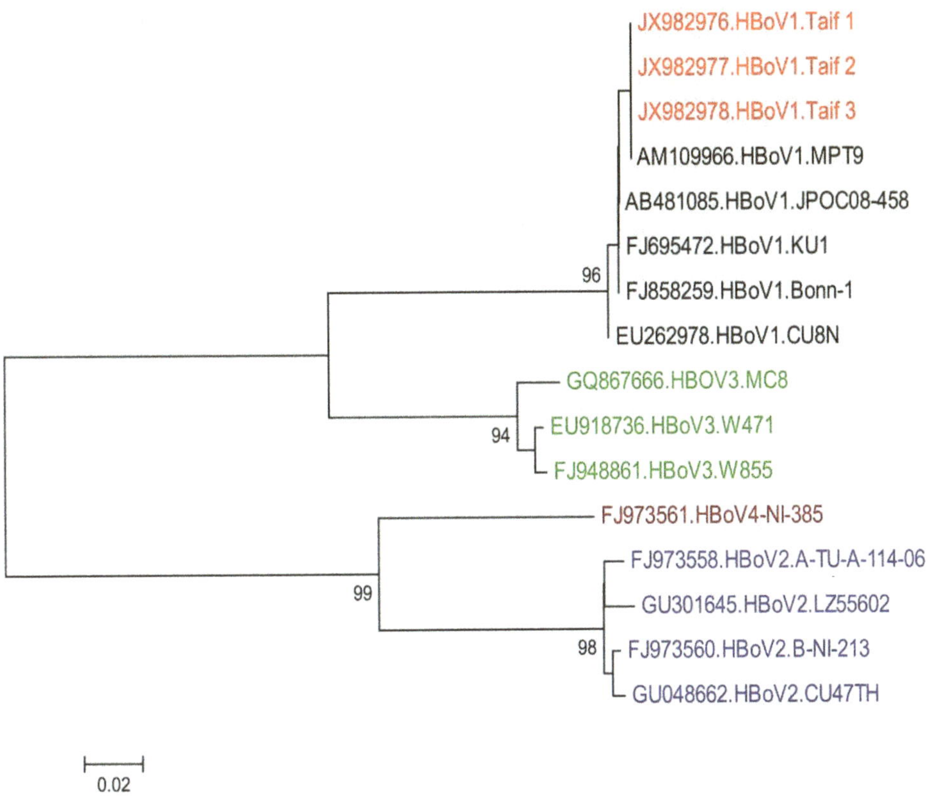

Figure 1. Phylogenetic analysis of Saudi HBoV1 isolates. The phylogenetic tree with 1,000 bootstrap replicates was generated using the Clustal W program in the MEGA 4.0 software package and based on partial NP-1 sequences of the HBoV strains. Samples obtained in the current study from children with acute respiratory distress in Saudi Arabia are in red. HBoV1 strains are presented in black, HBoV 2 strains are presented in blue, HBoV3 strains are presented in green while HBoV4 isolate is presented in brown.

Real Time Polymerase Chain Reaction (RT PCR)

The real-time PCR assay was performed using commercial, TaqMan hydrolysis probe based, real time PCR bocavirus detection Kit (Liferiver, Shanghai, China) in Eppendorf Mastercycler® ep realplex^2. The detection of the amplified amplicon was performed in fluorimeter channel FAM with the fluorescent quencher BHQ1. Amplification reactions were performed in a volume of 25 µl containing 2.5 µl of DNA template, 21.5 µl reaction mix, 0.4 µl enzyme mix, 1 µl internal control according to the manufacturer's instructions. The thermal cycling conditions were as follows: 2 min at 37°C, an initial denaturation of 2 min at 94°C and 40-cycles of 15 sec at 93°C and annealing/elongation step of 1 min at 60°C. HBoV positive samples were screened for the presence of respiratory syncytial virus (RSV), influenza A virus (IAV), parinfluenza virus 1(PIV-1) and parainfluenza virus 3(PIV-3), as well as respiratory enteric virus (AdenV) using real-time PCR Kits (Shanghai ZJ Bio-tech Co., Ltd).

HBoV Genotyping

PCR amplification of a 354–base pair fragment of the NP1 was performed as described previously [1]. The reaction mix contained 20 pmol of each primer and DNA master mix (Koma Bioteck, Inc., Seoul, Korea). The thermal cycling conditions were as follows: an initial denaturation of 5 min at 94°*C*, 35 cycles of 1 min at 94°C, 1 min at 54°C and 2 min at 72°C, final extension of 10 min at 72°C.Positive PCR products were purified using a QIAquick PCR purification kit (Qiagen) and were sequenced commercially (Macrogen Inc., Seoul, Korea).

Sequence Analysis

The nucleotide sequences of the NS1 gene were compared with those of HBoV strains available at the GenBank site. Phylogenetic analyses were conducted with MEGA, version 4.1. The 3/18 partial sequences of the NS1 gene were submitted to GenBank (accession numbers JX982976–JX982978).

Author Contributions

Conceived and designed the experiments: ASA. Performed the experiments: ASA MMK ASAG MIRA. Analyzed the data: ASA MMK. Contributed reagents/materials/analysis tools: ASA MMK ASAG MIRA. Wrote the paper: ASA.

References

1. Allander T, Tammi MT, Eriksson M, Bjerkner A, Tiveljung-Lindell A, et al. (2005) Cloning of a human parvovirus by molecular screening of respiratory tract samples. Proc Natl Acad Sci USA 102: 12891–12896.
2. Kapoor A, Simmonds P, Slikas E, Li L, Bodhidatta Let al. (2010) Human bocaviruses are highly diverse, dispersed, recombination prone, and prevalent in enteric infections. J Infect Dis 201: 1633–1643.
3. Claude M, Fauquet MAM, Maniloff J, Desselberger U, Ball LA (2004) Virus Taxonomy: The Eighth Report of the International Committee on Taxonomy of Viruses. Academic Press.
4. Cheng WX, Li JS, Huang CP, Yao DP, Liu N, et al. (2010) Identification and nearly full-length genome characterization of novel porcine bocaviruses. PLoS One 5: e13583.

5. Kapoor A, Mehta N, Esper F, Poljsak-Prijatelj M, Quan PL, et al. (2010) Identification and characterization of a new bocavirus species in gorillas. PLoS One 5: e11948.
6. Sharp CP, LeBreton M, Kantola K, Nana A, Diffo Jle D, et al. (2010) Widespread infection with homologues of human parvoviruses B19, PARV4, and human bocavirus of chimpanzees and gorillas in the wild. J Virol 84: 10289–10296.
7. Li L, Shan T, Wang C, Côté C, Kolman J, et al. (2011) The fecal viral flora of California sea lions. J Virol 85(19): 9909–9917.
8. Lau SK, Woo PC, Yeung HC, Teng JL, Wu Y, et al. (2012) Identification and characterization of bocaviruses in cats and dogs reveals a novel feline bocavirus and a novel genetic group of canine bocavirus. J Gen Virol 93: 1573–1582.
9. Ma X, Endo R, Ishiguro N, Ebihara T, Ishiko H, et al. (2006) Detection of human bocavirus in Japanese children with lower respiratory tract infections. J Clin Microbiol 44: 1132–1134.
10. Manning A, Russell V, Eastick K, Leadbetter GH, Hallam N, et al. (2006) Epidemiological profile and clinical associations of human bocavirus and other human parvoviruses. J Infect Dis 194: 1283–1290.
11. Vicente D, Cilla G, Montes M, Perez-Yarza EG, Perez-Trallero E (2007) Human bocavirus, a respiratory and enteric virus. Emerg Infect Dis 13: 636–637.
12. Cheng WX, Jin Y, Duan ZJ, Xu ZQ, Qi HM, et al. (2008) Human bocavirus in children hospitalized for acute gastroenteritis: a case-control study. Clin Infect Dis 47(2): 161–167.
13. Arthur JL, Higgins GD, Davidson GP, Givney RC, Ratcliff RM (2009) A novel bocavirus associated with acute gastroenteritis in Australian children. PLoS Pathog 2009, 5: e1000391.
14. Kapoor A, Slikas E, Simmonds P, Chieochansin T, Naeem A, et al. (2009) A newly identified bocavirus species in human stool. J Infect Dis 199: 196–200.
15. Foulongne V, Olejnik Y, Perez V, Elaerts S, Rodiere M, et al. (2006) Human bocavirus in French children. Emerg Infect Dis 12: 1251–1253.
16. Maggi F, Andreoli E, Pifferi M, Meschi S, Rocchi J, et al. (2007) Human bocavirus in Italian patients with respiratory diseases. J Clin Virol 38: 321–325.
17. Regamey N, Frey U, Deffernez C, Latzin P, Kaiser L (2007) Isolation of human bocavirus from Swiss infants with respiratory infections. Pediatr Infect Dis J 26: 177–179.
18. Bastien N, Brandt K, Dust K, Ward D, Li Y (2006) Human Bocavirus infection, Canada. Emerg Infect Dis 12: 848–850.
19. Kesebir D, Vazquez M, Weibel C, Shapiro ED, Ferguson D, et al. (2006) Human bocavirus infection in young children in the United States: molecular epidemiological profile and clinical characteristics of a newly emerging respiratory virus. J Infect Dis 194: 1276–1282.
20. Lin F, Zeng A, Yang N, Lin H, Yang E, et al. (2007) Quantification of human bocavirus in lower respiratory tract infections in China. Infect Agent Cancer 2: 3.
21. Arden KE, McErlean P, Nissen MD, Sloots TP, Mackay IM (2006) Frequent detection of human rhinoviruses, paramyxoviruses, coronaviruses, and bocavirus during acute respiratory tract infections. J Med Virol 78: 1232–1240.
22. Sloots TP, McErlean P, Speicher DJ, Arden KE, Nissen MD, et al. (2006) Evidence of human coronavirus HKU1 and human bocavirus in Australian children. J Clin Virol 35: 99–102.
23. Smuts H, Hardie D (2006) Human bocavirus in hospitalized children, South Africa. Emerg Infect Dis 12: 1457–1458.
24. Kaplan NM, Dove W, Abu-Zeid AF, Shamoon HE, Abd-Eldayem SA, et al. (2006) Human bocavirus infection among children, Jordan. Emerg Infect Dis 12: 1418–1420.
25. Bonzel L, Tenenbaum T, Schroten H, Schildgen O, Schweitzer-Krantz S, et al. (2008) Frequent detection of viral coinfection in children hospitalized with acute respiratory tract infection using a real-time polymerase chain reaction. Pediatr Infect Dis J 27: 589–594.
26. Kupfer B, Vehreschild J, Cornely O, Kaiser R, Plum G, et al. (2006) Severe pneumonia and human bocavirus in adult. Emerg Infect Dis 12: 1614–1616.
27. Xu L, He X, Zhang DM, Feng FS, Wang Z, et al. (2012) Surveillance and genome analysis of human bocavirus in patients with respiratory infection in guangzhou, china. PLoS One 7(9): e44876.
28. Lindner J, Karalar L, Zehentmeier S, Plentz A, Pfister H, et al. (2008) Humoral immune response against human bocavirus VP2 virus-like particles. Viral Immunol 21: 443–449.
29. Allander T, Jartti T, Gupta S, Niesters HG, Lehtinen P, et al. (2007) Human bocavirus and acute wheezing in children. Clin Infect Dis 44: 904–910.
30. Ghietto LM, Cámara A, Zhou Y, Pedranti M, Ferreyra S, et al. (2012) High prevalence of human bocavirus 1 in infants with lower acute respiratory tract disease in Argentina, 2007–2009. Braz J Infect Dis 16(1): 38–44.
31. Christensen A, Nordbø SA, Krokstad S, Rognlien AG, Døllner H (2008) Human bocavirus commonly involved in multiple viral airway infections. J Clin Virol 41: 34–37.

21

Epstein Barr Virus and *Helicobacter pylori* Co-Infection are Positively Associated with Severe Gastritis in Pediatric Patients

María G. Cárdenas-Mondragón, Ricardo Carreón-Talavera, Margarita Camorlinga-Ponce, Alejandro Gomez-Delgado, Javier Torres, Ezequiel M. Fuentes-Pananá*

Unidad de Investigación Médica en Enfermedades Infecciosas y Parasitarias (UIMEIP), Hospital de Pediatría, CMN Siglo-XXI, Instituto Mexicano del Seguro Social (IMSS), Mexico City, Mexico

Abstract

Background: *H. pylori* infection is acquired during childhood and causes a chronic inflammatory response in the gastric mucosa, which is considered the main risk factor to acquire gastric cancer (GC) later in life. More recently, infection by Epstein-Barr virus (EBV) have also been associated with GC. The role of EBV in early inflammatory responses and its relationship with *H. pylori* infection remains poorly studied. Here, we assessed whether EBV infection in children correlated with the stage of gastritis and whether co-infection with *H. pylori* affected the severity of inflammation.

Methodology/Principal Findings: 333 pediatric patients with chronic abdominal pain were studied. From them, gastric biopsies were taken and inflammation graded according to the Sydney system; peripheral blood was drawn and antibodies against EBV (IgG and IgM anti-VCA) and *H. pylori* (IgG anti-whole bacteria and anti-CagA) were measured in sera. We found that children infected only by EBV presented mild mononuclear (MN) and none polymorphonuclear (PMN) cell infiltration, while those infected by *H. pylori* presented moderate MN and mild PMN. In contrast, patients co-infected with both pathogens were significantly associated with severe gastritis. Importantly, co-infection of *H. pylori* CagA+/EBV+ had a stronger association with severe MN (PR 3.0) and PMN (PR 7.2) cells than cases with single *H. pylori* CagA+ infection.

Conclusions/Significance: Co-infection with EBV and *H. pylori* in pediatric patients is associated with severe gastritis. Even single infections with *H. pylori* CagA+ strains are associated with mild to moderate infiltration arguing for a cooperative effect of *H. pylori* and EBV in the gastric mucosa and revealing a critical role for EBV previously un-appreciated. This study points out the need to study both pathogens to understand the mechanism behind severe damage of the gastric mucosa, which could identified children with increased risk to present more serious lesions later in life.

Editor: Yoshio Yamaoka, Veterans Affairs Medical Center (111D), United States of America

Funding: This study was partially supported by grant FIS/IMSS/PROT/G2011/941 (to M.G. Cárdenas-Mondragón) from the Fondo de Investigación en Salud (FIS)-IMSS, and grants 178199 (to MGC-M) and 69450 (to J. Torres) from CONACYT. The funders had no role in study design, data collection and analysis, decision to publish, or preparation of the manuscript.

Competing Interests: The authors have declared that no competing interests exist.

* E-mail: empanana@yahoo.com

Introduction

Persistent infections often lead to chronic inflammation, a well documented cancer risk factor. Gastric cancer (GC) generally starts with an inflammatory process mainly associated with infection by *Helicobacter pylori* (*H. pylori*) [1]. GC is the fourth most common type of cancer and the second cause of death by cancer world-wide, affecting particularly Asian and Latin American countries [2]. More recently, GC has also been associated with Epstein-Barr virus (EBV) but the role of the viral infection in early inflammatory gastric responses remains poorly studied.

H. pylori infects over 50% of the world population, with a higher prevalence in developing countries. Infection is usually acquired early in life; in Mexico, about 50% of children are infected by the age of 10 [3]. Inflammation after infection in children is usually associated with a low level of polymorphonuclear (PMN) and mononuclear (MN) cells infiltrating the gastric mucosa [4]. It has been suggested than the earlier the infection, the greater the risk to present GC later in life, conceivable because of a long lasting (decades) chronic inflammatory reaction to the infection [5].

Only a fraction of *H. pylori* infected individuals develop gastroduodenal disease: <15% peptic ulcer, <3% GC and <1% MALT lymphoma [6]. The outcome of *H. pylori* infection depends also on environmental, host and bacterial factors. Among the most important bacterial virulence factors is the pathogenicity island (CagPAI), which encodes a type IV secretion system (T4SS) that translocates the effector protein CagA into epithelial cells [7]. CagA activates multiple signaling pathways triggering cellular phenotypes associated with oncogenic transformation [7]. Moreover, transgenic mice expressing CagA develop adenocarcinomas of the digestive tract. Based on these data, CagA has been recognized as the first known bacterial oncoprotein [8,9].

Table 1. Characteristics of the333 children studied.

Variable	Value
Age (mean±SD) Median	10.1±3.8 10
Sex, male/female (ratio)	136/197 (0.69)
EBV positive, n (%)	214 (64.3)
H. pylori positive, n (%)	178 (53.4)
H. pylori CagA+	112 (33.6)
Gastric mucosa cell infiltration	
MN infiltration (Inflammation):	
Mild, n (%)	260 (78)
Moderate, n (%)	48 (14.4)
Severe, n (%)	25 (7.5)
PMN infiltration (Activity):	
None, n (%)	250 (75.1)
Mild, n (%)	52 (15.6)
Moderate, n (%)	16 (4.8)
Severe, n (%)	15 (4.5)

EBV infection has been consistently associated with several types of lymphoma, nasopharyngeal carcinoma (NPC) [10,11] and more recently to GC [12,13,14]. EBV infection also occurs early in childhood and usually persists in B cells, with most infected individuals carrying the virus asymptomatically in a latent stage in these cells. It is not clear when EBV infects the gastric mucosa and whether infection induces an inflammatory reaction, as observed with *H. pylori*. EBV reactivation from infected B cells has been proposed to facilitate infection of the epithelial basolateral face [15]. In that scenario, the titer of anti-EBV antibodies against structural proteins has been proposed to correlate with the level of viral reactivation and as a prognostic marker in NPC [10,16,17].

To our knowledge, no studies have previously addressed whether EBV infection in children is associated with inflammation in the gastric mucosa or whether there exists a cooperative effect between EBV and *H. pylori* correlating with the severity of the inflammatory reaction. In this study, we analyzed antibodies against EBV and *H. pylori* in sera of pediatric patients with chronic abdominal pain. Our results strongly suggest that single infection by either EBV or *H. pylori* is associated with a mild to moderate inflammatory response in the gastric mucosa; however, co-infection with both pathogens is significantly associated with severe gastritis. Even infection with *H. pylori* cagA+ strains is not associated with severe inflammatory responses in the absence of EBV. These data argue for a previously unknown critical role of EBV infection in the induction of an inflammatory response in the gastric mucosa of children.

Materials and Methods

Ethics Statement

The IMSS National Research Ethics Committee approved this project. Parents or guardians of the patients were informed on the nature of the study and those willing to participate signed a written informed consent prior to specimen collection.

Overview

Study population. The study included 333 pediatric patients (0–17 years old) attended because of recurring abdominal pain at the Gastroenterology unit, Pediatric Hospital of the Centro Medico Nacional SXXI, Instituto Mexicano del Seguro Social (IMSS), in Mexico City, between September 1994 and October 2001. Children were subjected to endoscopy and gastric biopsies were taken from antrum and corpus for histopathological diagnosis. Peripheral blood was also drawn and sera were stored at $-80^{\circ}C$ until tested for antibodies.

Data collected. Socio-demographic data and clinical information was registered in questionnaires at time of inclusion. The information collected included age, gender, clinical symptoms and clinical diagnosis based on endoscopy, histology and clinical presentation. Patients with antibiotic, proton pump inhibitor or antiacid treatments three weeks previous to sample collection were excluded from the study.

Laboratory Methods

Histopathological examination. Two biopsy specimens were obtained from de antrum and two from the gastric corpus. One biopsy was used for *H. pylori* culture and the second was used for histologic examination. One biopsy from the antrum and one from the corpus were fixed in formaline, paraffin-embedded and stained with hematoxylin and eosin (HE). The inflammatory response was graded according to the Sydney system [18] by a single experienced pathologist. The parameters evaluated were *H. pylori* positivity, polymorphonuclear and mononuclear cell infiltration, which were graded comparing with published diagrams (analogue scales). Infiltration by polymorphonuclear and mononuclear cells was graded from absent to severe in both corpus and antrum, and the site with the higher infiltration was considered as the end result.

Collection of blood. A sample of venous blood (4 ml) was drawn from all patients. Stored serum samples were used to analyze IgG and IgM antibodies against EBV viral capsid protein (VCA), as well as IgG antibodies against *H. pylori* whole-cell extracts and against CagA protein by enzyme-linked immunosorbent assay (ELISA).

Table 2. Degree of infiltration of MN and PMN cells in the gastric mucosa of children according to infection with EBV and *H. pylori*.

Groups	Total	MN infiltration, n (%)			PMN infiltration, n (%)		
		Mild	Moderate	Severe	None	Mild	Moderate-severe
EBV positive	214	162 (75.7)	31 (14.5)	21 (9.8)	157 (73.4)	29 (13.6)	28 (13.1)
H. pylori positive	178	110 (61.8)	43 (24.1)	25 (14.0)	105 (58.9)	43 (24.1)	30 (16.9)
H. pylori CagA positive	112	54 (48.2)	37 (33)	21 (18.8)	55 (49.1)	30 (26.8)	27 (24.1)
EBV & *H. pylori* neg	66	63 (95.5)	3 (4.5)	0	61 (92.4)	5 (7.6)	0

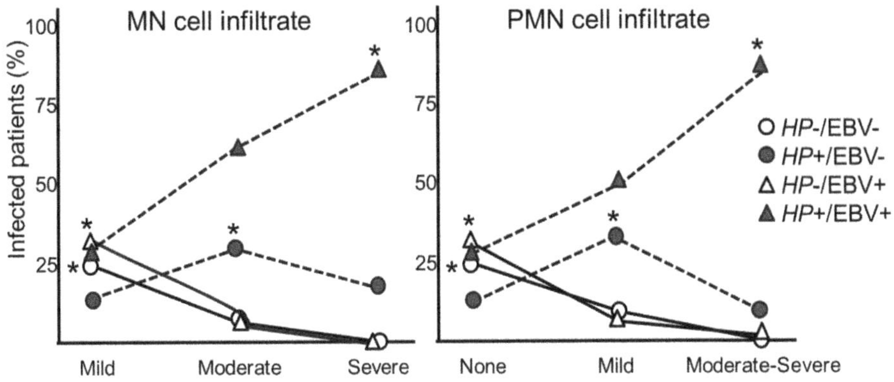

Figure 1. *H. pylory* and EBV infection frequencies in pediatric patients with gastritis according to the different grades of mononuclear (inflammation) and polymorphonuclear (activity) cell infiltration. Asterisks denote associations with statistical significance: *HP*−/EBV− and *HP*−/EBV+ groups with mild MN and no PMN (open circle and triangle), *HP*+/EBV− (grey circle) with moderate MN and mild PMN, and *HP*+/EBV+ (grey triangle) with severe MN and moderate-severe PMN.

Determination of Anti-EBV VCA antibodies. Anti-EBV VCA antibodies were determined using ELISA commercial kits (HUMAN; Wiesbaden, Germany), for IgG anti-VCA (catalog 51204) and for IgM anti-VCA (catalog 51104) following manufacturer instructions. Briefly, 100 µl of the appropriate patient-serum dilution (1:100 for IgM and 1:20 for IgG) were deposited on the corresponding well with the VCA antigen already attached, and incubated for 1 hour (IgG) or 30 min (IgM) at 25°C. Next, the wells were washed four times with washing buffer, and 100 µl of peroxidase-conjugated anti-human IgG or IgM rabbit antibody were added and incubated for 30 min at 25°C. Plates were then washed five times and 100 µl of substrate reagent (3,3′,5,5′ tetramethylbenzidin (TMB) – hydrogen peroxide) were added and incubated for 15 min a 25°C in the dark. The reaction was then stopped with 100 µl of stop solution (sulphuric acid 0.5 mol/L) and the plates were read in an ELISA reader (Thermoscientific, multiskan ascent) to an absorbance of 450 nm. The reported value is the average of two independent assays. A subgroup of samples was done in quadruplicate using different lots of the ELISA kit to check for reproducibility. Calculations for antibody titers were done according to the manufacturer's instructions and the values are reported as HU units/ml. A patient was considered EBV seropositive when sera tested positive for either IgG and/or IgM antibodies.

Determination of antibodies anti-whole *H. pylori* extracts and anti-CagA. IgG antibodies against *H. pylori* and CagA were determined using ELISA tests previously validated in a Mexican population [19]. Wells were coated either with a sonicated extract of a mixture of three *H. pylori* strains isolated from Mexican patients (0.5 µg/well in 100 µl of carbonate buffer pH 9.6) or with recombinant CagA (0.1 µg/well in same buffer as above) and incubated at 4° overnight. Next, the plates were blocked with 200 µl of PBS-gelatin (0.1%) for *H. pylori* whole-extract and with PBS-milk (2.5%) for CagA and incubated at 4° overnight. The sera were diluted 1:1000 for *H. pylori* and 1:200 for CagA and 100 µl were added per well and incubated for one hour at 37°C. One hundred µl of a 1:1000 dilution of the anti-human IgG antibody-conjugated to alkaline phosphatase were added and plates were incubated for 30 min at room temperature, followed by 100 µl of p-nitrophenylphosphate substrate (Sigma; St. Louis MO USA. No. 2770) in glycine-MgCl2-ZnCl buffer. Plates were read in an ELISA reader at an absorbance of 405 nm. All samples were analyzed in duplicate and each plate included four positive and four negative sera samples. Patients were considered positive

Table 3. Degree of infiltration of mononuclear (MN) and polymorphonuclear (PMN) cells in the gastric mucosa of children according to co-infection with EBV and *H. pylori* (*HP*).

		MN infiltration, n (%)			PMN infiltration, n (%)		
Groups	**Total**	**Mild**	**Moderate**	**Severe**	**None**	**Mild**	**Moderate-severe**
H. pylori and EBV groups	333	260	48	25	250	52	31
HP−/EBV−	66 (19.8)	63 (24.2)	3 (6.3)	0	61 (24.4)	5 (9.6)	0
HP+/EBV−	53 (15.9)	35 (13.5)	14 (29.2)	4 (16)	32 (12.8)	18 (34.6)	3 (9.7)
HP−/EBV+	89 (26.7)	87 (33.5)	2 (4.2)	0	84 (33.6)	4 (7.7)	1 (3.2)
HP+/EBV+	125 (37.5)	75 (28.8)	29 (60.4)	21 (84)	73 (29.2)	25 (48.1)	27 (87.1)
CagA and EBV groups	178	110	43	25	105	43	30
HP CagA−/EBV−	19 (10.7)	16 (14.5)	2 (4.7)	1 (4)	13 (34.2)	5 (11.6)	1 (3.3)
HP CagA+/EBV−	34 (19.1)	19 (17.3)	12 (27.9)	3 (12)	19 (18.1)	13 (30.2)	2 (6.7)
HP CagA−/EBV+	47 (26.4)	40 (36.4)	4 (9.3)	3 (12)	37 (35.2)	8 (18.6)	2 (6.7)
HP CagA+/EBV+	78 (43.8)	35 (31.8)	25 (58.1)	18 (72)	36 (34.2)	17 (39.5)	25 (83.3)

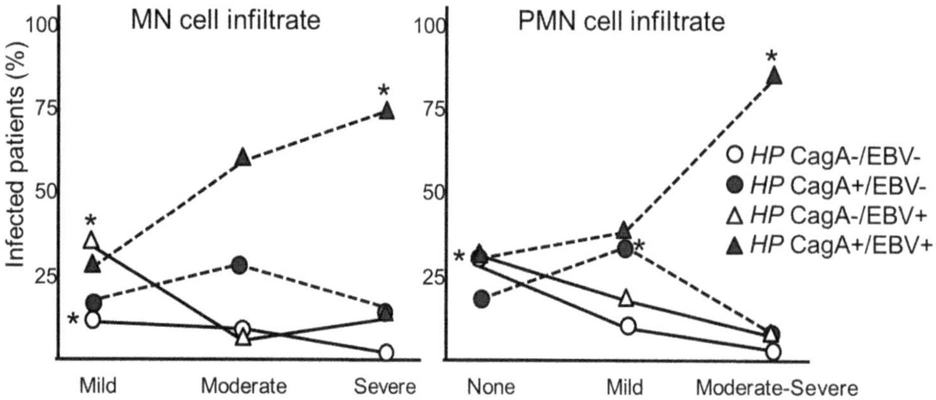

Figure 2. Infection frequencies and gastritis severity related to the presence of CagA. Asterisks denote associations with statistical significance: *HP* CagA−/EBV− and *HP* CagA−/EBV+ groups with mild MN and no PMN (open circle and triangle), *HP* CagA+/EBV− (grey circle) with mild PMN, and *HP* CagA+/EBV+ (grey triangle) with severe MN and moderate-severe PMN.

for *H. pylori* antibodies when ELISA units were ≥1.0, and for CagA when ELISA units were ≥1.5, according to the validated cut-offs [19].

Statistical Analysis

The statistical differences of continuous variables between patient's groups were determined with the Student's *t* test or with the Mann-Whitney U test for non-normally distributed variables. Differences among three or more continuous variables were compared by one-way ANOVA, followed by Bonferroni test, or by the Kruskal-Wallis one-way test, followed by the Mann-Whitney U test. The differences between categorical variables were estimated using the Chi square (X^2) test with Yate's continuity correction or the Fisher's exact test for small samples. Variables with more than two categories were analyzed using Mantel-Haenszel X^2 with linear tendency. Statistical significance was set at $p \leq 0.05$. The strength of associations between the inflammation grade's groups and IgG anti-VCA were estimated using prevalence ratios (PRs) and 95% confidence intervals (CIs).

Table 4. Age adjusted PR values for severe MN and moderate-severe PMN infiltration when compared between co-infected children against without infection or with single *H. pylori* infection.

Groups	No./total	PR (95% CI)	p
H. pylori and EBV MN, severe			
HP+/EBV+ vs HP−/EBV−	21/125 *vs* 0/66	Undefined	0.0004
HP+/EBV+ vs HP+/EBV−	21/125 *vs* 4/53	2.23 (0.7–5.8)	0.15
PMN, moderate-severe			
HP+/EBV+ vs HP−/EBV−	27/125 *vs* 0/66	Undefined	0.00004
HP+/EBV+ vs HP+/EBV−	27/125 *vs* 3/53	4.1 (1.2–23.5)	0.01
CagA and EBV MN, severe			
CagA+/EBV+ *vs HP* CagA−/EBV−	18/78 *vs* 1/19	5.4 (0.7–43.3)[a]	0.08
CagA+/EBV+ *vs HP* CagA+/EBV−	18/78 *vs* 3/34	3.0 (0.8-11.1)	0.08
PMN, moderate-severe			
CagA+/EBV+ *vs HP* CagA−/EBV−	25/78 *vs* 1/19	8.5 (1.1–67.2)[a]	0.01
CagA+/EBV+ *vs HP* CagA+/EBV−	25/78 *vs* 2/34	7.2 (1.6–31.7)	0.003

[a]This estimation could not be adjusted by age because there are 0 cases of severe MN or moderate-severe PMN infiltration in the ≤10 years of age group.

Results

Characteristics of the patients studied

333 gastric samples from pediatric patients with chronic abdominal pain were studied, 197 (59.2%) were female and 136 (40.8%) male with an average and median age of 10.1±3.7 (mean ± SD) and 10 years, respectively (***Table 1***). All patients were diagnosed with non atrophic gastritis (NAG) through histological examination; the morphology of the epithelial cells was not atypical and no glandular atrophy was found. The frequency of infection by EBV was 64.3% and by *H. pylori* 53.4%, whereas 33.9% presented antibodies against CagA. In most children the gastric mucosa presented with a mild infiltration of MN (78%) and no infiltration of PMN (75%); only 7.5% presented a severe infiltration of MN and 4.5% of PMN cells (***Table 1***). Because of the low number of samples with severe activity, samples with a diagnostic of moderate and severe gastritis were combined for the rest of the analysis. The seroprevalence to *H. pylori* and EBV in the studied children according to age is described in ***Table S1***.

Degree of inflammation and infection with either EBV or *H. pylori*

We identified 214 children with EBV infection [179 were IgG and 35 were IgM positive (7 only IgM and 28 IgM and IgG)], 9.8% of these cases showed a severe MN infiltration, and 13.1% a moderate-severe PMN infiltration (***Table 2***). All of the 35 children (28+7) positive for IgM were considered in primary infection and presented mild inflammation and none activity. On the other hand, 178 children were infected with *H. pylori* and of those 14% showed severe MN infiltration and 16.9% moderate-severe PMN infiltration. Among the 112 children infected with *H. pylori cagA*+ strains 18.8% had severe MN infiltration and 24.1% moderate-severe PMN infiltration. Whereas, none of the 66 children without infection presented severe MN nor PMN infiltration.

Significantly higher titers of anti-EBV antibodies were found only in mild PMN infiltration, suggesting that higher anti-EBV antibody titers are not indicative of more severe inflammation in pediatric gastritis (***Table S2***). On the other hand, a positive correlation of *H. pylori* antibody titers and the gastritis severity was observed as it has been previously reported [20,21].

Degree of inflammation related to the interaction between infection with EBV and *H. pylori*

We next addressed whether there was any interaction between infection with both *H. pylori* and EBV, and this analysis is presented in ***Table 3*** (see also **Figure 1**). We found that most of the children with no infection (*HP*−/EBV−) and children with only EBV infection (*HP*−/EBV+) had a mild MN infiltration and no PMN in the gastric mucosa. Cases with moderate MN and mild PMN cells were more frequent in patients with only *H. pylori* infection (*HP*+/EBV−) and with both *H. pylori* and EBV infection (*HP*+/EBV+). In contrast, over 80% of the cases with severe MN and moderate-severe PMN infiltration occurred in patients with co-infection (*HP*+/EBV+).

Positive interactions between *H. pylori* CagA and EBV according to the degree of inflammation were also analyzed and a similar result was observed (***Table 3***), only *H. pylori* CagA+/EBV+ double positive patients were significantly associated with severe inflammation for both MN and PMN infiltrate (**Figure 2**). These results argue that *H. pylori* infection alone is not sufficient to develop severe gastritis.

To further confirm the combined effect of mixed EBV and *H. pylori* infection, we determined the significance of the association of co-infection with the cases showing a severe MN or moderate-severe PMN infiltration (***Table 4***). In this analysis, to assess whether the observed association of EBV and *H. pylori* infection with severe gastritis could be influenced by age, patients were divided into two groups of age according to the median: ≤ 10 (group 1) and >10 (group 2), and prevalence ratios (PR) were adjusted by these age groups. When patients with co-infection (*HP*+/EBV+) were compared against patients with no infection (*HP*−/EBV−) PR values for severe MN and PMN infiltration were undefined because none of the uninfected children (*HP*−/EBV−) had severe MN or PMN infiltration. When patients with co-infection (*HP*+/EBV+) were compared against patients with single *H. pylori* infection (*HP*+/EBV−) PR's for severe infiltration were 2.2 for MN and 4.1 for PMN; this latter with statistical significance ($p = 0.01$).

When cases with co-infection (CagA+/EBV+) were compared against cases of only *H. pylori* infection (*HP* CagA−/EBV−) PR's were 5.4 for MN and 8.5 for PMN. Similarly, when patients with co-infection (CagA+/EBV+) were compared against cases with single *H. pylori* CagA+ infection (CagA+/EBV−PR's were 3.0 for MN and 7.2 for PMN (***Table 4***). The level of PMN infiltration also showed statistical significance supporting that co-infection is necessary to develop severe gastritis in children, and thus pointing out for a critical role for EBV that cannot be provided even by the CagA virulence factor ($p = 0.003$).

Discussion

H. pylori infection is acquired early in life during childhood, and the presence of the bacteria induces an inflammatory reaction in the gastric mucosa which in most cases causes no disease. However, in some individuals the chronic long lasting inflammation triggers serious damage to the gastric epithelium increasing the risk to develop precancerous lesions, which in turn increase the risk to end up with a life threatening GC.

Some of the co-factors that promote a more severe inflammatory reaction may present early on during childhood. The inflammatory nature of GC denotes a critical role for an immunogenic agent and in accordance with this, GC is a cancer primarily of infectious etiology. While the association of *H. pylori* with GC and early inflammatory lesions is well documented, only a few studies have analyzed the participation of EBV infection in patients with gastritis, three of them in adults over 40 years old [22,23,24] and two case reports in young women of 18 [25] and 17 years old [26]. To our knowledge, the latter is the only case of EBV and gastritis reported to date in a pediatric patient in which high serum levels of anti-VCA antibodies (IgG and IgM) were found. Other studies have examined the presence of EBV sequences in gastritis samples. A recent report found EBV sequences by quantitative PCR in 15/50 and 5/6 of pediatric and adult gastritis, respectively [27]. Another recent study in adults found that about 90% (12/13) of chronic atrophic gastritis present EBV sequences [28]. Taken together these data support an important role for EBV in early inflammatory reactions of the gastric mucosa.

Studies in adults with NPC have found that disease progression correlates with increased antibodies against EBV reactivation antigens [10,16,17]. We hypothesized that a similar phenomenon may occur in GC and that the study of children with EBV infection may help identify patients with severe inflammation in the gastric mucosa, potentially at higher risk to develop precancerous lesions. Antibodies against proteins of the EBV lytic cycle could reflect higher levels of infection of the upper digestive tract epithelia and thus serve as a marker for the lesion progression. However, when we analyzed EBV infection in children, we did not observe the expected correlation with severe gastritis, and higher levels of anti-EBV antibodies either IgG or IgM, reflecting acute or chronic infections, were found preferentially in cases with mild gastritis. Thus, EBV single infection does not explain the cases of severe gastritis.

Until now, studies have been limited to *H. pylori* infection and have shown that in children it is usually associated with a mild to moderate inflammation (MN cell infiltration) and a mild to absent activity (PMN cell infiltration), although a severe inflammation and activity is observed in a few cases. When we analyzed co-infection with both *H. pylori* and EBV we found that children infected with both pathogens had the strongest association with severe gastritis, as measured by severe infiltration of MN (inflammation) and PMN cells (activity) in the gastric mucosa. In contrast, patients *HP*−/EBV+ preferentially presented mild inflammation (MN cell infiltration) and no activity (absence of PMN cells); while those *HP*+/EBV− presented moderate inflammation and mild activity. Our results suggest that co-infection with EBV and *H. pyori* is necessary to cause severe gastritis, supporting an important role for EBV, at least in pediatric patients. This increased effect was also true for patients infected with *H. pylori* CagA+ strains, already known to be associated with greater virulence and increased risk for GC. In our analyses, children co-infected with CagA+/EBV+ showed a significantly stronger association with severe gastritis than infected with CagA+/EBV−, further supporting the need of EBV to cause severe gastritis even in the presence of highly pathogenic *H. pylori* CagA+ strains. Interestingly, co-infection by EBV and *H. pylori* CagA negative strains did not trigger severe stages of gastritis, arguing against EBV complementing the pathogenesis of less virulent CagA negative *H. pylori* strains and thus still supporting the importance of CagA.

It is postulated that in order to infect epithelial cells, EBV must exit first from B cell latency, a step triggered by expression of transcriptional factor Zta, which is the main orchestrator of the lytic cycle. However, the extracellular signals in the upper digestive tract that trigger Zta expression are unknown. CagA is an oncoprotein that among many documented functions induces loss of polarity in epithelial cells, allowing the transport of basolateral proteins towards the apical face [29]. It might be possible that CagA signaling could function as trigger of the EBV lytic cycle, and CagA induced loss of cell polarity could also favor EBV tropism for epithelial cells. Arguing against the latter, we observed more pediatric patients infected with EBV (214 cases) than with *H. pylori* (178 cases), which might indicate that infection with the bacteria does not necessarily occur first.

It is important to address how EBV and *H. pylori* interact in the gastric mucosa in future studies. Two possible mechanisms are envisioned: one is simply through additive inflammatory responses causing increased damage to the tissue. A second mechanism is through more intimate interactions between EBV and *H. pylori* genes, *e.g.* the above-mentioned putative CagA and Zta co-operation. *H. pylori* infection has also been positively linked to MALT gastric lymphoma [30] supporting increased activation/signaling of B cells transiting through the gastric mucosa. In this scenario, one of the main inducers of Zta expression and the EBV lytic cycle in B cell cultures is protein kinase C (PKC) [31,32], and CagA is a known activator of this kinase [33]. Ectopic expression of CagA in transgenic mice supports that this protein is the first described bacterial oncoprotein and as such it behaves similarly to viral oncoproteins [8,9]. Interestingly, CagA and EBV oncogenes LMP1 and LMP2A trigger activation of NFκB and MAP Kinases, important signaling pathways for increased cell survival and proliferation during oncogenic transformation [34,35]. The common activation of signaling pathways by both pathogens suggests a common mechanism of infection/transformation of the gastric epithelium.

Although our data supports that co-infection of EBV with *H. pylori* is necessary to cause severe gastric inflammation and activity, EBV requirement seems to be greater for induction of severe activity in the gastric mucosa. Severe activity is given by a large infiltrate of polymorphonuclear cells permeating the lamina propria and the gastric glands, which in turn activate and secrete more pro-inflammatory mediators, thus enhancing and perpetuating the local inflammatory reaction and increasing the risk for severe and permanent damage to the gastric mucosa. In *H. pylori* infection, IL-8 seems to be the main neutrophil attracting cytokine [4,36,37]. IL-1β has been found overexpressed in NPC tumor samples, an important cytokine for PMN recruiting [38]. It is possible that the combined role of IL-8 and IL-1β results in the increased activity observed in EBV and *H. pylori* co-infected patients.

In conclusion, our results strongly suggest that EBV is involved in the pathophysiology of severe gastric lesions in children infected with *H. pylori*. Our results also suggest that in the absence of EBV infection, *H. pylori* is not sufficient to trigger severe gastritis in children. This study points out the need to study both pathogens jointly to understand the mechanism behind severe damage of the gastric mucosa early in life, which could have implications for the correct disease diagnosis and treatment; also, it could help to identify children with increased risk to present more serious lesions later in life.

Author Contributions

Conceived and designed the experiments: MC-P JT EMF-P. Performed the experiments: MGC-M RC-T. Analyzed the data: MGC-M AG-D JT EMF-P. Contributed reagents/materials/analysis tools: MGC-M MC-P JT EMF-P. Wrote the paper: MGC-M JT EMF-P.

References

1. IARC (1994) Schistosomes, liver flukes and Helicobacter pylori. IARC Working Group on the Evaluation of Carcinogenic Risks to Humans. Lyon, 7–14 June 1994. IARC Monogr Eval Carcinog Risks Hum 61: 1–241.
2. Thun MJ, DeLancey JO, Center MM, Jemal A, Ward EM (2010) The global burden of cancer: priorities for prevention. Carcinogenesis 31: 100–110.
3. Torres J, Leal-Herrera Y, Perez-Perez G, Gomez A, Camorlinga-Ponce M, et al. (1998) A community-based seroepidemiologic study of Helicobacter pylori infection in Mexico. J Infect Dis 178: 1089–1094.
4. Camorlinga-Ponce M, Aviles-Jimenez F, Cabrera L, Hernandez-Pando R, Munoz O, et al. (2003) Intensity of inflammation, density of colonization and interleukin-8 response in the gastric mucosa of children infected with Helicobacter pylori. Helicobacter 8: 554–560.
5. Recavarren-Arce S, Gilman RH, Leon-Barua R, Salazar G, McDonald J, et al. (1997) Chronic atrophic gastritis: early diagnosis in a population where Helicobacter pylori infection is frequent. Clin Infect Dis 25: 1006–1012.
6. Peek RM Jr., Blaser MJ (2002) Helicobacter pylori and gastrointestinal tract adenocarcinomas. Nat Rev Cancer 2: 28–37.
7. Hatakeyama M (2008) SagA of CagA in Helicobacter pylori pathogenesis. Curr Opin Microbiol 11: 30–37.
8. Ohnishi N, Yuasa H, Tanaka S, Sawa H, Miura M, et al. (2008) Transgenic expression of Helicobacter pylori CagA induces gastrointestinal and hematopoietic neoplasms in mouse. Proc Natl Acad Sci U S A 105: 1003–1008.
9. Miura M, Ohnishi N, Tanaka S, Yanagiya K, Hatakeyama M (2009) Differential oncogenic potential of geographically distinct Helicobacter pylori CagA isoforms in mice. Int J Cancer 125: 2497–2504.
10. Li S, Deng Y, Li X, Chen QP, Liao XC, et al. (2010) Diagnostic value of Epstein-Barr virus capsid antigen-IgA in nasopharyngeal carcinoma: a meta-analysis. Chin Med J (Engl) 123: 1201–1205.
11. Akiba S, Koriyama C, Herrera-Goepfert R, Eizuru Y (2008) Epstein-Barr virus associated gastric carcinoma: epidemiological and clinicopathological features. Cancer Sci 99: 195–201.
12. Camargo MC, Murphy G, Koriyama C, Pfeiffer RM, Kim WH, et al. (2011) Determinants of Epstein-Barr virus-positive gastric cancer: an international pooled analysis. Br J Cancer 105: 38–43.
13. Shibata D, Weiss LM (1992) Epstein-Barr virus-associated gastric adenocarcinoma. Am J Pathol 140: 769–774.
14. Chang MS, Kim WH (2005) Epstein-Barr virus in human malignancy: a special reference to Epstein-Barr virus associated gastric carcinoma. Cancer Res Treat 37: 257–267.
15. Faulkner GC, Burrows SR, Khanna R, Moss DJ, Bird AG, et al. (1999) X-Linked agammaglobulinemia patients are not infected with Epstein-Barr virus: implications for the biology of the virus. J Virol 73: 1555–1564.
16. Fachiroh J, Paramita DK, Hariwiyanto B, Harijadi A, Dahlia HL, et al. (2006) Single-assay combination of Epstein-Barr Virus (EBV) EBNA1- and viral capsid antigen-p18-derived synthetic peptides for measuring anti-EBV immunoglobulin G (IgG) and IgA antibody levels in sera from nasopharyngeal carcinoma patients: options for field screening. J Clin Microbiol 44: 1459–1467.
17. Gu AD, Xie YB, Mo HY, Jia WH, Li MY, et al. (2008) Antibodies against Epstein-Barr virus gp78 antigen: a novel marker for serological diagnosis of nasopharyngeal carcinoma detected by xMAP technology. J Gen Virol 89: 1152–1158.
18. Dixon MF, Genta RM, Yardley JH, Correa P (1996) Classification and grading of gastritis. The updated Sydney System. International Workshop on the Histopathology of Gastritis, Houston 1994. Am J Surg Pathol 20: 1161–1181.
19. Camorlinga-Ponce M, Torres J, Perez-Perez G, Leal-Herrera Y, Gonzalez-Ortiz B, et al. (1998) Validation of a serologic test for the diagnosis of Helicobacter pylori infection and the immune response to urease and CagA in children. Am J Gastroenterol 93: 1264–1270.
20. Camorlinga-Ponce M, Flores-Luna L, Lazcano-Ponce E, Herrero R, Bernal-Sahagun F, et al. (2008) Age and severity of mucosal lesions influence the performance of serologic markers in Helicobacter pylori-associated gastroduodenal pathologies. Cancer Epidemiol Biomarkers Prev 17: 2498–2504.

21. Yamamoto I, Fukuda Y, Mizuta T, Fukada M, Nishigami T, et al. (1995) Serum anti-Helicobacter pylori antibodies and gastritis. J Clin Gastroenterol 21 Suppl 1: S164–168.
22. Kitayama Y, Honda S, Sugimura H (2000) Epstein-Barr virus-related gastric pseudolymphoma in infectious mononucleosis. Gastrointest Endosc 52: 290–291.
23. Zhang Y, Molot R (2003) Severe gastritis secondary to Epstein-Barr viral infection. Unusual presentation of infectious mononucleosis and associated diffuse lymphoid hyperplasia in gastric mucosa. Arch Pathol Lab Med 127: 478–480.
24. Chen ZM, Shah R, Zuckerman GR, Wang HL (2007) Epstein-Barr virus gastritis: an underrecognized form of severe gastritis simulating gastric lymphoma. Am J Surg Pathol 31: 1446–1451.
25. Owens SR, Walls A, Krasinskas A, Rund CR (2008) Epstein-Barr virus gastritis: rare or rarely sampled? A case report. Int J Surg Pathol.
26. Hisamatsu A, Nagai T, Okawara H, Nakashima H, Tasaki T, et al. (2010) Gastritis associated with Epstein-Barr virus infection. Intern Med 49: 2101–2105.
27. Ryan JL, Shen YJ, Morgan DR, Thorne LB, Kenney SC, et al. (2012) Epstein-Barr virus infection is common in inflamed gastrointestinal mucosa. Dig Dis Sci 57: 1887–1898.
28. Hirano A, Yanai H, Shimizu N, Okamoto T, Matsubara Y, et al. (2003) Evaluation of Epstein-Barr virus DNA load in gastric mucosa with chronic atrophic gastritis using a real-time quantitative PCR assay. Int J Gastrointest Cancer 34: 87–94.
29. Saadat I, Higashi H, Obuse C, Umeda M, Murata-Kamiya N, et al. (2007) Helicobacter pylori CagA targets PAR1/MARK kinase to disrupt epithelial cell polarity. Nature 447: 330–333.
30. Sagaert X, Van Cutsem E, De Hertogh G, Geboes K, Tousseyn T (2010) Gastric MALT lymphoma: a model of chronic inflammation-induced tumor development. Nat Rev Gastroenterol Hepatol 7: 336–346.
31. Baumann M, Mischak H, Dammeier S, Kolch W, Gires O, et al. (1998) Activation of the Epstein-Barr virus transcription factor BZLF1 by 12-O-tetradecanoylphorbol-13-acetate-induced phosphorylation. J Virol 72: 8105–8114.
32. Lee HH, Chang SS, Lin SJ, Chua HH, Tsai TJ, et al. (2008) Essential role of PKCdelta in histone deacetylase inhibitor-induced Epstein-Barr virus reactivation in nasopharyngeal carcinoma cells. J Gen Virol 89: 878–883.
33. Brandt S, Wessler S, Hartig R, Backert S (2009) Helicobacter pylori activates protein kinase C delta to control Raf in MAP kinase signalling: role in AGS epithelial cell scattering and elongation. Cell Motil Cytoskeleton 66: 874–892.
34. Tegtmeyer N, Wessler S, Backert S Role of the cag-pathogenicity island encoded type IV secretion system in Helicobacter pylori pathogenesis. FEBS J 278: 1190–1202.
35. Dawson CW, Port RJ, Young LS (2012) The role of the EBV-encoded latent membrane proteins LMP1 and LMP2 in the pathogenesis of nasopharyngeal carcinoma (NPC). Semin Cancer Biol 22: 144–153.
36. Kabir S (2011) The role of interleukin-17 in the Helicobacter pylori induced infection and immunity. Helicobacter 16: 1–8.
37. Zhang QB, Etolhi G, Dawodu JB, Husain A, Gemmell CG, et al. (1998) Relationship between mucosal levels of interleukin 8 and toxinogenicity of Helicobacter pylori. Inflammopharmacology 6: 109–117.
38. Chen LC, Wang LJ, Tsang NM, Ojcius DM, Chen CC, et al. (2012) Tumour inflammasome-derived IL-1beta recruits neutrophils and improves local recurrence-free survival in EBV-induced nasopharyngeal carcinoma. EMBO Mol Med 4: 1276–1293.

Host Immune Transcriptional Profiles Reflect the Variability in Clinical Disease Manifestations in Patients with *Staphylococcus aureus* Infections

Romain Banchereau[1]*, Alejandro Jordan-Villegas[1], Monica Ardura[3], Asuncion Mejias[3], Nicole Baldwin[2], Hui Xu[2], Elizabeth Saye[4], Jose Rossello-Urgell[2], Phuong Nguyen[2], Derek Blankenship[2], Clarence B. Creech[4], Virginia Pascual[2], Jacques Banchereau[2,5], Damien Chaussabel[2,6], Octavio Ramilo[3]

1 UT Southwestern Medical Center, Dallas, Texas, United States of America, **2** Baylor Institute for Immunology Research, Dallas, Texas, United States of America, **3** Nationwide Children's Hospital, Columbus, Ohio, United States of America, **4** Vanderbilt University School of Medicine, Nashville, Tennessee, United States of America, **5** Hoffmann-Laroche, Nutley, New Jersey, United States of America, **6** Benaroya Research Institute, Seattle, Washington, United States of America

Abstract

Staphylococcus aureus infections are associated with diverse clinical manifestations leading to significant morbidity and mortality. To define the role of the host response in the clinical manifestations of the disease, we characterized whole blood transcriptional profiles of children hospitalized with community-acquired *S. aureus* infection and phenotyped the bacterial strains isolated. The overall transcriptional response to *S. aureus* infection was characterized by over-expression of innate immunity and hematopoiesis related genes and under-expression of genes related to adaptive immunity. We assessed individual profiles using modular fingerprints combined with the molecular distance to health (MDTH), a numerical score of transcriptional perturbation as compared to healthy controls. We observed significant heterogeneity in the host signatures and MDTH, as they were influenced by the type of clinical presentation, the extent of bacterial dissemination, and time of blood sampling in the course of the infection, but not by the bacterial isolate. System analysis approaches provide a new understanding of disease pathogenesis and the relation/interaction between host response and clinical disease manifestations.

Editor: Michael Otto, National Institutes of Health, United States of America

Funding: This work was supported by the National Institute of Allergy and Infectious Diseases; the National Institutes of Arthritis and Musculo-Skeletal and Skin Diseases; and the Baylor Healthcare System Foundation [grant numbers U01 AI082110, U19 AI089987, R01 ARO50770, U19 AI057234]. The funders had no role in study design, data collection and analysis, decision to publish, or preparation of the manuscript.

Competing Interests: J. Banchereau is affiliated with F. Hoffmann-La Roche Ltd. This does not alter the authors' adherence to all the PLoS ONE policies on sharing data and materials.

* E-mail: romain.banchereau@utsouthwestern.edu

Introduction

Staphylococcus aureus has emerged as one of the most frequent cause of community-acquired invasive bacterial infections, with significant morbidity and mortality. Just in 2005 in the United States, 18,650 deaths were reported due to methicillin-resistant *S. aureus* (MRSA) [1,2,3,4,5,6]. The spectrum of community-associated (CA) *S. aureus* disease is wide and patients can present with a variety of clinical illness, ranging from mild soft tissue infections to invasive disease such as bacteremia, pneumonia, or osteoarticular infections [1,7,8]. The emergence of multidrug resistant *S. aureus* strains worldwide [9,10] combined with limited therapeutic options demand novel approaches to further elucidate host-pathogen interactions, and especially host responses to *S. aureus* infection. Circulating leukocytes represent an accessible source of molecular information, which can be studied by analyzing the whole blood genome-wide transcriptome. The value of blood microarray analysis has been illustrated in infection, cancer and autoimmunity [11,12,13,14], leading to diagnostic and therapeutic advances [14].

We have previously used microarray analysis to characterize the differences in host responses to different microbial pathogens [11] including *S. aureus* (Ardura et al, 2009) by analyzing peripheral blood mononuclear cells (PBMC) from pediatric patients hospitalized with acute infections. The neutrophil depletion from PBMC may result in the loss of key information in the systemic characterization of bacterial infections [15]. As new research tools became available we performed whole blood microarray profiling –including neutrophils – in a new cohort of 99 pediatric patients with *S aureus* infection. Using this large cohort we now defined: a) the common host response to *S aureus* infection; and b) the differences in host response patterns depending on the site of infection and the clinical presentation of the disease. The main objective of this analysis was to determine whether the transcriptional profiles reflect the variation of clinical disease manifestations and to provide new insights in disease pathogenesis by defining the differences in host responses among patients with different clinical presentations.

Results

S. aureus induces a distinct and robust transcriptional signature in whole blood

To define the whole blood biosignature of *S. aureus* infection in children, 99 patients and 44 healthy controls were assigned to two independent groups of subjects, to serve as "training" and "test" sets. The training set was used to identify the signature of *S. aureus* infection. This signature was validated in the independent test set by assessing its capacity to separate the patients from healthy controls by hierarchical clustering. The training set included 40 patients with *S. aureus* infection and 22 healthy controls, matched for age, sex and race (Table 1). Statistical group comparison yielded 1,422 differentially regulated transcripts. Hierarchical clustering of these transcripts grouped them according to similarities in gene expression patterns (Figure 1A). This signature was validated in the independent test set of 59 patients and 22 healthy controls (Figure 1B). Hierarchical clustering of these 1,422 transcripts grouped 52 out of 59 patients from the test set together. The seven patients who clustered with controls presented with either mild or moderate disease, and were closer to recovery and hospital discharge compared with all other patients.

S. aureus infection activates innate immunity and suppresses the adaptive immune response

To better understand the whole blood response to *S. aureus* infection and the immune pathways activated, we used an analytical framework of 62 transcriptional modules that group together genes with shared expression pattern and similar biological function across independent blood transcriptional datasets [16]. Module maps were derived independently for the training (Figure 1C) and test sets (Figure 1D), using their respective healthy control group as reference. Patients with acute *S. aureus* infection demonstrated significant over-expression of modules linked to the myeloid lineage (M3.2, M4.6, M4.13, M4.14, M6.6), and inflammation (M4.2, M5.1, M6.13) confirming our earlier findings in PBMC. Further-

Table 1. Demographic and laboratory characteristics of patients and healthy controls in training and test sets.

Parameter	TRAINING SET			TEST SET		
	Patients	*Controls*	p^a	*Patients*	*Controls*	p^a
Count	40	22		59	22	
Age (years)	8.00 [0.15–17]	7.0 [4–18]	0.865	6.50 [0.06–16]	3 [0.17–14.00]	0.03
Race	19AA,12H,9C	6AA,11H,4C,1O	0.156	19AA,18H,15C,7O	1AA,13H,6C,2O	0.018
Gender	20M,20F	12M,10F	0.795	34M,25F	11M,11F	0.805
WBC (10^3/mm^3)	9.3 [4.1–28.1]	6.8[3.40–12.6]	0.006	10.10[3.20–33.3]	9.1 [4.20–16.0]	0.065
Neutrophils (%)	52.0 [15–87]	50.7 [34.7–59.8]	0.536	55.00[12.0–84]	35.0 [10.0–55.00]	<0.001
Neutrophils (10^3/mm^3)	5.20 [1.16–22.4]	3.58[1.46–6.94]	0.025	5.63[0.74–18.1]	3.0 [0.84–7.76]	<0.001
Lymphocytes (%)	28.50 [5–67]	37.0 [29.4–53.8]	0.073	33.00 [5.00–72.0]	55.0[33.2–81.0]	<0.001
Lymphocytes (10^3/mm^3)	2.70[0.93–11.0]	2.72 [1.29–4.36]	0.721	3.42 [0.44–13.3]	5.3 [1.44–11.2]	0.016
Monocytes (%)	7.50[1–21]	7.30[5.00–10.6]	0.775	8.0 [2–17]	5.6 [2.00–9.0]	0.096
Monocytes (10^3/mm^3)	0.83 [0.08–3.40]	0.48 [0.19–0.72]	0.036	0.75 [0.14–3.49]	0.44 [0.30–0.98]	0.01
RBC (10^6/mm3)	3.92 [2.6–4.7]	3.90[3.40–4.03]	0.507	4.05 [1.27–5.65]	no data	
Hemoglobin	10.5 [7.3–13.7]	8.80[7.90–11.40]	0.1	10.60 [3.4–13.7]	12.60*	
Hematocrit (%)	31.70 [22.1–38.6]	27.25[25.90–33.30]	0.13	31.70[11.1–40.3]	36.6*	
MCV (um^3)	80.90 [70.7–88.9]	73.50[67.00–86.00]	0.083	81.00 [56.8–97.6]	no data	
MCH (pg)	27.30 [22.9–29.8]	23.75[20.40–29.30]	0.03	27.00 [17.9–33.4]	no data	
MCHC (g/dL)	33.6 [31–35.7]	32.05[30.40–34.20]	0.015	33.5 [30.6–35.9]	no data	
RDW (%)	13.40[11.8–19.4]	12.75[11.50–14.90]	0.337	13.30 [11.6–17.6]	no data	
MPV	9.30 [7.7–15]	7.80[6.50–10.00]	0.009	9.50 [7.8–12.4]	no data	
Platelets (10^3/mm^3)	412 [83–880]	261.00[214.00–288.00]	0.005	414.00 [136–833]	335.00*	
ESR	67.00 [15–142]	no data		68.00 [8–135]	no data	
CRP (mg/dL)	5.95 [0.1–37.4]	no data		4.30 [0.1–42.8]	no data	
Hospitalization Duration	11.00 [5–98]	n/a		9.00 [1–53.00]	n/a	
Draw Day	5.00 [2–16]	n/a		5.00 [1–35]	n/a	
Draw Index	0.43 [0.04–1]	n/a		0.50 [0.08–1]	n/a	

Median values [min-max range]; AA = African-American, C = Caucasian, H = Hispanic, O = Other; M = Male, F = Female; WBC = White Blood Count; RBC = Red Blood Cell count; MCV = Mean Corpuscular Volume; MCH = Mean Corpuscular Hemoglobin; MCHC = Mean Corpuscular Hemoglobin Concentration; RDW = Red blood cell Distribution Width; MPV = Mean Platelet Volume; ESR = Erythrocyte Sedimentation Rate; CRP = C-reactive Protein;
*only 1 sample.
Statistics: for categorical variables, Fisher's exact test is used; for continuous variables, Mann-Whitney test is used.

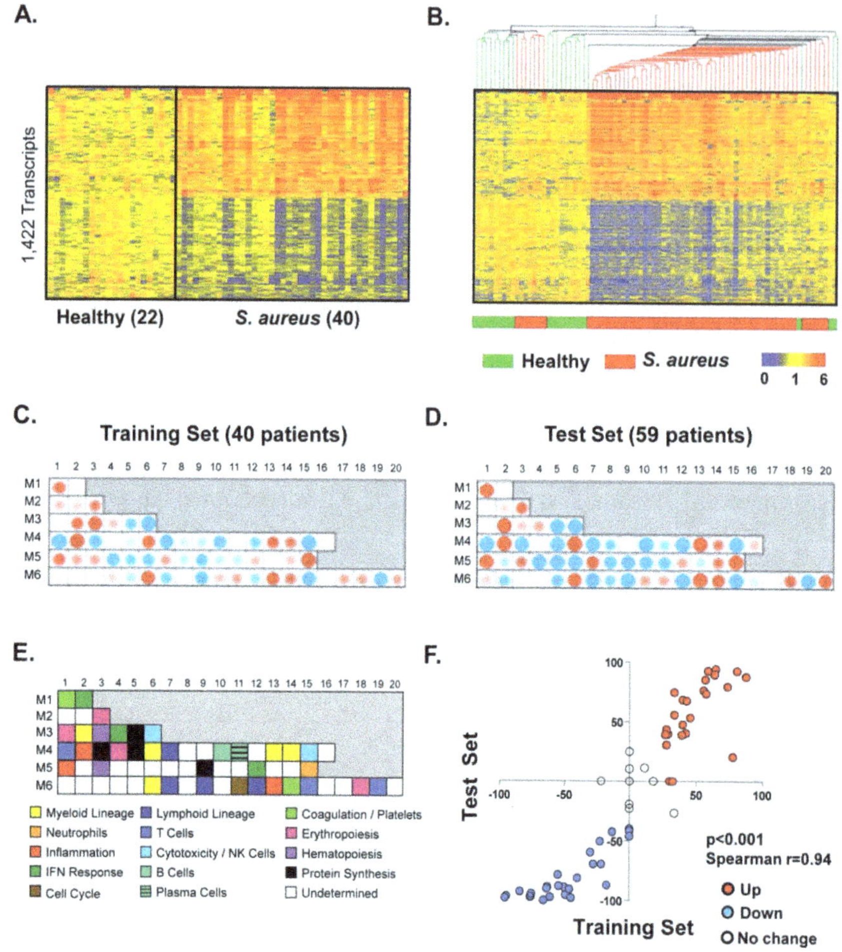

Figure 1. The *S. aureus* infection whole blood transcriptional signature is characterized by over-expression of myeloid lineage transcripts and under-expression of lymphoid lineage transcripts. A. Statistical group comparison between 22 healthy subjects and 40 patients with acute *S. aureus* infection (non-parametric test, $\alpha = 0{\cdot}01$, Benjamini-Hochberg multiple testing correction, 1·25 fold change) yielded 1,422 differentially expressed transcripts. Transcripts were organized by hierarchical clustering (Spearman) according to similarities in expression profiles. Each row represents a transcript and each column an individual subject. Normalized log ratio levels are indicated by red (over-expressed) or blue (under-expressed), as compared to the median of healthy controls. **B.** The same 1,422 transcript list and hierarchical clustering were applied to an independent test set of 22 healthy controls and 59 patients with acute *S. aureus* infection. Sample hierarchical clustering (Spearman) was performed on the 1,422 transcript list in the test set. **C.** Average modular transcriptional fingerprrint for *S. aureus* patients as compared to healthy controls in the training set. **D.** Average modular transcriptional profile for *S. aureus* patients as compared to healthy controls in the test set. **E.** Module functional annotations legend. **F.** Scatter plot comparing module expression between training (x-axis) and test (y-axis) sets. Spearman correlation was applied.

more, patients displayed over-expression of modules linked to the coagulation cascade (M1.1), hematopoietic precursors (M3.3 and M5.3), and neutrophils (M5.15). Conversely, they demonstrated significant under-expression of modules linked to T cells (M4.1, M6.15 and M6.19), cytotoxicity/NK cells (M3.6 and M4.15), B cells (M4.10), and lymphoid lineage (M4.7 and M6.9). Transcript composition of these modules is summarized online (http://www.biir.net/public_wikis/module_annotation/V2_Trial_8_Modules). These findings were confirmed in the test set as shown by significant correlation of module expression between training and test sets (Figure 1F, $p<0{\cdot}0001$, Spearman $R=0{\cdot}94$) demonstrating the consistency of these observations.

The blood signature of *S. aureus* infection demonstrates significant heterogeneity

As the clinical presentation of individual patients was diverse, once we defined the global whole blood response to *S. aureus* infection, we then aimed to characterize how the variation in anatomical site, dissemination of the infection and bacterial isolate (Table 2) affect the signatures. Because the training and test sets yielded similar modular fingerprints (Figure 1F), they were merged into one dataset for subsequent analysis.

Our initial step was to examine the heterogeneity in the signatures and then determine which factors could be associated with such variation. To this end, we first calculated the molecular distance to health, or MDTH for each individual patient. The MDTH is a score that measures the global transcriptional perturbation in each patient compared to the median of healthy controls. Thus by summarizing the overall transcriptional activity in one score, the MDTH facilitates the correlation with clinical parameters [12,17]. Overall, as expected, the median MDTH of patients was significantly higher than that of healthy controls (Figure 2A, $p<0{\cdot}001$). However, 25 patients had MDTH scores that were within the range of healthy controls MDTH (3–259). These patients were flagged as transcriptionally quiescent (TQ) and separated from transcriptionally active patients ($n=74$). Unsupervised hierarchical clustering of the 10,972 transcripts expressed in at least one of the 143 subjects grouped these quiescent patients with healthy controls (Figure 2B). When analyzed from a clinical perspective the majority of these patients presented with mild and local infections with low C-reactive protein (CRP) and the samples were obtained late in the course of the infection as reflected by an elevated mean draw index (0.64) (see methods).

To assess the qualitative heterogeneity of transcriptionally active patients (n = 74; MDTH scores >259), individual modular fingerprints were derived and k-means clustering was used to further identify modular expression patterns. Four major transcriptional active patient clusters (C1 to C4) were identified (Figure 2C, Figure 2D) [18] (Figure S3). Group module expression was derived for each cluster (Figure S4). Cluster C1 included 13 patients with a high mean MDTH (3,003) and strong over-expression of myeloid (M3.2, M4.6, M4.13, M6.6) and inflammation (M4.2, M5.1, M6.13) modules. Cluster C2 comprised 31 patients with a signature qualitatively similar to C1, but quantitatively dimmer as supported by the lower mean MDTH (973). Cluster C3 regrouped 12 patients with high MDTH (2,395) and low inflammatory signature, but over-expression of modules linked to erythropoiesis (M2.3, M3.1, M4.4, M6.18) and hematopoiesis (M5.3). C1 and C3 both displayed significant down-regulation of transcripts linked to B and T cells (Figure S5). Gene level analysis (Figure S6A) combined with PANTHER [19] ontology ranking (http://www.pantherdb.org) supported this observation as heme biosynthesis (Figure S6B) and porphyrin metabolism (Figure S6C) were the most enriched pathways in C3 versus C1. The top 100 transcripts differentially expressed between C1 and C3 are displayed in Table S4 and Figure S6D. Finally, cluster C4 was comprised 18 patients with lower mean MDTH (699). Interestingly, 11 of them displayed an IFN signature, although only one patient had concomitant CMV infection detected by viral culture.

The median values for different clinical findings and laboratory parameters were calculated for each cluster (Figure 2E, Table S5). In addition, we assessed whether the differences observed at the modular level were related to the time of sample collection in relation to the length of stay (draw index). Cluster C1 displayed a lower draw index, indicating that blood samples were collected at an earlier stage of hospitalization. Patients from C1 required a longer duration of hospitalization than other patients. Additionally, patients from C1 had significantly higher CRP, WBC, neutrophil and monocyte counts. Thus, these routine laboratory markers of inflammation corroborated the over-expression of myeloid and inflammatory modules.

The C3 patients showed decreased hemoglobin, hematocrit, and MCHC (Figure S6F, Table S5), suggesting an anemic state that might trigger erythropoiesis as indicated by the signature. The C3 erythropoietic signature overlapped with transcripts from CD71+ early erythroid precursors [20] (Figure S6D).

Then, we analyzed how infection site, clinical presentation, and type of bacterial strain were distributed among clusters (Figure 2F, Table S6). All patients in cluster C1 had invasive or disseminated disease, and a higher proportion of patients with pneumonia. Clusters C4 and TQ (transcriptionally quiescent) included most patients with skin and soft tissue abscesses, confirming the association between low MDTH and mild presentation.

Bacterial factors had limited influence on the host expression profiles

Finally, to determine whether heterogeneity in bacterial virulence factors was associated with clustering patterns, the isolates from 63 patients were characterized (Figure S1). The majority (87%) of isolates tested were PVL-positive. Both clusters C1 and C3 displayed a higher percentage of MRSA isolates (100% and 92%) than the overall mean (67%), suggesting that clones of CA-MRSA USA300 might induce a stronger host response than the currently circulating MSSA clones. No difference in other bacterial characteristics such as agr locus type or genetic relatedness was observed between the four clusters. (Table 3, Table S7).

Elements of the molecular signature correlate with laboratory parameters

We then asked whether patient's molecular profiles correlated with clinical laboratory parameters commonly used to assess clinical disease status (Table S8). The MDTH positively correlated with neutrophil counts, white blood cell counts, C-reactive protein, band neutrophil counts, red blood cell distribution width, and monocyte counts. MDTH inversely correlated with relative lymphocyte counts, red blood cell count, hemoglobin concentration, mean corpuscular hemoglobin (MCH) concentration, and hematocrit. Correlations were assessed on a module-by-module basis (Figure 3A). Inflammatory modules positively correlated with neutrophil counts, CRP and WBC while modules linked to adaptive immunity negatively correlated with these parameters. Hematopoiesis (M3.3) and cell cycle (M6.11) modules correlated

Table 2. Infection localization and clinical presentation distribution for training and test sets.

		Definition	Training (n = 40)	Test (n = 59)	Total (n = 99)
Localization	Local	SST abscess or cellulitis	0 (0%)	10 (16.9%)	10 (10%)
	Invasive	Bacteremia, pneumonia, osteomyelitis, meningitis	33 (82.5%)	41 (69.5%)	74 (74.8%)
	Disseminated	Bacteremia+2 sites of infection	5 (12.5%)	8 (13.6%)	13 (13%)
	Unclassified		2 (5%)	0 (0%)	2 (2%)
Clinical Presentation	SST Abscess	Skin abscess, no bacteremia	0 (0%)	10 (16.9%)	10 (10%)
	Osteoarticular	Bacteremia and osteomyelitis or suppurative arthritis	29 (72.5%)	27 (45.8%)	56 (56.6%)
	Pneumonia		6 (15%)	5 (8.5%)	11 (11.1%)
	Unclassified		5 (12.5%)	17 (28.8%)	23 (23.2%)

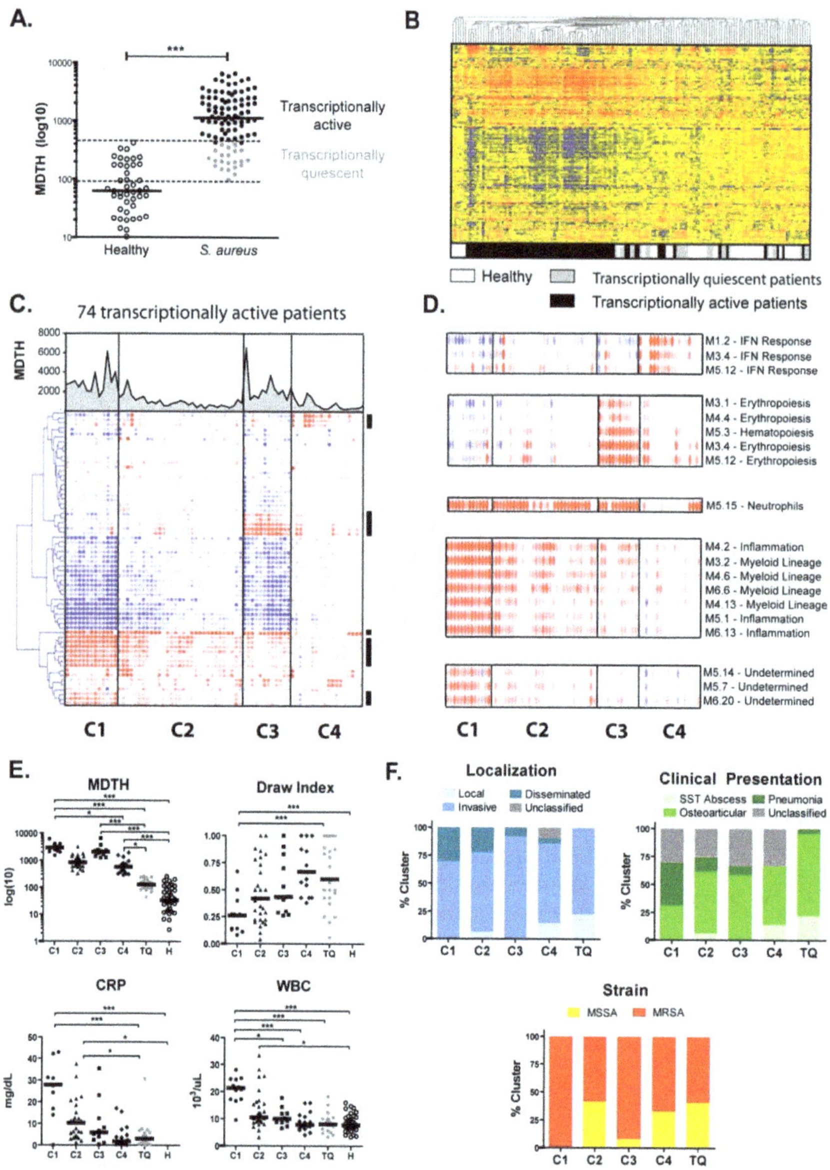

Figure 2. Individual analysis identifies heterogeneous components of the blood signature to *S. aureus*. A. Column scatter plot representing the distribution of individual molecular distance to health (MDTH) in healthy controls and *S. aureus* patients. The list of all transcripts composing the modules was used as reference to calculate individual MDTH (***: p<0·001, Mann-Whitney). Horizontal bars represent the group median. Patients with MDTH within healthy range (n = 25) were categorized as transcriptionally quiescent (TQ) and represented in grey. **B.** Unsupervised hierarchical clustering of the 10,972 transcripts expressed in at least one of the 143 samples (2-fold normalized, 100 difference in raw data) from the combined training and test sets. **C.** The modular signature was derived for individual transcriptionally active patients (n = 74) as compared to the median of the healthy control group for the corresponding patient set (training or test). Four major clusters (C1 through C4) of patients were obtained by K-means clustering and reorganized into a single heatmap, with modules in rows and patients in columns. Molecular distance to health for individual samples is represented as a line chart on top of the heatmap. **D.** Zoom on modules with specific over-expression patterns across the four clusters. **E.** MDTH and clinical lab measurements distribution by cluster. Five or six-group non-parametric ANOVA (Kruskal-Wallis) with Dunn's post-hoc test was applied. (*: p<0·05, **: p<0·01, ***: p<0·001). **F.** Bar charts representing the percent distribution of infection localization, clinical presentation and bacterial strain for the five clusters of patients identified.

with absolute band (immature neutrophils) count. Significant correlations between clinical nodes and molecular nodes are summarized as a network (Figure 3B).

Time of blood sampling, infection dissemination, and clinical presentation influence the transcriptional signature

To determine whether the type and dissemination of the disease as well as time of sample collection influenced the genomic fingerprint, a supervised analysis was conducted to compare transcriptional signatures according to: 1) time in the course of the infection as defined by draw index quarters; 2) infection site; and 3) types of invasive clinical presentations. Three myeloid lineage and three inflammation related modules were differentially regulated from quarter to quarter (Figure 4A). The MDTH also displayed a decreasing trend (Figure 4B) that was paralleled by the decrease in CRP (Figure 4C). MDTH increased as the infection became more disseminated (Figure 4D), which was most evident during the first

Table 3. Distribution of bacterial isolate characteristics by infection localization, presentation and cluster.

			Infection Dissemination		Clinical Presentation		Cluster	
			Fisher's Exact Test		Fisher's Exact Test		Fisher's Exact Test	
			Table Probability (P)	Pr<=P	Table Probability (P)	Pr<=P	Table Probability (P)	Pr<=P
	# Patients		-	-	-	-	-	-
	# Isolates		-	-	-	-	-	-
Antibiotic Resistance	MRSA		0.07	**>0.05**	0.06	**>0.05**	0.0016	**>0.05**
	MSSA							
Agr Type	agr I		0.08	**>0.05**	0.11	**>0.05**	2.60E-03	**>0.05**
	agr II							
	agr III							
Genetic Relatedness	USA 200		0.01	**>0.05**	0.02	**>0.05**	2.20E-07	**>0.05**
	USA 300							
	USA 400							
	USA 500							
	USA 700							
	USA 1100							
Toxin Production	PVL	+	0.12	**>0.05**	0.16	**>0.05**	1.40E-02	**>0.05**
		–						
	TSST/SEA/SEB/SEC	+	0.15	**>0.05**	0.17	**>0.05**	0.028	**>0.05**
		–						
	SEH/SEG	+	0.09	**>0.05**	0.18	**>0.05**	0.0019	**>0.05**
		–						

TQ: Transcriptionally Quiescent.

half of the hospitalization period (Figure S7A, Figure S7B), and was paralleled by increased CRP and hospitalization duration (Table S9).

Next, we analyzed patients according to the type of clinical presentation. Patients with pneumonia had a higher median MDTH than patients with osteoarticular infections as well higher WBC, neutrophil and monocyte counts (Figure 4E, Figure S8A, and Table S10).

Patients with osteoarticular infections display transcripts linked to activated blood coagulation that are not present in patients with pneumonia

To assess transcriptional differences between patients with distinct clinical presentations we selected nine patients with osteoarticular infection and compared them to nine patients with pneumonia matched for MDTH (Figure S8B). Eighteen healthy controls (nine from each training and test sets) were used as reference. Module fingerprints identified over-expression of the coagulation cascade (M1.1) and platelet adhesion (M6.14) in patients with osteoarticular infection but not pneumonia (Figure 5A). From the 385 genes differently expressed (Figure 5B), PANTHER analysis for pathway enrichment (Figure 5C) identified blood coagulation as the most significant pathway over-expressed in osteoarticular infection, and cholesterol biosynthesis over-expressed in pneumonia. No significant correlations were observed between bacterial isolates (Table S7) and clinical presentation.

Discussion

This study is the first analysis of whole blood transcriptional profiles in pediatric patients with acute community-associated *S. aureus* infections. Both conserved and heterogeneous elements of the transcriptional signature were identified, which correlate with time elapsed since hospitalization, bacterial dissemination, and the type of clinical presentation. Supporting our earlier study on PBMC [21], the whole blood signature was characterized by significant over-expression of myeloid lineage and inflammation transcripts, and under-expression of lymphoid lineage transcripts. This may reflect the large expansion of circulating neutrophils and monocytes during the acute phase of infection.

While all patients share a global signature to *S. aureus* infection, analysis of fingerprints of individual patients revealed heterogeneous elements of the molecular signature. The major transcriptional patterns identified included a pro-inflammatory myeloid signature, linked to sampling early in the course of infection, high neutrophil and monocyte counts, and elevated CRP (C1). Some patients displayed an erythropoiesis fingerprint with limited myeloid components (C3), which likely represents an increased release of hematopoietic precursors from the bone marrow during acute infection [22]. This erythropoiesis signature was observed in systemic onset juvenile idiopathic arthritis (SOJIA) [20] and was proposed to reflect the expansion of immature precursor cells and ineffective erythropoiesis. The latter results in accumulation of iron in tissues [23], which supports bacterial survival. It was suggested that erythropoietin (EPO) inhibits NF-kB and TNFa-mediated pro-inflammatory pathways [24], which could explain

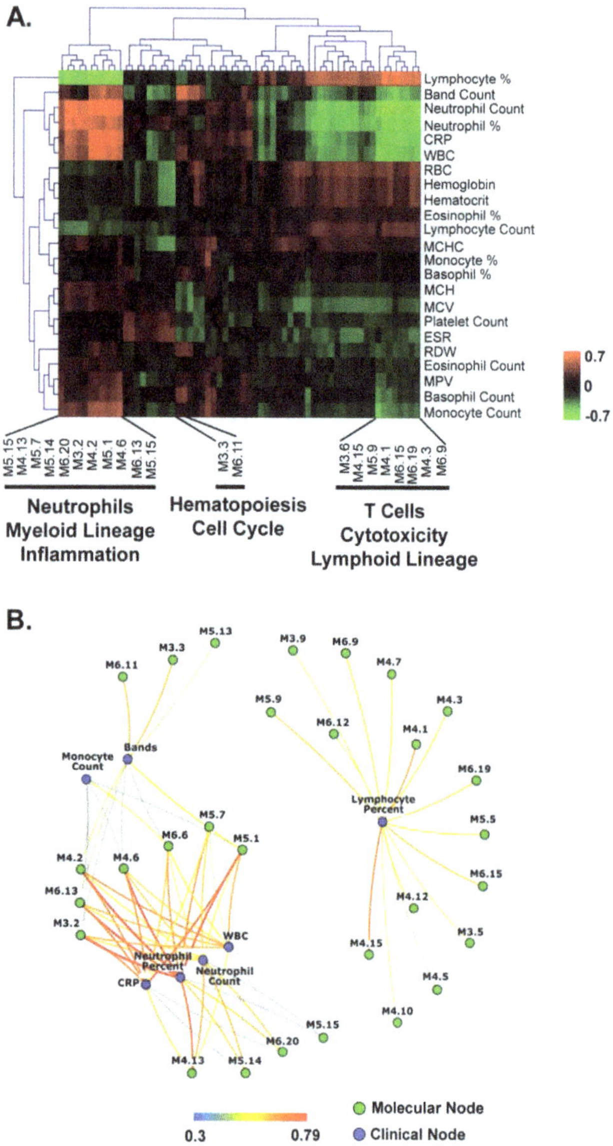

Figure 3. Specific module subsets correlate with laboratory results. A. Heatmap representing correlation (Spearman R) between module percent expression in columns and continuous laboratory parameters in rows. Hierarchical clustering (Euclidian distance) was applied in both dimensions. **B.** Connection network representing correlation between molecular nodes (modules) in blue and clinical nodes (laboratory parameters) in green. Spearman R correlation greater than 0·3 are represented.

why C3 patients displayed limited pro-inflammatory signature. This could represent a bacterial survival mechanism, whereby increased erythropoiesis would prevent the development of an adequate pro-inflammatory response and subsequent bacterial clearance. Despite increased numbers of neutrophils, we did not detect consistent changes in transcripts linked to the interferon response, as previously observed in patients with active pulmonary tuberculosis [12]. Fifteen out of 99 patients displayed over-expression of the three IFN modules but tested negative for concomitant viral infections. It may reflect IFN activation to counter arrest the bacteria-induced pro-inflammatory milieu [25] in the later stages of infection.

Currently, there are no established laboratory markers that either objectively define the extent of clinical disease severity in patients with *S. aureus* infections or monitor the spread of the infection to multiple organs [8]. Transcriptional profiling highlighted global quantitative differences between patients with local or disseminated disease, supporting the value of microarrays and the quantitative MDTH genomic score to monitor the spread of infection.

Additionally, the signatures provided unique transcriptional information on the pathogenesis of different clinical syndromes. Patients with osteoarticular infections displayed over-expression of transcripts linked to blood coagulation, a finding possibly related with the increased systemic coagulation and deep venous thrombosis observed in patients with musculoskeletal infections [26]. Additionally, patients with pneumonia displayed over-expression of genes involved in cholesterol synthesis, which might be involved in neutrophil recruitment to the lung [27]. Importantly, the location and extent of disease dissemination impacted transcriptional profiles to a greater extent than molecular characteristics of the *S. aureus* strains. This suggests that either: 1) the early innate response is directed towards features of *S. aureus* conserved across strains; 2) the human response is specifically tailored to the infection site; 3) staphylococcal gene expression differs based on the site of disease.

Despite the qualitative variability of the host response, the intensity of the signature decreases as patients get closer to discharge, regardless of the localization of the infection or the type of clinical presentation, suggesting that this assay has potential to monitor the clinical course of infection. Future studies should focus on the diagnostic and prognostic value of this approach in identifying patients at risk for infection dissemination and eventually determine its value in guiding therapeutic decisions.

Materials and Methods

Ethics Statement

This study was conducted according to the principles expressed in the Declaration of Helsinki. The study was approved by the Institutional Review Boards of the University of Texas Southwestern Medical Center and Children's Medical Center of Dallas (IRB #0802-447) and Baylor Institute of Immunology Research (BIIR, IRB # 002-141). Informed written consent was obtained from legal guardians and informed assent was obtained from patients 10 years of age and older prior to any study-related procedure.

Patient characteristics

Blood samples from 99 patients hospitalized with community-acquired *S. aureus* infection and 44 healthy controls were collected in tempus tubes (Applied Biosystems, PN 4342792). Patients represented the clinical spectrum of acute *S. aureus* infection, including skin and soft tissue infection, bacteremia, osteomyelitis, suppurative arthritis, pyomyositis, pneumonia with empyema, and disseminated disease defined as bacteremia and the involvement of 2 different anatomical sites. Patients with a diagnosis of toxic shock syndrome, polymicrobial infections, or treated with corticosteroids in the preceding four weeks were excluded. Viral direct fluorescent antibody testing and/or culture of the nasopharynx was performed in all patients and healthy controls to exclude concomitant viral infections. Patient demographic data and clinical characteristics are summarized in Table S1 and Table S2. The median duration of hospitalization was ten days (range: 1–98 days). The median time from patient hospitalization to blood sample acquisition was five days (range: 1–35 days).

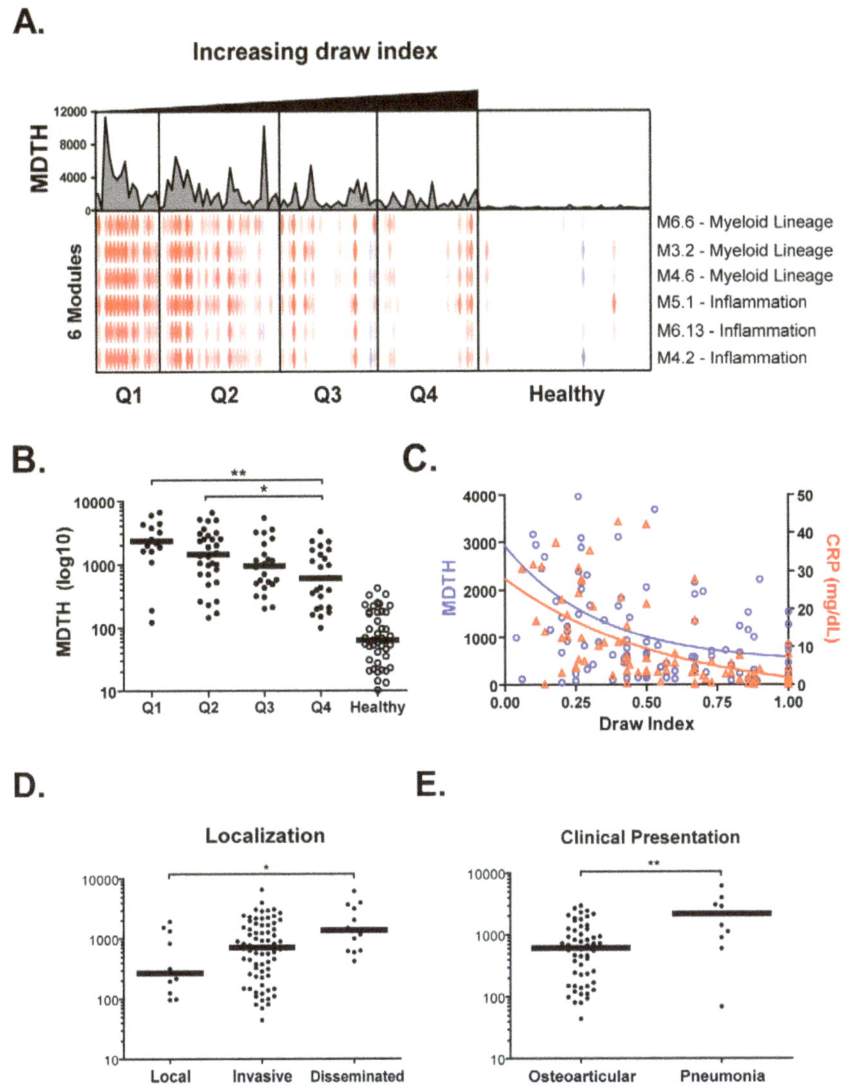

Figure 4. Patient signature varies with blood draw index, dissemination and clinical presentation. A. Patients were organized in four quarters Q1 through Q4 based on blood draw index (ratio draw day/hospitalization duration). A low draw index signifies proximity to hospital admission while a high draw index signifies proximity to discharge. Transcripts differently expressed between the four draw index quarters were selected by non-parametric ANOVA (Kruskal-Wallis, $p<0.01$, Benjamini-Hochberg false discovery rate) and represented as a heatmap (red, yellow, blue). The same statistical filter was applied at the module level (red, white, blue heatmap below). Individual MDTH was represented above as a line chart. **B.** Column scatter plot of individual MDTH per blood draw index quartile. Horizontal bars represent group median. Non-parametric ANOVA (Kruskal-Wallis) with Dunn's post-hoc test was applied. **C.** Non-linear regression model (one-phase decay) of MDTH (left Y-axis) and CRP (right Y-axis) as a function of blood draw index. **D.** Column scatter plot of individual MDTH per infection localization group. **E.** Column scatter plot of individual MDTH per clinical presentation group. Horizontal bars represent the median value for each group. Non-parametric ANOVA (Kruskal-Wallis) with Dunn's post-hoc test was applied between patient groups.

Patient classification

The study cohort of 99 patients and 44 healthy controls was divided into independent training (40 patients, 22 healthy controls) and test sets (59 patients, 22 healthy controls) (Table 1). Patients were categorized according to three schemes (Table 2) based on assessment by an independent clinician who was blinded to the transcriptional data: i) by localization of infection, defined as local ($n=10$), invasive ($n=74$) or disseminated ($n=13$); ii) by clinical presentation, separating patients with skin and soft tissue infection with negative blood culture ($n=10$), patients with osteoarticular infections ($n=56$), and patients with pneumonia ($n=11$).

Sampling time: Draw index and hospitalization quarter

This cross-sectional study included samples drawn at different days during hospitalization. To assess the influence of the time the sample was obtained during the course of the infection we calculated a draw index, a numeric score between 0 and 1 calculated as the ratio of the blood draw day over the duration of hospitalization. Accordingly, samples were classified according to the hospitalization quarter ($0\leq$Quarter $1<0{\cdot}25\leq$Quarter $2<0{\cdot}50\leq$Quarter $3<0{\cdot}75\leq$Quarter 4).

Characterization of Bacterial Isolates

Bacterial isolates from 63 patients were recovered from blood culture, synovial fluid, or abscesses. Single colonies were selected

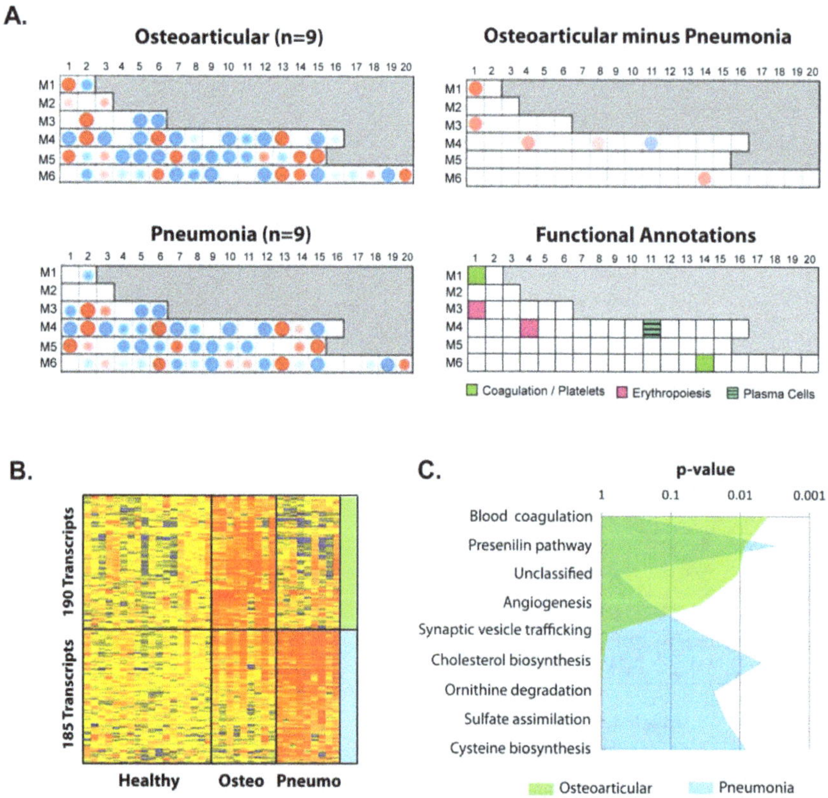

Figure 5. The osteoarticular infection signature displays increased blood coagulation. We compared the transcriptional signatures from patients with pneumonia and patients with osteoarticular infections. To properly balance osteoarticular and pneumonia groups, patients with pneumonia with a draw index less than 0·75 (nine patients) were selected (active disease). Nine patients with osteoarticular infection were selected with matching MDTH so that global quantitative signature was equivalent between the two groups. Nine healthy controls were selected from the training and nine from the test set (18 healthy controls in total) as reference. **A. Top left panel:** mean module map for the nine patients with osteoarticular infections compared to the 18 healthy controls. **Bottom left panel:** mean module map for the 9 patients with staphylococcal pneumonia compared to the 18 healthy controls. **Top right panel:** substraction map of osteoarticular infections minus pneumonia. Only differences greater than 40% are represented. **Bottom right panel**: Annotation legend for modules identified. **B.** Heatmap representing genes differentially expressed (t-test, <0·05, no correction) between osteoarticular infections and pneumonia (hierarchical clustering, Pearson). 190 genes were upregulated 1·5-fold or more in osteoarticular infections versus pneumonia and healthy controls. 185 genes were upregulated 1·5-fold or more in pneumonia versus osteoarticular infections and healthy controls. **C.** Area chart representing PANTHER comparison for pathway enrichment between the two lists from C.

and sub-cultured. *S. aureus* was confirmed by nuclease PCR and isolates were tested for methicillin resistance by mecA PCR. SCCmec typing of MRSA isolates was performed by classifying the ccr and mec complexes [28]. agr locus typing was performed and genetic relatedness was determined by repetitive-element, sequence-based PCR (rep-PCR). Gene encoding of toxins was detected by traditional PCR [28,29] (Figure S1, Table S3).

RNA Preparation and Microarray Hybridization

RNA was processed as described elsewhere [12]. The data are deposited in the NCBI Gene Expression Omnibus (GEO, http://www.ncbi.nlm.nih.gov/geo, GEO Series accession number GSE30119).

Batch Correction

To prevent batch effect between training and test sets, principal variance component analysis (PVCA) was conducted using JMP Genomics (SAS Institute, Cary, NC) to identify sources of batch effect. Cohort number accounted for 58% of the variability observed (Figure S2A) and scatter plot visualization (Figure S2B) with ellipsoids (Figure S2C) revealed strong segregation of samples based on cohort. The batch correction algorithm CombatR [30] was used on the cohort variable to reduce its contribution to the global variance. The batch effect from the cohort was reduced to approximately 0% (Figure S2D, Figure S2E and Figure S2F).

Module Framework Development

This analysis strategy has been described elsewhere [16]. A set of 62 transcriptional modules derived from 410 whole blood gene expression profiles was applied to the dataset described herein. Modules were annotated with Ingenuity Pathway Analysis (IPA) (Ingenuity Systems, Redwood City, CA), Pubmed, iHOP, and Novartis Gene Atlas (http://biogps.gnf.org) databases. Module transcript content and annotations are available online (http://www.biir.net/public_wikis/module_annotation/V2_Trial_8_Modules).

Module-level Analysis

Gene expression levels were compared between patients and healthy controls on a module-by-module basis. The percentage of transcripts showing significant differences (Mann-Whitney, $p<0•05$) in expression was used as an indicator of module activity. Modules containing transcripts with increased expression were represented on a red scale while those containing transcripts with decreased expression were represented on a blue scale. Modules with 15% or less transcripts with significant change in abundance compared to healthy controls were not displayed.

Supporting Information

Figure S1 Characterization of the 63 clinical bacterial isolates. A. Pie charts representing distribution of methicillin resistance, agr locus type and genetic relatedness for the 63 bacterial isolates isolated from culture. **B.** Bar chart representing the percentage of isolates positive for the measured toxins.

Figure S2 Batch correction for the two cohorts of patients used as training and test sets. A. Pie chart of percent contribution of individual parameter to variance from principal variance component analysis (PVCA) before CombatR correction. **B.** Scatter plot representing the segregation of sample by cohort before CombatR correction. **C.** Elliptical fit of scatter plot data from B. **D.** Pie chart of individual parameter's percent contribution to variance from PVCA after CombatR correction for cohort. **E.** Scatter plot representing the segregation of sample by cohort after CombatR correction. **F.** Elliptical fit of scatter plot data from E.

Figure S3 Determination of the best number of K-means clusters from individual patient module expression. An appropriate K was chosen for clustering this dataset using an information theoretic approach called the "jump method". First, the data was clustered for all K 1 to 5, inclusive. **A.** The distortion of each clustering was calculated. In this instance, we chose to approximate the covariance matrix with the identity matrix so the distortion is simply the mean squared error. **B.** Next, the transformed distortion for each K is calculated by raising the distortion to a power of -(# of dimensions/2). **C.** Finally, the Jump at each K is calculated as follows: Jump_K = -TransformedDistortion_K - TransformedDistortion_K-1. The maximum Jump is used to select K, in this case, K = 4.

Figure S4 Module signature per cluster of patients. Module signature was derived for each cluster of molecularly active patients (C1 to C4) and the group of transcriptionally quiescent (TQ) patients as compared to the combined 44 healthy controls.

Figure S5 Cluster of under-expressed modules in the 74 molecularly active patients with *S. aureus* infection.

Figure S6 Cluster C3 displays an erythropoiesis signature. A. Heatmap representing the 680 transcripts differentially expressed between clusters C1 and C3. Statistical comparison between C1 and C3 yielded 680 differentially expressed transcripts (non-parametric test, $\alpha = 0{\cdot}01$, Benjamini-Hochberg multiple testing correction, 2× fold change). Of these, 246 transcripts were over-expressed in C1 and 434 transcripts were over-expressed in C3. **B.** Area chart representing pathways significantly enriched ($p<0{\cdot}05$) in the two gene lists identified in A according to PANTHER (http://www.pantherdb.org). **C.** Area chart representing biological processes significantly enriched ($p<0{\cdot}01$) in the two gene lists identified in A according to PANTHER. **D.** Heatmap representing the top 100 transcripts over or under-expressed in C3 versus C1. **E.** Heatmap representing the expression of 87 transcripts specifically expressed in CD71+ erythroid precursors in the four patient clusters. **F.** Scatter plot of various CBC measurements for patients organized by transcriptionally active clusters C1 through C4 and transcriptionally quiescent (TQ) patients. The green rectangle represents the range of values for healthy children (two months to 18 years) recorded at Childrens Hospital, Dallas.

Figure S7 *S. aureus* patient molecular distance to health varies with infection localization, clinical presentation and blood draw index. A. MDTH as a function of blood draw index for patients grouped by disease localization. B. MDTH as a function of blood draw index for patients grouped by disease presentation. A non-linear regression statistical model (one-phase decay) was applied.

Figure S8 Selection of osteoarticular infection and pneumonia patients for comparison. A. Dot plot of neutrophil counts for patients grouped by clinical presentation. Horizontal bars represent the median value for each group. Non-parametric ANOVA (Kruskal-Wallis) with Dunn's post-hoc test was applied. **B.** Column scatter plot of individual MDTH for patients selected for comparison. Horizontal bars represent the median value for each group. Non-parametric testing (Mann-Whitney) was applied between the two groups of patients.

Table S1 Training set subjects characteristics.

Table S2 Test set subjects characteristics.

Table S3 Characterization of bacterial isolates from 63 patients.

Table S4 Top 50 over-expressed genes in C1 vs. C3 (left) and C3 vs. C1 (right).

Table S5 Clinical parameters for patients grouped by transcriptional clustering.

Table S6 Disease localization, clinical presentation and strain distribution by cluster.

Table S7 Distribution of bacterial isolates characteristics by infection localization, clinical presentation and cluster.

Table S8 Spearman correlations between molecular distance to health (MDTH) and clinical laboratory parameters.

Table S9 Clinical parameters for patients grouped by infection localization.

Table S10 Clinical parameters for patients grouped by clinical presentation.

Acknowledgments

We thank our patients and their parents for agreeing to participate in the study. We thank Evelyn Torres, RN and Juanita Lozano, MD for their efforts in patient enrollment and Gordon Hayward for IT support.

Author Contributions

Conceived and designed the experiments: RB OR DC AJV AM MA CC. Performed the experiments: RB AJV ES PN. Analyzed the data: RB NB HX JRU DB. Contributed reagents/materials/analysis tools: NB ES CC. Wrote the paper: RB AM VP JB DC OR.

References

1. Klevens RM, Morrison MA, Nadle J, Petit S, Gershman K, et al. (2007) Invasive methicillin-resistant Staphylococcus aureus infections in the United States. JAMA: the journal of the American Medical Association 298: 1763–1771.
2. Wallin TR, Hern HG, Frazee BW (2008) Community-associated methicillin-resistant Staphylococcus aureus. Emergency medicine clinics of North America 26: 431–455, ix.
3. Crum NF (2005) The emergence of severe, community-acquired methicillin-resistant Staphylococcus aureus infections. Scandinavian journal of infectious diseases 37: 651–656.
4. Vandenesch F, Naimi T, Enright MC, Lina G, Nimmo GR, et al. (2003) Community-acquired methicillin-resistant Staphylococcus aureus carrying Panton-Valentine leukocidin genes: worldwide emergence. Emerging infectious diseases 9: 978–984.
5. Carleton HA, Diep BA, Charlebois ED, Sensabaugh GF, Perdreau-Remington F (2004) Community-adapted methicillin-resistant Staphylococcus aureus (MRSA): population dynamics of an expanding community reservoir of MRSA. The Journal of infectious diseases 190: 1730–1738.
6. Begier EM, Frenette K, Barrett NL, Mshar P, Petit S, et al. (2004) A high-morbidity outbreak of methicillin-resistant Staphylococcus aureus among players on a college football team, facilitated by cosmetic body shaving and turf burns. Clinical infectious diseases: an official publication of the Infectious Diseases Society of America 39: 1446–1453.
7. Rubinstein E (2008) Staphylococcus aureus bacteraemia with known sources. International journal of antimicrobial agents 32 Suppl 1: S18–20.
8. Vander Have KL, Karmazyn B, Verma M, Caird MS, Hensinger RN, et al. (2009) Community-associated methicillin-resistant Staphylococcus aureus in acute musculoskeletal infection in children: a game changer. Journal of pediatric orthopedics 29: 927–931.
9. Deleo FR, Otto M, Kreiswirth BN, Chambers HF (2010) Community-associated meticillin-resistant Staphylococcus aureus. Lancet 375: 1557–1568.
10. Appelbaum PC (2006) The emergence of vancomycin-intermediate and vancomycin-resistant Staphylococcus aureus. Clinical microbiology and infection: the official publication of the European Society of Clinical Microbiology and Infectious Diseases 12 Suppl 1: 16–23.
11. Ramilo O, Allman W, Chung W, Mejias A, Ardura M, et al. (2007) Gene expression patterns in blood leukocytes discriminate patients with acute infections. Blood 109: 2066–2077.
12. Berry MP, Graham CM, McNab FW, Xu Z, Bloch SA, et al. (2010) An interferon-inducible neutrophil-driven blood transcriptional signature in human tuberculosis. Nature 466: 973–977.
13. Bullinger L, Dohner K, Bair E, Frohling S, Schlenk RF, et al. (2004) Use of gene-expression profiling to identify prognostic subclasses in adult acute myeloid leukemia. The New England journal of medicine 350: 1605–1616.
14. Allantaz F, Chaussabel D, Stichweh D, Bennett L, Allman W, et al. (2007) Blood leukocyte microarrays to diagnose systemic onset juvenile idiopathic arthritis and follow the response to IL-1 blockade. The Journal of experimental medicine 204: 2131–2144.
15. DeLeo FR, Diep BA, Otto M (2009) Host defense and pathogenesis in Staphylococcus aureus infections. Infectious disease clinics of North America 23: 17–34.
16. Chaussabel D, Quinn C, Shen J, Patel P, Glaser C, et al. (2008) A modular analysis framework for blood genomics studies: application to systemic lupus erythematosus. Immunity 29: 150–164.
17. Pankla R, Buddhisa S, Berry M, Blankenship DM, Bancroft GJ, et al. (2009) Genomic transcriptional profiling identifies a candidate blood biomarker signature for the diagnosis of septicemic melioidosis. Genome biology 10: R127.
18. Sugar CA, James GM (2003) Finding the number of clusters in a dataset: An information-theoretic approach. Journal of the American Statistical Association 98: 750–763.
19. Thomas PD, Campbell MJ, Kejariwal A, Mi H, Karlak B, et al. (2003) PANTHER: a library of protein families and subfamilies indexed by function. Genome research 13: 2129–2141.
20. Hinze CH, Fall N, Thornton S, Mo JQ, Aronow BJ, et al. (2010) Immature cell populations and an erythropoiesis gene-expression signature in systemic juvenile idiopathic arthritis: implications for pathogenesis. Arthritis research & therapy 12: R123.
21. Ardura MI, Banchereau R, Mejias A, Di Pucchio T, Glaser C, et al. (2009) Enhanced monocyte response and decreased central memory T cells in children with invasive Staphylococcus aureus infections. PloS one 4: e5446.
22. Scumpia PO, Kelly-Scumpia KM, Delano MJ, Weinstein JS, Cuenca AG, et al. (2010) Cutting edge: bacterial infection induces hematopoietic stem and progenitor cell expansion in the absence of TLR signaling. Journal of immunology 184: 2247–2251.
23. Tanno T, Miller JL (2010) Iron Loading and Overloading due to Ineffective Erythropoiesis. Advances in hematology 2010: 358283.
24. Nairz M, Schroll A, Moschen AR, Sonnweber T, Theurl M, et al. (2011) Erythropoietin contrastingly affects bacterial infection and experimental colitis by inhibiting nuclear factor-kappaB-inducible immune pathways. Immunity 34: 61–74.
25. Nagai T, Devergne O, Mueller TF, Perkins DL, van Seventer JM, et al. (2003) Timing of IFN-beta exposure during human dendritic cell maturation and naive Th cell stimulation has contrasting effects on Th1 subset generation: a role for IFN-beta-mediated regulation of IL-12 family cytokines and IL-18 in naive Th cell differentiation. Journal of immunology 171: 5233–5243.
26. Gonzalez BE, Teruya J, Mahoney DH, Jr., Hulten KG, Edwards R, et al. (2006) Venous thrombosis associated with staphylococcal osteomyelitis in children. Pediatrics 117: 1673–1679.
27. Balamayooran G, Batra S, Fessler MB, Happel KI, Jeyaseelan S (2010) Mechanisms of neutrophil accumulation in the lungs against bacteria. American journal of respiratory cell and molecular biology 43: 5–16.
28. Thomsen I, McKenna BD, Saye EJ, Jimenez N, Edwards KM, et al. (2011) Molecular distinctions exist between community-associated methicillin-resistant Staphylococcus aureus colonization and disease-associated isolates in children. The Pediatric infectious disease journal 30: 418–421.
29. Campbell SJ, Deshmukh HS, Nelson CL, Bae IG, Stryjewski ME, et al. (2008) Genotypic characteristics of Staphylococcus aureus isolates from a multinational trial of complicated skin and skin structure infections. Journal of clinical microbiology 46: 678–684.
30. Chen C, Grennan K, Badner J, Zhang D, Gershon E, et al. (2011) Removing batch effects in analysis of expression microarray data: an evaluation of six batch adjustment methods. PloS one 6: e17238.

23

MicroRNA-146a and Ets-1 Gene Polymorphisms are Associated with Pediatric Uveitis

Lin Wei[1]ⓢ, Qingyun Zhou[1]ⓢ, Shengping Hou[1], Lin Bai[1], Yunjia Liu[1], Jian Qi[1], Qin Xiang[1], Yan Zhou[1], Aize Kijlstra[2], Peizeng Yang[1]*

1 The First Affiliated Hospital of Chongqing Medical University, Chongqing Key Laboratory of Ophthalmology and Chongqing Eye Institute, Chongqing, P. R. China, **2** University Eye Clinic Maastricht, Maastricht, The Netherlands

Abstract

Background: MicroRNA-146a (miR-146a) was a key negative regulator of autoimmunity. V-Ets oncogene homolog 1 (Ets-1) was demonstrated to bind to the miR-146a promoter region and markedly affects miR-146a promoter activity. This study aimed to investigate the association of miR-146a and Ets-1 gene polymorphisms with pediatric uveitis in a Han Chinese population.

Methodology/Principal Findings: A total of 520 patients and 1204 healthy controls were included in the present study. Five single-nucleotide polymorphisms (SNPs), miR-146a/rs2910164, miR-146a/rs57095329, miR-146a/rs6864584, ets-1/rs1128334 and ets-1/rs10893872 were genotyped using a polymerase chain reaction-restriction fragment length polymorphism assay. The expression of Ets-1 in peripheral blood mononuclear cells from genotyped healthy controls was tested by real-time PCR. Two SNPs (rs2910164 and rs10893872) were associated with pediatric uveitis in this study. The frequencies of the rs2910164 GG genotype and G allele were significantly increased ($P_c = 3.11 \times 10^{-4}$; $P_c = 2.75 \times 10^{-6}$) while the CC genotype and C allele were significantly decreased ($P_c = 0.001$; $P_c = 2.75 \times 10^{-6}$) in patients compared with normal controls. The frequencies of the rs10893872 CC genotype and C allele were significantly increased ($P_c = 3.89 \times 10^{-4}$; $P_c = 0.01$) while the CT genotype and T allele were significantly decreased ($P_c = 0.004$; $P_c = 0.01$) in patients compared with normal controls. The SNP rs2910164 GG genotype and G/C allele were also associated with the presence of microvascular leakage as detected by fundus fluorescein angiography in pediatric uveitis ($P_c = 0.01$; $P_c = 0.005$, respectively). Ets-1 expression in rs10893872 CC carriers was significantly higher than in CT and TT individuals ($P_c = 0.013$). There was no association of the other three SNPs with pediatric uveitis.

Conclusions: This study shows that miR-146a and Ets-1 are both associated with pediatric uveitis in Han Chinese. SNP rs10893872 may affect the genetic predisposition to pediatric uveitis by modulating expression of Ets-1.

Editor: Nanette H. Bishopric, University of Miami School of Medicine, United States of America

Funding: This work was supported by National Basic Research Program of China (973 Program)(2011CB510200), Key Project of Natural Science Foundation(81130019), Research Fund for the Doctoral Program of Higher Education of China (20115503110002), Clinic Key Project of Ministry of Health, Basic Research program of Chongqing, Chongqing Key Laboratory of Ophthalmology (CSTC, 2008CA5003), Key Project of Health Bureau of Chongqing(2012-1-003) and Fund for PAR-EU Scholars Program. The authors have declared that no competing interests exist. The funders had no role in study design, data collection and analysis, decision to publish, or preparation of the manuscript.

Competing Interests: The authors have declared that no competing interests exist.

* E-mail: peizengycmu@126.com

ⓢ These authors contributed equally to this work.

Introduction

Uveitis is a potentially sight threatening disease and one of the important causes of blindness in the world. It may occur due to an infection or may be due to an autoimmune etiology [1–3]. Children account for 5%~10% of all uveitis patients [4,5]. Although uveitis is less common in children than in adults, patients with pediatric uveitis more often develop serious complications such as cataract and glaucoma that result in visual loss [4]. Epidemiologic studies indicate that idiopathic uveitis (28.8%) is the most common subtype of pediatric uveitis, followed by juvenile idiopathic arthritis (JIA)-associated uveitis (20.9%) and pars planitis (17.1%) [6]. Fundus fluorescein angiography (FFA), rheumatoid factor (RF) and anti-nuclear antibody (ANA) are considered as important markers for pediatric uveitis [7]. Genetic factors have been reported to be involved in the pathogenesis of pediatric uveitis and a study of 316 Caucasian children demonstrated that human leukocyte antigen (HLA)-A19, HLA-B22 and HLA-DR9 increased the susceptibility of JIA-associated uveitis whereas HLA-DR1 was protective for uveitis development [8]. Other HLA alleles have also been reported to be associated with JIA-associated uveitis such as HLA-DRw5, HLA-DRB1*1104, HLA-DRB1*1301 [8–10]. It is suggested that the genetic factors play important role in pediatric uveitis and investigating proper genetic factors is imperative for pediatric uveitis.

MicroRNAs (miRNAs) are endogenous ~22 nt non-coding RNA molecules that function as negative regulators by targeting mRNAs for cleavage or translational repression, playing critical roles in diverse biologic processes, such as infection, immune response, inflammation and tumorigenesis [11,12]. The microRNA-146a (miR-146a) was reported as a negative regulator of innate immunity in systemic lupus erythematosus (SLE) patients and a key negative regulator of inflammation [13,14]. It was also indicated to be a vital regulator during viral infection [15,16].

The Ets1 transcription factor is a member of the Ets gene family and is highly conserved throughout evolution. It is known to regulate a number of important biological processes in normal cells and in tumors and associated with regulation of immune cell function and with an aggressive behavior in tumors [19,20]. Moreover, Ets1 can bind to the miR-146a promoter region and markedly affects miR-146a promoter activity in vitro. Knockdown of Ets-1 impaired the induction of miR-146a, whereas overexpression of Ets-1 enhanced the induction of miR-146a [21].

Single nucleotide polymorphisms (SNPs), located either in the pre-miRNAs or within miRNA-binding sites, have been shown to affect miRNA target expression, thereby possibly contributing to disease susceptibility [17,18]. Luo et al. identified 12 variants of miR-146a, 9 of which were already reported in the dbSNP database Build 130 [21]. Three variants of these 9 had a minor allele frequency (MAF)>1% (rs2910164, rs57095329, and rs6864584). A recent study showed that SNPs rs1128334 and rs10893872 located in the 3′UTR of Ets-1 were on putative miRNA binding sites and were both associated with SLE in Asian populations [22].

Considering the role of miR-146a in the development of autoimmune diseases and the role of Ets-1 as a regulator of miR-146a expression, we investigated the association of miR-146a/rs2910164, miR-146a/rs57095329, miR-146a/rs6864584, ets-1/rs1128334 and ets-1/rs10893872 with pediatric uveitis in a Han Chinese population. We showed a significant association between both miR-146a and Ets-1 gene polymorphisms and pediatric uveitis in our study population.

Materials and Methods

Study population

The study group comprised 520 consecutive Han Chinese pediatric uveitis patients and 1204 unselected, consecutive, ethnically and geographically matched normal controls. The blood samples of patients and controls were obtained from the Uveitis Study Center of the Sun Yat-sen University (Guangzhou, P.R. China) and the First Affiliated Hospital of Chongqing Medical University (Chongqing, P.R. China). Pediatric uveitis was defined as uveitis first occurring in a child under 16 years old. Children with Behcet's disease, Vogt-Koyanagi-Harada syndrome or with definite infectious uveitis were excluded. JIA was defined as arthritis of unknown etiology presenting in children younger than 16 years old and persisting for at least 6 weeks according to the criteria of International League of Associations for Rheumatology [23]. The study was approved by the Local Ethics Research Committee of the First Affiliated Hospital of Chongqing Medical University. The written informed consent from the guardians on the behalf of minor participants and adult subjects involved in the study were obtained. We adhered to the tenets of the Declaration of Helsinki during all procedures of this study.

Clinical and laboratory observations

Pediatric uveitis patients underwent a uveitis screening protocol encompassing ANA (n = 34; positive rate was 17.8%), RF (n = 32; positive rate was 15.5%), and FFA (n = 192; microvascular leakage rate detected by FFA was found in 62.1% of tested patients). An ANA titer above 1:100 and an RF level above 20.0 IU/ml were considered positive. FFA was considered a positive result when dye leakage from a retinal vessel was observed. All these tests were performed in the First Affiliated Hospital of Chongqing Medical University (Chongqing, P.R. China).

DNA extraction and genotyping

Genomic DNA of patients and healthy controls was extracted by the QIAamp DNA Blood Mini Kit (Qiagen, Hilden, Germany). Amplification of the target DNA sequence was analyzed by polymerase chain reaction (PCR) and the primers used herein are shown in Table 1. Each PCR reaction was carried out in a 10 μl reaction volume containing 5 μl Premix Taq (Ex Taq Version; TaKaRa Biotechnology Co. Ltd., Dalian, China), 20 pmol primers, 0.2 μg genomic DNA and proper sterile purified water. Genotyping of the five tested SNPs was carried out by PCR-restriction fragment length polymorphism (RFLP) analysis. PCR products were digested with 2 U of restriction enzymes which are listed in Table 1. The digestion products were separated on 4% agarose gels and stained with GoldView (SBS Genetech Beijing, China). Moreover, 10% of the samples were randomly selected to confirm the PCR-RFLP results using direct sequencing (Invitrogen Biotechnology Co., Guangzhou, China).

RNA extraction and real-time RCR

Peripheral blood mononuclear cells (PBMCs) were isolated from venous blood of healthy controls by Ficoll-Hypaque density-gradient centrifugation. Total RNA was extracted from PBMCs using TRIzol (Invitrogen, San Diego, California, USA), and then it was reverse transcribed by transcriptase kit (Applied Biosystems, ABI, Foster City, California, USA). Real-time PCR was performed to detect the quantity of Ets-1 mRNA using the Applied Biosystems 7500 Real-Time PCR System (Applied Biosystems, Foster City, CA) with the following primers Ets-1F: 5′-GCAGCCAGTCATCTTTCAACAGCC-3′; Ets-1R: 5′-TCAGCACGGTCCCGCACATA-3′. The β-actin (β-actinF: 5′-GGATGCAGAAGGAGATCACTG-3′ β-actinR: 5′-CGATCCACACGGAGTACTTG-3′) and GAPDH (F: 5′-GGGTGTGAACCATGAGAAGT-3′; R: 5′-GGCATGGACTGTGGTCATGA-3′) were chosen as dual internal reference genes to normalize the expression of Ets-1. Relative expression levels were calculated using the $2^{-\Delta\Delta Ct}$ method.

Statistical analysis

A Hardy–Weinberg equilibrium (HWE) calculation was performed to ensure a balance in genotype and allele distribution between patients and normal controls. HWE was tested in the subjects using the χ^2 test. Genotype and allele frequencies were compared between patients and controls by χ^2 test using SPSS version 17.0 (SPSS, Inc., Chicago, IL). The P values were corrected (Pc) with the Bonferroni correction by multiplying with the number of analyses performed. The odds ratio (OR) was used to determine whether a particular SNP is a risk factor for pediatric uveitis patients, and to compare the magnitude of various SNPs for pediatric uveitis patients (OR = 1: Exposure does not affect odds of pediatric uveitis; OR>1: Exposure associated with higher odds of pediatric uveitis; OR<1: Exposure associated with lower odds of pediatric uveitis) [24]. The independent-samples T test was used to compare Ets-1 expression among three genotype groups. P values <0.05 were considered to be statistically significant.

Table 1. Primers and restriction enzymes used in RFLP analysis.

SNP	Primers	Tm (°C)	Restriction enzymes
rs2910164	5′-ATGGGTTGTGTCAGTGTCAGACAT-3′	58	HSP92II
	5′-TGCCTTCTGTCTCCAGTCTTCCAA-3′		
rs17057381	5′-GTGCTCAGTTACTGTCCATGCACTT-3′	60	AflII
	5′-CAGGCATAGAGGAAGGGGAGATTA-3′		
rs57095329	5′-GGGGCTGCGGAGAGTACCG-3′	60	MspI
	5′-GGACCCTCTTGCAGCACGTGTC-3′		
rs6864584	5′-CGATAAAGCTCTCGGGATTTC-3′	56	ApaI
	5′-TCTTATTTGCTGGGGTAGAGGA-3′		
rs1128334	5′-TATTGTGTTTGACTATTTTCCAACAT-3′	55	HSP92II
	5′-ACTTACATCGCTACATCTCT-3′		
rs10893872	5′-ATCCCAGACCAAACCCAGTA-3′	60	TSP509I
	5′-TGGGCAGTAACAGGCTCTTT-3′		

RFLP, restriction fragment length polymorphism; SNP, single nucleotide polymorphism.

Results

Clinical features of pediatric uveitis patients and normal controls

Detailed clinical findings of the enrolled pediatric uveitis patients and normal controls were presented in Table 2. Age and gender distribution in pediatric uveitis patients and normal controls were also described in Table 2. Only category of JIA-associated uveitis (n = 70) can be confirmed in our study. Other cases cannot be confirmed in which category of pediatric uveitis.

Genotype and allele frequencies of SNPs in patients and controls

A total of 5 SNPs of miR-146a and Ets-1 were successfully genotyped in 520 pediatric uveitis patients and 1204 normal controls. The distribution of genotype frequencies of 5 SNPs were accorded with HWE in the controls. Altogether we found two SNPs (rs2910164 and rs10893872) that were associated with pediatric uveitis (Table 3). The frequencies of the rs2910164 CC genotype and C allele in pediatric uveitis patients were significantly lower than that in normal controls ($P = 8.93\times10^{-5}$, $P_c = 0.001$, OR = 0.646; $P = 5.50\times10^{-7}$, $P_c = 2.75\times10^{-6}$, OR = 0.686, respectively). While the frequencies of the rs2910164 GG genotype and G allele were significantly higher in pediatric uveitis patients compared to normal controls ($P = 2.07\times10^{-5}$, $P_c = 3.11\times10^{-4}$, OR = 1.773; $P = 5.50\times10^{-7}$, $P_c = 2.75\times10^{-6}$, OR = 1.457, respectively). In SNP rs10893872, the frequencies of the CC genotype and C allele were significantly increased ($P = 2.59\times10^{-5}$, $P_c = 3.89\times10^{-4}$, OR = 1.582; P = 0.002, $P_c = 0.01$, OR = 1.259) in patients compared to controls while the CT genotype and T allele were significantly decreased in patients compared to controls ($P = 2.63\times10^{-4}$, $P_c = 0.004$, OR = 0.680; P = 0.002, $P_c = 0.01$, OR = 0.794). There was no statistically significant difference concerning the genotype and allele of the other three SNPs between pediatric uveitis patients and controls (Table 3).

Table 2. Age, gender and clinical features distribution in pediatric uveitis patients and controls.

Clinical features	%	
Pediatric uveitis patients	n = 520	
Age	9.6±3.6	
Male	242	46.5
Female	278	53.5
Uveitis	520	100
Pediatric uveitis with JIA	70	13.5
FFA(+)	192(309 tested)	62.1
ANA(+)	34(191 tested)	17.8
RF(+)	32(206 tested)	15.5
Controls	n = 1204	
Mean age	34.8±11.4	
Male	545	45.3
Female	659	54.7

JIA, juvenile idiopathic arthritis; FFA, fundus fluorescein angiography; ANA, anti-nuclear antigen; RF, rheumatoid factor.

We subsequently studied the associations of the 5 SNPs with clinical and laboratory observations of pediatric uveitis including FFA, RF and ANA. An association was found between rs2910164 and patients with microvascular leakage as detected by FFA (FFA^+). The GG genotype and G allele frequencies of rs2910164 were significantly increased in FFA^+ patients compared to controls ($P = 6.84\times10^{-4}$, $P_c = 0.01$, OR = 1.899; $P = 9.41\times10^{-4}$, $P_c = 0.005$, OR = 1.441) while the C allele frequency was significantly decreased ($P = 9.41\times10^{-4}$, $P_c = 0.005$, OR = 0.694) (Table 4). No statistically significant association was found between the other four SNPs and FFA^+ patients. Moreover, there was no statistically significant association between the five SNPs and patient groups that were subdivided according to their RF or ANA status or whether they had JIA or not (data not shown).

The influence of rs10893872 on Ets-1 expression

Because a significant association was found between SNP rs10893872 and pediatric uveitis patients, we further tested the expression of Ets-1 in PBMCs obtained from 32 healthy individuals with a known genotype for this SNP. The mean

Table 3. Frequencies of genotypes and alleles of microRNA (miR)-146a and Ets-1 polymorphisms in pediatric uveitis patients and controls.

SNP	Genotyp Allele	Pediatric uveitis (n = 520)	Controls (n = 1204)	χ2	p value	pc value	OR (95% CI)
rs2910164	GG	113(0.217)	163(0.135)	18.127	2.07×10^{-5}	3.11×10^{-4}	1.773 (1.359–2.313)
	GC	248(0.477)	553(0.459)	0.453	0.501	NS	1.073(0.873–1.319)
	CC	159(0.306)	488(0.405)	15.350	8.93×10^{-5}	0.001	0.646(0.519–0.805)
	G	474(0.456)	879(0.365)	25.080	5.50×10^{-7}	2.75×10^{-6}	1.457(1.257–1.688)
	C	566(0.544)	1529(0.635)	25.080	5.50×10^{-7}	2.75×10^{-6}	0.686(0.592–0.796)
rs57095329	AA	317(0.609)	801(0.665)	4.937	0.026	NS	0.786(0.635–0.972)
	AG	184(0.354)	372(0.309)	3.347	0.067	NS	1.225(0.985–1.522)
	GG	19(0.037)	31(0.026)	1.502	0.220	NS	1.435(0.803–2.564)
	A	818(0.787)	1974(0.820)	5.206	0.023	NS	0.810(0.676–0.971)
	G	222(0.213)	434(0.180)	5.206	0.023	NS	1.234 (1.030–1.479)
rs6864584	CC	2(0.004)	5(0.004)	0.008	0.927	NS	0.926(0.179–4.788)
	CT	39(0.075)	112(0.093)	1.476	0.224	NS	0.791(0.541–1.156)
	TT	479(0.921)	1087(0.903)	1.466	0.226	NS	1.257(0.867–1.823)
	C	43 (0.041)	122(0.051)	1.384	0.239	NS	0.808(0.566–1.153)
	T	997(0.959)	2286(0.949)	1.384	0.239	NS	1.237(0.867–1.766)
rs1128334	AA	64(0.123)	145(0.120)	0.024	0.877	NS	1.025(0.749–1.403)
	AG	253(0.487)	544(0.452)	1.760	0.185	NS	1.150(0.936–1.413)
	GG	203(0.390)	515(0.428)	2.085	0.149	NS	0.857(0.694–1.057)
	A	381(0.366)	834(0.346)	1.273	0.259	NS	1.091(0.938–1.270)
	G	659(0.634)	1574(0.654)	1.273	0.259	NS	0.916(0.788–1.066)
rs10893872	CC	209(0.402)	359(0.298)	17.695	2.59×10^{-5}	3.89×10^{-4}	1.582(1.277–1.960)
	CT	218(0.419)	620(0.515)	13.320	2.63×10^{-4}	0.004	0.680(0.552–0.837)
	TT	93(0.179)	225(0.187)	0.156	0.693	NS	0.948(0.726–1.238)
	C	636(0.612)	1338(0.556)	9.270	0.002	0.01	1.259(1.085–1.460)
	T	404(0.388)	1070(0.444)	9.270	0.002	0.01	0.794(0.685–0.921)

pc, Bonferroni corrected p value; OR, odds ratio; NS, not significant; SNP, single nucleotide polymorphism.

Table 4. Genotype and allele frequency analysis of rs2910164 polymorphism in FFA positive pediatric uveitis patients.

SNP	Genotyp Allele	FFA^+ pediatric uveitis (n = 192)	Controls (n = 1204)	χ2	p value	pc value	OR (95% CI)
rs2910164	GG	44(0.229)	163(0.135)	11.533	6.84×10^{-4}	0.01	1.899(1.305–2.762)
	GC	86(0.448)	553(0.459)	0.086	0.769	NS	0.955(0.703–1.297)
	CC	62(0.323)	488(0.405)	4.709	0.030	NS	0.700(0.506–0.967)
	G	174(0.453)	879(0.365)	10.941	9.41×10^{-4}	0.005	1.441(1.160–1.791)
	C	210(0.547)	1529(0.635)	10.941	9.41×10^{-4}	0.005	0.694(0.558–0.862)

pc, Bonferroni corrected p value; OR, odds ratio; NS, not significant; SNP, single nucleotide polymorphism.

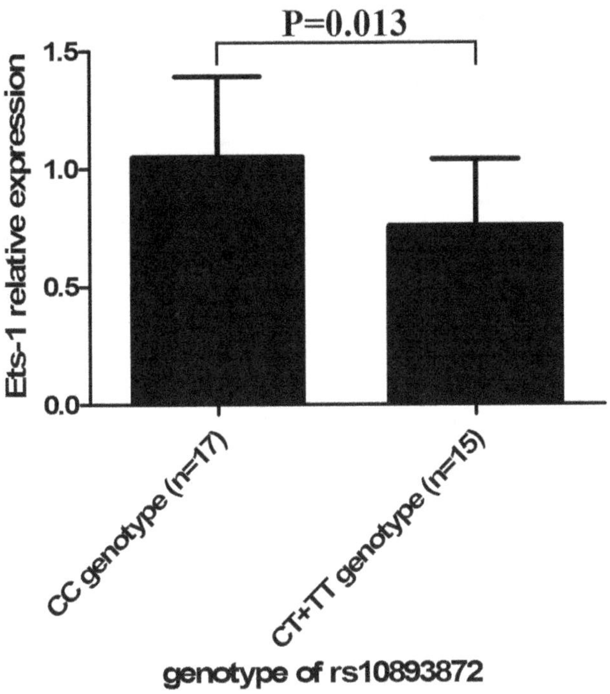

Figure 1. The relative expression of Ets-1. Ets-1 expression with three different genotypes of single nucleotide polymorphism (SNP) rs10893872 in peripheral blood mononuclear cells obtained from genotyped healthy controls (PBMCs). Real-time PCR analysis of Ets-1 expression in PBMCs derived from healthy individuals of SNP rs10893872 CC, CT and TT genotypes. The y axis represents relative Ets-1 expression level by real-time PCR of each genotype of SNP rs10893872. Data are shown as mean±SD.

expression of Ets-1 in CC carriers was 1.39-fold higher than that in CT and TT carriers (P = 0.013) (Figure 1).

Discussion

In the present study, we investigated the association of five SNPs of miR-146a and the transcription factor Ets-1 with pediatric uveitis patients in a Chinese Han population. To the best of our knowledge, this is the first study to investigate the possible associations of miR-146a and Ets-1 polymorphisms with pediatric uveitis. It was found that rs2910164 of miR-146a and rs10893872 of Ets-1 were both associated with pediatric uveitis. The expression of Ets-1 in individuals carrying the rs10893872 CC genotype was increased compared to the CT and TT genotype, suggesting a functional explanation for the observed association.

The frequencies of the rs2910164 CC genotype and C allele were significantly decreased in patients as compared to normal controls while the GG genotype and G allele were significantly increased. It was suggested that miR-146a might be a susceptibility factor for pediatric uveitis. Recently, we studied the miR-146a rs2910164 polymorphisms in acute anterior uveitis patients with ankylosing spondylitis and found a similar association as shown in the present work for pediatric uveitis patients [25]. Several similar results were also reported in ocular Behçet's disease [26], asthma [27] and various types of carcinoma [28–30]. Nevertheless, three SNPs of miR-146a/rs2910164, ets-1/rs1128334, and ets-1/rs10893872 were genotyped in Han Chinese patients with Fuchs uveitis syndrome (FUS), and no significant difference could be found between patients and the normal controls [31]. This is different with results found herein. Moreover, afunctional analysis performed in our previous study showed that carriers of the protective CC genotype showed a decreased expression of miR-146a and certain proinflammatory cytokines such as IL-17, TNF-α and IL-1β [26]. These results suggest that the rs2910164 CC genotype and C allele and GG genotype and G allele are common predisposing factors for pediatric uveitis despite the fact that the pathogenic mechanisms underlying cancer and pediatric uveitis are totally different.

We also identified an association between SNP rs10893872 of Ets-1 and pediatric uveitis in the present study. The CC genotype and C allele frequencies of this SNP were significantly increased in patients compared to controls while the frequencies of the CT genotype and T allele were significantly decreased, indicating that the CC genotype and C allele were predisposing factors for pediatric uveitis. Based on this association, we further designed a study to investigate whether this SNP (rs10893872) affected the expression of Ets-1. Our study demonstrated that the Ets-1 expression was significantly upregulated in healthy individuals carrying the CC genotype of rs10893872. We performed this assay in healthy individuals since immunosuppressive treatment in the patient group could possibly alter gene expression. SNP rs10893872 of Ets-1 was found to be highly associated with SLE [22,32]. Differently, there was no significant association of SNP rs10893872 of Ets-1 found in ocular Behçet's disease, Vogt–Koyanagi–Harada syndrome, and Fuchs uveitis syndrome in Chinese Han patients with previous works [26,31].

The transcription factor Ets-1, originally discovered as an oncogene (v-ets) within the genome of the avian leukemia virus [33], shows a dual nature in autoimmune diseases [34]. It was reported to be overexpressed in rheumatoid arthritis (RA) synovial membrane and to be involved in the destructive pathway of RA [35]. Nevertheless, the expression of Ets-1 in SLE was lower in PBMCs as compared with that of healthy subjects [36]. Ets-1 also plays important roles in regulating the differentiation of T helper cell subsets, cytotoxic T cells, B cells and other cell types, and controlling the expression of cytokine and chemokine genes in a wide variety of different cellular contexts [37]. The regulatory T cell (Treg) lineage is a key player maintaining peripheral self-tolerance and modulating almost any type of immune responses. Julia K. Polansky *et. al.* have proposed that Ets-1 binds to the CpG-rich Treg specific demethylated region only in its demethylated state, thereby restricting stable Foxp3 expression to the Treg lineage [38]. Concerning the important roles of Ets-1, the increased frequency of the rs10893872 CC genotype in patients and the increased expression of Ets-1 in CC genotype carriers suggest that Ets-1 is a predisposing factor in pediatric uveitis.

It is worthwhile to mention that there are several limitations in the present study. The sample of patients in our study is relatively small and only Han Chinese cohorts are included. Therefore, the results observed in this study need to be confirmed using a large sample size and should include other ethnic populations. We have not investigated whether the SNP rs10893872 influencing Ets-1 expression can also affect the production of cytokines importantly involved in pediatric uveitis development. Further studies are needed to clarify this issue.

In conclusion, our study has identified the associations of rs2910164 (miR-146a) and rs10893872 (Ets-1) with pediatric uveitis. Furthermore, our study has suggested that SNP rs10893872 may affect the genetic predisposition to this disease possibly through modulating the expression of Ets-1.

Acknowledgments

The authors would like to thank all donors enrolled in the present study.

Author Contributions

Conceived and designed the experiments: LW QZ PY. Performed the experiments: LW LB YL. Analyzed the data: LW SH JQ. Contributed reagents/materials/analysis tools: YZ QX. Wrote the paper: LW PY AK.

References

1. Babu K, Mahendradas P (2013) Medical Management of Uveitis–Current Trends. Indian journal of ophthalmology 61: 277.
2. Clarke LA, Guex-Crosier Y, Hofer M (2013) Epidemiology of uveitis in children over a 10-year period. Clin Exp Rheumatol 31: 633–637.
3. Lerman MA, Burnham JM, Chang PY, Daniel E, Foster CS, et al. (2013) Response of pediatric uveitis to tumor necrosis factor-alpha inhibitors. J Rheumatol 40: 1394–1403.
4. Cunningham J, Emmett T (2000) Uveitis in children. Ocular immunology and inflammation 8: 251–261.
5. Päivönsalo-Hietanen T, Tuominen J, Matti Saari K (2000) Uveitis in children: Population-based study in Finland. Acta ophthalmologica Scandinavica 78: 84–88.
6. Smith JA, Mackensen F, Sen H, Leigh JF, Watkins AS, et al. (2009) Epidemiology and course of disease in childhood uveitis. Ophthalmology 116: 1544–1551. e1541.
7. Tugal-Tutkun I (2011) Pediatric uveitis. Journal of Ophthalmic & Vision Research 6: 259.
8. Zulian F, Martini G, Falcini F, Gerloni V, Zannin ME, et al. (2002) Early predictors of severe course of uveitis in oligoarticular juvenile idiopathic arthritis. The Journal of rheumatology 29: 2446–2453.
9. Melin-Aldana H, Giannini EH, Taylor J, Lovell DJ, Levinson JE, et al. (1992) Human leukocyte antigen-DRB1* 1104 in the chronic iridocyclitis of pauciarticular juvenile rheumatoid arthritis. The Journal of pediatrics 121: 56–60.
10. Zeggini E, Packham J, Donn R, Wordsworth P, Hall A, et al. (2006) Association of HLA-DRB1* 13 with susceptibility to uveitis in juvenile idiopathic arthritis in two independent data sets. Rheumatology 45: 972–974.
11. Bartel DP (2004) MicroRNAs: genomics, biogenesis, mechanism, and function. Cell 116: 281–297.
12. Bushati N, Cohen SM (2007) microRNA functions. Annu Rev Cell Dev Biol 23: 175–205.
13. Boldin MP, Taganov KD, Rao DS, Yang L, Zhao JL, et al. (2011) miR-146a is a significant brake on autoimmunity, myeloproliferation, and cancer in mice. The Journal of experimental medicine 208: 1189–1201.
14. Tang Y, Luo X, Cui H, Ni X, Yuan M, et al. (2009) MicroRNA-146a contributes to abnormal activation of the type I interferon pathway in human lupus by targeting the key signaling proteins. Arthritis & Rheumatism 60: 1065–1075.
15. Hou J, Wang P, Lin L, Liu X, Ma F, et al. (2009) MicroRNA-146a feedback inhibits RIG-I-dependent Type I IFN production in macrophages by targeting TRAF6, IRAK1, and IRAK2. The Journal of Immunology 183: 2150–2158.
16. Cameron JE, Yin Q, Fewell C, Lacey M, McBride J, et al. (2008) Epstein-Barr virus latent membrane protein 1 induces cellular MicroRNA miR-146a, a modulator of lymphocyte signaling pathways. Journal of virology 82: 1946–1958.
17. Clop A, Marcq F, Takeda H, Pirottin D, Tordoir X, et al. (2006) A mutation creating a potential illegitimate microRNA target site in the myostatin gene affects muscularity in sheep. Nature genetics 38: 813–818.
18. Yu Z, Li Z, Jolicoeur N, Zhang L, Fortin Y, et al. (2007) Aberrant allele frequencies of the SNPs located in microRNA target sites are potentially associated with human cancers. Nucleic acids research 35: 4535–4541.
19. Dittmer J (2003) The biology of the Ets1 proto-oncogene. Mol Cancer 2: 29.
20. Garrett-Sinha LA (2013) Review of Ets1 structure, function, and roles in immunity. Cell Mol Life Sci 70: 3375–3390.
21. Luo X, Yang W, Ye D-Q, Cui H, Zhang Y, et al. (2011) A functional variant in microRNA-146a promoter modulates its expression and confers disease risk for systemic lupus erythematosus. PLoS Genetics 7: e1002128.
22. Yang W, Shen N, Ye D-Q, Liu Q, Zhang Y, et al. (2010) Genome-wide association study in Asian populations identifies variants in ETS1 and WDFY4 associated with systemic lupus erythematosus. PLoS Genetics 6: e1000841.
23. Petty RE, Southwood TR, Manners P, Baum J, Glass DN, et al. (2004) International League of Associations for Rheumatology classification of juvenile idiopathic arthritis: second revision, Edmonton, 2001. The Journal of rheumatology 31: 390.
24. Szumilas M (2010) Explaining odds ratios. Journal of the Canadian Academy of Child and Adolescent Psychiatry 19: 227.
25. Qi J, Hou S, Zhang Q, Liao D, Wei L, et al. (2013) A functional variant of pre-miRNA-196a2 confers risk for Behcet's disease but not for Vogt–Koyanagi–Harada syndrome or AAU in ankylosing spondylitis. Human genetics: 1–10.
26. Zhou Q, Hou S, Liang L, Li X, Tan X, et al. (2012) MicroRNA-146a and Ets-1 gene polymorphisms in ocular Behçet's disease and Vogt–Koyanagi–Harada syndrome. Annals of the rheumatic diseases.
27. Jiménez-Morales S, Gamboa-Becerra R, Baca V, Río-Navarro D, López-Ley D, et al. (2012) MiR-146a polymorphism is associated with asthma but not with systemic lupus erythematosus and juvenile rheumatoid arthritis in Mexican patients. Tissue Antigens 9999.
28. Guo H, Wang K, Xiong G, Hu H, Wang D, et al. (2010) A functional varient in microRNA-146a is associated with risk of esophageal squamous cell carcinoma in Chinese Han. Familial cancer 9: 599–603.
29. Jazdzewski K, Murray EL, Franssila K, Jarzab B, Schoenberg DR, et al. (2008) Common SNP in pre-miR-146a decreases mature miR expression and predisposes to papillary thyroid carcinoma. Proceedings of the National Academy of Sciences 105: 7269–7274.
30. Zhou F, Zhu H, Luo D, Wang M, Dong X, et al. (2012) A Functional Polymorphism in Pre-miR-146a Is Associated with Susceptibility to Gastric Cancer in a Chinese Population. DNA and Cell Biology 31: 1290–1295.
31. Zhou Q, Kijlstra A, Hou S, Yu H, Zhang X, et al. (2012) Lack of association of miR-146a and Ets-1 gene polymorphisms with Fuchs uveitis syndrome in Chinese Han patients. Mol Vis 18: 426–430.
32. Zhang J, Zhang Y, Zhang L, Yang J, Ying D, et al. (2013) Epistatic Interaction between Genetic Variants in Susceptibility Gene ETS1 Correlates with IL-17 Levels in SLE Patients. Annals of human genetics.
33. Nunn MF, Seeburg PH, Moscovici C, Duesberg PH (1983) Tripartite structure of the avian erythroblastosis virus E26 transforming gene.
34. Leng R-X, Pan H-F, Chen G-M, Feng C-C, Fan Y-G, et al. (2011) The dual nature of Ets-1: focus to the pathogenesis of systemic lupus erythematosus. Autoimmunity reviews 10: 439–443.
35. Redlich K, Kiener HP, Schett G, Tohidast-Akrad M, Selzer E, et al. (2001) Overexpression of transcription factor Ets-1 in rheumatoid arthritis synovial membrane: Regulation of expression and activation by interleukin-1 and tumor necrosis factor α. Arthritis & Rheumatism 44: 266–274.
36. LI Y, SUN L-D, LU W-S, HU W-L, GAO J-P, et al. (2010) Expression analysis of ETS1 gene in peripheral blood mononuclear cells with systemic lupus erythematosus by real-time reverse transcription PCR. Chinese medical journal 123: 2287–2288.
37. Russell L, Garrett-Sinha LA (2010) Transcription factor Ets-1 in cytokine and chemokine gene regulation. Cytokine 51: 217–226.
38. Polansky JK, Schreiber L, Thelemann C, Ludwig L, Krüger M, et al. (2010) Methylation matters: binding of Ets-1 to the demethylated Foxp3 gene contributes to the stabilization of Foxp3 expression in regulatory T cells. Journal of molecular medicine 88: 1029–1040.

Campylobacter Infection in Children in Malawi is Common and is Frequently Associated with Enteric Virus Co-Infections

Jenifer Mason[1], Miren Iturriza-Gomara[1], Sarah J. O'Brien[1], Bagrey M. Ngwira[2], Winifred Dove[1], Martin C. J. Maiden[3], Nigel A. Cunliffe[1]*

1 Institute of Infection and Global Health, University of Liverpool, Liverpool, United Kingdom, 2 Department of Community Health, College of Medicine, University of Malawi, Blantyre, Malawi, 3 Department of Zoology, University of Oxford, Oxford, United Kingdom

Abstract

Background: *Campylobacter* species are the most common cause of bacterial gastroenteritis in the developed world. However, comparatively few studies have determined the epidemiological features of campylobacteriosis in resource-poor settings.

Methods: A total of 1,941 faecal specimens collected from symptomatic (diarrhoeic) children and 507 specimens from asymptomatic (non-diarrhoeic) children hospitalised in Blantyre, Malawi, between 1997 and 2007, and previously tested for the presence of rotavirus and norovirus, was analysed for *C. jejuni* and *C. coli* using a real time PCR assay.

Results: *Campylobacter* species were detected in 415/1,941 (21%) of diarrhoeic children, with *C. jejuni* accounting for 85% of all cases. The median age of children with *Campylobacter* infection was 11 months (range 0.1–55 months), and was significantly higher than that for children with rotavirus and norovirus (6 months and 7 months respectively; $P<0.001$). Co-infection with either rotavirus or norovirus was noted in 41% of all cases in the diarrhoeic group. In contrast, the detection rate of *Campylobacter* in the non-diarrhoeic group was 14%, with viral co-infection identified in 16% of children with *Campylobacter*. There was no association between *Campylobacter* detection rate and season over the 10 year period.

Discussion: Using molecular detection methodology in hospitalised Malawian children, we have demonstrated a high prevalence of *Campylobacter* infection, with frequent viral co-infection. The burden of *Campylobacter* infection in young African children may be greater than previously recognised.

Editor: Georgina L. Hold, University of Aberdeen, United Kingdom

Funding: The study was funded by the University of Liverpool. The funders had no role in study design, data collection and analysis, decision to publish, or preparation of the manuscript.

Competing Interests: The authors have declared that no competing interests exist.

* E-mail: N.A.Cunliffe@liverpool.ac.uk

Introduction

It is estimated that 3.552 million children under the age of five years die each year in Africa; diarrhoeal disease accounts for 11% of these deaths [1]. Diarrhoea also contributes to childhood morbidity, particularly malnutrition and growth stunting [2,3]. The introduction of intervention strategies, such as provision of oral rehydration therapy, has had a positive impact on reducing childhood diarrhoea mortality, with an estimated annual reduction of diarrhoeal deaths in Africa since 2000 of 3.7% [1]; however diarrhoea remains a leading cause of child mortality and morbidity in this region. The importance of pathogens such as rotavirus and enterotoxigenic *Escherichia coli* in the aetiology of severe childhood diarrhoea in developing countries is well recognised [4,5]. However the role of *Campylobacter* is less well understood.

Campylobacter is a fastidious gram negative bacterium and *C. jejuni* and *C. coli* are considered the most common cause of bacterial gastroenteritis in the developed world. The clinical presentation ranges from mild watery to severe inflammatory diarrhoea which may be complicated by post infectious sequelae such as Guillain-Barré Syndrome [6]. Using bacterial culture methodology, estimates of the prevalence of *Campylobacter* infection in young children with diarrhoea in Sub Saharan Africa range from 1.5% to 18% [7,8,9,10,11]. While molecular techniques have been developed and employed for *Campylobacter* detection in epidemiological studies in developed countries, such methods have not been widely adopted in Sub Saharan Africa. Where molecular detection (notably PCR) was used to examine for *Campylobacter* species in adults and children with diarrhoea in South Africa the prevalence estimates of *C. jejuni*, *C. coli* and *C. concisus* were 12%, 7.5% and 2.7% respectively; however only 34 of the 255 samples analysed were from children <5 years of age [12].

As part of a long-term research programme investigating viral gastroenteritis in children in Malawi, we have collected stool samples since 1997 from children <5 years of age admitted to the Queen Elizabeth Central Hospital (QECH), Blantyre, Malawi with moderate to severe diarrhoea [5]. We have now examined stored faecal specimens using a real time PCR assay to determine the prevalence and epidemiological features of *Campylobacter* infection in this population.

Methods

Ethics Statement

Written, informed consent was obtained from the child's parent or guardian prior to enrolment. Ethical approval was obtained from the Malawi National Health Sciences Research Committee.

Study Site

The QECH is a large government run tertiary referral hospital in the southern Malawian city of Blantyre, which has a population of approximately 1 million living in urban and peri-urban settlements.

Specimen Collection

Enrolment and data collection procedures have previously been described in detail [5]. Briefly, children age <5 years admitted to the QECH with ≥3 loose or watery stools within a 24 hour period for <14 days, were eligible for inclusion. Children were enrolled Monday to Friday, 9 am to 5 pm, from 1st July 1997 to 30th June 2007. A second group of children <5 years of age without diarrhoea, who were admitted to the QECH with conditions such as malaria and respiratory infections, were enrolled between 1997 and 1999. A single faecal specimen was obtained from each child. Clinical data (illness severity, blood in stools etc.) were not routinely gathered. Following EIA testing for rotavirus [5], remaining samples were shipped to the University of Liverpool and stored at −80°C until testing for norovirus by real time PCR [13] and for *Campylobacter* (this study).

Campylobacter Testing

Of 2,458 faecal specimens collected from hospitalised diarrhoeic children in the primary study [5], 1,941 were available for testing for *Campylobacter* infection, together with 507 samples from children admitted to hospital without diarrhoea. DNA was extracted from all samples using an automated extractor (Qiasymphony, Qiagen). The presence of a 95 base pair fragment of the *mapA* gene of *C. jejuni* and a 103 base pair fragment of the *ceuE* gene of *C. coli* were detected using a real time PCR method [14].

Statistical Analysis

Data were analysed using "IBM SPSS Statistics Data Editor" version 11. Categorical data were analysed using Chi^2 test and continuous data using paired T-tests. A *p*-value of <0.05 was considered significant.

Results

Characteristics of the Study Population

In total 2,448 samples was analysed; 1,941 from diarrhoeic children and 507 from non-diarrhoeic children. The median age of children in the diarrhoeic group was 9 months (range 0–55 months) and in the non-diarrhoeic group was 6 months (range 1–50 months). The diarrhoeic group contained 55% males and the non-diarrhoeic group 52% males.

Prevalence

Over the 10 year study period (1997–2007) *Campylobacter* was detected in 415/1941 (21%) of diarrhoeic specimens. For the two year period (1997–1999) in which faecal specimens from non-diarrhoeic children were collected, the detection rate of *Campylobacter* was significantly higher in the diarrhoeic specimens than the non-diarrhoeic specimens (28% vs. 14%; $p<0.001$) (Table 1). Of the *Campylobacter* species detected between 1997 and 1999, *C. coli* comprised 10% and 4% of all *Campylobacter* from diarrhoeic and non-diarrhoeic specimens respectively ($p<0.001$). There was no statistical difference in the *Campylobacter* cycle threshold values obtained from diarrhoeic vs. non-diarrhoeic specimens (data not shown).

Age Distribution

The median age of children with diarrhoea in whom *Campylobacter* was detected was 11 months (range 0.1–55 months) which was higher than the age of children with rotavirus or norovirus (median age 6 months and 7 months respectively ($p<0.001$)). The detection rate of *Campylobacter* was relatively constant across all age groups, in contrast to the detection rate of rotavirus and norovirus which decreased with age (Figure 1). The median age of non-diarrhoeic children with *Campylobacter* infection was 11 months (range 1–34 months); the detection rate increased from 5% of children in the 0–2 month age group to 20% of children age >18 months (Table 1).

Viral Co-infections

In the diarrhoeic group 40% of children with *Campylobacter* had an enteric virus co-infection. These co-infections occurred predominantly in children <1 year of age with 50% of all *Campylobacter* cases in this age group also having either rotavirus or norovirus in the specimen. In the non-diarrhoeic group 16% of children with *Campylobacter* in the specimen also had a viral co-infection (Table 1). Although the overall prevalence of *Campylobacter* was significantly higher in the diarrhoeic than in the non-diarrhoeic group, when single infections were considered (i.e. in the absence of either rotavirus or norovirus) this difference is less pronounced (*Campylobacter* detection rate of 16% in the diarrhoeic vs. 11% in the non-diarrhoeic group, $p=0.02$).

Seasonality

The detection rate of *Campylobacter* did not vary consistently by month or season of specimen collection during the 10 year study period. In total 49% of *Campylobacter* positive specimens in the diarrhoeic group occurred in the dry season (May to October) and 51% in the wet season (November to April). In the non-diarrhoeic group 41% and 59% of positive specimens occurred in the dry and wet season respectively ($p=0.89$; data not shown).

Discussion

In this large study of *Campylobacter* infection in Malawian children, using a sensitive molecular assay we documented *Campylobacter* in 21% of specimens obtained from children <5 years of age hospitalised with diarrhoea. There are no previous data describing the prevalence of *Campylobacter* infection in Malawi. Estimates of the prevalence of *Campylobacter* infection in hospitalised children <5 years of age with diarrhoea in Sub Saharan Africa range from 1.5% in Botswana [12], 1.7% in Mozambique [8], 9% in Uganda [7], 11% in The Central African Republic [9] to 18% in Tanzania [10]. In community settings the detection rate of *Campylobacter* in diarrhoeal faecal specimens among children <5 years of age has been estimated at 15.9% in The Central African Republic [15], 3.3% in Djibouti [16] and 0.8% in Guinea-Bissau [17]. This variation in detection rate across Sub Saharan Africa may reflect the technical difficulties of isolating *Campylobacter*

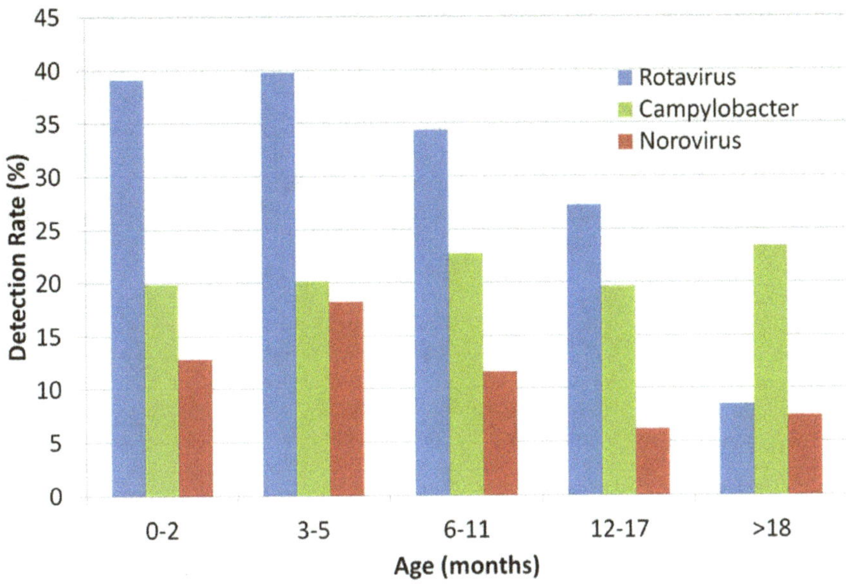

Figure 1. Age distribution of *Campylobacter*, rotavirus and norovirus infections in Malawian children with acute diarrhoea, 1997–2007.

species in resource poor settings because of its fastidious growth requirements and/or the relative insensitivity of some culture techniques.

Comparing culture and PCR in the detection of *C. jejuni* and *C. coli* in diarrhoeal faecal specimens in Ireland suggested that culture alone detected only 55% of all cases [18]. In the UK, *Campylobacter* detection rates in community diarrhoea cases increased from 4.0% by direct culture, to 5.0% after a faecal enrichment procedure was added, to 15% by PCR [19]. A study in South Africa of 255 adults and children with diarrhoea and 67 children without diarrhoea, demonstrated similar overall rates of *Campylobacter* using PCR to those reported in the current Malawi study (19.6% in symptomatic patients and 11% in asymptomatic patients) [12]; however the prevalence in children <5 years of age with diarrhoea was 11% compared with 21% in the current study. Thus our data suggest that the detection rate of *C. jejuni* and *C. coli* using a sensitive and specific PCR assay in faecal specimens of children <5 years of age hospitalised with diarrhoea in Sub Saharan Africa may be higher than previously reported.

Of note, we documented a relative over-representation of *C. coli* compared with *C. jejuni* in the faecal specimens of diarrhoeic compared with non-diarrhoeic children. A similar pattern was reported in Tanzania where *C. coli* was present in 20% of diarrhoeic and 6% of non-diarrhoeic specimens from adults and

Table 1. Age Distribution of *Campylobacter* infection.

	Age Group	Total	*Campylobacter* positive	*Campylobacter*+virus	*Campylobacter* alone
Diarrhoeic (1997–2007)	0–2 months	156	31 (20%)	20 (13%)	11 (7%)
	3–5 months	412	83 (20%)	43 (10%)	40 (10%)
	6–11 months	673	153 (23%)	70 (10%)	83 (12%)
	12–17 months	418	82 (20%)	28 (7%)	54 (13%)
	>18 months	282	66 (23%)	7 (2%)	59 (21%)
	Total : 1997–1999	738	206 (28%)	87 (12%)	119 (16%)
	Total: 1997–2007	1941	415 (21%)	168 (9%)	247 (13%)
Non-diarrhoeic (1997–1999)	0–2 months	140	7 (5%)	0	7 (5%)
	3–5 months	104	14 (13%)	0	14 (13%)
	6–11 months	81	15 (19%)	6 (7%)	9 (11%)
	12–17 months	80	12 (15%)	2 (3%)	10 (13%)
	>18 months	102	21(21%)	3 (3%)	18 (18%)
	Total: 1997–1999	507	69 (14%)	11 (2%)	58 (11%)
χ^2 (Diarrhoeic vs. non-diarrhoeic 1997–1999)			35.7	38.3	5.4
***p* value**			<0.001	<0.001	0.02

children [10]. In the developed world *C. coli* is particularly associated with chicken [20] and the over-representation of *C. coli* in children with diarrhoea raises the possibility that poultry may be a particularly important source of infection in this group. *Campylobacter spp.* other than *C. jejuni* and *C. coli*, which require either non-selective culture or specific molecular techniques for their optimal detection, are reported to be common in some studies. For example in South Africa *C. concisus* and *C. upsaliensis* accounted for 23%, and *C. coli* for 3%, of all *Campylobacter* and related species isolated [21] and in Ireland using PCR *C. ureolyticus* accounted for 22.3% of all *Campylobacter* species detected [22]. Although both *C. jejuni* and *C. coli* were commonly detected among hospitalised Malawian children with diarrhoea, the contribution of other *Campylobacter* species has not yet been determined.

The prevalence of *Campylobacter* remained relatively constant in children up to 5 years of age in the current study suggesting that unlike viral infections, *Campylobacter* may make a relatively greater contribution to diarrhoeal disease in children aged >12 months. It is possible that repeated exposure to *Campylobacter* species from environmental sources throughout childhood may explain the relatively high prevalence in children >1 year of age; however further clinical, epidemiological, and immunological studies are required to confirm the sources of transmission, environmental reservoirs and the role of *Campylobacter* infection in diarrhoeal disease in this setting. Where detailed age related prevalence rates have been determined in children in Sub Saharan Africa similar patterns have been observed, for example a large cohort study in The Central African Republic reported an average *Campylobacter* detection rate of 9.5% across all age groups [9]. Although deaths in children secondary to diarrhoea are decreasing worldwide, diarrhoea morbidity remains constant, particularly in older children [23]. Given the association of childhood diarrhoea with growth stunting in this population [24] the contribution of *Campylobacter* to the burden of diarrhoeal disease children >1 year of age requires further elucidation.

A significant proportion of diarrhoeal specimens in which *Campylobacter* was detected also contained norovirus or rotavirus, particularly in children <12 months of age. Given the high prevalence of *Campylobacter* in non-diarrhoeic specimens, its detection in diarrhoeic specimens may represent "flushing out" of organisms in diarrhoeal episodes caused by a viral pathogen. We do not have data on the presence of other bacterial or parasitic organisms. We are therefore unable to ascertain which, if any, pathogen is the causative agent of the diarrhoeal episode, although we speculate that *Campylobacter* when detected alone in older children may be more likely to be the causative agent of disease. Furthermore, although there was a significant difference in the rate of detection of *Campylobacter* in isolation between the diarrhoeic and non-diarrhoeic groups (16% vs. 11% respectively), further case control studies are required to confirm this finding. Mixed infections involving *Campylobacter* have been described previously; one large (n = 3,038) surveillance study of diarrhoea in hospitalised children <5 years of age in Bangladesh reported that 59% of all *Campylobacter* infections were associated with at least one other bacterial or protozoan pathogen [25]. Few studies have reported mixed infections of *Campylobacter* and viral pathogens; a cohort study in India demonstrated that rotavirus was associated with 11/18 *Campylobacter* infections in children <5 years of age [26]. Since data from in-vitro cell culture systems suggest that viral co-infection increases the adhesion and invasion of pathogenic *Campylobacter* species [27], further work should explore the clinical consequences of co-infection with viral enteric pathogens on the pathogenesis of *Campylobacter* infection.

Campylobacter was detected in 14% of non-diarrhoeic children who were recruited over a two-year period. Since no preceding clinical or microbiological data are available for these children, we are unable to determine whether this finding represents asymptomatic colonisation or extended excretion after resolution of a *Campylobacter* diarrhoeal episode. Asymptomatic colonisation appears to occur frequently in children in Sub Saharan Africa; one longitudinal study reported that 41.7% of all children in a community birth cohort were asymptomatically colonised with *Campylobacter* within the first 6 months of life [15]. This phenomenon does not appear to occur in the developed world with the exception of workers occupationally exposed to *Campylobacter* [28]. It is thought that regular exposure to *Campylobacter* within an abattoir or farm environment results in immune tolerance towards *Campylobacter* species and hence facilitates colonisation [29]. It is feasible that a similar response occurs in children in Sub Saharan Africa explaining the observed high rates of asymptomatic infection. Given the high sensitivity and specificity of the assay used in this study it is also possible that the detection rates seen in the control cohort could represent post excretion following a diarrhoeal episode as *Campylobacter* is known to be excreted for up to 12 weeks post infection [30].

This study highlights specific differences in the epidemiology of *Campylobacter* in developed compared to developing countries. Firstly, in the UK, the detection rate of *Campylobacter* in children with and without diarrhoea is less than that seen in children in Sub Saharan Africa (6.8% and 2% in diarrhoeal and non-diarrhoeal children in the UK respectively) [14]; secondly, there are age specific differences in detection rates in children in the UK with prevalence increasing throughout childhood [14]; and lastly there is a strong seasonal association in temperate climates with a peak in incidence occurring during the warmer months whereas no seasonal association was seen in Malawi [31]. These differences may be explained by a number of factors including differences in the routes of transmission between the two settings; in the developed world the majority of *Campylobacter* strains causing human infections can be epidemiologically linked to strains that colonise poultry, with the main route of transmission of the pathogen thought to be through the handling and consumption of contaminated meat [32]. Although there are no comparative epidemiological studies linking poultry and human strains in Sub Saharan Africa, up to 40% of commercial chickens in Senegal and 60% in South Africa are colonised with *Campylobacter* [33,34]. Furthermore, strains colonising chickens in Senegal are genetically similar to strains colonising chickens in the UK, The Netherlands and United States suggesting that the host association of *Campylobacter* genotypes transcends geographical boundaries [35]. Chicken is a widely consumed meat in Malawi and many families keep chicken flocks which are routinely housed within the human dwelling including in food preparation areas [36]. Thus in contrast to the developed world, there is increased potential for acquisition and spread of zoonotic and foodborne disease such as *Campylobacter* which may account for the higher prevalence rates reported in this and other studies.

In conclusion, this large study of children hospitalised with diarrhoea in Malawi suggests that the burden of *Campylobacter* is higher than previously appreciated, and is frequently identified in association with concomitant rotavirus and/or norovirus infection. Given the recent introduction of rotavirus vaccines into childhood immunisation programmes in Malawi and other parts of Sub Saharan Africa it is predicted that bacterial pathogens including *Campylobacter* could play a more prominent role in the aetiology of diarrhoeal disease in young children in this region in the future. An improved understanding of the clinical features, epidemiology, and pathogenesis of *Campylobacter* infection in Sub Saharan Africa will inform future prevention strategies against this foodborne zoonotic pathogen.

Acknowledgments

Dr. Jenifer Mason is a National Institute for Health Research (NIHR) Academic Clinical Fellow in Medical Microbiology.

Author Contributions

Conceived and designed the experiments: NC MIG BN JM. Performed the experiments: WD JM. Analyzed the data: JM MIG WD NC SOB. Contributed reagents/materials/analysis tools: BN NC MIG. Wrote the paper: JM MIG SOB MM NC.

References

1. Liu L, Johnson HL, Cousens S, Perin J, Scott S, et al. (2012) Global, regional, and national causes of child mortality: an updated systematic analysis for 2010 with time trends since 2000. Lancet 379: 2151–2161.
2. Lopez AD, Mathers CD, Ezzati M, Jamison DT, Murray CJL (2006) Global and regional burden of disease and risk factors, 2001: systematic analysis of population health data. Lancet 367: 1747–1757.
3. Checkley W, Buckley G, Gilman RH, Assis AM, Guerrant RL, et al. (2008) Multi-country analysis of the effects of diarrhoea on childhood stunting. Int J Epidemiol 37: 816–830.
4. Gupta SK, Keck J, Ram PK, Crump JA, Miller MA, et al. (2008) Part III. Analysis of data gaps pertaining to enterotoxigenic *Escherichia coli* infections in low and medium human development index countries, 1984–2005. Epidemiol Infect 136: 721–738.
5. Cunliffe NA, Ngwira BM, Dove W, Thindwa BD, Turner AM, et al. (2010) Epidemiology of rotavirus infection in children in Blantyre, Malawi, 1997–2007. J Infect Dis 202 Suppl: S168–174.
6. Hughes RAC, Cornblath DR (2005) Guillain-Barré syndrome. Lancet 366: 1653–1666.
7. Mshana SE, Joloba M, Kakooza A, Kaddu-Mulindwa D (2009) Campylobacter spp. among children with acute diarrhea attending Mulago hospital in Kampala - Uganda. Afr Health Sci 9: 201–205.
8. Mandomando IM, Macete EV, Ruiz J, Sanz S, Abacassamo F, et al. (2007) Etiology of diarrhea in children younger than 5 years of age admitted in a rural hospital of southern Mozambique. Am J Trop Med Hyg 76: 522–527.
9. Georges MC, Wachsmuth IK, Meunier DM, Nebout N, Didier F, et al. (1984) Parasitic, bacterial, and viral enteric pathogens associated with diarrhea in the Central African Republic. J Clin Microbiol 19: 571–575.
10. Lindblom GB, Ahren C, Changalucha J, Gabone R, Kaijser B, et al. (1995) Campylobacter jejuni/coli and enterotoxigenic *Escherichia coli* (ETEC) in faeces from children and adults in Tanzania. Scand J Infect Dis 27: 589–593.
11. Rowe JS, Shah SS, Motlhagodi S, Bafana M, Tawanana E, et al. (2010) An epidemiologic review of enteropathogens in Gaborone, Botswana: shifting patterns of resistance in an HIV endemic region. Plos One 5: e10924.
12. Samie A, Obi CL, Barrett LJ, Powell SM, Guerrant RL (2007) Prevalence of Campylobacter species, Helicobacter pylori and Arcobacter species in stool samples from the Venda region, Limpopo, South Africa: studies using molecular diagnostic methods. J Infect 54: 558–566.
13. Trainor E, Lopman B, Iturriza-Gomara M, Dove W, Ngwira BM, et al. (2013) Detection and molecular characterisation of noroviruses in hospitalised children in Malawi, 1997–2007. J Med Virol: In press.
14. Amar CF, East CL, Gray J, Iturriza-Gomara M, Maclure EA, et al. (2007) Detection by PCR of eight groups of enteric pathogens in 4,627 faecal samples: re-examination of the English case-control Infectious Intestinal Disease Study (1993–1996). Eur J Clin Microbiol Infect Dis 26: 311–323.
15. Georges-Courbot MC, Beraud-Cassel AM, Gouandjika I, Georges AJ (1987) Prospective study of enteric Campylobacter infections in children from birth to 6 months in the Central African Republic. J Clin Microbiol 25: 836–839.
16. Mikhall IA, Fox E, Haberberger Jr RL, Ahmed MH, Abatte EA (1990) Epidemiology of bacterial pathogens associated with infectious diarrhea in Djibouti. J Clin Microbiol 28: 956–961.
17. Molbak K, Wested N, Hojlyng N, Scheutz F, Gottschau A, et al. (1994) The etiology of early childhood diarrhea: a community study from Guinea-Bissau. J Infect Dis 169: 581–587.
18. Bessede E, Delcamp A, Sifre E, Buissonniere A, Megraud F (2011) New methods for detection of campylobacters in stool samples in comparison to culture. J Clin Microbiol 49: 941–944.
19. Tam CC, O'Brien SJ, Tompkins DS, Bolton FJ, Berry L, et al. (2012) Changes in causes of acute gastroenteritis in the United Kingdom over 15 years: microbiologic findings from 2 prospective, population-based studies of infectious intestinal disease. Clin Infect Dis 54: 1275–1286.
20. Mughini Gras L, Smid JH, Wagenaar JA, de Boer AG, Havelaar AH, et al. (2012) Risk factors for campylobacteriosis of chicken, ruminant, and environmental origin: a combined case-control and source attribution analysis. PLoS ONE 7: e42599.
21. Lastovica AJ, le Roux E (2000) Efficient isolation of campylobacteria from stools. J Clin Microbiol 38: 2798–2799.
22. Bullman S, Corcoran D, O'Leary J, O'Hare D, Lucey B, et al. (2011) Emerging dynamics of human campylobacteriosis in Southern Ireland. FEMS Immunol Med Microbiol 63: 248–253.
23. Walker CL, Black RE (2010) Diarrhoea morbidity and mortality in older children, adolescents, and adults. Epidemiol Infect 138: 1215–1226.
24. Weisz A, Meuli G, Thakwalakwa C, Trehan I, Maleta K, et al. (2011) The duration of diarrhea and fever is associated with growth faltering in rural Malawian children aged 6–18 months. Nutrition J 10: 25.
25. Glass RI, Stoll BJ, Huq MI, Struelens MJ, Blaser M, et al. (1983) Epidemiologic and clinical features of endemic *Campylobacter jejuni* infection in Bangladesh. J Infect Dis 148: 292–296.
26. Rajendran P, Babji S, George AT, Rajan DP, Kang G, et al. (2012) Detection and species identification of *Campylobacter* in stool samples of children and animals from Vellore, south India. Indian J Med Microbiol 30: 85–88.
27. Konkel ME, Joens LA (1990) Effect of enteroviruses on adherence to and invasion of HEp-2 cells by Campylobacter isolates. Infect Immun 58: 1101–1105.
28. Cawthraw SA, Lind L, Kaijser B, Newell DG (2000) Antibodies, directed towards *Campylobacter jejuni* antigens, in sera from poultry abattoir workers. Clin Exp Immunol 122: 55–60.
29. Havelaar AH, van Pelt W, Ang CW, Wagenaar JA, van Putten JP, et al. (2009) Immunity to Campylobacter: its role in risk assessment and epidemiology. Crit Rev Microbiol 35: 1–22.
30. Richardson N, Koornhof H, Bokkenheuser V, Maynet Z, Rosen E (1983) Age related susceptibility to *Campylobacter jejuni* infection in a high prevalence population. Arch Dis Child 58: 616–619.
31. Lal A, Hales S, French N, Baker MG (2012) Seasonality in human zoonotic enteric diseases: A systematic review. PLoS ONE 7: e31883.
32. Humphrey T, O'Brien S, Madsen M (2007) Campylobacters as zoonotic pathogens: A food production perspective. Int J Food Microbiol 117: 237–257.
33. Nierop W, Duse AG, Marais E, Aihara M, Thothobolo N, et al. (2004) Contamination of chicken carcasses in Gauteng, South Africa, by *Salmonella, Listeria monocytogenes* and *Campylobacter*. Int J Food Microbiol 99: 1–6.
34. Kinana AD, Cardinale E, Tall F, Bahsoun I, Sire JM, et al. (2006) Genetic diversity and quinolone resistance in *Campylobacter jejuni* isolates from poultry in Senegal. Appl Environ Microbiol 72: 3309–3313.
35. Sheppard SK, Colles F, Richardson J, Cody AJ, Elson R, et al. (2010) Host association of Campylobacter genotypes transcends geographic variation. Appl Environ Microbiol 76: 5269–5277.
36. Gondwe TN, Wollny CB (2007) Local chicken production system in Malawi: household flock structure, dynamics, management and health. Trop Anim Health Prod 39: 103–113.

25

Impact of Chest Radiography for Children with Lower Respiratory Tract Infection

Emmanuelle Ecochard-Dugelay[1], Muriel Beliah[2], Caroline Boisson[2], Francis Perreaux[2], Jocelyne de Laveaucoupet[3], Philippe Labrune[2,6], Ralph Epaud[4,7], Hubert Ducou-Lepointe[5,8], Jean Bouyer[1,6], Vincent Gajdos[1,2,6]*

1 Inserm, CESP Centre for research in Epidemiology and Population Health, U1018, Reproduction and Child Development Team, Le Kremlin Bicêtre, France, **2** APHP, Paediatric Department, Hopital Antoine Béclère, Clamart, France, **3** APHP, Radiology Department, Hopital Antoine Béclère, Clamart, France, **4** APHP, Paediatric Department, Centre Hospitalier Intercommunal, Créteil, France, **5** APHP, Paediatric Radiology Department, Hôpital Trousseau, Paris, France, **6** Université Paris Sud 11, Kremlin Bicêtre, France, **7** Université Paris Est, Créteil, Val de Marne, France, **8** Université Paris 6, Paris, France

Abstract

Background: Management of acute respiratory tract infection varies substantially despite this being a condition frequently encountered in pediatric emergency departments. Previous studies have suggested that the use of antibiotics was higher when chest radiography was performed. However none of these analyses had considered the inherent indication bias of observational studies.

Objective: The aim of this work was to assess the relationship between performing chest radiography and prescribing antibiotics using a propensity score analysis to address the indication bias due to non-random radiography assignment.

Methods: We conducted a prospective study of 697 children younger than 2 years of age who presented during the winter months of 2006–2007 for suspicion of respiratory tract infection at the Pediatric Emergency Department of an urban general hospital in France (Paris suburb). We first determined the individual propensity score (probability of having a chest radiography according to baseline characteristics). Then we assessed the relation between radiography and antibiotic prescription using two methods: adjustment and matching on the propensity score.

Results: We found that performing a chest radiography lead to more frequent antibiotic prescription that may be expressed as OR = 2.3, CI [1.3–4.1], or as an increased use of antibiotics of 18.6% [0.08–0.29] in the group undergoing chest radiography.

Conclusion: Chest radiography has a significant impact on the management of infants admitted for suspicion of respiratory tract infection in a pediatric emergency department and may lead to unnecessary administration of antibiotics.

Editor: Stephania Ann Cormier, University ofTennessee Health Science Center, United States of America

Funding: This work was supported by a research grant from the French Society of Pediatric. The funders had no role in study design, data collection and analysis, decision to publish or preparation of the manuscript.

Competing Interests: The authors have declared that no competing interests exist.

* E-mail: vincent.gajdos@abc.aphp.fr

Introduction

Lower respiratory tract infection (LRTI) is one of the most common conditions encountered in pediatric emergency departments (PED) during the winter months, and its management consumes substantial health-care resources.[1] There is substantial diversity in the management of LRTI reflecting the absence of a consensual treatment. Although combinations of clinical features have been proposed to distinguish viral (the most frequent cause) from bacterial diseases, none are sufficiently sensitive to be reliable or widely used.[2–4]. Prescription of chest radiography (CR) is common despite recent World Health Organization guidelines advising against its routine use.[5]

Although radiographic findings are often nonspecific, observational studies have reported a higher prevalence of prescription of antibiotics among children in whom CR has been performed.[6,7] However, the effects of CR may have been overestimated in these reports owing to a likely indication bias, as these children had not been randomly selected for radiography. To avoid such a bias, Rosenbaum and Rubin suggested using the *propensity score* (PS), defined as the probability of receiving a particular treatment or procedure conditional on the observed covariates: two subjects from the two groups compared (CR or no CR) with the same propensity score can be considered as if they had been randomly assigned to the two groups.[8]

The aim of this study was to assess the effects of CR on the likelihood of antibiotic therapy, using PS-based methods to minimize bias due to non-random radiography assignment.

Patients and Methods

Study design and clinical data collection

The ethics committee, Comité de Protection des Personnes Ile de France 3, reviewed this project and concluded that this research conformed to generally accepted scientific principles, and to French laws and regulations Informed oral consent was obtained from parents and refusal to participate did not alter the clinical care provided to the patients.

We conducted a prospective study in the PED of an urban general hospital in France (Paris suburb). All infants (less than 2 years of age) who presented for suspicion of LRTI between October 2006 and February 2007 were included. Suspicion of LRTI was defined as one or more of the following clinical findings: hypoxia (<95%), age-related tachypnea, signs of respiratory distress (retractions, nasal flaring, abdominal breathing) or abnormal breath sounds (wheezing, prolonged expiratory phase, or crackles) obtained by auscultation.

Physicians filled in a short questionnaire with a fixed-choice format, collecting information about demographics, case history, physical examination and management. Demographic data included age, gender, history of prematurity, known chronic illness, and previous wheezing episodes. Case history information included duration of symptoms, history of fever, feeding difficulties, and antibiotic use before PED admission. Physicians were also asked to report temperature at first evaluation, respiratory rate, oxygen saturation, retraction signs, auscultation findings, presence of acute otitis media, conjunctivitis or apparent toxicity. They also recorded the following details of the management: CR, antibiotic prescription, and decision about hospitalization. Patients who received antibiotics before admission were excluded from the study because prior antibiotic therapy undoubtedly affects final treatment decision. CR were interpreted by the emergency pediatrician.

Statistical methods

Descriptive and multivariate data analyses were performed with Stata 11.2 software (Statacorp. 2009. Stata Statistical Software. Release 11. College Station, TX: Statacorp LP).As recommended, the propensity score (PS), i.e. the probability to undergo CR, was calculated with a non-parsimonious multivariate logistic regression model (without an algorithm of selection of variables) with baseline characteristics at admission as independent covariates (14 variables included) and CR as the dependent dichotomized variable. These baseline characteristics were chosen because they were related to the prescription of both CR and antibiotics.[9] Some were dichotomous variables (history of prematurity, infantile asthma, presence of eating disorders, prolonged expiratory phase, crackles, wheezing, conjunctivitis, toxic appearance). Five quantitative variables were transformed into clinically relevant classes (temperature, oxygen saturation, duration of respiratory symptoms, respiratory rate from Liu classification score (*table 1*) and respiratory distress score by Silverman).[10,11] Three variables were left in continuous form. We studied their relationship with the variable of interest to choose from include linear form (arterial oxygen saturation temperature) or with fractional polynomials (age).[12] The area under the Receiver Operator Characteristic (ROC) curve was calculated to assess model discrimination.[13]

To study the association between CR and antibiotic prescription, and controlling for indication bias, we used two methods: adjustment for and matching on PS.[14]

The adjustment method consisted of including PS as a continuous adjustment variable in a logistic model with antibiotic prescription as the dependent variable and CR as an independent variable. To ensure that confounders are taken into account as best as possible, we also adjusted on a subset of nine covariates linked to antibiotic prescription, leading to a *double-robust* model as described by D'Agostino and al.[15] This method provided an odds-ratio (OR) for CR with 95% confidence interval (CI). Variables related to antibiotics prescription were selected by a stepwise procedure: fever, blood oxygen saturation, duration of respiratory symptoms, age, prematurity, prolonged expiratory phase, presence of crackles, conjunctivitis, toxic appearance.

The matching method consisted of matching two subjects on PS (one from each group, CR or no CR) so as to obtain pairs with the same set of baseline covariates.[16] We used a nearest-neighbor matching method that matched pairs of subjects with the nearest PS value. This method provided the difference between percentages of the two groups for which antibiotics were prescribed (with the 95% CI), after taking into account indication bias.

Missing data (less than 5% per variable) were imputed using a method based on multiple chained equations.[17]

Results

Study population

Demographic and clinical characteristics of the sample ($n = 697$) are shown in *table 2*. The mean age was 7.7 months (+/−5.8). Prematurity and a history of infant asthma were reported in 14% f and 21% of patients, respectively. Moderate respiratory distress was observed in 56% of the infants (respiratory distress score of 1), and 14% presented with more severe distress (score ≥2). In half of the patients, the duration of respiratory symptoms was short (less than 3 days) and 57% had a normal age-related respiratory rate. Most children (87.4%) had no hypoxia (oxygen saturation ≥95%). The mean observed temperature was 37.9°C (+/− 1). At triage, 58%, 9% and 48% of subjects presented wheezing, crackles and prolonged expiratory phase, respectively. Fifty-one percent of patients underwent CR. Thirty-one CR were considered to be abnormal (8.7%): 29 with alveolar condensation, one with lobar atelectasia and one with cardiomegaly. Antibiotics were prescribed in 31% of patients in the group with CR, and 8% of the group without CR.

Propensity score

Distributions of PS are displayed by group (CR or no CR) in *figure 1*. The mean PS was lower in the group without CR than in the group with CR. However, there was a wide overlapping area between distributions of both groups, thus allowing a high-quality matching. The area under ROC curve for propensity score was 0.84 [0.83–0.85], indicating a good discrimination capacity.

Effect of undergoing chest radiography on antibiotic use *(table 3)*

The crude OR between CR and antibiotic prescription was 4.9 (95CI [3.1–7.8], $p<0.001$).

After adjustment for PS and for the subset of nine covariates linked to antibiotic therapy, the association between CR and antibiotics prescription remained significant: OR 2.3 (95%CI [1.3–4.1], $p = 0.004$).

With the matching method, we found a significantly higher rate (18.6% higher) of antibiotic prescription in the group of patients with than in the group without CR (mean effect = 0.186, 95CI [0.08–0.29]).

Table 1. Age-related respiratory rate, from Liu et al. [10].

	Respiratory rate (/min)		
	1 point	2 points	3 points
Age < 2 months	≤60	61–69	≥70
Age 2 - 12 months	≤50	51–59	≥60
Age 12 - 24 months	≤40	41–44	≥45

Table 2. Demographics of the study population ($n = 697$).

Characteristics	All	CR group	no CR group
		n = 355	n = 342
Age, *N* (%), months			
≤ 3 m	160 (23.0)	99 (27.9)	61 (17,8)
> 3 m	537 (77.0)	256 (71.1)	281 (82.2)
Age, mean (se), m	7.7 (5.8)	6.4 (6.1)	6.9 (5.3)
Infant asthma (≥3 bronchiolitis), *N* (%)	143 (21.1)	75 (21.1)	68 (19.9)
Prematurity <37 weeks of gestation, *N* (%)	92 (14.0)	59 (16.6)	33 (9.6)
Duration of respiratory symptoms, mean (se), days	4 (5.4)	4.0 (5.6)	3.9 (5.2)
Duration of respiratory symptoms, *N* (%), days			
[0–2] jours	342 (49.9)	171 (48.9)	171 (51.0)
] 2–4] jours	182 (26.6)	103 (29.4)	79 (23.6)
] 4–30] jours	161 (23.5)	76 (21.7)	85 (25.4)
Feeding difficulties, *N* (%)	249 (36.6)	171 (49.3)	78 (23.4)
Maximum of temperature, mean (se), °C	37.9 (1.0)	38.1 (1.0)	37.6 (0.8)
Age-related respiratory rate (Liu (9)), *N* (%)			
1 point	366 (57.4)	157 (48.5)	209 (66.8)
2 points	89 (14.0)	48 (14.8)	41 (13.1)
3 points	182 (28.6)	119 (36.7)	63 (20.1)
Oxygen saturation, *N* (%)			
≥95%	587 (87.4)	270 (78.2)	317 (96.4)
[92–94]	52 (7.7)	43 (12.5)	9 (2.7)
<92	33 (4.9)	30 (8.8)	3 (0.9)
Respiratory distress score (Silverman), *N* (%)			
0	204 (30.0)	65 (18.9)	139 (41.5)
1	381 (56.0)	207 (60.0)	174 (51.9)
2	71 (10.4)	54 (15.6)	17 (5.1)
3	24 (3.5)	19 (5.5)	5 (1.5)
Wheezing, *N* (%)	401 (58.1)	202 (57.5)	199 (58.7)
Crackles, *N* (%)	63 (9.1)	59 (16.8)	4 (1.2)
Prolonged expiratory phase, *N* (%)	330 (47.8)	174 (49.6)	156 (46.0)
Otitis	62 (8.9)	34 (9.6)	28 (8.2)
Conjunctivitis, *N* (%)	25 (3.7)	13 (3.7)	12 (3.6)
Apparent toxicity, *N* (%)	27 (3.9)	6 (1.7)	21 (6.0)
Abnormal chest X-ray	31 (8.7)	31 (8.7)	-
alveolar condensation	29 (8.4)	29 (8.4)	-
lobar or segmental atelectasia	1(0.3)	1 (0.3)	-
Cardiomegaly	1(0.3)	1 (0.3)	-
Antibiotics, *N* (%)	136 (19.5)	108 (31.0)	28 (8.4)

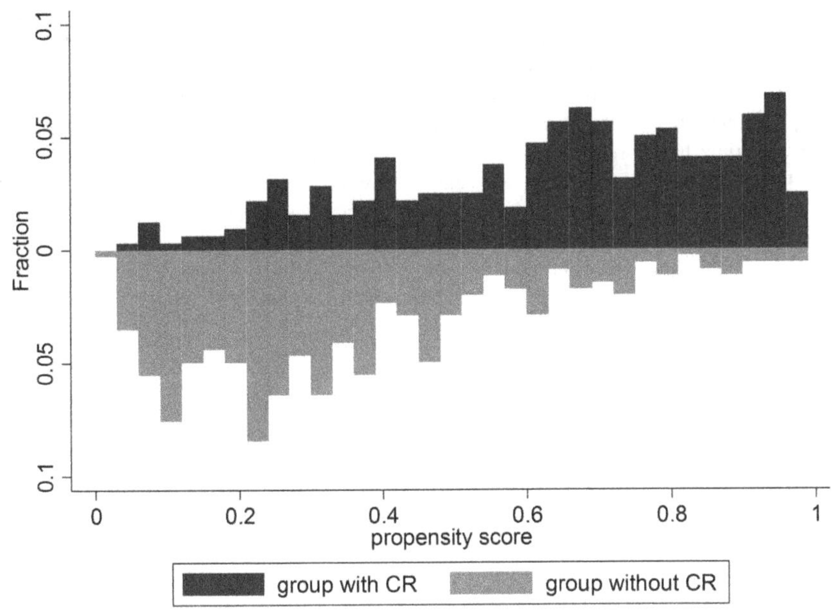

Figure 1. Histograms of propensity score values for the two groups (CR or no CR). The mean propensity score was lower in the group that did not have chest radiography, although there was a wide overlap between both groups.

Discussion

Our study showed that children presenting with LRTI to an emergency department were more likely to receive antibiotics if they underwent CR as part if their initial evaluation. Using PS, this association remained statistically significant after taking into account a possible indication bias. Indeed, antibiotics were prescribed in 18.6% more o infants with CR than in those without CR. This finding suggested that the management of two infants with identical LRTI prognostic baseline characteristics differed, depending on whether or not they had CR: therefore CR had a significant effect on care and might have lead to unnecessary antibiotic therapy. For the purpose of this study, CR images were independently reviewed by two radiologists who were blinded for clinical history. They were simply aware that the imaging was obtained as part of LRTI evaluation but were blinded to other clinical history and outcomes. The Emergency Department practitioners made clinical decisions based on their own interpretation of the CR. This was very important because one of the aim of our study was to determine if the prescription of CR influenced antibiotic prescription, especially without interpretation by a pediatric radiologist.

Our findings are consistent with previous studies. A randomized control trial published in 1998 reported that performing CR had consequences for both management and clinical outcome in 522 children who met the WHO case definition of pneumonia.[18] CR was randomly allocated. Although it was not the primary outcome measure in the study, antibiotic use was higher in the CR group (60.8% vs. 52.2%, p = 0.05). However, children with clinical signs of severity were excluded from this previous study, limiting the extrapolation of the results to LRTI of other causes. Other studies used observational data and did not consider indication bias. Shuh et al. studied 265 infants with typical bronchiolitis who underwent CR.[7] They reported more frequent prescription of antibiotics after CR (post-radiography scenario), relative to the PED physician's intention to treat before CR (pre-radiography scenario), with a percentage difference of 12 (95%CI [0.08–0.16]). However, asking the question may itself have affected physicians' responses before and after CR. Another study [6] showed that performing CR was associated with an increased likelihood of antibiotic use among children over 3 months old (OR 1.22, 95%CI [1.10–1.36], p<0.001); for children less than 3-months-old, there was a similar but not significant relationship (OR 1.11, 95%CI [0.96–1.28]).

Our study had two main strengths: the choice of the study population and the control of indication bias using PS. We analyzed a large sample of infants under two years with various clinical forms and severity scores of respiratory distress. Our study population was not selected, so it was likely to represent the population encountered in clinical practice. We focused on infants because clinical forms and causes of respiratory tract infections in children under 2 years of age are generally homogeneous and comparable. We had a CR rate of 51% that was consistent with rates reported in previous observational studies [6,19–21].

Using PS (i.e. the probability that a patient would have a CR) to adjust the association between CR and antibiotic use, we

Table 3. Effect of chest radiography on antibiotic use.

Crude odds-ratio (OR, 95%CI, p-value)	OR = 4.9; [3.1–7.8]; p<0.001
Adjustment method (OR, 95%CI, p-value)	OR = 2.3; [1.3–4.1]; p = 0.004
Matching method (percentage, 95%CI)	0.186; [0.08–0.29]

mimicked a "quasi-randomized" experiment in which two subjects with the same baseline characteristics are randomly assigned to two groups (CR or no CR). It can be shown that PS provides an unbiased estimate of the association between CR and antibiotic use, if all confounders are considered.[22] Therefore, we collected data for numerous baseline covariates and built PS according to current guidelines recommending the creation of a non parsimonious model to use all available data.[23,24] The continuous variables were modeled according to their linear gradient, or as categorical. All these considerations lead to a robust method for estimating the independent association between CR and antibiotic prescription from observational data.

There were several potential limitations to our study. Some relevant factors may have been unobserved or unmeasured. Consequently, our results were not as reliable as those of a randomized trial. Data were collected in only one PED such that extrapolation of the results to other centers or to infants consulting in private practice may be questionable. We also observed a higher rate of antibiotic use in the group that underwent CR (30.9%) than in another previous study reporting antibiotic therapy in 15% of the CR group.[7] However, the total rate of antibiotic therapy was low (20%), compared to values reported in the literature (between 30 and 60%).[6]

Finally, we stressed that CR prescriptions must be limited for several reasons, other than reducing the rate of unnecessary antibiotic therapy. Although the radiation dose associated with CR is small (0.02 mSv, to be compared to natural exposure estimated to be about 0.05 mSv per week), a recent report on exposure of the French population to ionizing radiation related to acts of medical diagnosis reported a mean of 0.2 CR per year per child under one year old (approximately 160,000 procedures per year for a country with 800,000 births annually).[25] Furthermore, in a cost-effectiveness analysis, Yong et al. concluded that omission of routine CR in infants with bronchiolitis saved $59 per patient (due to savings in radiography and hospitalization costs) without compromising diagnostic accuracy of alternate diagnosis and associated pneumonia.[26] However, in some particular situations (ie when clinical signs are difficult to be interpreted), CR may be essential in order to eliminate bacterial infection requiring antibiotics.

Conclusion

Our study confirmed the previously observed increase of antibiotic use among children undergoing CR, even when indication bias was taken into account. We can assume that part of this antibiotherapy was unnecessary, in the context of an emergency room. Guidelines should be updated to reduce CR prescriptions in PED for children with suspected LRTI.

Author Contributions

Conceived and designed the experiments: VG JB PL RE. Performed the experiments: EED MB CB FP JDL HDL. Analyzed the data: EED JB VG. Contributed reagents/materials/analysis tools: EED PL RE VG. Wrote the paper: EED PL JB VG.

References

1. Hall CB, Weinberg GA, Iwane MK, Blumkin AK, Edwards KM, et al. (2009) The burden of respiratory syncytial virus infection in young children. N Engl J Med 360: 588–598.
2. Mathews B, Shah S, Cleveland RH, Lee EY, Bachur RG, et al. (2009) Clinical predictors of pneumonia among children with wheezing. Pediatrics 124: e29–36.
3. Neuman MI, Monuteaux MC, Scully KJ, Bachur RG (2011) Prediction of pneumonia in a pediatric emergency department. Pediatrics 128: 246–253.
4. Rothrock SG, Green SM, Fanelli JM, Cruzen E, Costanzo KA, et al. (2001) Do published guidelines predict pneumonia in children presenting to an urban ED? Pediatr Emerg Care 17: 240–243.
5. American Academy of Pediatrics (2006) Diagnosis and management of bronchiolitis. Pediatrics 118: 1774–1793.
6. Christakis DA, Cowan CA, Garrison MM, Molteni R, Marcuse E, et al. (2005) Variation in inpatient diagnostic testing and management of bronchiolitis. Pediatrics 115: 878–884.
7. Schuh S, Lalani A, Allen U, Manson D, Babyn P, et al. (2007) Evaluation of the utility of radiography in acute bronchiolitis. J Pediatr 150: 429–433.
8. Rosenbaum PR, Rubin DB (1983) The central role of the propensity score in observationnal studies for causal effects. Biometrika 70: 41–55.
9. Austin PC (2011) A Tutorial and Case Study in Propensity Score Analysis: An Application to Estimating the Effect of In-Hospital Smoking Cessation Counseling on Mortality. Multivariate Behav Res 46: 119–151.
10. Liu LL, Gallaher MM, Davis RL, Rutter CM, Lewis TC, et al. (2004) Use of a respiratory clinical score among different providers. Pediatr Pulmonol 37: 243–248.
11. Dabbous IA, Tkachyk JS, Stamm SJ (1966) A double blind study on the effects of corticosteroids in the treatment of bronchiolitis. Pediatrics 37: 477–484.
12. Royston P, Sauerbrei W (2008) Multivariable model-building. A pragmatic approach to regression analysis based on fractional polynomials for modelling continuous variables: Chichester: John Wiley & Sons.
13. Metz CE (1978) Basic principles of ROC analysis. Semin Nucl Med 8: 283–298.
14. Austin PC, Mamdani MM (2006) A comparison of propensity score methods: a case-study estimating the effectiveness of post-AMI statin use. Stat Med 25: 2084–2106.
15. D'Agostino RB Jr (1998) Propensity score methods for bias reduction in the comparison of a treatment to a non-randomized control group. Stat Med 17: 2265–2281.
16. Austin PC (2008) A critical appraisal of propensity-score matching in the medical literature between 1996 and 2003. Stat Med 27: 2037–2049.
17. Van Buuren S, Boshuizen H, Knook D (1999) Multiple imputation of missing blood pressure covariates in survival analysis. Statistics in Medicine 18: 681–694.
18. Swingler GH, Hussey GD, Zwarenstein M (1998) Randomised controlled trial of clinical outcome after chest radiograph in ambulatory acute lower-respiratory infection in children. Lancet 351: 404–408.
19. Brand PL, Baraldi E, Bisgaard H, Boner AL, Castro-Rodriguez JA, et al. (2008) Definition, assessment and treatment of wheezing disorders in preschool children: an evidence-based approach. Eur Respir J 32: 1096–1110.
20. Willson DF, Horn SD, Hendley JO, Smout R, Gassaway J (2001) Effect of practice variation on resource utilization in infants hospitalized for viral lower respiratory illness. Pediatrics 108: 851-855.
21. Plint AC, Johnson DW, Wiebe N, Bulloch B, Pusic M, et al. (2004) Practice variation among pediatric emergency departments in the treatment of bronchiolitis. Acad Emerg Med 11: 353–360.
22. Kwiatkowski F, Slim K, Verrelle P, Chamorey E, Kramar A (2007) [Propensity score: interest and limits]. Bull Cancer 94: 680–686.
23. Blackstone EH (2002) Comparing apples and oranges. J Thorac Cardiovasc Surg 123: 8–15.
24. Weitzen S, Lapane KL, Toledano AY, Hume AL, Mor V (2004) Principles for modeling propensity scores in medical research: a systematic literature review. Pharmacoepidemiol Drug Saf 13: 841–853.
25. Etard C, Sinno-Tellier S, Aubert B (2010) Exposition de la population française aux rayonnements ionisants liésaux axtes de diagnostic médical en 2007. Institut de veille sanitaire.
26. Yong JH, Schuh S, Rashidi R, Vanderby S, Lau R, et al. (2009) A cost effectiveness analysis of omitting radiography in diagnosis of acute bronchiolitis. Pediatr Pulmonol 44: 122–127.

26

Bloodstream Infection among Children Presenting to a General Hospital Outpatient Clinic in Urban Nepal

Rahul Pradhan[1]*, Umesh Shrestha[1], Samir C. Gautam[1], Stephen Thorson[1], Kabindra Shrestha[1], Bharat K. Yadav[2], Dominic F. Kelly[3], Neelam Adhikari[1], Andrew J. Pollard[3], David R. Murdoch[4]

1 Pediatric Research Unit, Pediatric Department, Patan Academy of Health Sciences, Lalitpur, Nepal, **2** General Practice and Emergency Medicine, Patan Academy of Health Sciences, Lalitpur, Nepal, **3** Oxford Vaccine Group, Department of Pediatrics, University of Oxford; and the NIHR Oxford Biomedical Research Centre, Oxford, United Kingdom, **4** Department of Pathology, University of Otago, Christchurch, New Zealand; and Microbiology Unit, Canterbury Health Laboratories, Christchurch, New Zealand

Abstract

Background: There are limited data on the etiology and characteristics of bloodstream infections in children presenting in hospital outpatient settings in South Asia. Previous studies in Nepal have highlighted the importance of murine typhus as a cause of febrile illness in adults and enteric fever as a leading bacterial cause of fever among children admitted to hospital.

Methods: We prospectively studied a total of 1084 febrile children aged between 2 months and 14 years presenting to a general hospital outpatient department in Kathmandu Valley, Nepal, over two study periods (summer and winter). Blood from all patients was tested by conventional culture and by real-time PCR for *Rickettsia typhi*.

Results: Putative etiological agents for fever were identified in 164 (15%) patients. *Salmonella enterica* serovar Typhi (*S.* Typhi) was identified in 107 (10%), *S. enterica* serovar Paratyphi A (*S.* Paratyphi) in 30 (3%), *Streptococcus pneumoniae* in 6 (0.6%), *S. enterica* serovar Typhimurium in 2 (0.2%), *Haemophilus influenzae* type b in 1 (0.1%), and *Escherichia coli* in 1 (0.1%) patient. *S.* Typhi was the most common organism isolated from blood during both summer and winter. Twenty-two (2%) patients were PCR positive for *R. typhi*. No significant demographic, clinical and laboratory features distinguished culture positive enteric fever and murine typhus.

Conclusions: Salmonella infections are the leading cause of bloodstream infection among pediatric outpatients with fever in Kathmandu Valley. Extension of immunization programs against invasive bacterial disease to include the agents of enteric fever and pneumococcus could improve the health of children in Nepal.

Editor: Niko Speybroeck, Université Catholique de Louvain, Belgium

Funding: This work was supported by a part of the grant for invasive bacterial diseases surveillance to the University of Oxford by PneumoADIP (Pneumococcal Vaccines Accelerated Development and Introduction Plan) and Hib Initiative at Johns Hopkins University. PneumoADIP and the Hib initiative are funded in full by Global Alliance for Vaccine and Immunisation and the Vaccine Fund. The funders had no role in study design, data collection and analysis, decision to publish, or preparation of the manuscript.

Competing Interests: The authors have declared that no competing interests exist.

* E-mail: philiprahul@hotmail.com

Introduction

Although febrile illness is one of the most common reasons for seeking medical care in Nepal, information on the clinical importance of invasive bacterial infections is often unavailable due to limited diagnostic microbiological facilities. This is especially true of patients who present to hospital outpatient departments and do not need admission, as these patients are rarely investigated.

We have previously shown that vaccine-preventable bacterial infections are important causes of hospitalization in Nepali children [1,2]. In particular, there is a high burden of enteric (typhoid) fever, which has also been demonstrated in adults [3,4]. However, the spectrum and burden of invasive bacterial infections among children seen in outpatient clinics remain poorly defined. The hospital outpatient clinic functions as a primary care facility in urban Nepal and it is in this setting that the majority of pediatric febrile illness is managed.

The importance of *Rickettsia typhi* as a cause of febrile illness in South Asia has been increasingly appreciated [3,4,5,6], but there are limited data from pediatric studies. Recently, relatively high rate of murine typhus was reported among febrile adults in Nepal [7], and serological studies performed in various countries outside the region highlight the importance of this disease in children [8,9,10,11].

We describe the etiology and burden of bloodstream infections and murine typhus in febrile children presenting to the pediatric outpatient department of a large district general hospital in Kathmandu Valley, Nepal. In order to address seasonal variations, the study was conducted over two study periods during summer and winter.

Materials and Methods

Setting

Nepal is a low income country with an under five year old mortality rate of 50/1000 live births [12]. Kathmandu Valley, the main urban center of Nepal with three districts, has a population of 2.1 million (average population density: 2372/km^2) of which 29% are under 15 years of age [13]. Situated at an average altitude of 1616 m, the Valley has a sub-tropical cool temperate climate with a hot summer/monsoon season (June to September; average maximum temperature 29°C; rainfall 1200 mm/year) and cool, dry winters (December to February; average minimum temperature 2°C). Overcrowding, insufficient water supply, inadequate sanitation, and pollution are significant problems in Kathmandu Valley. In summer there is a heavy burden of water-borne diseases and in winter respiratory tract infections are predominant. Enteric fever is endemic in the city.

At the time of the study, Patan Hospital was one of only two large hospitals in Kathmandu Valley with a sizeable pediatric department. Patan Hospital accepts patients from all over the Valley. Annually the Pediatric Department cares for over 50,000 outpatients (21% of all hospital outpatient attendances) and accepts approximately 2,700 inpatient admissions. Only 10% of the patients reside outside Kathmandu Valley.

During the study period, pneumococcal conjugate vaccines were not available in the country. Vaccines against *Haemophilus influenzae* type b and typhoid were available within the private market, but they were not widely used.

Patients

To capture the seasonal spectrum of infectious diseases, the study was conducted during two periods. The summer study took place between April 30 and August 22, 2006, and the winter study between December 15, 2006, and February 27, 2007. Consecutive children between 2 months and 14 years of age presenting to our hospital outpatient clinics with axillary temperature of ≥38°C (recorded in the clinic at the time of presentation) were offered enrollment in the study. Written informed consent was obtained from parents or caregivers of all patients included in the study. Any patient who was hospitalized within 24 hours after their outpatient visit was excluded.

Data were recorded on case report forms and then computerized. Irrespective of severity of disease, blood was drawn from all patients for blood culture, complete blood count and *Rickettsia typhi* PCR. Other tests were performed as indicated by the patient's clinical condition. The case report forms and laboratory results for all patients were reviewed by one of two senior pediatricians, and a final diagnosis was assigned.

Laboratory Methods

Blood samples were inoculated into BACTEC™ PEDS PLUS™/F blood culture bottles (Becton Dickinson, USA), incubated at 35°C and processed manually. All bottles were checked twice daily for turbidity and had subcultures performed, irrespective of turbidity, at 12–24 hours and after five days of incubation. Bacterial identification was done by standard microbiological methods and antibiotic susceptibility testing was by disc diffusion using Clinical and Laboratory Standards Institute guidelines [14]. Isolates were sent to Canterbury Health Laboratories, Christchurch, New Zealand, for further confirmation. Complete blood count was performed on the day of the patient's visit using automatic blood cell counter (PCE-210, Erma Particle Counter). Whole blood samples (stored at −70°C) were tested by real-time PCR for *R. typhi* at Canterbury Health Laboratories using an assay described elsewhere [7].

Nutritional Status

Weight for age Z-scores were calculated for each subject (EpiInfo 2002). Moderate or severe malnutrition was defined as a Z-score <−2 and severe malnutrition was defined as a Z-score <−3.

Statistical Analysis

Data from patients with enteric fever were compared with other patients using the chi-square test or Fisher exact test for dichotomous and ordinal variables, and 2-sided Wilcoxon rank sum test and the Student t test for continuous variables. We used multivariable logistic regression analysis to further evaluate variables associated with enteric fever. Enteric fever was the outcome variable in the final model; other variables were those associated with the outcome with $p<0.1$ on bivariable analysis. Likelihood ratio tests were used to compare models with and without interaction terms. Collinearity was tested by a correlation matrix. Data were analyzed using Stata version 11.0 (StataCorp, College Station, TX).

Ethics Statement

Ethics approval to conduct this study was obtained from Nepal Health Research Council (Ref. no. 686, 46) and Oxford Tropical Research Ethics Committee (OXTREC 026-04, 032-06).

Results

During the two study periods, 1084 (845 in summer and 239 in winter) febrile children less than 15 years of age were enrolled (Table 1). Of the total, 649 (60%) were male and 227 (21%) had reported taking antibiotics within 48 hours before presentation. Over the entire study period, upper respiratory tract infection and enteric fever were the most common initial clinical diagnoses. Enteric fever was the most common initial diagnosis in summer and respiratory tract infection in the winter.

Diagnostic Testing

Whole blood for culture was received from all the enrolled patients and the average blood volume drawn was 2.3 mL. Only 4% had blood volume <1 mL. Only five (0.5%) of the blood cultures yielded an isolate thought to be a contaminant. Whole blood specimens were available from all of the patients for testing by PCR for *R. typhi*.

As presented in Table 2, putative etiological agents for fever were identified in 164 (15%) patients. *Salmonella enterica* serovar Typhi (*S.* Typhi) was the most common organism isolated from blood during both seasons. The median age of patients for bacteremia differed by pathogen (Table 3). The median age for *S.* Typhi, *S.* Paratyphi A and *R. typhi* infection was above five years and for *S. pneumoniae* was below five years.

Twenty-two (2%) patients had positive *R. typhi* PCR results. Five patients in summer, who were positive for *R. typhi* PCR, also had bacterial isolates in blood culture. Four of these patients had *S.* Typhi and one had *S.* Paratyphi A. There were no dual etiological diagnoses in winter.

Antimicrobial Susceptibility Testing

Among the 107 isolates of *S.* Typhi, 60 (56%) were resistant to nalidixic acid and, of these, only 3 showed intermediate resistance to ciprofloxacin. Among the 30 *S.* Paratyphi A isolates, 27 (90%) were resistant to nalidixic acid and, of these, 3 showed intermediate resistance to ciprofloxacin. One of the two *S.* Typhimurium isolates showed resistance to nalidixic acid and gentamicin. None of the six *S. pneumoniae* was resistant to penicillin but three were resistant to cotrimoxazole and one showed intermediate resistance to chloramphenicol. The single *H. influenzae* type b isolate was resistant to amoxicillin.

Table 1. Clinical characteristics of febrile children presenting to the Pediatric Outpatient Department at Patan Hospital, Nepal, during the summer and winter study periods.

Characteristics	Summer (n = 845)	Winter (n = 239)
Age (years), median (range)	4 (2 months–14 years)	4 (2 months–14 years)
Male	502 (59%)	147 (62%)
Recruitment rate (no./day)	10	4
Duration of fever (days), median (range)	3 (<1–30)	2 (<1–9)
Temperature at presentation (°C), median (range)	38.3 (38–42)	38.5 (38–40)
Antibiotic use reported within 48 hours before presentation	186 (22%)	41 (17%)
Clinical diagnosis at presentation		
Enteric fever	311 (37%)	23 (10%)
Lower respiratory tract infection	125 (15%)	25 (10%)
Upper respiratory tract infection	216 (26%)	159 (67%)
Acute gastroenteritis/Dysentery	24 (3%)	4 (2%)
Urinary tract infection	28 (3%)	2 (1%)
Viral fever (without obvious focus of infection)	106 (13%)	16 (7%)

Clinical Associations

Enteric fever. Out of the total 1084 patients, 137 (13%) had culture-confirmed enteric fever. Among 600 total children under five years of age, 42 (7%) had culture-confirmed enteric fever (36 positive for *S.* Typhi and 6 positive for *S.* Paratyphi A). Whereas among 484 total children ≥5 years of age, 95 (20%) had culture-confirmed enteric fever (71 positive for *S.* Typhi and 24 positive for *S.* Paratyphi A).

Compared with all the other patients in the cohort, the patients with culture-confirmed enteric fever were more likely to be older, have fever for more than three days at presentation, present in the summer, be moderately or severely malnourished, and were more likely to have headache, abdominal pain, diarrhea and splenomegaly (Table 4). These children were also less likely to present with cough or rhinorrhea. No significant differences were found between culture positive typhoid and paratyphoid fever cases.

On multivariable analysis, culture-confirmed enteric fever was only independently associated with increasing age, diarrhea, duration of fever more than three days, and inversely associated with cough, leukocytosis, and (in winter only) rhinorrhea (Table 5).

Among blood culture positive patients, those who had leukocyte count $<5000/mm^3$ were all positive for *S.* Typhi or *S.* Paratyphi A. Among the culture-confirmed enteric fever patients, fifteen (11%) had leukocyte count $\leq 5000/mm^3$ and four (3%) patients had a leukocyte count $\geq 20{,}000/mm^3$ with ≥50% polymorphonuclear cells; all these four patients were below five years of age.

Nine (2%) of 375 patients who were presumed to have upper respiratory tract infection at presentation, had *S.* Typhi or *S.* Paratyphi A in their blood cultures. Among the patients with duration of fever with rhinorrhea more than five days, 12/46 (26%) had culture-confirmed enteric fever.

Murine typhus. There were 22 patients (2%) who were PCR positive for *R. typhi*. Of these, 13 (59%) were male and the median age was 6.4 years. Enteric fever was the most common clinical diagnosis (45%) at presentation for these patients. Compared with all the other patients in the cohort, these patients were more likely to present with nausea or vomiting (50% versus 29.4%; $p = 0.04$) and diarrhea (31.8% versus 8.1%; $p < 0.001$), and were less likely to present with cough (36.4% vs. 62.2%, $p = 0.01$). No demographic, clinical and laboratory features distinguished these patients from

Table 2. Etiological agents identified in febrile children presenting to the Pediatric Outpatient Department at Patan Hospital, Nepal, during the summer and winter study periods.

Bacterial pathogen	Summer (n = 845)	Winter (n = 239)
Bloodstream isolates (Blood culture)	131 (16%)	16 (7%)
Salmonella enterica serovar Typhi	95 (11%)	12 (5%)
Salmonella enterica serovar Paratyphi A	29 (3%)	1 (0.4%)
Salmonella enterica serovar Typhimurium	2 (0.2%)	0 (0%)
Streptococcus pneumoniae	3 (0.4%)	3 (1%)
Haemophilus influenzae type b	1 (0.1%)	0 (0%)
Escherichia coli	1 (0.1%)	0 (0%)
PCR		
Rickettsia typhi	17† (2%)	5 (2%)

†4 *R. typhi* PCR positive patients had *S.* Typhi and 1 had *S.* Paratyphi A in blood culture.

Table 3. Pathogens responsible for blood stream infections according to age group*.

Pathogen†	Isolates	Age Groups (Total patients = 1084)				Median age (IQR)‡
		2 - <6 mo (n = 20)	6 mo - <1 yr (n = 77)	1 - <5 yr (n = 503)	5–14 yr (n = 484)	
Gram-positive						
Streptococcus pneumoniae	6 (4)	0	0	4 (9)	2 (2)	41 (31–67)
Gram-negative						
Salmonella enterica serotype Typhi	107 (73)	0	1 (33)	35 (74)	71 (73)	76 (45–118)
Salmonella enterica serotype Paratyphi A	30 (20)	0	0	6 (13)	24 (25)	117 (71–139)
Salmonella enterica serotype Typhimurium	2 (1)	0	1 (33)	1 (2)	0	16 (12–19)
Haemophilus influenzae type b	1 (1)	0	0	1 (2)	0	32
Escherichia coli	1 (1)	0	1 (33)	0	0	10
Total bacterial isolates by blood culture	147 (100)	0	3	47	97	79 (45–121)
Rickettsia (PCR)						
Rickettsia typhi	22	1	1	6	14	78 (30–112)
Total microbiological diagnosis	169††	1	4	53	111	78 (44–121)

*Data are no. (%) or no. unless stated otherwise. Percents shown for column totals only for bacterial isolates by blood culture.
†Pathogens isolated by blood culture unless indicated otherwise.
‡Median age in months.
††4 patients with *S.* Typhi and 1 patient with *S.* Paratyphi A were PCR positive for *R. typhi.*

patients with culture-confirmed enteric fever. None of these patients presented with rash.

Pneumonia. Of the 192 (18%) patients with pneumonia as a final diagnosis, only seven (4%) had positive blood cultures (six with *S. pneumoniae* and one with *H. influenzae* type b). All of these seven patients had neutrophil count >11,000/mm^3 and presented with duration of illness of less than five days.

Discussion

To our knowledge, this is the first study in the Indian subcontinent to examine bloodstream infections among children up to 14 years of age presenting to an outpatient clinic, the only inclusion criteria for whom was documented fever ≥38°C. In our study, all febrile children were studied rather than a subset of more severely ill children. Every child enrolled had a blood culture performed irrespective of severity of disease. Studies conducted in South Asia that included children either concentrated on pneumonia or acute respiratory infections [15,16,17], included more severe patients [18,19], collected data based on blood cultures received in the laboratory [20,21], or focused on patients diagnosed with specific disease syndromes such as typhoid fever [22,23]. Two studies [24,25] which looked at typhoid and paratyphoid bacteremia are similar to our study; however, they were community-based studies and only the bacteremia rate from patients under five years from one of the two studies can be compared with our results (see below).

Even though we excluded patients severe enough to be hospitalized, some 15% of children with febrile illness who were managed in the outpatient setting in our study had documented bacteremia. This was largely driven by the burden of enteric fever, but we also documented the presence of invasive pneumococcal and *H. influenzae* type b infections. This study also confirms that murine typhus, previously unrecognized as an important pathogen among children in Nepal, is endemic in Kathmandu Valley. We found that distinguishing between enteric fever and murine typhus is clinically difficult.

Enteric fever is an important cause of illness and death in south-central and south-east Asia, particularly among children and adolescents [26]. In this study, *S.* Typhi and *S.* Paratyphi A were the most common bloodstream isolates, comparable to the results found in the Nepal study in adults [4]. Culture-confirmed enteric fever was also relatively common in children aged less than five years, which has been noted in other Asian studies [20,25,27]. In children less than five years, *S.* Typhi isolation rate was 6% compared to 4.4% in the study conducted in Bangladesh [24], which had similar inclusion criteria to our study but only for children under five years. However, *S.* Paratyphi A isolation rate in our study was 1% compared to 0.2% in the Bangladesh study. During the last decade, salmonella bacteremia in our hospital patients has more than doubled, and *S.* Paratyphi A as a proportion of all salmonella isolates has risen significantly [28]. The latter has been attributed to the emergence of a single clone of *S.* Paratyphi A in South Asia [29].

In our study, the clinical presentations of *S.* Typhi and *S.* Paratyphi A infections were similar. This is consistent with studies from Indonesia [30] and among adult Nepalis [31] that showed these two infections were clinically indistinguishable and had equal severity. Compared with other patients in the study, children with culture-confirmed enteric fever were more likely to be older, have diarrhea, and have a more prolonged duration of fever, and were less likely to have a raised leukocyte count or cough. While the odds of enteric fever were considerably reduced in children with rhinorrhea during the winter period, one-quarter of all patients with fever and rhinorrhea lasting more than five days were culture-positive for *S.* Typhi or *S.* Paratyphi A. This finding is clinically important as standard practice here has been to avoid blood cultures in outpatients with obvious upper respiratory infections.

Nalidixic acid resistance was more common in *S.* Paratyphi A isolates compared with *S.* Typhi (90% vs 56%). This is in concordance with other studies undertaken in our hospital [31] and in India [32]. Nalidixic acid resistance is a marker of reduced susceptibility to the fluoroquinolone group [33,34,35,36] which may be associated with increased clinical virulence [37] and

Table 4. Demographic, clinical and laboratory features of patients with culture-confirmed enteric fever and their comparison with all the other patients in the cohort*.

Variable	*S.* Typhi/*S.* Paratyphi A bacteremia (n = 137)	Others (n = 947)	*p* value
Demographics			
Age, months, median (range)	81.3 (10.9–167.8)	48.4 (2.6–208)	<0.001
Male sex	74 (54)	575 (61)	0.14
Summer Season	124 (91)	721 (76)	<0.001
Duration of fever, days, median (range)	4 (1–22)	3 (0–30)	<0.001
Duration of fever >3 days	76 (55)	309 (33)	<0.001
Antibiotics taken within 48 hours before presentation	41/125 (33)	186/762 (24)	0.05
Symptoms			
Cough	55/137 (40)	613/946 (65)	<0.001
Shortness of breath	0/137 (0)	7/944 (0.7)	0.31
Nausea/vomiting	49/137 (36)	274/947 (29)	0.10
Diarrhea	21/137 (15)	72/944 (8)	0.003
Abdominal pain	76/131 (58)	311/766 (41)	<0.001
Headache	92/130 (71)	355/710 (50)	<0.001
Joint pain	1/130 (0.8)	10/703 (1)	0.55
Muscle pain	0/130 (0)	23/702 (3)	0.04
Baseline Observations			
Temperature, °C, mean (SD)	38.8 (0.7)	38.3 (1.3)	0.01
Pulse rate (per minute), mean (SD)	121 (15)	124 (19)	0.05
Respiratory rate, breaths per minute, mean (SD)	29 (9)	32 (11)	0.004
Hepatomegaly	16/137 (12)	72/940 (8)	0.11
Splenomegaly	21/137 (15)	77/940 (8)	0.007
Rhinorrhea	28/137 (20)	427/943 (45)	<0.001
Moderate or severe malnutrition	46/110 (42)	242/784 (31)	0.02
Laboratory findings			
Hematocrit, %, mean (SD)	36 (4.5)	35.6 (4.9)	0.38
Leukocyte count, total count/mm^3, median (IQR)	7250 (6000–9050)	9750 (7100–13600)	<0.001
Leukocyte count >11000/mm^3	17/136 (13)	368/947 (39)	<0.001

*Data are no. (%) unless stated otherwise. SD, standard deviation; IQR, interquartile range.

Table 5. Associations with *S.* Typhi/*S.* Paratyphi A bacteremia on multivariable analysis.

Variable	OR	95% CI	*p* value
Age group<1 year	1.0		
1–5 years	5.49	0.73 to 41.30	0.10
>5 years	10.94	1.46 to 81.85	0.02
Cough	0.48	0.30 to 0.75	0.001
Diarrhea	2.22	1.18 to 4.17	0.01
Duration of fever >3 days	1.64	1.04 to 2.57	0.03
Splenomegaly	1.05	0.55 to 2.01	0.88
Rhinorrheasummer	0.70	0.39 to 1.27	0.24
Winter	0.13	0.03 to 0.64	0.01
WBC >11,000/mm^3	0.33	0.18 to 0.59	<0.001
Moderate/severe malnutrition	1.36	0.86 to 2.14	0.18

treatment failure [38,39,40]. Widespread use of ciprofloxacin/ofloxacin in Nepal may have driven this increase in fluoroquinolone resistance and alternative approaches to management may be needed, such as azithromycin or gatifloxacin [41].

We did not have any multidrug-resistant salmonella in our study. Nevertheless, there have been reports of extended-spectrum β-lactamase-producing *S.* Typhi in Asia [42,43] and from travelers returning from Asia [44,45]. Multidrug-resistant extended-spectrum β-lactamase-producing *S.* Paratyphi A has also been reported from blood isolates in Nepal [46], leading to further concerns about optimal management of the condition where third generation cephalosporins have been widely used for hospitalized cases. Effective typhoid vaccines [47,48] should be considered for programmatic use in Kathmandu Valley, and paratyphoid vaccines are urgently needed following the emergence of *S.* Paratyphi A as a major cause of enteric fever in the region [28,46]. Health education, adequate sanitation and the use of chlorinated water will greatly help to reduce the public health burden both now and in the future, but the scale of the problem means that this cannot be resolved rapidly in Kathmandu Valley and immunization is the only intervention which could have a rapid impact.

There is growing interest in the importance of murine typhus in Nepal following the findings of recent studies in adults [3,7] and given the frequent contact between humans and rodents in urban areas. Rats and other rodents are the natural reservoirs for *R. typhi*, with the rat flea being the transmission vector to humans. Since *R. typhi* antibodies can persist for several months to years following infection [49] and serological detection is non-specific and cross-reactive [4,50], (and in the absence of convalescent sera), we tested blood samples by real-time PCR assays for *R. typhi* using a recently developed sensitive and specific method [51]. We detected *R. typhi* DNA in the blood from 22 (2%) patients, with a similar prevalence across both seasons. This contrasts with the earlier adult study in Kathmandu Valley that showed an overall prevalence of 7% and winter predominance [7]. This adult study had similar patient inclusion criteria to ours (although hospitalized patients were included) and used real-time PCR for *R. typhi* detection. The other serological study conducted in Nepal [3] among a subset of febrile patients used indirect microimmunofluorescence assay for detection of antibodies to *R. typhi*; this study showed that 26% of their patients were positive for *R. typhi* IgM antibody.

Five of our patients who were positive for *R. typhi* also had positive blood cultures for other bacteria making the significance of the *R. typhi* results uncertain. The collective evidence of recent studies suggests that murine typhus is endemic in Kathmandu Valley, but further focused studies are needed to more precisely determine the burden of disease in children and the clinical significance of a positive PCR in suitable controls. This is especially important given its clinical similarity with enteric fever as this pediatric study and the adult study [7] emphasize the similar clinical features of blood culture positive enteric fever and murine typhus. The absence of rash has been consistently reported in murine typhus from Nepal [7]. Murine typhus should be considered as an alternative diagnosis in patients suspected with enteric fever in Nepal, especially in those not responding to first-line antimicrobial drug therapy to enteric fever [7].

This study has several limitations. For practical reasons we could only conduct the study during two brief periods to capture the seasonal variation of infectious diseases in the Valley. Consequently, we lack data over a complete year or over multiple years to account for annual variation in disease rates. We did not follow-up patients for the study purpose and, therefore, have no data on outcomes once they were sent home from the clinic. We did not test for HIV infection given the low seroprevalence among children admitted with febrile illness in Nepal. Of 485 serum samples tested from admitted febrile children around the same time, only one (0.2%) was positive for HIV antibodies [1]. Other possible pathogens detected by serological diagnoses such as *Leptospira* spp., *Orientia tsutsugamushi*, dengue viruses, as shown in the adult population [3,4], were not included in this study because of limited resources and blood volumes.

However, this study has highlighted the burden of enteric fever among children in Kathmandu Valley, including children considered well enough to be managed in an outpatient/primary care setting. Sentinel studies like this in resource poor settings can define the burden, pattern and treatment of infectious diseases and alter healthcare delivery. However, since the spectrum of pathogens, incidence of diseases and antimicrobial susceptibility change over time, the data should be monitored continuously to allow an appropriate clinical response and healthcare planning. The data show that immunization programmes against invasive bacterial disease could improve the health of children in Kathmandu Valley and that there is a pressing need for effective vaccines against the agents of enteric fever.

Acknowledgments

We are grateful to all the staff at Patan Hospital, especially Kundu Yangzom, Dinesh Kumar BK, Chandra M Kharel, Sabina Dangol, Rita Bajracharya, Sher Bahadur Thapa, Durga Baral, Prashanna Shah, and late Uttar KC, and David Hammer, Trevor Anderson and Anja Werno from Canterbury Health Laboratories.

DFK and AJP are supported by the NIHR Oxford Biomedical Research Centre and AJP is a Jenner Investigator and James Martin Senior Fellow.

Author Contributions

Conceived and designed the experiments: RP US SCG ST KS BKY DFK NA AJP DRM. Performed the experiments: RP US SCG KS. Analyzed the data: RP ST BKY DFK NA AJP DRM. Wrote the paper: RP US SCG ST KS BKY DFK NA AJP DRM.

References

1. Kelly DF, Thorson S, Maskey M, Mahat S, Shrestha U, et al. (2011) The burden of vaccine-preventable invasive bacterial infections and pneumonia in children admitted to hospital in urban Nepal. Int J Infect Dis 15: e17–e23.
2. Williams EJ, Thorson S, Maskey M, Mahat S, Hamaluba M, et al. (2009) Hospital-based surveillance of invasive pneumococcal disease among young children in urban Nepal. Clin Infect Dis 48: S114–S122.
3. Blacksell SD, Sharma NP, Phumratanaprapin W, Jenjaroen K, Peacock SJ, et al. (2007) Serological and blood culture investigations of Nepalese fever patients. Trans Roy Soc Trop Med Hyg 101: 686–690.
4. Murdoch DR, Woods CW, Zimmerman MD, Dull PM, Belbase RH, et al. (2004) The etiology of febrile illness in adults presenting to Patan Hospital in Kathmandu, Nepal. Am J Trop Med Hyg 70: 670–675.
5. Kularatne SA, Edirisingha JS, Gawarammana IB, Urakami H, Chenchittikul M, et al. (2003) Emerging rickettsial infections in Sri Lanka: the pattern in the hilly Central Province. Trop Med Int Health 8: 803–811.
6. Mathai E, Lloyd G, Cherian T, Abraham OC, Cherian AM (2001) Serological evidence for the continued presence of human rickettsioses in southern India. Ann Trop Med Parasitol 95: 395–398.
7. Zimmerman MD, Murdoch DR, Rozmajzl PJ, Basnyat B, Woods CW, et al. (2008) Murine typhus and febrile illness, Nepal. Emerg Infect Dis 14: 1656–1659.
8. Hidalgo M, Salguero E, de la Ossa A, Sánchez R, Vesga JF, et al. (2008) Murine typhus in Caldas, Colombia. Am J Trop Med Hyg 78: 321–322.
9. Nogueras MM, Cardeñosa N, Sanfeliu I, Muñoz T, Font B, et al. (2006) Serological evidence of infection with *Rickettsia typhi* and *Rickettsia felis* among the human population of Catalonia, in the northeast of Spain. Am J Trop Med Hyg 74: 123–126.
10. Shalev H, Raissa R, Evgenia Z, Yagupsky P (2006) Murine typhus is a common cause of febrile illness in Bedouin children in Israel. Scand J Infect Dis 38: 451–455.
11. Purcell K, Fergie J, Richman K, Rocha L (2007) Murine typhus in children, South Texas. Emerg Infect Dis 13: 926–927.
12. UNICEF Nepal Statistics Basic Indicator. Available: http://www.unicef.org/infobycountry/nepal_nepal_statistics.html. Accessed 2012 May 24.
13. Sharma NK, Joshi SR, Bhandari H (2007) District profile of Nepal 2007/2008 (A socio-economic development database of Nepal). Kathmandu: Intensive Study and Research Center.
14. Clinical and Laboratory Standards institute (CLSI) CaLSI (2006) Performance standards for antimicrobial susceptibility testing; sixteenth informational supplement. CLSI document M100-S16. Wayne, PA: CLSI.
15. Owais A, Tikmani SS, Sultana S, Zaman U, Ahmed I, et al. (2010) Incidence of pneumonia, bacteremia, and invasive pneumococcal disease in Pakistani children. Trop Med Int Health 15: 1029–1036.
16. Nizami SQ, Bhutta ZA, Hasan R (2006) Incidence of acute respiratory infections in children 2 months to 5 years of age in periurban communities in Karachi, Pakistan. J Pak Med Assoc 56: 163–167.
17. Ghafoor A, Nomani NK, Ishaq Z, Zaidi SZ, Anwar F, et al. (1990) Diagnoses of acute lower respiratory tract infections in children in Rawalpindi and Islamabad, Pakistan. Rev Infect Dis 12: S907–S914.
18. Owais A, Sultana S, Zaman U, Rizvi A, Zaidi AK (2010) Incidence of typhoid bacteremia in infants and young children in southern coastal Pakistan. Pediatr Infect Dis J 29: 1035–1039.
19. Factor SH, Schillinger JA, Kalter HD, Saha S, Begum H, et al. (2001) Diagnosis and management of febrile children using the WHO/UNICEF guidelines for IMCI in Dhaka, Bangladesh. Bull World Health Organ 79: 1096–1105.

20. Saha SK, Baqui AH, Hanif M, Darmstadt GL, Ruhulamin M, et al. (2001) Typhoid fever in Bangladesh: implications for vaccination policy. Pediatr Infect Dis J 20: 521–524.
21. Amatya NM, Shrestha B, Lekhak B (2007) Etiological agents of bacteraemia and antibiotic susceptibility pattern in Kathmandu Model Hospital. JNMA J Nepal Med Assoc 46: 112–118.
22. Sharma N, Koju R, Karmacharya B, Tamang MD, Makaju R, et al. (2004) Typhoid fever in Dhulikhel hospital, Nepal. Kathmandu Univ Med J (KUMJ) 2: 188–192.
23. Khan MI, Sahito SM, Khan MJ, Wassan SM, Shaikh AW, et al. (2006) Enhanced disease surveillance through private health care sector cooperation in Karachi, Pakistan: experience from a vaccine trial. Bull World Health Organ 84: 72–77.
24. Naheed A, Ram PK, Brooks WA, Hossain MA, Parsons MB, et al. (2010) Burden of typhoid and paratyphoid fever in a densely populated urban community, Dhaka, Bangladesh. Int J Infect Dis 14: e93–e99.
25. Sinha A, Sazawal S, Kumar R, Sood S, Reddaiah VP, et al. (1999) Typhoid fever in children aged less than 5 years. Lancet 354: 734–737.
26. Crump JA, Mintz ED (2010) Global trends in typhoid and paratyphoid fever. Clin Infect Dis 50: 241–246.
27. Ochiai RL, Acosta CJ, Danovaro-Holliday MC, Baiqing D, Bhattacharya SK, et al. (2008) A study of typhoid fever in five asian countries: disease burden and implications for controls. Bull World Health Org 86: 260–268.
28. Maskey AP, Basnyat B, Thwaites GE, Campbell JI, Farrar JJ, et al. (2008) Emerging trends in enteric fever in Nepal: 9124 cases confirmed by blood culture 1993–2003. Trans Roy Soc Trop Med Hyg 102: 91–95.
29. Woods CW, Murdoch DR, Zimmerman MD, Glover WA, Basnyat B, et al. (2006) Emergence of *Salmonella enterica* serotype Paratyphi A as a major cause of enteric fever in Kathmandu, Nepal. Trans Roy Soc Trop Med Hyg 100: 1063–1067.
30. Vollaard AM, Ali S, Widjaja S, Asten HAGH, Visser LG, et al. (2005) Identification of typhoid fever and paratyphoid fever cases at presentation in outpatient clinics in Jakarta, Indonesia. Trans Roy Soc Trop Med Hyg 99: 440–450.
31. Maskey AP, Day JN, Tuan PQ, Thwaites GE, Campbell JI, et al. (2006) *Salmonella enterica* serovar Paratyphi A and *S. enterica* serovar Typhi cause indistinguishable clinical syndromes in Kathmandu, Nepal. Clin Infect Dis 42: 1247–1253.
32. Joshi S, Amarnath SK (2007) Fluoroquinolone resistance in *Salmonella typhi* and *S. paratyphi* A in Bangalore, India. Trans Roy Soc Trop Med Hyg 101: 308–310.
33. Kumar Y, Sharma A, Mani KR (2009) High level of resistance to nalidixic acid in *Salmonella enterica* serovar Typhi in Central India. J Infect Dev Ctries 3: 467–469.
34. Parry CM (2004) The treatment of multidrug-resistant and nalidixic acid-resistant typhoid fever in Viet Nam. Trans Roy Soc Trop Med Hyg 98: 413–422.
35. Krishnan P, Stalin M, Balasubramanian S (2009) Changing trends in antimicrobial resistance of *Salmonella enterica* serovar typhi and *Salmonella enterica* serovar paratyphi A in Chennai. Indian J Pathol Microbiol 52: 505–508.
36. Renuka K, Kapil A, Kabra SK, Wig N, Das BK, et al. (2004) Reduced susceptibility to ciprofloxacin and gyra gene mutation in North Indian strains of *Salmonella enterica* serotype Typhi and serotype Paratyphi A. Microb Drug Resist 10: 146–153.
37. Kadhiravan T, Wig N, Renuka K, Kapil A, Kabra SK, et al. (2008) Is nalidixic acid resistance linked to clinical virulence in *Salmonella enterica* serovar Typhi infections? J Med Microbiol 57: 1046–1048.
38. Dimitrov T, Udo EE, Albaksami O, Kilani AA, Shehab E-DMR (2007) Ciprofloxacin treatment failure in a case of typhoid fever caused by *Salmonella enterica* serotype Paratyphi A with reduced susceptibility to ciprofloxacin. J Med Microbiol 56: 277–279.
39. Nkemngu N, Asonganyi E, Njunda A (2005) Treatment failure in a typhoid patient infected with nalidixic acid resistant *S. enterica* serovar Typhi with reduced susceptibility to Ciprofloxacin: a case report from Cameroon. BMC Infect Dis 5: 49.
40. Rupali P, Abraham OC, Jesudason MV, John TJ, Zachariah A, et al. (2004) Treatment failure in typhoid fever with ciprofloxacin susceptible *Salmonella enterica* Serotype Typhi. Diagn Microbiol Infect Dis 49: 1–3.
41. Dolecek C, Phi La TT, Rang NN, Phuong LT, Vinh H, et al. (2008) A multi-center randomised controlled trial of gatifloxacin versus azithromycin for the treatment of uncomplicated typhoid fever in children and adults in Vietnam. PLoS ONE 3: e2188.
42. Rotimi VO, Jamal W, Pal T, Sovenned A, Albert MJ (2008) Emergence of CTX-M-15 type extended-spectrum β-lactamase-producing *Salmonella* spp. in Kuwait and the United Arab Emirates. J Med Microbiol 57: 881–886.
43. Ahmed D, Hoque A, Mazumder R, Nahar K, Islam N, et al. (2012) *Salmonella enterica* serovar Typhi strain producing extended-spectrum β-lactamases in Dhaka, Bangladesh. J Med Microbiol 61: 1032–1033.
44. Al Naiemi N, Zwart B, Rijnsburger MC, Roosendaal R, Debets-Ossenkopp YJ, et al. (2008) Extended-spectrum-beta-lactamase production in a *Salmonella enterica* serotype Typhi Strain from the Philippines. J Clin Microbiol 46: 2794–2795.
45. Pfeifer Y, Matten J, Rabsch W (2009) *Salmonella enterica* serovar Typhi with CTX-M beta-lactamase, Germany. Emerg Infect Dis 15: 1533–1535.
46. Pokharel BM, Koirala J, Dahal RK, Mishra SK, Khadga PK, et al. (2006) Multidrug-resistant and extended-spectrum beta-lactamase (ESBL)-producing *Salmonella enterica* (serotypes Typhi and Paratyphi A) from blood isolates in Nepal: surveillance of resistance and a search for newer alternatives. Int J Infect Dis 10: 434–438.
47. Sur D, Ochiai RL, Bhattacharya SK, Ganguly NK, Ali M, et al. (2009) A cluster-randomized effectiveness trial of Vi typhoid vaccine in India. N Engl J Med 361: 335–344.
48. WHO (2008) Typhoid vaccines: WHO position paper. Wkly Epidemiol Rec 83: 49–59.
49. Halle S, Dasch GA (1980) Use of a sensitive microplate enzyme-linked immunosorbent assay in a retrospective serological analysis of a laboratory population at risk to infection with typhus group rickettsiae. J Clin Microbiol 12: 343–350.
50. Kelly DJ, Chan CT, Paxton H, Thompson K, Howard R, et al. (1995) Comparative evaluation of a commercial enzyme immunoassay for the detection of human antibody to *Rickettsia typhi*. Clin Diagn Lab Immunol 2: 356–360.
51. Henry KM, Jiang J, Rozmajzl PJ, Azad AF, Macaluso KR, et al. (2007) Development of quantitative real-time PCR assays to detect *Rickettsia typhi* and *Rickettsia felis*, the causative agents of murine typhus and flea-borne spotted fever. Mol Cell Probes 21: 17–23.

27

Surveillance of Airborne Adenovirus and *Mycoplasma pneumoniae* in a Hospital Pediatric Department

Gwo-Hwa Wan[1*], Chung-Guei Huang[2,3], Yhu-Chering Huang[4,5], Ju-Ping Huang[1], Su-Li Yang[2], Tzou-Yien Lin[4,5], Kuo-Chien Tsao[2,3]

1 Department of Respiratory Therapy, College of Medicine, Chang Gung University, Tao-Yuan, Taiwan, **2** Department of Laboratory Medicine, Chang Gung Memorial Hospital, Tao-Yuan, Taiwan, **3** Department of Biotechnology and Laboratory Science, Research Center for Emerging Viral Infections, Chang Gung University, Tao-Yuan, Taiwan, **4** Division of Pediatric Infectious Diseases, Chang Gung Memorial Hospital, Tao-Yuan, Taiwan, **5** College of Medicine, Chang Gung University, Tao-Yuan, Taiwan

Abstract

This investigation evaluated the distributions of airborne adenovirus and *Mycoplasma pneumoniae* in public areas in the pediatric department of Children's Hospital in northern Taiwan. The airborne viral and bacterial concentrations were evaluated twice a week for a year using filter sampling with an airflow rate of 12 liters per minute for eight hours in the pediatric outpatient department and 24 hours in the pediatric emergency room. Real-time polymerase chain reaction assays were conducted for analysis. Approximately 18% of the air samples from the pediatric emergency room were found to contain adenovirus. Approximately forty-six percent of the air samples from the pediatric outpatient department contained *Mycoplasma pneumoniae* DNA products. High detection rates of airborne adenovirus DNA were obtained in July and August in the pediatric public areas. Airborne *Mycoplasma pneumoniae* was detected only in July in the pediatric emergency room and the peak levels were found from August to January in the pediatric outpatient department. Airborne particles that contained adenovirus and *Mycoplasma pneumoniae* were the most prevalent in the pediatric public areas. The potential relationship between these airborne viral/bacterial particles and human infection should be examined further. Keywords: adenovirus; *Mycoplasma pneumoniae*; filter sampling; real-time polymerase chain reaction; hospital; pediatric public areas.

Editor: Benjamin J. Cowling, University of Hong Kong, Hong Kong

Funding: The authors would like to thank the Chang Gung Memorial Hospital, Taiwan, for financially supporting this research under grant CMRPD170831. The funder had no role in study design, data collection and analysis, decision to publish, or preparation of the manuscript.

Competing Interests: The authors have declared that no competing interests exist.

* E-mail: ghwan@mail.cgu.edu.tw

These authors contributed equally to this work.

Introduction

Viral respiratory infection is the most common infectious disease. The viruses, such as enterovirus, influenza virus, and adenovirus, were most often isolated from the pediatric outpatients [1]. Adenovirus causes acute respiratory tract infections in children younger than 5 years old. *Mycoplasma pneumoniae* is a common causative pathogen of community-acquired pneumonia (CAP) in children and young adults. In Taiwan, *Mycoplasma pneumoniae* was reported to account for 20–30% of CAP cases [2,3]. Airborne viruses are known to be associated with larger particles and aggregate in nature [4]. Most aerosolized droplet nuclei are between 0.58 and 5.42 µm in diameter [5]. One investigation found 53% of detectable influenza virus particles in the respiratory aerosol fraction (1–4 µm) [6].

Three primary factors - the virus concentration in the air, the collection efficiency of the air sampler, and the sensitivity of the analytical assay to the target pathogen - determine the probability of detecting airborne viral pathogens [7]. Previous studies have found that sampling devices such as the all-glass impinger 30, the SKC BioSampler and a frit bubbler are unsuited to collect viral particles [8]. Filtration was used to collect airborne particles that contain viruses, including rhinovirus [9,10], severe acute respiratory syndrome (SARS) coronavirus [11–13], RSV [14], enterovirus, adenovirus, and influenza A virus [15]. PCR analysis amplifies nucleic acids exponentially, and is particularly sensitive to airborne infectious agents, such as rhinovirus [9,10], RSV [14], enterovirus, adenovirus, influenza A virus [15], SARS coronavirus [11–13], and measles virus [16]. No standard protocol had been established for collecting and detecting specific viral particles in the air.

Until recently, few studies have examined the long-term distributions of airborne viral and bacterial aerosols in health-care settings in the subtropical region of Taiwan using filter sampling with pathogen-specific PCR assays. Accordingly, in this investigation, airborne adenovirus and bacterial (*Mycoplasma pneumoniae*) concentrations at the pediatric emergency room and pediatric outpatient department of the Children's Hospital in northern Taiwan were evaluated for one year.

Materials and Methods

Sampling location

A medical center, Chang Gung Memorial Hospital with 3,500 beds located in north Taiwan, was selected in this study. This hospital contains many departments (such as department of medicine, department of surgery, department of pediatrics, department of gynecology and obstetric, department of Chinese medicine, etc.). The sampling site was the pediatric public areas including the pediatric emergency room and the pediatric outpatient department. In the sampling periods, the air in the pediatric public areas was conditioned without heating. No local source of industrial air pollution was close to the hospital. The study protocol was approved by the institutional review board of the hospital.

Air Sampling

Air samplers were placed in the center of the pediatric outpatient department and the pediatric emergency room for 8 hours (from 9 am to 5 pm) and 24 hours, respectively, randomly selected twice weekly (Monday to Saturday) for a year (February 2009 to January 2010). Sampling was performed 1.2–1.5 m above the floor, in the human breathing zone. The indoor air was filtered through a closed-face, three-piece disposable plastic cassette with a 0.2 μm polytetrafluoroethylene filter at an airflow rate of 12 L/min (LPM) for bioaerosol sampling. A total of 186 filter samples (93 samples from the pediatric outpatient department and 93 samples from the pediatric emergency room) were collected and the filters were immediately stored at −70°C until they were analyzed.

The air quality indices (air temperature, relative humidity (RH), carbon dioxide (CO_2) and suspended particular matter) in the pediatric public areas of the hospital were evaluated during the study period. The indoor temperature, RH and CO_2 concentration were determined using a digital psychrometer (TSI incorporated 500 Cardigan Road, Shoreview, MN 55126, USA). The portable DUSTcheck monitor (Grimm, model 1.108, Germany) was used to measure the mass concentrations of particulate matters.

Preparation of filter sample extracts and DNA extraction

One thousand and five hundred microliters aliquots of phosphate-buffered saline (PBS) were pipetted into 60 mm diameter petri dishes that each contained a filter, and these petri dishes were then placed on an orbital tabletop shaker at a speed of 150 rpm for 60 minutes at room temperature. All samples were stored at −80°C until DNAs were extracted.

The DNA was extracted using the Qiagen DNA mini kit (Qiagen, Hilden, Germany) according to the manufacturer's directions. Briefly, 500 μL of the sample was extracted and the nucleic acid was eluted in a final volume of 30 μL. All eluted samples were stored at −80°C until analysis. In the negative controls, sterile distilled water was added in place of the samples.

Real-time quantitative PCR assay

Table 1 presented the sequences of the primers and probes for adenovirus and *Mycoplasma pneumoniae*. The adenovirus and *Mycoplasma pneumoniae* in the filter samples were quantitatively measured as previously described [17]. Concentrations of calibration standards ranged from 10 to 10^6 copies/μL for adenovirus and 10 to 10^4 copies/μL for *Mycoplasma pneumoniae*. For the tested adenovirus and *Mycoplasma pneumoniae*, the known amounts of plasmid cDNA yielded cycle threshold (Ct) values ranging between 19.46 and 36.58 cycles. The correlation coefficient (r) values of the calibration curves were 0.99 for adenovirus and *Mycoplasma pneumoniae*.

Statistical analysis

SPSS (Statistical Package for Social Science) version 13.0 (SPSS Inc., Chicago, USA) was used for the statistical analyses. The level of significance was set to 0.05. The figures were constructed using GraphPad Prism 5.0 software. A two-sample *t* test was used to assess the differences of detection rates between adenovirus and *Mycoplasma pneumoniae* in the pediatric emergency room and pediatric outpatient department, respectively.

Results

During the study period, the air temperatures and relative humidity were 16.1–26.6°C and 42.5–77.7%, respectively, in the pediatric emergency room, and 13.7–24.8°C and 50.4–84.7% in the pediatric outpatient department. The CO_2 concentrations were 404–704 ppm in the pediatric emergency room and 372–2,575 ppm in the pediatric outpatient department. The mean concentrations of ≤10 μm (PM_{10}) and ≤1 μm (PM_1) particles were 8.9 μg/m^3 and 17.0 μg/m^3, respectively, in the pediatric emergency room, and approximately 105 μg/m^3 and 167 μg/m^3, respectively, in the pediatric outpatient department.

Filter samples without airflow passage were selected as negative controls. The adenovirus and *Mycoplasma pneumoniae* were not found in the blank filters. Also, PCR positive rates of the positive controls containing adenovirus or *Mycoplasma pneumoniae* in the sampling filters are 100%. The monthly detection rate (18.3%) of the adenovirus in the air samples of the pediatric emergency room of the medical center was clearly higher than that of *Mycoplasma pneumoniae* (0.9% of the air samples) ($p = 0.009$) (Fig. 1). Around 45.8% of the air samples from the pediatric outpatient department contained *Mycoplasma pneumoniae*. Other pathogen, adenovirus (9.8% of the air samples), was also found in the pediatric outpatient department.

In this study, airborne particles that contained adenovirus were detected in the pediatric emergency room throughout the year except in March to May, and October (Fig. 2A). Detection rates of airborne adenovirus DNA products in the filter samples in the

Table 1. The sequences of primers and probes of adenovirus and *Mycoplasma Pneumoniae*.

Oligo Names	Sequences(5′→3′)	Genes	Reference
Adenovirus		Hex	-
Ad-s	GCCCCAGTGGGCTTACATGCACATC		
Ad-as	ATTGAAGTAGGTGTCTGTGGCGCGGG		
Ad-probe	FAM-AACTGCACCAGACCCGGGCTCAGGTACTCC-TAMRA		
Mycoplasma pneumoniae		P1	17
MP-TM1	CCAACCAAACAACAACGTTCA		
MP-TM2	ACCTTGACTGGAGGCCGTTA		
MP-probe	VIC-ATCCGAATAACGGTGACTT-MGB		

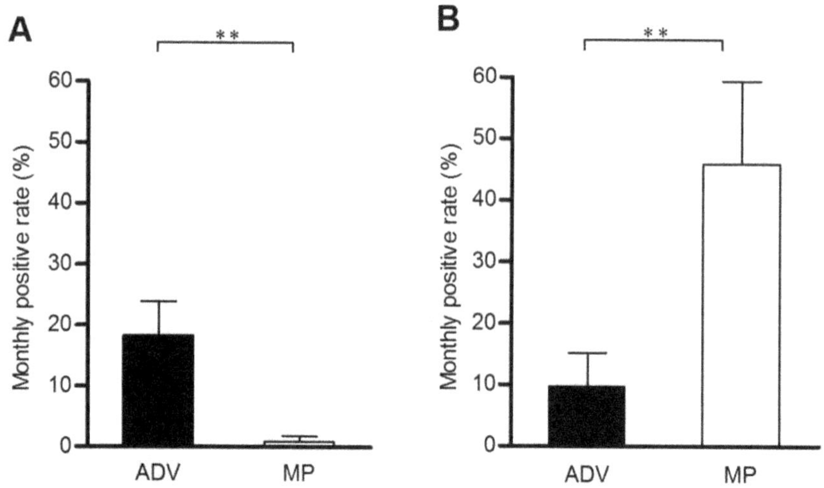

Figure 1. Airborne adenovirus and *Mycoplasma pneumoniae* in the pediatric public areas. The monthly positive rates (mean±se) of airborne particles containing adenovirus (ADV) and *Mycoplasma pneumoniae* (MP) in the pediatric emergency room (ER) (A) and pediatric outpatient department (OPD) (B). **: $p<0.01$.

pediatric emergency room were high in July (33.3%) and August (66.7%). The airborne *Mycoplasma pneumoniae* DNA products were detected in the pediatric emergency room only in July (11.1% of the air samples). The airborne particles that contained adenovirus concentrations ranged between <10 copies/m^3 and 104 copies/m^3 in the pediatric emergency room. The median concentration of airborne adenovirus DNA was highest in December. Only one air sample in the pediatric emergency room was positive for *Mycoplasma pneumoniae* DNA product (645 copies/m^3).

The detection rate of adenovirus-containing particles in the air samples in the pediatric outpatient department peaked in July (66.7%) (Fig. 2B). However, airborne particles that contained *Mycoplasma pneumoniae* were found in the pediatric outpatient department throughout the year except in February to June. High detection rates of airborne *Mycoplasma pneumoniae* DNA products in the filter samples were found in August (83.3%), September (100%), October (88.9%), and November (100%), and January (100%). The detected concentrations of adenovirus in the air in the pediatric outpatient department ranged from 48.4 copies/m^3 to 461 copies/m^3, and the median concentration was highest in March. The concentrations of *Mycoplasma pneumoniae* in airborne particles ranged between 114 copies/m^3 and 9.9×10^4 copies/m^3 in the pediatric outpatient department. The median concentration of *Mycoplasma pneumoniae* DNA product in the air of the pediatric outpatient department was highest in October.

Discussion

This study is the first to examine the long-term variation of the distribution of airborne adenoviral particles and *Mycoplasma pneumoniae* in the pediatric emergency room and pediatric outpatient department of the Children's Hospital in Taiwan. The detection rate of airborne adenovirus DNA products in the pediatric emergency room clearly exceeded those of *Mycoplasma pneumoniae* DNA products. Airborne *Mycoplasma pneumoniae* DNA products were detected in around 46% of samples from the pediatric outpatient department of the hospital. The distribution of microbial species in the pediatric public areas warrants further attention from the department of environmental safety and health to reduce the risk of microbial exposure in humans. The possibility of adenovirus and *Mycoplasma pneumoniae* that transmitted by the airborne route also warrants further investigation.

In this study, the detection rates of airborne adenovirus DNA products peaked in summer in the pediatric outpatient department and the pediatric emergency room, respectively. Furthermore, airborne *Mycoplasma pneumoniae* were frequently detected in the pediatric outpatient department and the detection rates were highest in autumn and winter seasons. This results suggest that the ventilation rate in pediatric public areas (including the emergency room and outpatient department) of hospitals should be increased during the peak seasons of adenovirus and *Mycoplasma pneumoniae* contamination to reduce the airborne bioaerosol levels. The limitation of this study was lack of environmental characteristics measurement along with airborne adenovirus and *Mycoplasma pneumoniae* sampling. Further study will enable the relationship between indoor environmental characteristics (including temperature, relative humidity and CO_2 concentration) and the airborne adenovirus/*Mycoplasma pneumoniae* to be elucidated.

The air sampling time in the pediatric outpatient department was shorter than that in the pediatric emergency room. The main reason was that the pediatric outpatient department of the hospital was close at nighttime. The monthly detection rate of airborne adenovirus DNA products in the filter samples in the pediatric outpatient department was lower than that in the pediatric emergency room, but the measured viral concentrations in March, May, June, and July in the pediatric outpatient department considerably exceeded those measured in the pediatric emergency room. Additionally, *Mycoplasma pneumoniae* exhibited not only a higher detection rate but also higher concentrations in the pediatric outpatient department than in the pediatric emergency room. The possible cause may be the indoor unfair ventilation and more patients with *Mycoplasma pneumoniae* infection in the pediatric outpatient department. The results demonstrate that the mean CO_2 concentration in the pediatric outpatient department exceeded that in the pediatric emergency room. Therefore, the ventilation system should be adjusted periodically and the air change rate should be increased during peak seasons with high viral concentrations in the pediatric public areas. Also, high-efficiency particulate air (HEPA) filters should perhaps be installed in the ventilation systems in the pediatric public areas of hospitals

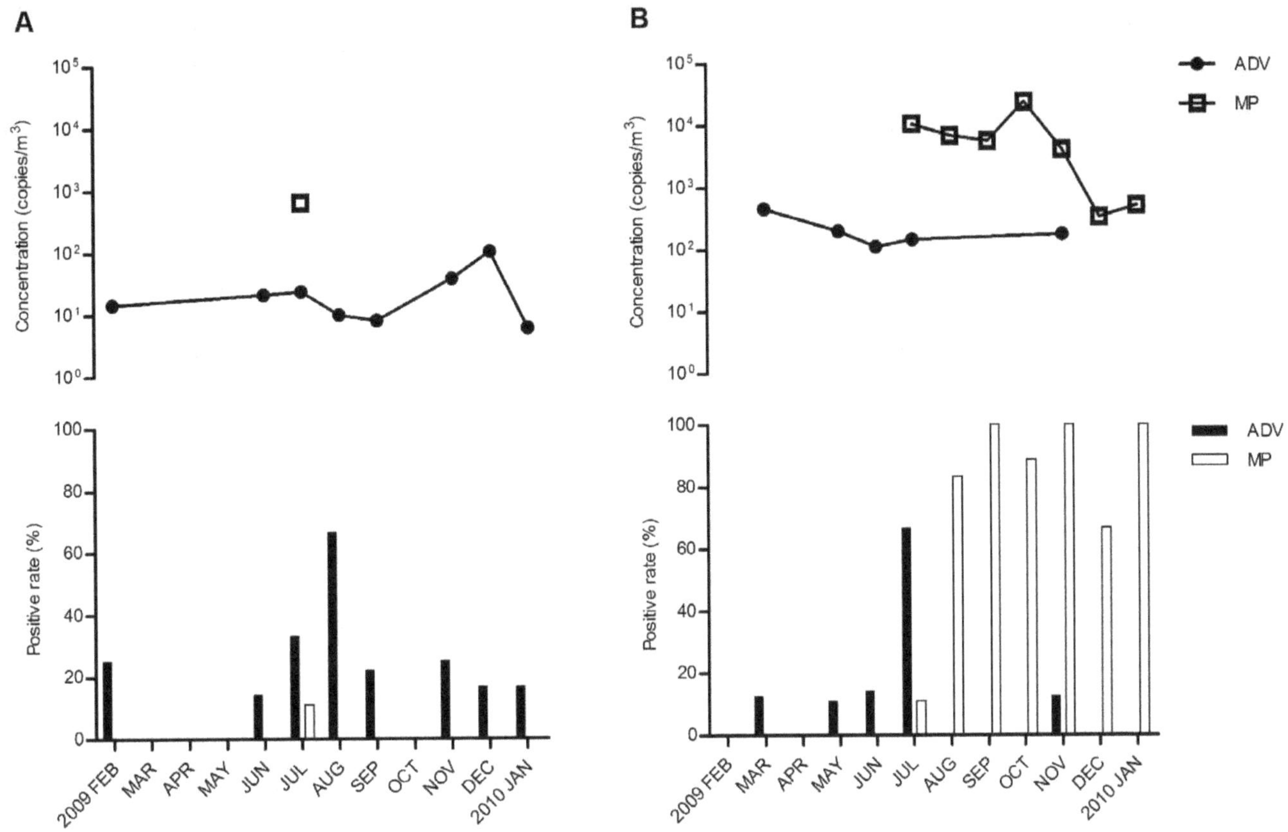

Figure 2. Monthly distributions of airborne ADV and MP in the pediatric ER (A) and OPD (B). Monthly distributions of the detection rates of airborne ADV and MP in the filter samples and the median concentration distributions of ADV and MP in the air of the pediatric public areas.

to maintain indoor air quality. In addition, the results indicated that monthly distributions of detection rates of adenovirus and *Mycoplasma pneumoniae* in the air samples were inconsistent with the median concentration distributions of airborne adenovirus and *Mycoplasma pneumoniae* in the pediatric public areas. The possible reason might be included: 1) the air samples in the pediatric public areas were only collected twice in a week; 2) the exact number of infected patients in the pediatric public areas was unknown.

A previous investigation found that the number of patients with influenza was closely correlated with the number of air samples that contained influenza A RNA ($r = 0.77$) [18]. Tseng et al. study indicated that the influenza A virus concentrations in the air were significantly correlated with the number of patients with low respiratory tract infections ($r = 0.43$, $p = 0.02$), but no correlation occurred between the viral concentrations and the number of patients with upper respiratory tract infections ($r = 0.33$, $p = 0.06$) [15]. During the study period, there was not outbreak occurrence of adenovirus and *Mycoplasma pneumoniae* infections in the hospital. There were a great number of patients and visitors in the hospital, and not all of patients with respiratory tract infection were tested for adenovirus or *Mycoplasma pneumoniae* infections, so it would be underestimated the number of patients with adenovirus or *Mycoplasma pneumoniae* infection in the pediatric public areas. The relationship between the number of infected patients and the number of air samples with detected certain pathogens warrants further investigation.

Indoor air quality is important to prevent infection and thereby protect patients and health care workers in hospitals. The quality of indoor air depends on heating ventilation and air conditioning (HVAC) systems, the number of persons, human activity and other factors (i.e., the outdoor air quality) [19,20]. Until recently, no standard method had been established for detecting specific viral aerosol particles. Tolerable levels of airborne viruses in hospitals have not yet been established. Airborne particle concentration has been suggested to be an indicator of microbial contamination [21]. In this study, PM_{10} and PM_1 levels were higher in the pediatric outpatient department than in the pediatric emergency room. Hence, further investigations must be performed to characterize the relationship between particulate matter levels, such as PM_{10} and PM_1, and the concentrations of airborne viruses and bacteria.

Acknowledgments

The authors thank Yueh-Hsiang Chen and Ted Knoy for their assistance during this investigation.

Author Contributions

Conceived and designed the experiments: G-HW C-GH. Performed the experiments: C-GH J-PH Y-CH T-YL. Analyzed the data: J-PH S-LY K-CT. Wrote the paper: G-HW.

References

1. Centers for Disease Control and Prevention, Department of Health, R.O.C. (Taiwan). (2010) Statistics of Communicable Diseases and Surveillance Report 2009. pp 60–65.
2. Yen MY, Hu BS, Chen YS, Lee SS, Lin YS, et al. (2005) A prospective etiologic study of community-acquired pneumonia in Taiwan. J Formos Med Assoc 104: 724–730.

3. Chang YT, Yang YH, Chiang BL (2006) The significance of a rapid cold hemagglutination test for detecting mycoplasma infections in children with asthma exacerbation. J Microbiol Immunol Infect 39: 28–32.
4. Aller JY, Kuznetsova MR, Jahns CJ, Kemp PF (2005) The sea surface microlayer as a source of viral and bacterial enrichment in marine aerosols. J Aerosol Sci 36: 801–812.
5. Yang S, Lee GW, Chen CM, Wu CC, Yu KP (2007) The size and concentration of droplets generated by coughing in human subjects. J Aerosol Med 20: 484–494.
6. Blachere FM, Lindsley WG, Pearce TA, Anderson SE, Fisher M, et al. (2009) Measurement of airborne influenza virus in a hospital emergency department. Clin Infect Dis 48: 438–440.
7. Hermann JR, Hoff SJ, Yoon KJ, Burkhardt AC, Evans RB, et al. (2006) Optimization of a sampling system for recovery and detection of airborne porcine reproductive and respiratory syndrome virus and swine influenza virus. Appl Environ Microbiol 72: 4811–4818.
8. Hogan CJ, Kettleson EM, Lee MH, Ramaswami B, Angenent LT, et al. (2005) Sampling methodologies and dosage assessment techniques for submicrometre and ultrafine virus aerosol particles. J Appl Microbiol 99: 1422–1434.
9. Myatt TA, Johnston SL, Rudnick S, Milton DK (2003) Airborne rhinovirus detection and effect of ultraviolet irradiation on detection by a semi-nested RT-PCR assay. BMC Public Health 3: 5.
10. Myatt TA, Johnston SL, Zuo Z, Wand M, Kebadze T, et al. (2004) Detection of airborne rhinovirus and its relation to outdoor air supply in office environments. Am J Respir Crit Care Med 169: 1187–1190.
11. Wan GH, Tsai YH, Wu YK, Tsao KC (2004) A large-volume nebulizer would not be an infectious source for severe acute respiratory syndrome (SARS). Infect Control Hosp Epidemiol 25: 1113–1115.
12. Booth TF, Kournikakis B, Bastien N, Ho J, et al. (2005) Detection of airborne severe acute respiratory syndrome (SARS) coronavirus and environmental contamination in SARS outbreak units. J Infect Dis 191: 1472–1477.
13. Tsai YH, Wan GH, Wu YK, Tsao KC (2006) Airborne SARS Coronavirus concentrations in a negative pressure isolation room containing a mechanically ventilated patient with SARS. Infect Control Hosp Epidemiol 27: 523–525.
14. Aintablian N, Walpita P, Sawyer MH (1998) Detection of Bordetella pertussis and respiratory syncytial virus in air samples from hospital rooms. Infect Control Hosp Epidemiol 19: 918–923.
15. Tseng CC, Chang LY, Li CS (2010) Detection of airborne viruses in a pediatrics department measured using real-time qPCR coupled to an air-sampling filter method. J Environ Health 73: 22–28.
16. Pyankov OV, Agranovski IE, Pyankova O, Mokhonova E, Mokhonov V, et al. (2007) Using a bioaerosol personal sampler in combination with real-time PCR analysis for rapid detection of airborne viruses. Environ Microbiol 9: 992–1000.
17. Weltia M, Jatona K, Altweggb M, Sahlia R, Wengera A, et al. (2003) Development of a multiplex real-time quantitative PCR assay to detect *Chlamydia pneumoniae*, *Legionella pneumophila* and *Mycoplasma pneumoniae* in respiratory tract secretions. Diagn Microbiol Infect Dis 45: 85–95.
18. Lindsley WG, Blachere FM, Davis KA, Pearce TA, Fisher MA, et al. (2010) Distribution of airborne influenza virus and respiratory syncytial virus in an urgent care medical clinic. Clin Infect Dis 50(5): 693–698.
19. Spengler JD, Saxton K (1983) Indoor air pollution: a public health perspective. Science 221: 9–17.
20. Samet JM, Marbury MC, Spengler JD (1987) Health effects and sources of indoor air pollution. Am Rev Respir Dis 136: 1486–1508.
21. Dharan S, Pittet D (2002) Environmental controls in operating theatres. J Hosp Infect 51: 79–84.

Molluscum Contagiosum in a Pediatric American Indian Population: Incidence and Risk Factors

Andrea M. McCollum[1,2]*, Robert C. Holman[1], Christine M. Hughes[1], Jason M. Mehal[1], Arianne M. Folkema[1], John T. Redd[3], James E. Cheek[3], Inger K. Damon[1], Mary G. Reynolds[1]

1 Division of High-Consequence Pathogens and Pathology, National Center for Emerging and Zoonotic Infectious Diseases, Centers for Disease Control and Prevention, Atlanta, Georgia, United States of America, **2** Epidemic Intelligence Service, Scientific Education and Professional Development Program Office, US Centers for Disease Control and Prevention, Atlanta, Georgia, United States of America, **3** Division of Epidemiology and Disease Prevention, Office of Public Health Support, Indian Health Service, Albuquerque, New Mexico, United States of America

Abstract

Background: Molluscum contagiosum virus (MCV) causes an innocuous yet persistent skin infection in immunocompetent individuals and is spread by contact with lesions. Studies point to atopic dermatitis (AD) as a risk factor for MCV infection; however, there are no longitudinal studies that have evaluated this hypothesis.

Methods: Outpatient visit data from fiscal years 2001–2009 for American Indian and Alaska Native (AI/AN) children were examined to describe the incidence of molluscum contagiosum (MC). We conducted a case-control study of patients <5 years old at an Indian Health Service (IHS) clinic to evaluate dermatological risk factors for infection.

Results: The incidence rate for MC in children <5 years old was highest in the West and East regions. MC cases were more likely to have a prior or co-occurring diagnosis of eczema, eczema or dermatitis, impetigo, and scabies ($p<0.05$) compared to controls; 51.4% of MC cases had a prior or co-occurring diagnosis of eczema or dermatitis.

Conclusions: The present study is the first demonstration of an association between AD and MC using a case-control study design. It is unknown if the concurrent high incidence of eczema and MC is related, and this association deserves further investigation.

Editor: Ravi Jhaveri, University of North Carolina School of Medicine, United States of America

Funding: Funding was provided for by the Centers for Disease Control and Prevention, Atlanta, Georgia. The findings and conclusions in this report are those of the author(s) and do not necessarily represent the views of the Centers for Disease Control and Prevention or the Indian Health Service. The funders had no role in study design, data collection and analysis, decision to publish, or preparation of the manuscript.

Competing Interests: The authors have declared that no competing interests exist.

* Email: amccollum@cdc.gov

Introduction

Molluscum contagiosum (MC) is a skin disease caused by molluscum contagiosum virus (MCV), a poxvirus. The infection causes firm, small, papular lesions, often with an umbilicated center. Lesions may have a region of erythema and can be found anywhere on the body. Lesions may remain for many weeks to months before resolving without treatment; however, in immunocompromised individuals, infection with MCV can cause giant lesions and a large number of lesions that require treatment. Diagnosis is usually made upon visual inspection of the lesions. Although rarely pursued, laboratory confirmation is available. There are several approaches to treating MC lesions, including physical destruction (cryotherapy, curettage, laser therapy) or use of immunomodulatory medicines (topical imiquimod) [1,2].

MCV is spread by contact with lesion material from an affected individual. Recommendations to prevent the spread of MCV on an individual's body or to others may include keeping the lesions covered and not sharing clothing, linens, or items that may contain lesion exudate with others [3]. Also, avoiding any behavior that would open the lesion and spread the material, such as shaving [4], scratching, and electrolysis [5], is recommended to prevent spread of the virus. An association between swimming pool use and MCV infection has been reported [6,7], but robust scientific data do not exist to firmly support this association. Although benign, MC can have an adverse effect on patients' and their families' lives, causing emotional concern and anxiety about physical manifestations of the infection [8].

There have been notable clinical cases of patients who present with atopic dermatitis (AD, including eczema) and have concurrent extensive MC lesions [9,10]. One clinical review of 284 children noted more lesions and a greater extent of surrounding eczema in patients presenting with MC and AD compared to those patients presenting with MC alone [11]. Indeed, there are indications that AD may be a risk factor for acquisition of MCV and that patients with AD may suffer a more extensive course of MC illness [12], but, to date, there are no case-control studies to evaluate these hypotheses.

Although MCV infection occurs in individuals of all ages, the infection is seen most often in children [13–15]. Publications often associate MC with tropical environments, the developing world, and poor living conditions, but infections are seen worldwide in a multitude of climates [8,13,16,17]. An analysis of Indian Health Service (IHS) outpatient visit data showed a higher incidence of MC in American Indian/Alaska Native (AI/AN) children aged 1–4 years old compared to other age groups, and this rate was particularly high in the IHS West region [15]. This increased incidence and disparity seen among IHS AI/AN patients, specifically those in the West region, warranted further investigation of cases and their potential risk factors.

We present a study designed to determine potential dermatological risk factors of MCV infection among AI/AN children seen in IHS facilities with a high incidence of MC. Furthermore, we investigated the occurrence of those risk factors in patients with MC.

Materials and Methods

Incidence of MC at IHS outpatient facilities

The national Indian Health Service (IHS) direct and contract care outpatient visit data for fiscal years 2001–2009 were obtained from the IHS National Patient Information Reporting System (NPIRS) [18]. These data consist of all outpatient visit records from IHS-operated, tribally-operated and community hospitals and facilities that are contracted with the IHS or with tribes to provide healthcare services to eligible AI/AN persons [19]. The IHS administrative areas were classified into regions as described by the IHS: Alaska, East (Nashville), Northern Plains East (Bemidji), Northern Plains West (Aberdeen and Billings), Southern Plains (Oklahoma), Southwest (Albuquerque, Navajo, Phoenix, and Tucson), and West (California and Portland). Outpatient visit records were selected for AI/AN children <5 years of age listing the International Classification of Diseases, 9th Revision, Clinical Modification (ICD-9-CM) code for MC (078.0) [20].

The outpatient visit records for AI/AN children <5 years of age with a MC diagnosis were examined by sex, age group (<1 and 1–4 years) and IHS region. The IHS West region, a region with a high incidence of MC [15], was further analyzed by Service Unit to identify those Service Units with the highest MC incidence. Annual and average annual MC-associated incidence rates per 10,000 children <5 years of age from the corresponding group were calculated for the study period using the annual number of patients with a MC diagnosis and the corresponding annual fiscal year IHS user population as the denominator. The IHS user population includes all registered AI/AN persons who have received IHS-funded health care services at least once during the preceding three years [19].

Case-control study

A case-control study was conducted to identify clinical characteristics of dermatological conditions among children <5 years of age that may be associated with the occurrence of MC using chart review at Facility B. Facility B is contained within Service Unit B, a service unit with a high annual incidence of MC in children <5 years of age (Table 1). The MC outpatient cases were identified as described below. Controls were randomly selected as children <5 years of age with outpatient visits during the same time period as cases, and did not list a current or prior MC diagnosis. Complete medical charts were abstracted for 84 cases and 109 controls at Facility B. Data from MC case patients were abstracted if the specific diagnosis of MC was listed on the medical chart. The specific dermatological conditions abstracted from medical charts included candidiasis; dermatitis; dry skin; eczema; hand, foot, and mouth disease; impetigo; rash; ringworm; scabies; varicella; viral exanthem; and viral warts. The diagnoses for additional conditions were captured as either co-occurring with the MC diagnosis and/or occurring prior to the MC diagnosis. A univariate analysis was conducted to identify clinical characteristics associated with MC. We refer to these significant characteristics as 'risk factors' noting that this analysis does not identify causation, but rather an association of a characteristic with MC.

Characteristics of MC cases at two outpatient clinics

Two IHS facilities (Facilities A and B) in the northwest United States were identified from IHS Service Units A and B, respectively, with a high incidence of MC among AI/AN children <5 years of age (Table 1). A chart review of records was conducted for all MC-associated outpatients <5 years of age during fiscal years 2001–2009 at the two facilities. A data collection form was developed to extract demographic and clinical information from medical records for these patients.

The ICD-9-CM code diagnosis of MC was validated by a healthcare provider's noted diagnosis entered on the medical record, and patients meeting these criteria were considered MC cases. Data were abstracted from a total of 175 cases (97.2% of identified ICD-9-CM diagnoses) from Facility A and 84 cases (81.6% of identified ICD-9-CM diagnoses) from Facility B. Data were not abstracted from all of the ICD-9-CM diagnosed cases because of missing medical records (n = 24, 8.5%) or misdiagnoses (n = 8, 2.8%). Age in months at first visit was compared using the Wilcoxon rank-sum test [21]. Statistical significance was considered at the $p<0.05$ level for all analyses.

Ethics Statement

The chart review at the two health facilities was determined to be public health non-research by CDC and exempt from review by the Portland Area IHS Human Subjects Institutional Review Board. Patient data was de-identified and anonymized prior to analysis.

Results

Incidence of MC at IHS outpatient facilities nationwide

The incidence of MC infections was calculated from IHS outpatient visit records for AI/AN children <5 years of age (Table 1). The overall incidence rate was 68.5 per 10,000 children, and the rate was similar amongst males and females. Children aged 1–4 years had an incidence rate four times higher than the rate for children <1 year old. The incidence rate was highest in the West (132.9) and East (121.5) IHS regions. Service Units A and B (including corresponding Facilities A and B) had particularly high incidence rates of 188.4 and 222.8, respectively. At Service Unit B, the incidence rate for children aged 1–4 years old was eight times that of children <1 year old.

Dermatological risk factors for MCV infection

Patient charts were reviewed from 175 cases (67.6%) at Facility A and 84 cases (32.4%) at Facility B. There were slightly more female (52.1%) than male patients (47.9%) (Table 2). The average age of patients at their first diagnosis of MC was 35 months with a median of 36 months. Approximately 95% of MC patients were one year of age or older (Table 2).

Table 1. Incidence rates[a] of molluscum contagiosum in American Indian children <5 years of age, fiscal years 2001–2009.

	Overall	Sex		Age (years)	
		Male	Female	<1	1–4
Service Unit A	188.4	179.2	198.7	45.1	212.7
Service Unit B	222.8	198.5	247.7	31.9	265.3
IHS Overall	68.5	67.4	69.6	19.2	77.6
Region					
Alaska	83.2	77.7	89.1	24.4	96.6
East	121.5	132.5	119.4	40.5	135.3
Northern Plains East	77.8	75.0	80.7	19.4	87.1
Northern Plains West	71.4	67.0	75.8	19.9	81.0
Southern Plains	51.1	53.2	48.9	16.5	56.7
Southwest	48.3	48.4	48.2	13.3	55.2
West	132.9	129.6	136.4	35.1	148.2

[a]Incidence rates are reported as per 10,000 children <5 years of age.

Data were collected for each visit where MC was diagnosed, including multiple visits. The majority of cases (68.7%) had only one diagnosis of MC. However, a substantial proportion of patients had multiple diagnoses over time: 19% of patients had a MC diagnosis for two visits, 9.7% for three visits, 1.9% for four visits, and 0.8% (2 patients) for five visits. Common descriptions for lesion presentation included characteristic 'pitted' or 'umbilicated' lesions (49.3%), 'colorless' (44.8%), 'red' or 'pink' (17.2%), erythema (16.4%), and pruritus (25.4%).

A case-control study to evaluate potential dermatological risk factors for MCV infection was conducted using medical records obtained at Facility B. The gender distribution was similar among MC cases and controls, and controls were significantly younger than case patients ($p<0.0001$, Table 2). Control patients presented to the clinic with a variety of chief complaints, whereas the chief compliant for most of the visits for case patients was self-described bumps or rash (84.3%).

Dermatological conditions were examined as potential risk factors for MCV infection at three different time periods relative to the visit - a) prior dermatological conditions, b) co-occurring dermatological conditions, and c) a combination of prior and co-occurring conditions. Considering prior dermatological conditions only, cases were more likely to have had a prior diagnosis of eczema (OR = 2.51, 95% CI 1.10–6.01), eczema or dermatitis (OR = 2.09, 95% CI 1.16–3.81), impetigo (OR = 2.88, 95% CI 1.40–6.10), or scabies (OR = 3.72, 95% CI 1.04–17.40) compared to controls ($p<0.05$) (Table 3). Considering co-occurring conditions only, cases were more likely to have diagnoses of eczema (OR = 5.71, 95% CI 1.98–20.66), eczema or dermatitis (OR = 2.97, 95% CI 1.24–7.69), or impetigo (OR = 4.86, 95% CI 1.14–33.24) than controls ($p<0.05$) (Table S1 in File S1). Grouping past and co-occurring conditions together, eczema (OR = 3.58, 95% CI 1.77–7.52), eczema or dermatitis (OR = 2.28, 95% CI 1.28–4.11), impetigo (OR = 3.40, 95% CI 1.73–6.92), and scabies (OR = 3.72, 95% CI 1.04–17.40) were more likely to occur in MC cases compared to controls ($p<0.05$) (Table S2 in File S1).

The frequencies of these risk factors in MC patients at both facilities and for the three time periods examined are shown in Figure 1. In considering any time period, 30.9% of MC cases had a diagnosis of eczema and 51.4% had a diagnosis of eczema or dermatitis. Also, 26.6% and 8.1% of MC cases had a diagnosis of impetigo or scabies, respectively.

Table 2. Demographic characteristics of American Indian molluscum contagiosum case and control patients <5 years old by facility.

	Facility A	Facility B	
	Cases[a]	Cases[a]	Controls[a]
Total	175 (100)	84 (100)	109 (100)
Sex			
Male	87 (50)	37 (44)	50 (46)
Female	88 (50)	47 (56)	59 (54)
Age (years)			
<1	9 (5)	5 (6)	40 (37)
1–4	166 (95)	79 (94)	69 (63)

[a]Number of patients (%).

Table 3. Univariate analysis of prior dermatological conditions for American Indian molluscum contagiosum (MC) cases and control patients <5 years of age at facility B.[a]

Condition	Case N (%)	Control N (%)	OR (95% CI)	p-value
Eczema				
No	67 (79.8)	99 (90.8)	Reference	
Yes	17 (20.2)	10 (9.2)	2.51 (1.10–6.01)	0.029
Eczema or Dermatitis[b]				
No	44 (52.4)	76 (69.7)	Reference	
Yes	40 (47.6)	33 (30.3)	2.09 (1.16–3.81)	0.014
Impetigo				
No	59 (70.2)	95 (87.2)	Reference	
Yes	25 (29.8)	14 (12.8)	2.88 (1.40–6.10)	0.004
Scabies				
No	76 (90.5)	106 (97.2)	Reference	
Yes	8 (9.5)	3 (2.8)	3.72 (1.04–17.40)	0.043

[a]Significant variables (conditions) are shown here. Non-significant variables were candidiasis; dermatitis; dry skin; hand, foot, and mouth disease; rash; ringworm; varicella; viral exanthem; and viral warts.[b]This variable includes diagnoses of eczema or dermatitis.

Discussion

Published data show a higher incidence of MC in AI/AN children <5 years of age, specifically amongst children aged 1–4 years [15]; and the more recent measures here show the same trend across IHS regions, with the West region having the highest incidence. Moreover, this age distribution has been noted previously in children <5 years old [13,22–24]. Some authors have hypothesized that children in this age range have behaviors and activities that facilitate close contact with affected individuals,

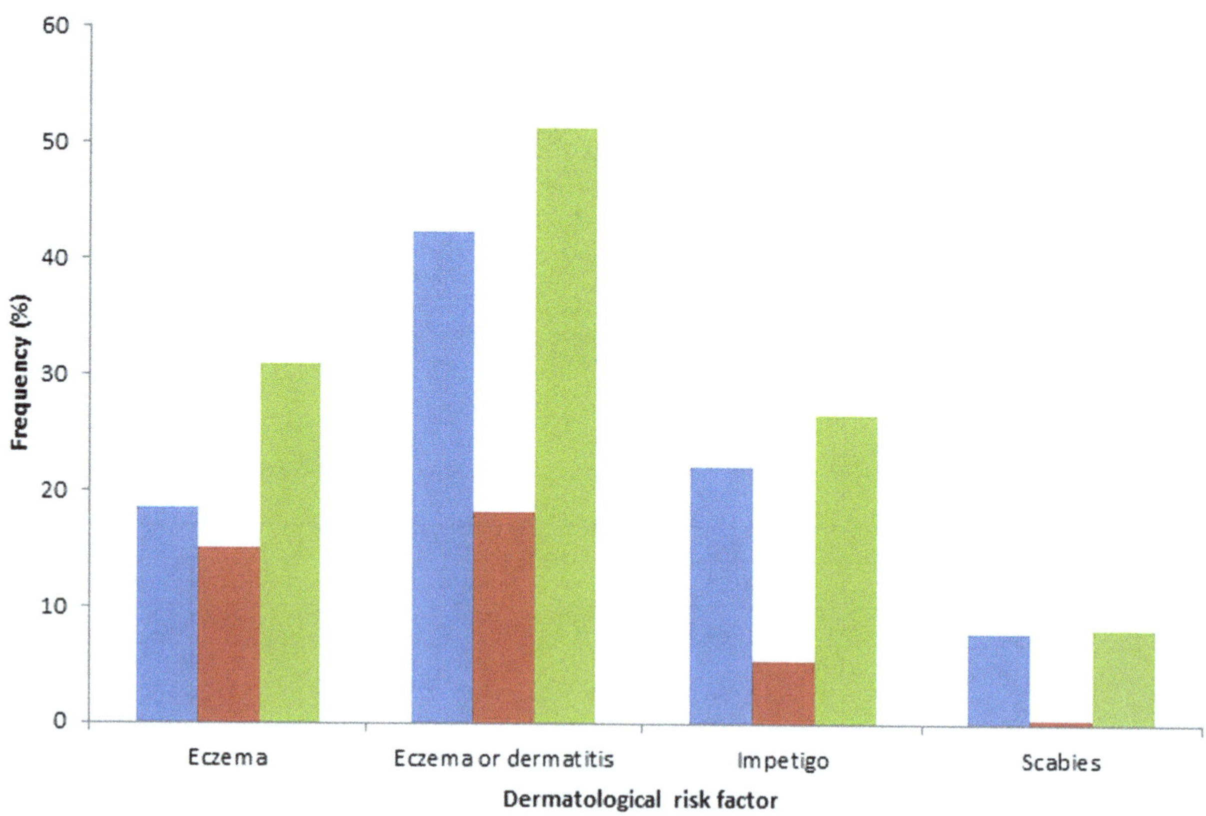

Figure 1. The frequency of dermatological risk factors in MC case patients at three time periods relative to the initial visit where MC was diagnosed - a) prior dermatological conditions (blue), b) co-occurring dermatological conditions (red), and c) a combination of prior and co-occurring conditions (green). MC cases include those from Facilities A and B.

thereby facilitating the spread of MCV to others [23,25], and others have suggested that maternal antibodies may protect newborn infants from infection [23]. Cases from the two IHS facilities examined in the present study had a slight predominance of female patients versus male. There are no consistent data in the literature to suggest one gender is overrepresented by MCV infections [8].

The majority of MC cases in the present study were noted to have a MC diagnosis only once, but over 30% of cases had MC on multiple healthcare center visit records. The duration of illness lasted for several months for many patients and up to one year for one patient. MC is known to persist for months to years, eventually resolving without treatment for many patients [3].

In this population of pediatric AI/AN patients with a high burden of MC, there was an association between MC and prior or co-occurring diagnosis of eczema, eczema or dermatitis, impetigo, and scabies. Prior research has suggested a purported association between patients with AD or eczema and MC [25–27], but this study is the first to quantify this relationship. AD patients are known to have an increased susceptibility to many dermatologic infections and are at risk for severe complications from poxviral infections, notably *Orthopoxviruses* including vaccinia virus [22,28,29]. A study that utilized parent recall of prior dermatological conditions in pediatric patients did not find an association between MC illness and prior history of AD [30], but this approach has the limitation of dependence on recall of clinical diagnosis. Here, we utilized documented clinical diagnoses of MC and concurrent or prior diagnosis of several dermatological skin conditions. All of the significant conditions (eczema, eczema or AD, impetigo, scabies) can compromise the integrity of the external epidermal surface, providing portals of entry for the establishment of viral infections. Eczema and AD can also be considered manifestations of immune deficits or disregulation, and this may yield a propensity to develop infections [22].

A recent study of pediatric health survey data suggested that approximately 10% of all children <17 years old in the United States have had a prior diagnosis of eczema, and children <4 years old have the highest incidence of eczema. Also, the incidence of eczema differed geographically, with the western United States having a notably high incidence (although, high incidence rates were is not observed exclusively in the western United States) [31]. Over half of the pediatric MC patients in the present study had a diagnosis of eczema or dermatitis, a remarkably high frequency of diagnoses compared to national data. In a published chart review by Berger, et al., a high percentage of pediatric MC patients (37.2%) had a history of AD [28]. It is unknown if the co-occurring high incidence of eczema and MC are related.

The present study has several possible limitations, as well as, some unique attributes that contribute to the strength of our conclusions. Because the AI/AN populations studied are relatively isolated, the IHS clinic, which offers no-cost health care to eligible beneficiaries, is the source of the vast majority of health care for these populations. It is believed that the charts at Facilities A and B represented most of the clinical visits for an individual over their life to date (up to 5 years of age), so our ascertainment of prior dermatological conditions was likely to be complete. Also, this study was able to capture and review the majority of MC cases <5 years of age at the two outpatient clinics. However, clinical diagnoses (including those for impetigo and scabies) were based on clinical examination alone and never laboratory confirmed, which likely suggests that some diagnoses may have been inaccurate. Diagnostic laboratory testing was only requested for one MC case and the results were not listed in the chart. Similarly, in most diagnoses of AD there was no documentation of any additional laboratory evaluation or referral to a dermatologist for evaluation. Further, surrounding erythema is known to occur with some MC lesions and this was noted for 16.4% of MC cases reviewed here. It is unknown if the presence of erythema surrounding lesions was considered by the practitioners to be a presentation of MC or a presentation of atopy. Such possible misdiagnoses could lead to a misclassification bias in our study, although unless primary care providers systematically misdiagnosed MC for AD, there should not be a significant effect on our measures of association. Further, descriptive information was missing from some charts, particularly information relevant to the MC presentation.

The AI/AN population harbors a high burden of infectious diseases [32,33], and MC in the pediatric population is no exception. The present study affirms the association between AD and MC; however, the mechanisms of such an association are unknown and deserve further attention and study in additional patient populations. AI/AN pediatric populations would benefit from targeted outreach to prevent and mitigate the spread of MCV among children.

Acknowledgments

The authors thank Thomas Weiser, Barbara Strzelczyk, Phil Smith (IHS) for technical assistance and comments, and the staff at the two participating IHS care facilities. Funding was provided for by the Centers for Disease Control and Prevention, Atlanta, Georgia. The findings and conclusions in this report are those of the author(s) and do not necessarily represent the views of the Centers for Disease Control and Prevention or the Indian Health Service.

Author Contributions

Conceived and designed the experiments: AMM RCH AMF JTR JEC IKD MGR. Performed the experiments: AMM RCH CMH JMM AMF. Analyzed the data: AMM RCH JMM AMF. Contributed to the writing of the manuscript: AMM RCH JMM AMF MGR.

References

1. Janniger CK, Schwartz RA (1993) Molluscum contagiosum in children. Cutis 52: 194–196.
2. Nelson KC, Morrell DS (2007) Spreading bumps: molluscum contagiosum in the pediatric population. Pediatr Ann 36: 814, 816–818.
3. (2012) Red Book; Pickering LK, Baker, Kimberlin DW, Long SS, editors: American Academy of Pediatrics.
4. Lee B, Kang HY (2004) Molluscum folliculitis after leg shaving. J Am Acad Dermatol 51: 478–479.
5. Rich JD, Dickinson BP, Flaxman AB, Mylonakis E (1999) Local spread of molluscum contagiosum by electrolysis. Clin Infect Dis 28: 1171.
6. Castilla MT, Sanzo JM, Fuentes S (1995) Molluscum contagiosum in children and its relationship to attendance at swimming-pools: an epidemiological study. Dermatology 191: 165.
7. Niizeki K, Kano O, Kondo Y (1984) An epidemic study of molluscum contagiosum. Relationship to swimming. Dermatologica 169: 197–198.

8. Braue A, Ross G, Varigos G, Kelly H (2005) Epidemiology and impact of childhood molluscum contagiosum: a case series and critical review of the literature. Pediatr Dermatol 22: 287–294.
9. Ghura HS, Camp RD (2001) Scarring molluscum contagiosum in patients with severe atopic dermatitis: report of two cases. Br J Dermatol 144: 1094–1095.
10. Solomon LM, Telner P (1966) Eruptive molluscum contagiosum in atopic dermatitis. Can Med Assoc J 95: 978–979.
11. Seize MB, Ianhez M, Cestari Sda C (2011) A study of the correlation between molluscum contagiosum and atopic dermatitis in children. An Bras Dermatol 86: 663–668.
12. Wollenberg A, Wetzel S, Burgdorf WH, Haas J (2003) Viral infections in atopic dermatitis: pathogenic aspects and clinical management. The Journal of Allergy and Clinical Immunology 112: 667–674.
13. Koning S, Bruijnzeels MA, van Suijlekom-Smit LW, van der Wouden JC (1994) Molluscum contagiosum in Dutch general practice. Br J Gen Pract 44: 417–419.
14. Molino AC, Fleischer AB Jr, Feldman SR (2004) Patient demographics and utilization of health care services for molluscum contagiosum. Pediatr Dermatol 21: 628–632.
15. Reynolds MG, Holman RC, Yorita Christensen KL, Cheek JE, Damon IK (2009) The Incidence of Molluscum contagiosum among American Indians and Alaska Natives. PLoS One 4: e5255.
16. Overfield TM, Brody JA (1966) An epidemiologic study of molluscum contagiosum in Anchorage, Alaska. J Pediatr 69: 640–642.
17. Postlethwaite R, Watt JA, Hawley TG, Simpson I, Adam H (1967) Features of molluscum contagiosum in the north-east of Scotland and in Fijian village settlements. J Hyg (Lond) 65: 281–291.
18. (2010) Direct/CHS Inpatient data, Fiscal years 1998–2009. National Patient Information Reporting System. Albuquerque, NM: Indian Health Service.
19. (2009) Trends in Indian Health 2002–2003. Rockville, MD: Indian Health Service.
20. (2008) International classification of diseases, 9th revision, clinical modification (CD-ROM). Washington, DC: US Department of Health and Human Services; Public Health Service and Health Care Financing Administration.
21. Lehmann EL (1975) Nonparametrics: statistical methods based on ranks. San Francisco: Holden Day.
22. Boguniewicz M, Leung DY (2010) Recent insights into atopic dermatitis and implications for management of infectious complications. The Journal of Allergy and Clinical Immunology 125: 4–13.
23. Netchiporouk E, Cohen BA (2012) Recognizing and managing eczematous ID reactions to molluscum contagiosum virus in children. Pediatrics 129: e1072–1075.
24. Sturt RJ, Muller HK, Francis GD (1971) Molluscum contagiosum in villages of the West Sepik District of New Guinea. Med J Aust 2: 751–754.
25. Coloe J, Burkhart CN, Morrell DS (2009) Molluscum contagiosum: what's new and true? Pediatr Ann 38: 321–325.
26. Dohil MA, Lin P, Lee J, Lucky AW, Paller AS, et al. (2006) The epidemiology of molluscum contagiosum in children. J Am Acad Dermatol 54: 47–54.
27. Lee R, Schwartz RA (2010) Pediatric molluscum contagiosum: reflections on the last challenging poxvirus infection, Part 1. Cutis 86: 230–236.
28. Berger EM, Orlow SJ, Patel RR, Schaffer JV (2012) Experience with molluscum contagiosum and associated inflammatory reactions in a pediatric dermatology practice: the bump that rashes. Arch Dermatol 148: 1257–1264.
29. Vora S, Damon I, Fulginiti V, Weber SG, Kahana M, et al. (2008) Severe eczema vaccinatum in a household contact of a smallpox vaccinee. Clin Infect Dis 46: 1555–1561.
30. Hayashida S, Furusho N, Uchi H, Miyazaki S, Eiraku K, et al. (2010) Are lifetime prevalence of impetigo, molluscum and herpes infection really increased in children having atopic dermatitis? J Dermatol Sci 60: 173–178.
31. Shaw TE, Currie GP, Koudelka CW, Simpson EL (2011) Eczema prevalence in the United States: data from the 2003 National Survey of Children's Health. J Invest Dermatol 131: 67–73.
32. Holman RC, Curns AT, Cheek JE, Singleton RJ, Anderson LJ, et al. (2003) Infectious disease hospitalizations among American Indian and Alaska native infants. Pediatrics 111: E176–182.
33. Holman RC, Folkema AM, Singleton RJ, Redd JT, Christensen KY, et al. (2011) Disparities in infectious disease hospitalizations for American Indian/Alaska Native people. Public Health Rep 126: 508–521.

Time Trends in Pediatric Hospitalizations for Varicella Infection are Associated with Climatic Changes

Elena Critselis[1], Panagiotis T. Nastos[2], Kalliopi Theodoridou[3], Maria Theodoridou[3], Maria N. Tsolia[1], Christos Hadjichristodoulou[4], Vassiliki Papaevangelou[1]*

1 Second University Department of Pediatrics, "P. & A. Kyriakou" Children's Hospital, National and Kapodistrian University of Athens School of Medicine, Athens, Greece, **2** Laboratory of Climatology and Atmospheric Environment, Department of Geology and Geoenvironment, National and Kapodistrian University of Athens, Athens, Greece, **3** First University Department of Pediatrics, "Aghia Sophia" Children's Hospital, National and Kapodistrian University of Athens School of Medicine, Athens, Greece, **4** Department of Hygiene and Epidemiology, University of Thessaly School of Medicine, Thessaly, Greece

Abstract

Background/Aims: The transmission rate of air-borne infectious diseases may vary secondary to climate conditions. The study assessed time trends in the seasonality of hospitalized varicella cases in a temperate region in relation to climatic parameters prior to the implementation of universal varicella immunization.

Methods: A retrospective descriptive study was conducted among all pediatric and adolescent varicella patients (n = 2366) hospitalized at the "Aghia Sophia" Children's Hospital during 1982–2003 in Athens, Greece. Date of infection was computed based on hospital admission date. Seasonal and monthly trends in the epidemiology of varicella infection were assessed with time series analysis (ARIMA modeling procedure). The correlation between the frequency of varicella patients and the meteorological parameters was examined by the application of Generalized Linear Models with Gamma distribution.

Results: During 1982–2003, the occurrence of hospitalized varicella cases increased during summer ($p = 0.025$) and decreased during autumn ($p = 0.021$), and particularly in September ($p = 0.003$). The frequency of hospitalized varicella cases was inversely associated with air temperature ($p < 0.001$). In contrast, the occurrence of hospitalized varicella cases was positively associated with wind speed ($p = 0.009$).

Conclusions: Pediatric hospitalizations for varicella infection rates have increased during summer and decreased during autumn in the examined temperate region. Time trends in hospitalized varicella cases are associated with climatic variables.

Editor: D. William Cameron, University of Ottawa, Canada

Funding: The present work was funded by the Second University Department of Pediatrics, "P. & A. Kyriakou" Children's Hospital, of the National and Kapodistrian University of Athens School of Medicine. The funders had no role in study design, data collection and analysis, decision to publish, or preparation of the manuscript.

Competing Interests: The authors have declared that no competing interests exist.

* E-mail: vpapaev@med.uoa.gr

Introduction

Chickenpox, caused by the varicella zoster virus (VZV), constitutes a prevalent disease among pediatric populations, particularly in temperate regions [1,2]. Prior to the implementation of universal infant vaccination for varicella, more than 90% of children in temperate regions presented with varicella infection by mid-adolescence [3–6]. In Europe, the annual hospitalization rate attributed to varicella infection ranges between 12.9 to 28.0 per 100,000 children [1]. Although varicella is considered a mild disease, approximately 2–6% of varicella patients present with severe and potentially fatal complications, including respiratory and neurological complications, such as encephalitis and cerebellar ataxia [1,3].

VZV is primarily transmitted by direct contact and secondarily by airborne transmission [7]. The epidemiology of varicella infection is noted to be remarkably different between temperate and tropical regions, with incidence rates being lower in the latter [8,9]. Therefore, while varicella is a disease of preschool and school-aged children in temperate regions, in the tropics it often affects older age groups [1,10–12]. Moreover, in tropical regions the seroprevalence rate of VZV is higher in urban versus rural populations [12–14]. It has been postulated that ambient temperature and humidity negatively affect VZV transmission [10]. Moreover, in temperate European countries, the seropositivity rate of VZV is lower in those Mediterranean countries with the hottest climates of the region [1,15]. However, other factors such as population density, nursery attendance and socioeconomic development also may influence the epidemiology of VZV in areas where universal vaccination has not yet been implemented [16]. To date, the association between the epidemiological trends in varicella infection and climatic factors (temperature, rainfall, humidity) has mainly been studied in tropical regions [12,17–19]. Nowadays, while environmental factors are modified in temperate regions secondary to the ozone phenomenon, the investigation of a possible association with epidemiologic changes in varicella incidence may be vital for designing related evidence-based public health prevention strategies [20].

The study objectives were to assess the time trends in the epidemiology of hospitalized varicella cases in a temperate Mediterranean country during the pre-licensure period for the varicella vaccine when climate changes were notable [20]. In addition, the study objectives were to evaluate the association between the frequency of hospitalized varicella cases and climatic variables in the aforementioned study site.

Methods

Study Design and Population

A retrospective descriptive study was conducted in all pediatric patients aged ≤14 years hospitalized for varicella infection at the public tertiary "Aghia Sophia" Children's Hospital in Athens, Greece between Jan. 1, 1982 – Dec. 31, 2003. The study site is located in the Athens metropolitan area and serves approximately 650,000 children aged 0–14 years [21]. The study hypothesis was that the diminishment over time in hospitalized varicella cases could be associated with changes in climatic conditions in the region. Data was retrieved from the hospital admission data log records, rather than individual patient files. As a result, access to personal details, such as immigrant status, number of siblings, and/or nursery attendance, was not granted. Moreover, no exclusion criteria with respect to either socio-demographic variables and/or severity of disease manifestation were applied. The research protocol was approved by the Hospital Ethics Committee. Since no personal data was recorded for the purposes of the study, written informed consent for study participation was not required.

Data Collection

Hospital records were utilized to identify pediatric patients with varicella infection and demographic characteristics were recorded. In order to account for the incubation period and to consequently evaluate date of infection, the following assumptions were made: (1) varicella incubation period extends 10–14 days and admission occurs during the first four days of illness; and, (2) admission for cerebellar ataxia occurs one week later (8–11th day of illness). Thus, the following computations were applied to approximate the date of infection: (1) patients without cerebellar ataxia were infected 2 weeks prior to hospital admission; and, (2) patients with cerebellar ataxia were infected 3 weeks prior to hospital admission. The derived estimated date of varicella infection was utilized for all analyses.

The climatic variables examined were air temperature (°C), relative humidity (%), and wind speed (m/s). Mean monthly values of meteorological data were extracted from historical daily records for the period 1982–2003 from the meteorological station of the National Observatory of Athens which is located on the Hill of Nymphs near the centre of Athens ($\lambda = 23° 43'$ E, $\phi = 37° 58'$ N, h = 107 m a.m.s.l.).

Statistical Analysis

Time series analyses (ARIMA modeling procedure) were applied to assess time trends in the occurrence of hospitalized varicella cases according to both season and month, respectively. The correlation between the frequency of hospitalized varicella cases and climatic parameters was examined by the application of Generalized Linear Models (GLM) with Gamma distribution [22–23]. Varicella cases fitted well to the Gamma distribution, after being checked by the application of the Kolmogorov-Smirnov test (statistic d). The modeling procedure used as a dependent variable the mean monthly number of hospitalized varicella patients, while climatic parameters were included separately as independent covariates. The goodness-of-fit of the models was evaluated through deviance residuals [22]. A p-value (p) of ≤0.05 was considered as the criterion for statistical significance. Analyses were conducted with SPSS version 17.0.

Results

Time trends in pediatric hospitalizations for varicella infection

During 1982–2003, 2366 pediatric patients were hospitalized with varicella infection in the temperate region examined. Overall, no significant change in the occurrence of hospitalized varicella cases was observed during the study period.

The occurrence of hospitalized varicella cases was highest during spring, exceeding two fifths of all cases, and winter (Table 1). However, no significant changes in the frequency of hospitalized cases were observed during either of the aforementioned seasons. In contrast, the proportion of hospitalized varicella cases increased during summer ($p = 0.025$) and decreased during autumn ($p = 0.021$). In particular, the mean increase in the proportion of hospitalized varicella cases during summer was 0.49% per year, while the mean decrease in the proportion of cases during autumn was 0.56% per year. Also, an inverse trend with regard to hospitalized varicella cases was observed during the autumn months (Table 1), as they were reduced to approximately half upon the conclusion of the study period. This trend was primarily attributed to the diminishment in varicella infection rates during the September months (Table 2).

Hospitalizations for varicella infection and climatic factors

The overall intra-annual mean monthly variation of meteorological variables during the study period examined are presented in Figures 1a–1f. Mean monthly air temperature was inversely related with the frequency of hospitalized varicella cases (Figure 1a). However, when adjusted for seasonality and trend, mean air temperature was not significantly associated with the monthly frequency of hospitalized varicella patients (Figure 1d). Similar findings were observed for relative humidity (Figures 1b and Figure 1e). In contrast, mean monthly wind speed was positively correlated with the frequency in hospitalized varicella cases (Figure 1c), even following adjustment for seasonality (Figure 1f).

GLM with Gamma distribution (Kolmogorov-Smirnov statistical index $d = 0.08$) were applied using as the dependent variable the mean monthly number of hospitalized varicella patients and as independent covariates the individual climatic parameters. Thus, three GLM were constructed, each one including only one independent covariate, in order to examine the individual impact of each climatic covariate on varicella hospitalizations. The non-multicollinearity between the three independent variables was investigated by the application of the multicollinearity index VIF.

Table 1. Seasonal time trends in pediatric hospitalized varicella cases in Athens, Greece (n = 2366).

Year	1982–83 (n = 96) n (%)	1984–85 (n = 153) n (%)	1986–87 (n = 245) n (%)	1988–89 (n = 267) n (%)	1990–91 (n = 243) n (%)	1992–93 (n = 195) n (%)	1994–95 (n = 211) n (%)	1996–97 (n = 218) n (%)	1998–99 (n = 216) n (%)	2000–01 (n = 233) n (%)	2002–03 (n = 289) n (%)	p-value
Spring	33 (33.4)	62 (40.5)	122 (49.8)	130 (48.7)	90 (37.0)	89 (45.6)	101 (47.9)	88 (40.4)	92 (42.6)	104 (44.6)	107(37.0)	0.949
Summer	11 (11.4)	26 (17.0)	34 (13.9)	52 (19.5)	38 (15.6)	42 (21.5)	37 (17.5)	35 (16.0)	38 (17.6)	71 (30.5)	61 (21.1)	***0.025***
Fall	21 (21.9)	26 (17.0)	16 (6.5)	19 (7.1)	22 (9.0)	20 (10.3)	19 (9.0)	29 (13.3)	16 (7.4)	10 (4.3)	31 (10.7)	***0.021***
Winter	31 (32.3)	39 (25.5)	73 (29.8)	66 (24.7)	93 (38.3)	44 (22.6)	54 (25.6)	66 (30.3)	70 (32.4)	48 (20.6)	90 (31.1)	0.961

The term of non-multicollinearity between the three independent variables T, RH and V was fully fulfilled (Table 3).

The results of the GLM applied are presented in Table 4. A significant correlation between the mean monthly number of varicella hospitalised patients and the climatic parameters was established. Specifically, a decrease by an increment of 1°C in mean monthly air temperature was associated with a 3% increase in the number of hospitalized varicella cases. Furthermore, it is noteworthy that an increase by 1 m/s in mean monthly wind speed was associated with a 20% increase in the probability of hospitalization. On the other hand, no significant association was established between hospitalized varicella cases and relative humidity (Table 4).

Discussion

The present study evaluated the time trends in pediatric hospitalizations for varicella infection in a temperate region prior to the implementation of universal VZV immunization among infants and during which period climate changes were notable [20]. The study also evaluated the association between the occurrence of hospitalized varicella cases and climatic variables during the aforementioned study period. The main study findings indicate that the occurrence of pediatric hospitalized varicella cases increased notably in the summer and decreased in the autumn seasons during the period 1982–2003. In particular, the most notable effects were observed in the September months of the period examined. The evidence provided supports that modifications in hospitalized varicella cases during the period 1982–2003 in the examined temperate Mediterranean region were associated with climatic factors. Specifically, the occurrence of hospitalized varicella cases was inversely associated with air temperature ($p<0.001$) and positively associated with wind speed ($p=0.009$). No statistically significant relationship was revealed between hospitalized varicella cases and relative humidity.

Changes in the epidemiology of varicella infection, particularly in tropical regions, have been attributed to demographic changes, including increased population density and urbanization [2,14]. Seroprevalence rates of varicella infection have been observed to be higher among urban populations, regardless of the population"s age distribution [8,13]. It has been proposed that in urban tropical regions an elevated population density may partially overcome the transmission-interrupting effect of a tropical climate [12–13]. Specifically, urban settings may enable enhanced social interaction and population mobility, both within and between communities, and hence facilitate viral transmission [12]. Such evidence is corroborated by findings in temperate countries indicating that children with enhanced social interaction, such as that incurred by their attendance in nurseries, are more likely to contract varicella infection [15]. In the present reference population, a significant influx of immigrants was observed following the 1990′s. Immigrant children are more likely to be hospitalized for varicella complications [15]. However, as compared to Greek children, immigrant children have lower day care attendance rates and

Table 2. Monthly time trends in pediatric hospitalized varicella cases in Athens, Greece (n = 2366).

	1982–83 (n = 96) n (%)	1984–85 (n = 153) n (%)	1986–87 (n = 245) n (%)	1988–89 (n = 267) n (%)	1990–91 (n = 243) n (%)	1992–93 (n = 195) n (%)	1994–95 (n = 211) n (%)	1996–97 (n = 218) n (%)	1998–99 (n = 216) n (%)	2000–01 (n = 233) n (%)	2002–03 (n = 289) n (%)	p-value
Jan.	9 (9.4)	16 (10.4)	27 (11.0)	18 (6.7)	20 (8.2)	9 (4.6)	18 (8.5)	21 (9.6)	25 (11.6)	13 (5.6)	27 (9.3)	0.792
Feb.	8 (8.3)	10 (6.5)	29 (11.8)	27 (10.1)	23 (9.5)	20 (10.2)	25 (11.8)	20 (9.2)	28 (13.0)	18 (7.7)	42 (14.5)	0.476
Mar.	12 (12.5)	21 (13.7)	38 (15.5)	35 (13.1)	34 (14.0)	17 (8.7)	25 (11.8)	28 (12.8)	30 (13.9)	27 (11.6)	65 (22.5)	0.902
Apr.	10 (10.4)	23 (15.0)	43 (17.6)	37 (13.8)	21 (8.6)	26 (13.3)	34 (16.1)	24 (11.0)	24 (11.1)	30 (12.9)	28 (9.7)	0.933
May	11 (11.4)	18 (11.8)	41 (16.7)	58 (21.7)	35 (14.4)	46 (23.6)	42 (19.9)	36 (16.5)	38 (17.6)	47 (20.2)	14 (4.8)	0.799
Jun.	6 (6.2)	9 (5.9)	24 (9.8)	33 (12.4)	26 (10.7)	37 (19.0)	22 (10.4)	26 (11.9)	31 (14.4)	55 (23.6)	45 (15.6)	0.214
Jul.	4 (4.2)	11 (7.2)	9 (3.7)	12 (4.5)	8 (3.3)	4 (2.0)	12 (5.7)	5 (2.3)	7 (3.2)	15 (6.4)	14 (4.8)	0.482
Aug.	1 (1.0)	6 (3.9)	1 (0.4)	7 (2.6)	4 (1.6)	1 (0.5)	3 (1.4)	4 (1.8)	0 (0.0)	1 (0.4)	2 (0.7)	0.941
Sept.	4 (4.2)	6 (3.9)	3 (1.2)	5 (1.9)	7 (2.9)	1 (0.5)	1 (0.5)	4 (1.8)	3 (1.4)	2 (0.8)	6 (2.1)	***0.003***
Oct.	7 (7.3)	10 (6.5)	8 (3.3)	2 (0.7)	9 (3.7)	2 (1.0)	4 (1.9)	12 (5.5)	5 (2.3)	3 (1.3)	7 (2.4)	0.112
Nov.	10 (10.4)	10 (6.5)	5 (2.0)	12 (4.5)	6 (2.5)	17 (8.7)	14 (6.6)	13 (6.0)	8 (3.7)	5 (2.1)	18 (6.2)	0.063
Dec.	14 (14.6)	13 (8.5)	17 (6.9)	21 (7.9)	50 (20.6)	15 (7.7)	11 (5.2)	25 (11.5)	17 (7.9)	17 (7.3)	21 (7.3)	0.907

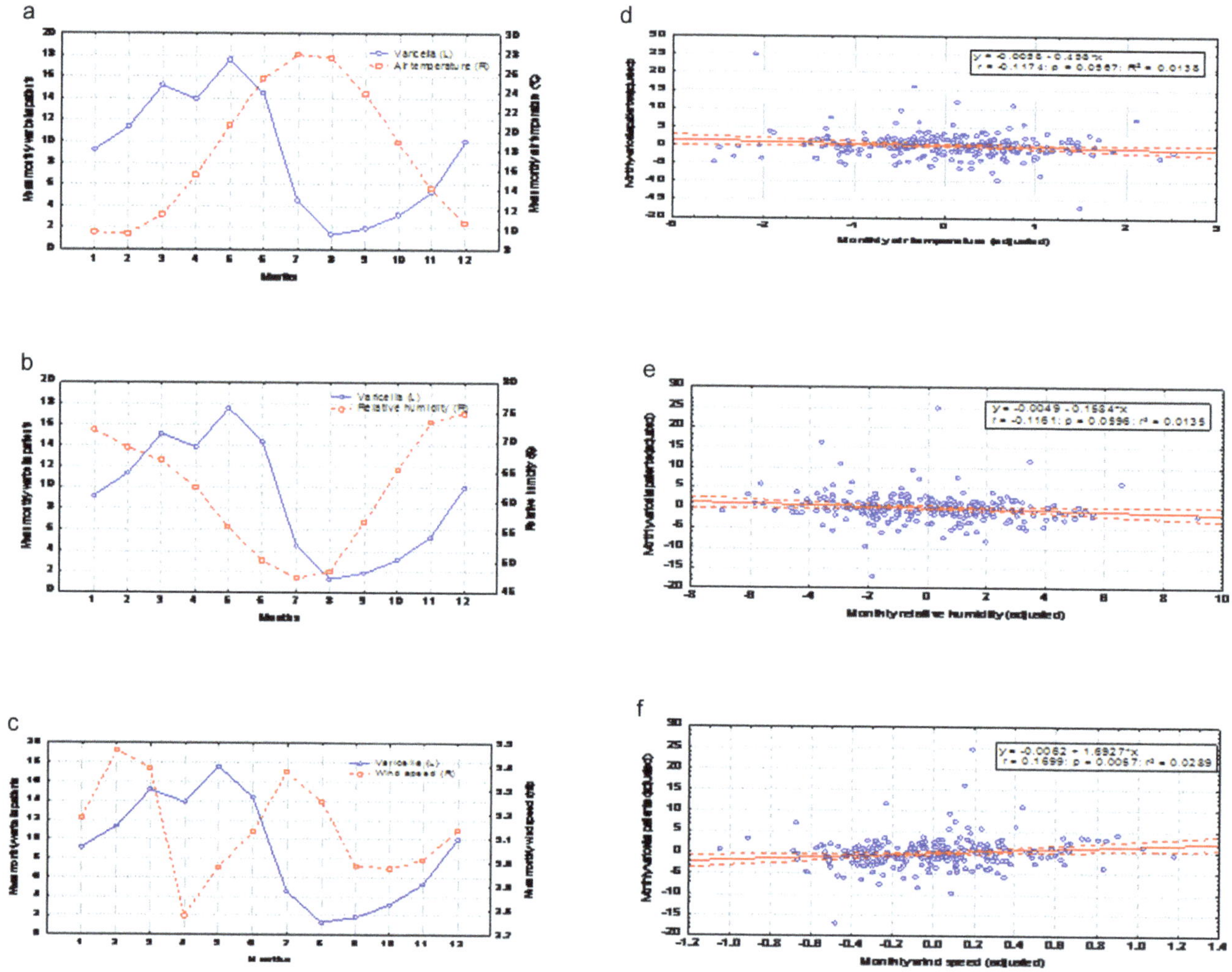

Figure 1. Association between climatic variables and hospitalization rates for varicella infection among children in a Greek tertiary care center (1982–2003). a. Intra annual variation of mean monthly air temperature and hospitalized varicella patients for the period 1982–2003. **b.** Intra annual variation of mean monthly relative humidity and hospitalized varicella patients for the period 1982–2003. **c.** Intra annual variation of mean monthly wind speed and hospitalized varicella patients for the period 1982–2003. **d.** Scatter plot between mean monthly varicella patients (adjusted for season and trend) and air temperature for the period 1982–2003. **e.** Scatter plot between mean monthly varicella patients (adjusted for season and trend) and relative humidity for the period 1982–2003. **f.** Scatter plot between mean monthly varicella patients (adjusted for season and trend) and wind speed for the period 1982–2003.

consequently contract varicella at an older age [15]. Since the mean age of hospitalized patients for varicella infection has not significantly changed during the study period [15], it is upheld that the aforementioned demographic changes did not markedly affect the epidemiological trends of hospitalizations for varicella infection in the population examined.

The study findings indicated that significant changes in the epidemiology of varicella infection have occurred during the seasons of summer and autumn. In particular, a diminishment in hospitalized varicella cases was observed during the September months. These findings corroborate with proposed hypotheses positing that changes in varicella infection rates in urban regions

Table 3. Non-multicollinearity test results between the three independent variables: air temperature (T), relative humidity (RH) and wind speed (V).

Combination of the independent variables	Square of multiple correlation coefficient (R^2)	VIF
T = f(RH, V)	0.166	1.20
RH = f(T, V)	0.173	1.21
V = f(T, RH)	0.219	1.28

Table 4. Generalized Linear Models (GLM) with Gamma distribution for assessing the association between mean monthly number of varicella patients and meteorological parameters.

Parameter	Estimate	Standard Error	p-value
Air temperature (°C)	−0.030	0.008	*<0.001*
Relative humidity (%)	−0.001	0.005	0.916
Wind speed (m/s)	0.181	0.070	*0.009*

may be attributed to the combined effects of atmospheric air pollution and ultraviolet radiation [24].

The present study findings indicated that the modifications in the occurrence of hospitalized varicella cases in the evaluated temperate Mediterranean region were associated with climatic variables. In particular, the occurrence of hospitalized varicella cases was inversely associated with air temperature. Moreover, the frequency of hospitalized varicella cases was proximally associated with wind speed. Interestingly, although during the summer months of the period 1982–2003 an increase in mean air temperature was documented in the evaluated region, a concomitant increase in hospitalized varicella cases was also observed. However, the GLM analysis indicated that the potential effect of wind speed upon the occurrence of hospitalized varicella cases is substantially greater than that of mean air temperature. This is corroborated by the origin of the Greek term for "chickenpox" ("anemevlogia") which is derived from the combination of the terms "anemos" (= wind) and "evlogia" (= small pox), indicating that the association between wind speed and varicella infection has been empirically suspected for several centuries. Therefore, it is upheld that the observed increase in hospitalized varicella cases in the summer months of the period 1982–2003 is more likely to be attributable to mean wind speed rather than mean air temperature.

Differential seroprevalence rates in varicella infection have been partly attributed to climatic factors, particularly in relation to temperature and humidity [10,25]. Correlations between varicella incidence rates with both temperature and rainfall have been observed [2]. In tropical regions, evidence supports that the mean of extreme minimum temperatures is most proximally associated with increases in VZV seroprevalence. Due to the heat sensitivity of VZV, the virus may be inactivated at higher temperatures [12]. Hence, the viral transmission potential may be markedly reduced in countries with elevated mean temperatures and humidity [8,14]. This has been primarily corroborated by the lower VZV seroprevalence rates observed in tropical regions [2].

Similarly, lower varicella seroprevalence rates in southern European countries have been attributed to the effects of the mild Mediterranean climate upon disease transmission potential [1]. It has been suggested that both the high levels of humidity and diminishment in the seasonal variations in temperature, particularly in countries proximal to the equator, may be associated with a uniform distribution of varicella cases throughout the year [8]. It is proposed that the observed epidemiological changes in the study region may be partly attributed to climatic changes which have resulted in the modifications of mean air temperature, relative humidity and, in particular, wind speed during the summer and autumn seasons [20]. However, mounting evidence exists supporting that the risk of infection by airborne viruses via aerosol transmission may be equivalent to that of direct transmission [26,27], particularly in settings with low humidity [28]. The study findings indicated that the peak incidence rate remained greatest during the spring season throughout the time period evaluated. This contrasts findings in tropical regions which indicate that the peak incidence of varicella infection occurs during the cooler months of the year [12]. Thus, it may be inferred that although climatic changes in the study region have potentially influenced the seasonal distribution of varicella infection, the disease epidemiology still concurs with that of other temperate countries.

The strengths of present study include that it is the first of its kind to examine time trends in the epidemiology of pediatric hospitalized varicella cases over an extended time period in a temperate Mediterranean country. Data collected include more than four fifths of all patients hospitalized with varicella infection during the study period in the region [21]. In addition, the study included children hospitalized for varicella infection prior to the introduction of universal VZV vaccination in 2004. Hence, any changes observed in the epidemiological trends of varicella infection cannot be attributed to the introduction of the VZV universal vaccination. However, due to the retrospective nature of the study design applied, the etiological association between climatic changes and varicella infection cannot be conclusively established. Moreover, the potential confounding effects of socioeconomic factors upon the association of interest could also not be evaluated due to the retrospective study design applied. Finally, the present study cannot account for varicella infection cases contracted through direct cutaneous contact, rather than through the transmission via aerosolized droplets. Additional longitudinal studies are necessary to evaluate the interactive effects between demographic, climatic, and epidemiological changes, respectively, of other airborne viral diseases upon infection rates among children in temperate regions.

In conclusion, in a temperate Mediterranean region where significant variations in seasonality occurred during the prelicensure period for the varicella vaccine (1982–2003), the occurrence of pediatric hospitalized varicella cases significantly increased during the summer and decreased during the autumn seasons. The observed epidemiological changes in the time trends of pediatric hospitalized varicella cases may be attributed to climatic changes in the region. It is hypothesized that time trends in the epidemiology of pediatric hospitalized cases for other infectious diseases which are similarly transmitted through indirect airborne transmission, such as influenza [29], may have also been affected by modifications in climatic variables [27,28]. Therefore, public health interventions targeted at diminishing such infectious diseases among pediatric populations in the region should also account for the potential notable effects of modification of climatic variables upon the epidemiology of disease attributable hospitalizations [26].

Acknowledgments

The preliminary findings of this work were presented at the 28th Annual Meeting of the European Society for Pediatric Infectious Diseases (ESPID) in Nice, France on May 10th, 2010.

Author Contributions

Conceived and designed the experiments: VP MT EC. Performed the experiments: PN KT VP EC. Analyzed the data: EC PN CH VP. Contributed reagents/materials/analysis tools: KT MT MNT PN VP EC. Wrote the paper: EC VP PN MT MNT CH.

References

1. Bonanni P, Breuer J, Gershon A, Gershon M, Hryniewicz W, et al. (2009) Varicella vaccination in Europe: taking the practical approach. BMC Med 7: 26. doi:10.1186/1741-7015-7-26.
2. O'Grady K, Merianos A, Patel M, Gilbert L (2000) High seroprevalence of antibodies to varicella zoster virus in adult women in a tropical climate. Tropical Med Int Health 5(10):732–736.
3. Centres for Disease Control and Prevention (CDC) (1996) Prevention of varicella: recommendations of the Advisory Committee on Immunization Practices (ACIP). MMWR 45:1–35.
4. de Melker H, Berbers G, Hahne S, Rümke H, van den Hof S, et al. (2006) The epidemiology of varicella and herpes zoster in the Netherlands: implications for varicella zoster virus vaccination. Vaccine 24: 3946–3952.
5. Khoshnood B, Debruyne M, Lancon F, Emery C, Fagnani F, et al. (2006) Seroprevalence of varicella in the French population. Pediatr Infect Dis J 25: 41–44.
6. Vyse AJ, Gay NJ, Hesketh LM, Morgan-Capner P, Miller E (2004) Seroprevalence of antibody to varicella zoster virus in England and Wales in children and young adults. Epidemiol Infect 132:1129–1134.
7. Red Book (2009) 2009 Report of the Committee on Infectious Diseases. 28th ed. Elk Grove Village, IL: American Academy of Pediatrics.
8. Liyanage NP, Fernando S, Malavige GN, Mallikahewa R, Sivayogan S, et al. (2007) Seroprevalence of varicella zoster infections in Colombo district, Sri Lanka. Indian J Med Sci 61(3): 128–134.
9. Tseng HF, Tan HF, Chang CK, Wang LY, Yang SE, et al. (2005) A seroepidemiology study of varicella among children aged 0-12 years in Taiwan. Southeast Asian J Trop Med Public Health 36(5): 1201–1207.
10. Garnett G, Cox M, Bundy D, Didier JM, St Catharine J (1993) The age of infection with varicella zoster virus in St. Lucia, West Indies. Epidemiol Infect 110: 361–372.
11. Lee BW (1998) Review of varicella zoster seroepidemiology in India and Southeast Asia. Trop Med Int Health. 3(11):886–90.
12. Lolekha S, Tanthiphabha W, Sornchai P, Kosuwan P, Sutra S, et al. (2001) Effect of climatic factors and population density on varicella zoster virus epidemiology within a tropical country. Am J Trop Med Hyg 64(3,4): 131–136.
13. Mandal BK, Mukherjee PP, Murphy C, Mukherjee R, Naik T (1998) Adult susceptibility to varicella in the tropics is a rural phenomenon due to the lack of previous exposure. J Infect Dis (suppl 1):S52–54.
14. Venkitaraman AR, Seigneurin J, Baccard M, Lenoir GM, John TJ (1984) Measurement of antibodies to varicella-zoster virus in a tropical population be enzyme-linked immunosorbent assay. J Clin Microb 20(3): 582–583.
15. Katsafadou A, Ferentinos G, Constantopoulos A, Papaevangelou V (2008) The epidemiology of varicella in school-aged Greek children before the implementation of universal vaccination. Eur J Clin Microb Infect Dis 27(3): 223–226.
16. Yawn BP, Yawn RA, Lydick E (1997) Community impact of childhood varicella infections. J Pediatr. 130(5):759–765.
17. Chan JY, Tian L, Kwan Y, Chan W, Leung C (2011) Hospitalizations for varicella in children and adolescents in a referral hospital in Hong Kong, 2004 to 2008: a time series study. BMC Public Health. 11:366.
18. Kokaze A, Yoshida M, Sekine Y, Ishikawa M, Kurokochi T, et al. (2001) The magnitude of variation in temperature within a year has an effect on the seasonal variations of chickenpox incidence in Japan. Epidemiol Infect. 126(2):269–277.
19. Wu PY, Li YC, Wu HD (2007) Risk factors for chickenpox incidence in Taiwan from a large-scale computerized database. Int J Dermatol. 46(4):362–366.
20. Nastos PT, Philandras CM, Founda D, Zerefos CS (2011) Air temperature trends related to changes in atmospheric circulation in the wider area of Greece. Int J Remote Sens 32(3):737–750.
21. Theodoridou M, Laina I, Hadjichristodoulou C, Syriopoulou V (2006) Varicella-related complications and hospitalizations in a tertiary paediatric medical center before vaccine introduction. Eur J Pediatr 165:273–274.
22. McGullagh P, Nelder JA (1997) Generalized Linear Models. 2nd Edition, London: Chapman & Hall.
23. Nedler JA, Wedderburn RWM (1972) Generalized linear models, J Roy Stat Soc Ser A. 135:370–384.
24. Zak-Prelich M, Borkowski JL, Alexander F, Norval M (2002) The role of solar ultraviolet irradiation in zoster. Epidemiol Infect. 129(3):593–597.
25. Sauerbrei A (2007) Differences in varicella-zoster virus seroepidemiology between temperate and tropical regions. Indian J Med Sci 61:123–124.
26. Gustin KM, Belser JA, Wadford DA, Pearce MB, Katz JM, et al. (2011) Influenza virus aerosol exposure and analytical system for ferrets. Proc Natl Acad Sci USA 108(20): 8432–8437.
27. Teunis PF, Brienen N, Kretzschmar ME (2010) High infectivity and pathogenicity of influenza A virus via aerosol and droplet transmission. Epidemics 2(4): 215–222.
28. Yang W, Marr LC (2011) Dynamics of airborne influenza A viruses indoors and dependence on humidity. PLoS One 6(6): e21481.
29. Knibbs LD, Morawska L, Bell SC (2012) The risk of airborne influenza transmission in passenger cars. Epidemiol Infect 140(3): 474–478.

30

A Molecular Epidemiology Survey of Respiratory Adenoviruses Circulating in Children Residing in Southern Palestine

Lina Qurei[1], Donald Seto[2], Zaidoun Salah[1], Maysa Azzeh[1]*

1 Virology Research Laboratory, Medical Research Center, Al-Quds University , East Jerusalem-Abu Dies, Palestine, 2 School of Systems Biology, George Mason University, Manassas, Virginia, United States of America

Abstract

A molecular epidemiology survey was performed in order to establish and document the respiratory adenovirus pathogen profiles among children in Southern Palestine. Three hundred and thirty-eight hospitalized pediatric cases with adenovirus-associated respiratory tract infections were analyzed. Forty four cases out of the 338 were evaluated in more detail for the adenoviruses types present. All of the children resided in Southern Palestine, that is, in city, village and refugee camp environments within the districts of Hebron and Bethlehem. Human adenoviruses circulated throughout 2005–2010, with major outbreaks occurring in the spring months. A larger percent of the children diagnosed with adenoviral infections were male infants. DNA sequence analysis of the hexon genes from 44 samples revealed that several distinct adenovirus types circulated in the region; these were HAdV-C1, HAdV-C2, HAdV-B3 and HAdV-C5. However, not all of these types were detected within each year. This is the first study ever conducted in Palestine of the genetic epidemiology of respiratory adenovirus infections.

Editor: Eric J. Kremer, French National Centre for Scientific Research, France

Funding: Support for this work came, in part, from the internal resources of the Virology Laboratory at the Medical Research Center. No additional external funding received for this study. The funders had no role in study design, data collection and analysis, decision to publish, or preparation of the manuscript.

Competing Interests: The authors have declared that no competing interests exist.

* E-mail: mazzeh@med.alquds.edu

Introduction

Human adenoviruses (HAdVs) are classified within the family Adenoviridae, genus Mastadenovirus. Based on their hemagglutination and serum neutralization properties, 51 serotypes of HAdVs were orginally identified [1]. However, a more recent and comprehensive understanding of HAdVs has been made possible by the use of genomics and bioinformatics. These approaches are used to identify and characterize novel human adenoviruses based on the whole genome sequence, extending beyond the hexon and fiber markers, and phylogenomics [2]. As a result, additional seven types have been identified, including several novel respiratory and ocular pathogens. These new HAdV genotypes were identified as either sequence-divergent and/or recombinant viruses of previously recognized types, and include HAdV-G52 [3]; HAdV-D53 [4]; HAdV-D54 [5]; HAdV-B55 [6]; HAdV-D56 [7]; HAdV-D57 [8]; and HAdV-D58 [9].

HAdVs were initially characterized as respiratory tract pathogens in the 1950s [10,11]. Although respiratory infections caused by HAdVs are mostly self-limiting, severe and even fatal infections may occur. HAdV infections in children predominantly involve the respiratory tract, with approximately 5–7% of respiratory illnesses in young children attributed to HAdVs [12,13]. Particular HAdV species and serotypes are correlated with specific diseases, epidemiologic settings and demographic risk groups [14]. Infections of the respiratory tract are predominantly caused by HAdV types of species B, C and E; however, severe acute respiratory disease is mainly caused by only few types, namely HAdV-B3, -E4, -B7, -B14, -B16, -B21 and -B55 [6,14,15,16,17]. In addition, HAdVs are also responsible for a wide spectrum of clinical diseases involving ocular, gastrointestinal and genitourinary tissues [14].

Presented in this report are data from the epidemiological analysis of 338 cases of HAdV isolated from nasal pharyngeal aspirates (NPAs). These were sampled from hospitalized pediatric patients who resided in Southern Palestine between 2005 and 2010. Of these, 44 samples were analyzed in detail using DNA sequence-based HAdV typing to illuminate the viruses circulating in Southern Palestine. For this, a nested PCR and DNA sequencing assay of the HAdV hexon gene HVR1–6, developed by Lu and Erdman [18] and successfully used by several researchers [19,20,21,22], was utilized. Our work reveals which HAdV types were circulating in southern Palestine during the study period, allowing for strategies in developing and applying potential vaccines.

Methods

Ethics Statement

Patients' data collection and archived patients' samples were approved specifically for this research by the Human Medical Research Committee of the Caritas Baby Hospital in a written approval letter dated March, 19th, 2010.

Study population

The respiratory pathogens were sampled from patients admitted to the Caritas Baby Hospital (CBH), which is located in Bethlehem. Accordingly, most of the children admitted came from the southern regions of Palestine, particularly the districts of Bethlehem and Hebron. These children represent a cross-section of diverse living conditions: cities, refugee camps and villages throughout the region. Figure 1 indicates the areas in which the children reside, for reference. Between January 2005 and December 2010, 8033 respiratory tract infection cases residing in southern Palestine were admitted to the CBH, 338 cases (4.2%) were caused by HAdV. The other cases were caused by other respiratory tract pathogens. The ages of the children ranged from a few days to seven years.

Demographics and medical records of patients

Data from all of the 338 pediatric patients in this study were subjected to statistical analysis, including the parameters of age, sex, residency and date of admission, as collected from the CBH records. Additionally, clinical data, including symptoms and other metadata, were collected from the medical charts of 150 children. All data were entered into a Microsoft Excel spreadsheet for statistical analysis. The statistical associations of the data were concluded using Pearson's Chi-squared test for independence. The analyses were performed using statistical package for social sciences (SPSS) software.

Nasopharyngeal aspirate specimen

The nasopharyngeal aspirates (NPAs) were collected at the CBH from the children between 2005 and 2010 and archived. These were tested for respiratory tract viruses, using a direct Immunofluorescence assay. This test was performed at the CBH clinical laboratory using Millipore Respiratory DFA Viral Screening & Identification Kit (Light Diagnostics; CA, USA). This kit identifies HAdV, Respiratory Synsytial Virus (RSV), Parainfluenza (1, 2 and 3) and Influenza (A and B). In this study, one hundred archived NPA samples, tested positive for HAdV, were subjected to the molecular genotyping of HAdV by DNA sequencing. These 100 NPA samples were selected randomly and represented 10–20 NPAs per year (2005–2010).

DNA extraction and PCR

DNA extraction from 100 NPA was performed using the QiaAmp DNA mini kit (Qiagen 51304), according to the manufacturer's instructions. AdhexF1/R1 and AdhexF2/R2 primer pairs [18] were used in one PCR reaction to amplify a ~750 bp of the hexon gene as followed: 94°C for 2 min, 35 cycles of 94°C for 1 min, 45°C for 1 min, and 72°C for 2 min with a final extension of 72°C for 5 min. PCR products were purified using the QiaAmp PCR Purification Kit according to the manufacturer's instructions (Qiagen 28004), and then subjected to DNA sequencing using Sanger chemistry (ABI 3130; Applied Biosystems, Inc., USA).

Sequence analysis and HAdV typing

Forty-four DNA sequences, representing 13% of the total HAdV cases which were distributed throughout the study years, were analyzed using the NCBI BLAST software (http://www.ncbi.nlm.nih.gov/blast/Blast.cgi?PAGE = Nucleotides) and the DNASTAR Lasergene MegAlign program (DNASTAR Inc., WI, USA) using reference sequences.

Results

Residency, sex and age distribution of HAdV-infected children

The pediatric patients were predominantly from villages (68%), while 21% were residents of refugee camps and 11% were from cities. A larger percentage of children diagnosed with HAdV respiratory tract infections were male (60%). The children, with ages ranging between a few days and one year (age group 0–1), showed the highest rate of HAdV infections (62%), followed by the age group 1.1–2 years (Fig. 2).

Yearly and seasonal HAdV infection

HAdV infections increased yearly, with 40 cases detected in 2005 and almost 100 cases noted in 2010. These infections occurred throughout the year, with a detectable increase of cases in the months ranging from March to May (Fig. 3). In 2010, the year with the highest recorded number of HAdV infections, however, most cases occurred in January. Pearson's Chi-squared test was used to test for an association between HAdV infection and season, the test was significant (P value$<$0.001).

Clinical observations

Metadata from the medical charts revealed 150 cases belonging to the group of children with the highest HAdV infection rate, that is, aged one year and younger. An average of 25 cases per year were distributed over the four seasons, with the majority of these cases sexed male (71%). A majority of the children (80%) suffered from fevers as a major sign of lower respiratory disease; whereas only 50% suffered from coughs. Thirty-three percent had severe symptoms, requiring mechanical ventilation. Bronchitis/broncho-pneumonia (33.3%) and upper respiratory tract infections (URTI) (24.7%) were the major presenting symptoms in the children upon admission. The following symptoms were also observed, with a lower frequency of 2–5%: sepsis, gastroenteritis, otitis media, meningitis, dehydration, tonsillitis, congenital heart disease (CHD), conjunctivitis, chronic renal failure, yellow skin and febril convulsion. In individual cases, the children presented with croup, skin rash, hypoglycemia, anemia, cystic leukomalacia and lung infection. None of the 150 charts recorded co-infection with another respiratory tract virus. Finally, 104 cases (69.3%) were treated with antibiotics as documented in the medical records. Of these, 70 children were indeed suffering from bacterial co-infections; therefore antibiotics should have not been prescribed in 34 cases (33% of those children who actually received antibiotics) as they had exclusively viral infection.

Genetic analysis of HAdV circulating in Southern Palestine

The most common HAdV types as revealed from comparing Palestinian sequences with reference data were HAdV-B3 and HAdV-C2, represented in 45.5% and 31.8% of the 44 sequenced samples respectively (Fig. 4). Less dominant were other types of C: HAdV-C1 and HAdV-C5, which were represented in 15.9% and 6.8% of the samples, respectively (Fig. 4). Overall, species C was the most common HAdV species among hospitalized children in Southern Palestine (54.5%).

Annual distribution of human adenovirus serotypes

The different types of HAdV were not present equally across the years. While HAdV-C2 was present throughout the years of the study, HAdV-C1 was present in all years except 2008; HAdV-B3 was present in all years except 2009, and HAdV-C5 was present

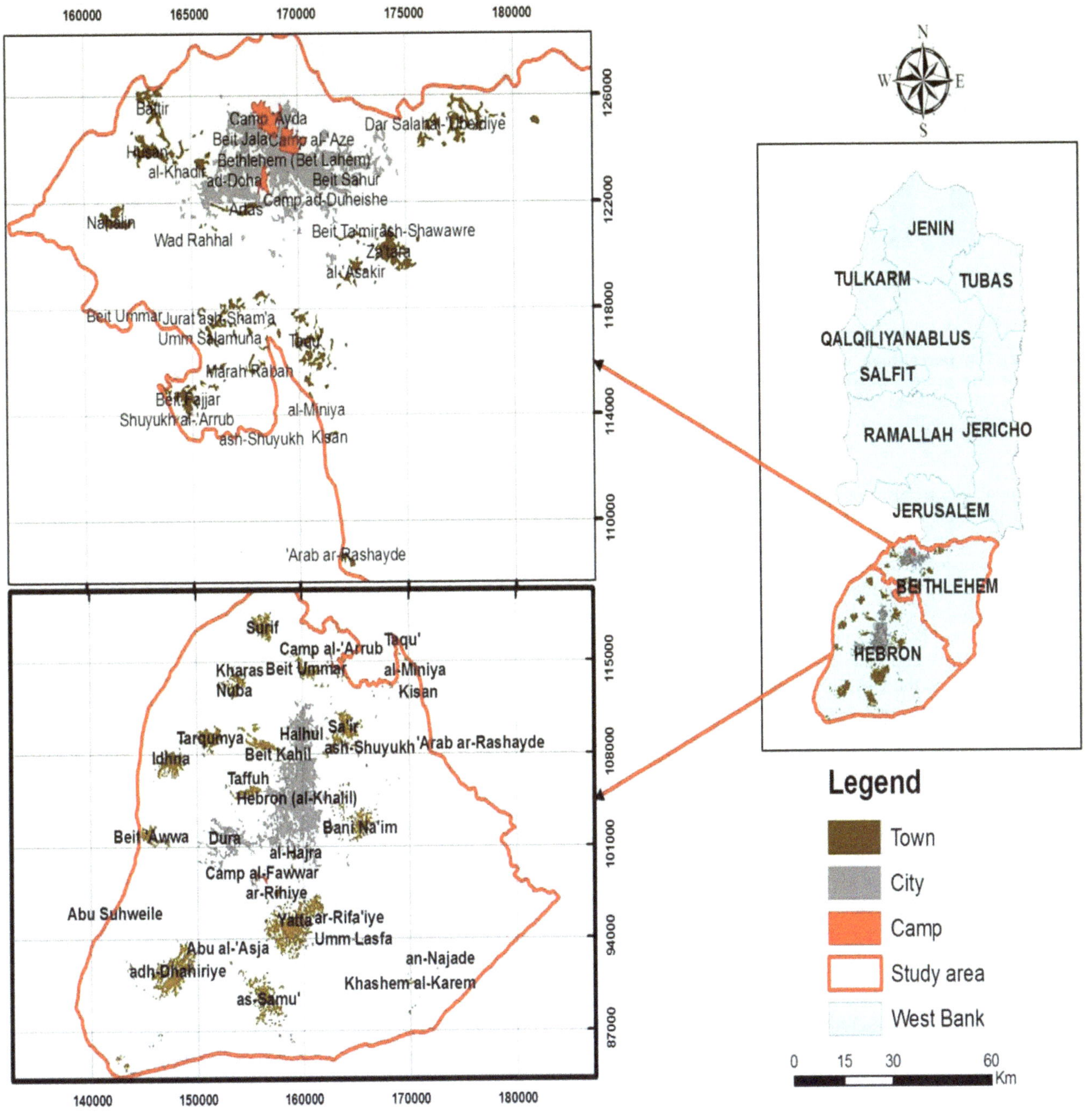

Figure 1. A map of the West Bank and a detailed map of Southern Palestine. The detailed maps of Southern Palestine on the left show the villages and refugee camps in the districts of Hebron and Bethlehem, where the children with respiratory tract infection caused by Adenovirus reside.

only in 2005 and 2006 (Table 1). HAdV-B3 was the most dominant type in 2005 and 2010, as it presented in 62% and 71% of the samples respectively. HAdV-C2 was dominant in 2009, occurring in 67% of the samples. In the other years, 2006–2008, no specific HAdV type seemed to dominate.

Discussion

Adenovirus is a significant causative agent of respiratory tract disease in pediatric and adult patients. Numerous outbreaks of acute respiratory disease caused by HAdV have been reported during the last decade in many countries [17,23,24,25,26,27,28,29,30,31,32,33]. Some outbreaks resulted in high morbidity and mortality in neonatal and pediatric units, in children admitted to hospitals [32,34,35,36,37,38], in schools [17] and most strikingly in military camps [26,39,40] and military hospitals [41]. Presented in this report are epidemiological and limited DNA sequence analyses of HAdV respiratory tract infections from hospitalized children, who resided in Southern Palestine between 2005 and 2010. The HAdV infection rate among other respiratory tract infections in this study population was 4.2%, in line with earlier reports [12,13]. The highest percentage (68%) of infections among children in this sample population with adenovirus was located in villages. This may be

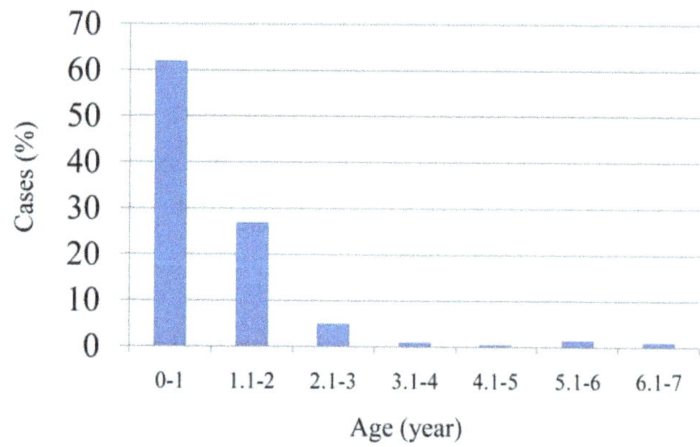

Figure 2. The percentage of pediatric cases suffering from HADV for age groups between a few days and 7 years. The percentage was calculated according to the 338 total number of HAdV cases investigated in this study.

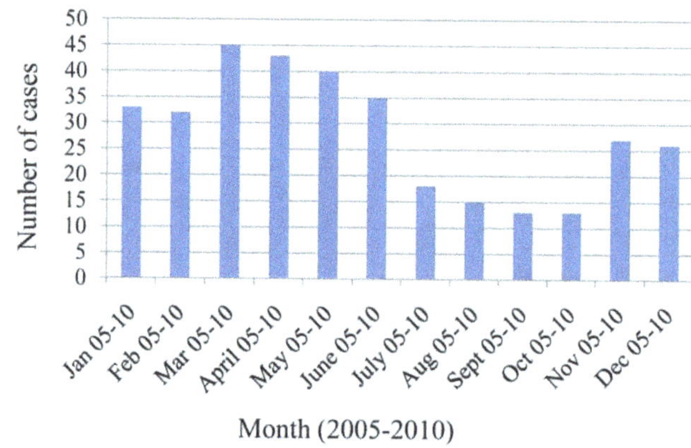

Figure 3. HAdV cases per month from 2005–2010. The actual number of cases each month and for each year is displayed along the y-axis.

due to population density and the living conditions coupled with the high potential for contact between children in the village community, along with their lower socioeconomic status. Adults and children of lower socioeconomic status are known to be at higher risk for a wide range of contagious infectious diseases, especially respiratory [42]. Surprisingly, the number of cases from refugee camps was the lowest in this study, which may be partially explained by the camp residents taking advantages of clinical services provided by the UN. Accordingly, Pearson's Chi-squared test for independence used to measure the association between adenovirus infection and district residency was not significant (P value>0.05). The higher rate of male infections of HAdV found in this study was previously described [43,44]. Interestingly, the lowest HAdV infection rate was among school age children (age group 6.1–7 years). This may suggest that they had already been exposed to the common endemic serotypes of adenovirus early in life and may have thereby established a protective immunity [43]. Children younger than two years of age were the most susceptible to respiratory tract infections of HAdV (89% of total cases). According to the Pearson's Chi-squared test for independence, a strong association between age and HAdV infection was present in our study (P value<0.001). Adenovirus outbreaks were more likely to occur in young children and infants, as confirmed by earlier reports [32,34,35,36,37,38].

The HAdV-associated respiratory diseases, as documented in medical charts, were bronchitis/bronchopneumonia (33.3%) as well as upper respiratory tract infections URTI (24.7%). Indeed, the most common clinical presentations of HAdV infections are pneumonia, bronchitis/bronchiolitis, conjunctivitis, pharyngoconjunctival fever and upper respiratory tract infections or common cold-like symptoms [25,26,34,45,46,47,48,49,50,51]. A significant association of symptoms was found between fevers and HAdV infection (P value<0.001), as well as cough and HAdV infections (P value<0.001). Coughs and fevers are common symptoms related to various respiratory tract infections [26] and respiratory tract infections of HAdV [43,49,52]. As antibiotics may be useful in some cases, in order to prevent further complications caused by bacterial co-infections due to weakened immunity during viral infections or in case of viral co-infection with bacterial agents [53,54], 34 children received these prophylactic antibiotics, despite the exclusive viral URTI assayed. In general, prescribing antibiotics before diagnosis or because an exact diagnosis is not possible is a common mistake made by most physicians, and is a practice that has led to more and more drug-resistant bacterial strains worldwide along with unexpected complications in patients [54,55,56,57]. Therefore, admittedly, the diagnostics of viral respiratory infections in medical laboratories in Palestine is substandard and is a major problem that could have global impact in this era of a "global village".

In conclusion, this study demonstrated that HAdV-C1, HAdV-C2, HAdV-B3 and HAdV-C5 were the most common HAdV types circulating among hospitalized children in Southern Palestine currently and recently. The different types were not equally distributed over all the years or all of the months in the year sampled. It has been shown earlier that some HAdV types correlated specifically to one or two months throughout the year, or were also found in some years but not in others [43]. Similar genetic epidemiological studies have shown that HAdV types, comprising HAdV-C1, -C2, -B3, -C5, -C6, and -B7 were mainly involved in respiratory tract infections in children living in Argentina, Iceland, Chile, Taiwan, Canada, China, Malaysia, Korea, Israel, Egypt and the USA, respectively [17,22,25,31,51,52,58,59,60,61,62]. HAdV types -C1, -C2 and -B3 were detected in most of these studies. HAdV-C5, however,

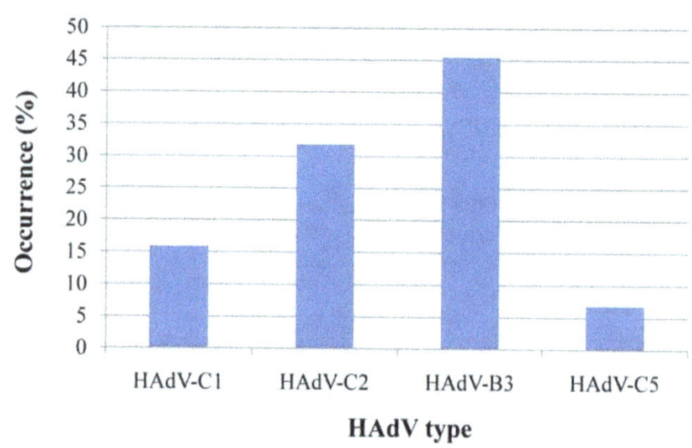

Figure 4. Circulating HAdV types in southern Palestine. HAdV types circulating in Southern Palestine from 2005 to 2010 were detected using nested PCR and DNA sequencing assay of the HAdV hexon gene HVR1–6 followed by sequencing and sequence analysis. The 44 sequences were assigned the GenBank accession numbers [JQ796022–JQ796065]. The percentage of each serotype was calculated relatively to the number of total sequenced samples (44 samples).

Table 1. Yearly presence of HAdV types in southern Palestine.

Serotypes	2005	2006	2007	2008	2009	2010
HAdV-C1	+	+	+	–	+	+
HAdV-C2	+	+	+	+	+	+
HAdV-B3	+	+	+	+	–	+
HAdV-C5	+	+	–	–	–	–

Viruses isolated from pediatrics patients in a six-year period were subjected to DNA sequencing of the hexon gene, with BLAST analysis using the NCBI software (http://www.ncbi.nlm.nih.gov/blast/Blast.cgi?PAGE = Nucleotides) and the DNASTAR program using reference sequences. Not all types are represented each year, with HAdV-C5 absent from 2007 onward.

was detected in Iceland, Taiwan, Korea, Egypt and according to a very recent study, also in Argentina [31,52,59,62,63]. Interestingly, the prevalence of HAdV-C5 in all of these studies was low, in line with our findings. With regards to the noted HAdV type predominance of HAdV-B3, followed by HAdV-C1, -C2 and -C5, our current study is consistent with a regional study reported in Egypt [62]. The most striking co-accordance between our study and the Egyptian one was the fact that HAdV-C5 was only detected in two out of four years of their study period [62].

Although most studies of HAdV infections were unable to show a clear evidence for seasonal distribution, specific types have been found to correlate to specific seasons [43,64]. Also presented in this report, HAdV-C2 and HAdV-B3 seem to occur more frequently in the spring and winter seasons. Nevertheless, this finding needs further confirmation by the analysis of a larger number of HAdV samples throughout the study years 2005–2010. Of all the HAdV types detected in Southern Palestine, only HAdV-B3 has been identified as well in numerous other studies to be responsible for respiratory disease outbreaks; for example, in the USA, Taiwan, Korea and Portugal [24,28,31,32]. Although there were no records of an equivalent outbreak in Southern Palestine, the adenovirus typing results show clearly that HAdV-B3 was the most common serotype over all the years with 45.5%, and presenting in 68% of the samples in the years 2005 and 2010. These data may provide evidence for a possible unrecorded and undocumented outbreak, since HAdV-B3 was also reported to be detected in both outbreaks and in sporadic cases [31]. In summary, this is the first study ever to provide an insight into the epidemiological characteristics and genotype profile of HAdV types in Palestine, including a breakdown of cities, refugee camps and villages throughout Southern Palestine. Detection of the circulating HAdV types contributing to respiratory tract infections in Palestine allows for future vaccination strategies in the region. Finally, the use of DNA sequencing-based techniques for typing viral infection agents and its application in Palestine presents a solid platform for investigating viral infections and will be very valuable in the case of respiratory outbreaks.

Acknowledgments

This work comprises, in part, Lina Qurei's master thesis in epidemiology (School of Public Health, Al-Quds University; East Jerusalem-Abu Dies, Palestine) which was performed at the Virology Laboratory-MRC, Al-Quds University. We would like to thank Dr. Amer Marei (Environmental Research Laboratory, Al-Quds University; East Jerusalem-Abu Dies, Palestine) for his generous help in providing the geographic map of the sampling regions. We would like to thank Professor Robert Stern (Division of Basic Medical Sciences, Touro College of Osteopathic Medicine; NY, USA) for the critical review of this manuscript and the clinical data specifically. Finally, we would like to thank Dr. Monjed Samuh (Department of Mathematics and Computer Science, Palestine Polytechnic University; Hebron, Palestine) for his contribution in performing the statistical analysis presented in this manuscript.

Author Contributions

Conceived and designed the experiments: LQ MA. Performed the experiments: LQ. Analyzed the data: LQ MA ZS. Contributed reagents/materials/analysis tools: MA. Wrote the paper: MA DS.

References

1. De Jong JC, Wermenbol AG, Verweij-Uijterwaal MW, Slaterus KW, Wertheim-Van Dillen P, et al. (1999) Adenoviruses from human immunodeficiency virus-infected individuals, including two strains that represent new candidate serotypes Ad50 and Ad51 of species B1 and D, respectively. J Clin Microbiol 37: 3940–3945.
2. Seto D, Chodosh J, Brister JR, Jones MS (2011) Using the whole-genome sequence to characterize and name human adenoviruses. J Virol 85: 5701–5702.
3. Jones MS, Harrach B, Ganac RD, Gozum MM, Dela Cruz WP, et al. (2007) New adenovirus species found in a patient presenting with gastroenteritis. J Virol 81: 5978–5984.
4. Walsh MP, Chintakuntlawar A, Robinson CM, Madisch I, Harrach B, et al. (2009) Evidence of molecular evolution driven by recombination events influencing tropism in a novel human adenovirus that causes epidemic keratoconjunctivitis. PLoS One 4: e5635.
5. Ishiko H, Aoki K (2009) Spread of epidemic keratoconjunctivitis due to a novel serotype of human adenovirus in Japan. J Clin Microbiol 47: 2678–2679.
6. Walsh MP, Seto J, Jones MS, Chodosh J, Xu W, et al. (2010) Computational analysis identifies human adenovirus type 55 as a re-emergent acute respiratory disease pathogen. Journal of clinical microbiology 48: 991–993.
7. Robinson CM, Singh G, Henquell C, Walsh MP, Peigue-Lafeuille H, et al. (2011) Computational analysis and identification of an emergent human adenovirus pathogen implicated in a respiratory fatality. Virology 409: 141–147.
8. Walsh MP, Seto J, Liu EB, Dehghan S, Hudson NR, et al. (2011) Computational analysis of two species C human adenoviruses provides evidence of a novel virus. J Clin Microbiol 49: 3482–3490.
9. Liu EB, Ferreyra L, Fischer SL, Pavan JV, Nates SV, et al. (2011) Genetic analysis of a novel human adenovirus with a serologically unique hexon and a recombinant fiber gene. PLoS One 6: e24491.
10. Rowe WP, Huebner RJ, Gilmore LK, Parrott RH, Ward TG (1953) Isolation of a cytopathogenic agent from human adenoids undergoing spontaneous degeneration in tissue culture. Proceedings of the Society for Experimental Biology and Medicine Society for Experimental Biology and Medicine 84: 570–573.
11. Hilleman MR, Werner JH (1954) Recovery of new agent from patients with acute respiratory illness. Proceedings of the Society for Experimental Biology and Medicine Society for Experimental Biology and Medicine 85: 183–188.
12. Piedra PA (1962) Enteroviruses/Adenoviruses In: Patrick CC, editor. Infections in immunocompromised infants and children. New York, NY: Churchill Livingstone, Inc. pp. 662–668.
13. Brandt CD, Kim HW, Vargosko AJ, Jeffries BC, Arrobio JO, et al. (1969) Infections in 18,000 infants and children in a controlled study of respiratory tract disease. I. Adenovirus pathogenicity in relation to serologic type and illness syndrome. American journal of epidemiology 90: 484–500.
14. Wold WSM, and Horwitz, M. S. (2007) Adenoviruses. In: Knipe DM, and Howley, P. M. ,editor. Fields Virology. fifth ed: Lippincott Williams & Wilkins. pp. 2396–2436.
15. Fu WY, Liang D, Zheng YC, Liu WM, Xu Z, et al. (1989) A study of molecular epidemiology of adenovirus of types 3 and 7 on infant pneumonia in northern China. Chinese medical journal 102: 857–861.
16. Zhang Q, Su X, Gong S, Zeng Q, Zhu B, et al. (2006) Comparative genomic analysis of two strains of human adenovirus type 3 isolated from children with acute respiratory infection in southern China. The Journal of general virology 87: 1531–1541.
17. Zhu Z, Zhang Y, Xu S, Yu P, Tian X, et al. (2009) Outbreak of acute respiratory disease in China caused by B2 species of adenovirus type 11. J Clin Microbiol 47: 697–703.
18. Lu X, Erdman DD (2006) Molecular typing of human adenoviruses by PCR and sequencing of a partial region of the hexon gene. Archives of virology 151: 1587–1602.
19. Gray GC, McCarthy T, Lebeck MG, Schnurr DP, Russell KL, et al. (2007) Genotype prevalence and risk factors for severe clinical adenovirus infection, United States 2004–2006. Clin Infect Dis 45: 1120–1131.

20. Zheng X, Lu X, Erdman DD, Anderson EJ, Guzman-Cottrill JA, et al. (2008) Identification of adenoviruses in specimens from high-risk pediatric stem cell transplant recipients and controls. Journal of clinical microbiology 46: 317–320.
21. Landry ML, Lebeck MG, Capuano AW, McCarthy T, Gray GC (2009) Adenovirus type 3 outbreak in connecticut associated with a novel variant. Journal of medical virology 81: 1380–1384.
22. Mandelboim M, Dror P, Azar R, Bromberg M, Mendelson E (2011) Adenovirus infections in hospitalized patients in Israel: epidemiology and molecular characterization. Journal of clinical microbiology 49: 597–601.
23. Harley D, Harrower B, Lyon M, Dick A (2001) A primary school outbreak of pharyngoconjunctival fever caused by adenovirus type 3. Communicable diseases intelligence 25: 9–12.
24. Ryan MA, Gray GC, Smith B, McKeehan JA, Hawksworth AW, et al. (2002) Large epidemic of respiratory illness due to adenovirus types 7 and 3 in healthy young adults. Clinical infectious diseases: an official publication of the Infectious Diseases Society of America 34: 577–582.
25. Palomino MA, Larranaga C, Villagra E, Camacho J, Avendano LF (2004) Adenovirus and respiratory syncytial virus-adenovirus mixed acute lower respiratory infections in Chilean infants. The Pediatric infectious disease journal 23: 337–341.
26. Chmielewicz B, Benzler J, Pauli G, Krause G, Bergmann F, et al. (2005) Respiratory disease caused by a species B2 adenovirus in a military camp in Turkey. Journal of medical virology 77: 232–237.
27. Mizuta K, Abiko C, Aoki Y, Murata T, Katsushima N, et al. (2006) A slow spread of adenovirus type 7 infection after its re-emergence in Yamagata, Japan, in 1995. Microbiology and immunology 50: 553–558.
28. Chang SY, Lee CN, Lin PH, Huang HH, Chang LY, et al. (2008) A community-derived outbreak of adenovirus type 3 in children in Taiwan between 2004 and 2005. Journal of medical virology 80: 102–112.
29. Esposito DH, Gardner TJ, Schneider E, Stockman LJ, Tate JE, et al. (2010) Outbreak of pneumonia associated with emergent human adenovirus serotype 14–Southeast Alaska, 2008. The Journal of infectious diseases 202: 214–222.
30. Kandel R, Srinivasan A, D'Agata EM, Lu X, Erdman D, et al. (2010) Outbreak of adenovirus type 4 infection in a long-term care facility for the elderly. Infection control and hospital epidemiology: the official journal of the Society of Hospital Epidemiologists of America 31: 755–757.
31. Lee J, Choi EH, Lee HJ (2010) Comprehensive serotyping and epidemiology of human adenovirus isolated from the respiratory tract of Korean children over 17 consecutive years (1991–2007). Journal of medical virology 82: 624–631.
32. Rebelo-de-Andrade H, Pereira C, Giria M, Prudencio E, Brito MJ, et al. (2010) Outbreak of acute respiratory infection among infants in Lisbon, Portugal, caused by human adenovirus serotype 3 and a new 7/3 recombinant strain. Journal of clinical microbiology 48: 1391–1396.
33. Ghanaiem H, Averbuch D, Koplewitz BZ, Yatsiv I, Braun J, et al. (2011) An outbreak of adenovirus type 7 in a residential facility for severely disabled children. The Pediatric infectious disease journal 30: 948–952.
34. Wu E, Martinez V, Alvarez AM, Larranaga C, Vela H (1990) [Fatal cases of adenovirus infection]. Revista chilena de pediatria 61: 177–184.
35. Pinto A, Beck R, Jadavji T (1992) Fatal neonatal pneumonia caused by adenovirus type 35. Report of one case and review of the literature. Archives of pathology & laboratory medicine 116: 95–99.
36. Mitchell LS, Taylor B, Reimels W, Barrett FF, Devincenzo JP (2000) Adenovirus 7a: a community-acquired outbreak in a children's hospital. The Pediatric infectious disease journal 19: 996–1000.
37. Carballal G, Videla C, Misirlian A, Requeijo PV, Aguilar Mdel C (2002) Adenovirus type 7 associated with severe and fatal acute lower respiratory infections in Argentine children. BMC pediatrics 2: 6.
38. Louie JK, Kajon AE, Holodniy M, Guardia-LaBar L, Lee B, et al. (2008) Severe pneumonia due to adenovirus serotype 14: a new respiratory threat? Clinical infectious diseases: an official publication of the Infectious Diseases Society of America 46: 421–425.
39. van der Veen J, Oei KG, Abarbanel MF (1969) Patterns of infections with adenovirus types 4, 7 and 21 in military recruits during a 9-year survey. The Journal of hygiene 67: 255–268.
40. Mantyjarvi R (1966) Adenovirus infections in servicemen in Finland. Annales medicinae experimentalis et biologiae Fenniae 44: Suppl 4:1–43.
41. Lessa FC, Gould PL, Pascoe N, Erdman DD, Lu X, et al. (2009) Health care transmission of a newly emergent adenovirus serotype in health care personnel at a military hospital in Texas, 2007. The Journal of infectious diseases 200: 1759–1765.
42. Cohen S (1999) Social status and susceptibility to respiratory infections. Annals of the New York Academy of Sciences 896: 246–253.
43. Cooper RJ, Hallett R, Tullo AB, Klapper PE (2000) The epidemiology of adenovirus infections in Greater Manchester, UK 1982–96. Epidemiology and infection 125: 333–345.
44. Schmitz H, Wigand R, Heinrich W (1983) Worldwide epidemiology of human adenovirus infections. Am J Epidemiol 117: 455–466.
45. Ruuskanen O, Nohynek H, Ziegler T, Capeding R, Rikalainen H, et al. (1992) Pneumonia in childhood: etiology and response to antimicrobial therapy. European journal of clinical microbiology & infectious diseases: official publication of the European Society of Clinical Microbiology 11: 217–223.
46. Singh-Naz N, Brown M, Ganeshananthan M (1993) Nosocomial adenovirus infection: molecular epidemiology of an outbreak. The Pediatric infectious disease journal 12: 922–925.
47. Hemming VG (1994) Viral respiratory diseases in children: classification, etiology, epidemiology, and risk factors. The Journal of pediatrics 124: S13–16.
48. Denny FW, Jr. (1995) The clinical impact of human respiratory virus infections. American journal of respiratory and critical care medicine 152: S4–12.
49. Munoz FM, Piedra PA, Demmler GJ (1998) Disseminated adenovirus disease in immunocompromised and immunocompetent children. Clinical infectious diseases: an official publication of the Infectious Diseases Society of America 27: 1194–1200.
50. Palomino MA, Larranaga C, Avendano LF (2000) Hospital-acquired adenovirus 7 h infantile respiratory infection in Chile. The Pediatric infectious disease journal 19: 527–531.
51. Yeung R, Eshaghi A, Lombos E, Blair J, Mazzulli T, et al. (2009) Characterization of culture-positive adenovirus serotypes from respiratory specimens in Toronto, Ontario, Canada: September 2007-June 2008. Virol J 6: 11.
52. Hsieh WY, Chiu NC, Chi H, Huang FY, Hung CC (2009) Respiratory adenoviral infections in Taiwanese children: a hospital-based study. Journal of microbiology, immunology, and infection = Wei mian yu gan ran za zhi 42: 371–377.
53. Franz A, Adams O, Willems R, Bonzel L, Neuhausen N, et al. (2010) Correlation of viral load of respiratory pathogens and co-infections with disease severity in children hospitalized for lower respiratory tract infection. Journal of clinical virology: the official publication of the Pan American Society for Clinical Virology 48: 239–245.
54. Shiley KT, Lautenbach E, Lee I (2010) The use of antimicrobial agents after diagnosis of viral respiratory tract infections in hospitalized adults: antibiotics or anxiolytics? Infection control and hospital epidemiology: the official journal of the Society of Hospital Epidemiologists of America 31: 1177–1183.
55. Rocholl C, Gerber K, Daly J, Pavia AT, Byington CL (2004) Adenoviral infections in children: the impact of rapid diagnosis. Pediatrics 113: e51–56.
56. Lautenbach E, Lee I, Shiley KT (2010) Treating viral respiratory tract infections with antibiotics in hospitals: no longer a case of mistaken identity. LDI issue brief 16: 1–4.
57. Pavia AT (2011) Viral infections of the lower respiratory tract: old viruses, new viruses, and the role of diagnosis. Clinical infectious diseases: an official publication of the Infectious Diseases Society of America 52 Suppl 4: S284–289.
58. Kajon AE, Wadell G (1992) Molecular epidemiology of adenoviruses associated with acute lower respiratory disease of children in Buenos Aires, Argentina (1984–1988). Journal of medical virology 36: 292–297.
59. Johansson ME, Ahrel-Andersson M, Gudnadottir S (1993) Molecular epidemiology of adenoviruses isolated in Iceland during 1988–1990. Journal of virological methods 42: 193–205.
60. Abd-Jamil J, Teoh BT, Hassan EH, Roslan N, Abubakar S (2010) Molecular identification of adenovirus causing respiratory tract infection in pediatric patients at the University of Malaya Medical Center. BMC pediatrics 10: 46.
61. Selvaraju SB, Kovac M, Dickson LM, Kajon AE, Selvarangan R (2011) Molecular epidemiology and clinical presentation of human adenovirus infections in Kansas City children. Journal of clinical virology: the official publication of the Pan American Society for Clinical Virology 51: 126–131.
62. Metzgar D, Osuna M, Yingst S, Rakha M, Earhart K, et al. (2005) PCR analysis of egyptian respiratory adenovirus isolates, including identification of species, serotypes, and coinfections. J Clin Microbiol 43: 5743–5752.
63. Barrero PR, Valinotto LE, Tittarelli E, Mistchenko AS (2012) Molecular typing of adenoviruses in pediatric respiratory infections in Buenos Aires, Argentina (1999–2010). J Clin Virol 53: 145–150.
64. Chew FT, Doraisingham S, Ling AE, Kumarasinghe G, Lee BW (1998) Seasonal trends of viral respiratory tract infections in the tropics. Epidemiology and infection 121: 121–128.

Permissions

All chapters in this book were first published in PLOS ONE, by The Public Library of Science; hereby published with permission under the Creative Commons Attribution License or equivalent. Every chapter published in this book has been scrutinized by our experts. Their significance has been extensively debated. The topics covered herein carry significant findings which will fuel the growth of the discipline. They may even be implemented as practical applications or may be referred to as a beginning point for another development.

The contributors of this book come from diverse backgrounds, making this book a truly international effort. This book will bring forth new frontiers with its revolutionizing research information and detailed analysis of the nascent developments around the world.

We would like to thank all the contributing authors for lending their expertise to make the book truly unique. They have played a crucial role in the development of this book. Without their invaluable contributions this book wouldn't have been possible. They have made vital efforts to compile up to date information on the varied aspects of this subject to make this book a valuable addition to the collection of many professionals and students.

This book was conceptualized with the vision of imparting up-to-date information and advanced data in this field. To ensure the same, a matchless editorial board was set up. Every individual on the board went through rigorous rounds of assessment to prove their worth. After which they invested a large part of their time researching and compiling the most relevant data for our readers.

The editorial board has been involved in producing this book since its inception. They have spent rigorous hours researching and exploring the diverse topics which have resulted in the successful publishing of this book. They have passed on their knowledge of decades through this book. To expedite this challenging task, the publisher supported the team at every step. A small team of assistant editors was also appointed to further simplify the editing procedure and attain best results for the readers.

Apart from the editorial board, the designing team has also invested a significant amount of their time in understanding the subject and creating the most relevant covers. They scrutinized every image to scout for the most suitable representation of the subject and create an appropriate cover for the book.

The publishing team has been an ardent support to the editorial, designing and production team. Their endless efforts to recruit the best for this project, has resulted in the accomplishment of this book. They are a veteran in the field of academics and their pool of knowledge is as vast as their experience in printing. Their expertise and guidance has proved useful at every step. Their uncompromising quality standards have made this book an exceptional effort. Their encouragement from time to time has been an inspiration for everyone.

The publisher and the editorial board hope that this book will prove to be a valuable piece of knowledge for researchers, students, practitioners and scholars across the globe.

List of Contributors

Penelope Koraka, Albert D. M. E. Osterhaus and Byron E. E. Martina
Department of Virology, Erasmus Medical Center, Rotterdam, The Netherlands

Eric C. M. van Gorp
Department of Virology, Erasmus Medical Center, Rotterdam, The Netherlands
Department of Internal Medicine, Slotervaart Hospital, Amsterdam, The Netherlands

Yow-Pin Lim and Michael D. Shin
ProThera Biologics, Inc., East Providence, Rhode Island, United States of America

Tatty E. Setiati and Augustinus Soemantri
Pediatric Department, Dr. Kariadi Hospital, Semarang, Indonesia

Albert T. A. Mairuhu
Department of Internal Medicine, Slotervaart Hospital, Amsterdam, The Netherlands
Division of Thrombosis and Haemostasis, Beth Israel Deaconess Medical Center, Boston, Massachusetts, United States of America

Romina A. Cutrullis, Guillermo F. Moscatelli, Samanta Moroni, Jaime M. Altcheh, Ricardo S. Corral, Héctor L. Freilij and Patricia B. Petray
Servicio de Parasitologíay Enfermedad de Chagas, Hospital de Niños Ricardo Gutiérrez, Buenos Aires, Argentina

Bibiana J. Volta and Rita L. Cardoni
Instituto Nacional de Parasitología Dr. M. Fatala Chabén, Administración Nacional de Laboratorios e Institutos de Salud Dr. C.G. Malbrán, Buenos Aires, Argentina

Stéphanie Boisson-Dupuis
St. Giles Laboratory of Human Genetics of Infectious Diseases, Rockefeller Branch, The Rockefeller University, New York, New York, United States of America
Laboratory of Human Genetics of Infectious Diseases, U980, Institut National de la Santé et de la Recherche Médicale (INSERM), Paris, France
Necker Medical School, University Paris Descartes, Paris, France

Jamila El Baghdadi
Genetics Unit, Military Hospital Mohamed V, Hay Riad Rabat, Morocco

Gonul Tanir
Dr. Sami Ulus Children's Health and Diseases Training and Research Center, Ankara, Turkey

Davood Mansouri
Division of Infectious Diseases and Clinical Immunology, National Research Institute of Tuberculosis and Lung Diseases, Shahid Beheshti University of Medical Sciences, Teheran, Iran

Rüdiger von Kries
Institut für Soziale Pädiatrie und Jugendmedizin, Ludwig-Maximilians-Universität, München, Germany

Gerhard Falkenhorst
Abteilung für Infektionsepidemiologie, Robert Koch-Institut, Berlin, Germany

Tobias Tenenbaum
Universitätskinderklinik, Universität Heidelberg, Mannheim, Germany

Hermann Girschick
Klinik für Kinder- und Jugendmedizin, Vivantes Klinikum im Friedrichshain, Berlin, Germany

Lynn Meurs and Katja Polman
Department of Biomedical Sciences, Institute of Tropical Medicine, Antwerp, Belgium

Maria Yazdanbakhsh
Department of Parasitology, Leiden University Medical Center, Leiden, The Netherlands

Lucja Labuda and Ayola Akim Adegnika
Department of Parasitology, Leiden University Medical Center, Leiden, The Netherlands
Medical Research Unit, Albert Schweitzer Hospital, Lambaréné, Gabon
Institute of Tropical Medicine, University of Tübingen, Tübingen, Germany

Ulysse Ateba Ngoa and Peter Gottfried Kremsner
Medical Research Unit, Albert Schweitzer Hospital, Lambaréné, Gabon
Institute of Tropical Medicine, University of Tübingen, Tübingen, Germany

Abena Serwaa Amoah and Daniel Adjei Boakye
Department of Parasitology, Noguchi Memorial Institute for Medical Research, Accra, Ghana

Moustapha Mbow, Souleymane Mboup and Tandakha Ndiaye Dièye
Laboratory of Immunology, Centre Hospitalier Universitaire Le Dantec, Dakar, Senegal

Adrian P. Mountford and Joseph D. Turner
Department of Biology, University of York, York, United Kingdom

Chih-Jung Chen, Tzou-Yien Lin and Yhu-Chering Huang
Divisions of Pediatric Infectious Diseases, Department of Pediatrics, Chang Gung Children's Hospital and Chang Gung Memorial Hospital, Taoyuan, Taiwan
Pediatric Research Center, Chang Gung Memorial Hospital, Taoyuan, Taiwan
College of Medicine, Chang Gung University, Taoyuan, Taiwan

Lin-Hui Su
College of Medicine, Chang Gung University, Taoyuan, Taiwan
Department of Laboratory Medicine, Chang Gung Memorial Hospital, Taoyuan, Taiwan

Elizabeth R. Sharp, Christian B. Willberg, Peter J. Kuebler and Douglas F. Nixon
Division of Experimental Medicine, Department of Medicine, University of California San Francisco, San Francisco, California, United States of America

Jacob Abadi, Glenn J. Fennelly, Joanna Dobroszycki, Andrew A. Wiznia and Michael G. Rosenberg
Jacobi Medical Center, Bronx, New York, United States of America

Laura Gosoniu, Christian Lengeler and Penelope Vounatsou
Department of Public Health and Epidemiology, Swiss Tropical and Public Health Institute, University of Basel, Switzerland

Amina Msengwa
Department of statistics, University of Dares Salaam, Dar es Salaam, Tanzania

Laurens Manning, Harin Karunajeewa and Timothy M. E. Davis
School of Medicine and Pharmacology, University of Western Australia, Fremantle Hospital, Fremantle, Western Australia, Australia

Moses Laman
School of Medicine and Pharmacology, University of Western Australia, Fremantle Hospital, Fremantle, Western Australia, Australia
Papua New Guinea Institute of Medical Research, Madang, Madang Province, Papua New Guinea

Irwin Law, Cathy Bona, Susan Aipit, David Teine, Jonathan Warrell, Anna Rosanas-Urgell, Enmoore Lin, Benson Kiniboro, Pascal Michon, Peter Siba and Ivo Mueller
Papua New Guinea Institute of Medical Research, Madang, Madang Province, Papua New Guinea

John Vince
School of Medicine and Health Sciences, University of Papua New Guinea, Boroko, Port Moresby, Papua New Guinea

Ilomo Hwaiwhanje
Department of Pediatrics, Goroka Base Hospital, Goroka, Eastern Highlands Province, Papua New Guinea

Adam L. Hersh
Pediatric Infectious Diseases, University of Utah, Salt Lake City, Utah, United States of America

Daniel J. Shapiro
Institute for Health Policy Studies, University of California San Francisco, San Francisco, California, United States of America

Jason G. Newland
Children's Mercy Hospital and Clinics, Kansas City, Missouri, United States of America

Philip M. Polgreen and Susan E. Beekmann
University of Iowa Carver College of Medicine, Iowa City, Iowa, United States of America

Samir S. Shah
Departments of Pediatrics and Biostatistics and Epidemiology and the Center for Clinical Epidemiology and Biostatistics, University of Pennsylvania School of Medicine, Philadelphia, Pennsylvania, United States of America
Division of Infectious Diseases, Center for Pediatric Clinical Effectiveness, The Children's Hospital of Philadelphia, Philadelphia, Pennsylvania, United States of America

Jia Hu and Joan Robinson
Department of Pediatrics, University of Alberta, Edmonton, Canada

Lisa Hartling and Lisa Tjosvold
Department of Pediatrics, University of Alberta, Edmonton, Canada
Alberta Research Centre for Health Evidence, University of Alberta, Edmonton, Canada

Karen Doucette
Department of Medicine, University of Alberta, Edmonton, Canada

Ana L. Egea, Alejandro J. Moyano, Ines Kevric, Claudia Sola and José L. Bocco
Centro de Investigaciones en Bioquímica Clínica e Inmunología (CIBICI-CONICET), Departamento de Bioquímica Clínica; Facultad de Ciencias Químicas, Universidad Nacional de Córdoba, Córdoba, Argentina

Hugo Paganini and Horacio Lopardo
Hospital de Pediatría "Prof. Dr.Juan P. Garrahan", Autonomous city of Buenos Aires (ACBA), Argentina

Analia Garnero and Catalina Culasso
Hospital de Niños de la Santísima Trinidad de Córdoba, Córdoba, Argentina

Ana Vindel
Laboratorio de Infecciones Nosocomiales, Instituto de Salud Carlos III, Centro Nacional de Microbiología, Majadahonda, Madrid, Spain

Brian C. Zanoni
The Ragon Institute of Massachusetts General Hospital, Massachusetts Institute of Technology and Harvard, Charlestown, Massachusetts, United States of America, Harvard Medical School, Boston, Massachusetts, United States of America
Sinikithemba Clinic and Philani Program, McCord Hospital, Durban, South Africa

Margaret E. Feeney
The Ragon Institute of Massachusetts General Hospital, Massachusetts Institute of Technology and Harvard, Charlestown, Massachusetts, United States of America, Division of Experimental Medicine, University of California San Francisco, San Francisco, California, United States of America

Thuli Phungula, Holly M. Zanoni and Holly France
Sinikithemba Clinic and Philani Program, McCord Hospital, Durban, South Africa

Lorenzo Isella, Ciro Cattuto, Vittoria Colizza and Wouter Van den Broeck
Complex Networks and Systems Group, Institute for Scientific Interchange (ISI) Foundation, Torino, Italy

Alain Barrat
Complex Networks and Systems Group, Institute for Scientific Interchange (ISI) Foundation, Torino, Italy
Centre de Physique Thé orique de Marseille, CNRS UMR 6207, Marseille, France

Mariateresa Romano, Francesco Gesualdo, Elisabetta Pandolfi and Lucilla Ravà and Alberto Eugenio Tozzi
Epidemiology Unit, Bambino Gesù Hospital, Rome, Italy

Caterina Rizzo
National Centre for Epidemiology, Surveillance and Health Promotion, Istituto Superiore di Sanità Rome, Rome, Italy

Inês Vitoriano, Kathy D. Saraiva-Pava and Mónica Roxo-Rosa
Faculdade de Engenharia, Universidade Católica Portuguesa, Rio de Mouro, Portugal

Alexandra Rocha-Gonçalves
Chymiotechnon, Departamento de Química, Universidade de Coimbra, Coimbra, Portugal

Andrea Santos and Mónica Oleastro
Departamento de Doenças Infecciosas, Instituto Nacional Saúde Dr. Ricardo Jorge, Lisboa, Portugal

Ana I. Lopes
Departamento de Pediatria, Hospital Universitário de Santa Maria/Faculdade de Medicina de Lisboa, Lisboa, Portugal

Anh Ha Lien Do, Thanh Hang thi Hoang, Quang Ha Do, Tan Le Van and Tan Thanh Tran
Oxford University Clinical Research Unit, Wellcome Trust Major Overseas Program, Ho Chi Minh City, Vietnam

H. Rogier van Doorn, Juliet E. Bryant, Bridget Wills and Jeremy Farrar
Oxford University Clinical Research Unit, Wellcome Trust Major Overseas Program, Ho Chi Minh City, Vietnam
Nuffield Department of Clinical Medicine, University of Oxford, Oxford, United Kingdom

Menno D. de Jong
Oxford University Clinical Research Unit, Wellcome Trust Major Overseas Program, Ho Chi Minh City, Vietnam
Nuffield Department of Clinical Medicine, University of Oxford, Oxford, United Kingdom
Department of Medical Microbiology, Academic Medical Center, University of Amsterdam, Amsterdam, The Netherlands

My Ngoc Nghiem, Vinh Chau van Nguyen, Minh Hien Vo, Cong Khanh Vo, Minh Dung Nguyen and Tinh Hien Tran
Hospital for Tropical Diseases, Ho Chi Minh City, Vietnam

Federica Giardina, Laura Gosoniu and Penelope Vounatsou
Department of Epidemiology and Public Health, Swiss Tropical and Public Health Institute, Basel, Switzerland
University of Basel, Basel, Switzerland

Lassana Konate and Ousmane Faye
Faculté des Sciences et Techniques, UCAD Dakar, Sénégal

Mame Birame Diouf
National Malaria Control Programme, Dakar, Sénégal

Robert Perry
Center for Global Health, Centers for Disease Control and Prevention, Atlanta, Georgia, United States of America

Oumar Gaye
Faculté de Médecine, Pharmacie et Odontologie, UCAD Dakar, Sénégal

Ingeborg Y. Bart, Yvonne Schabos and Esther de Vries
Department of Pediatrics, Jeroen Bosch Hospital's-Hertogenbosch, The Netherlands

Roeland W. N. M. van Hout
Department of Linguistics, Radboud University, Nijmegen, The Netherlands

Alexander C. A. P. Leenders
Department of Medical Microbiology, Jeroen Bosch Hospital's-Hertogenbosch, The Netherlands

Sandeep D. Patel
U. S. Indian Health Services, Belcourt, North Dakota, United States of America

Elysia Larson
American Schools of Public Health at U.S. Centers for Disease Control and Prevention, Pretoria, South Africa

Thobile Mbengashe
National Department of Health, Pretoria, South Africa

Thurma M. Golman, Jeffrey D. Klausner and Heidi O'Bra
Division of Global HIV/AIDS, U.S. Centers for Disease Control and Prevention, Pretoria, South Africa

J. W. Brown
U.S. Agency for International Development, Pretoria, South Africa

Abdullhamid S. Al-Ghamdi
College of Medicine, Taif University, Al-Taif, Saudi-Arabia

Ahmed S. Abdel-Moneim
College of Medicine, Taif University, Al-Taif, Saudi-Arabia
Department of Virology, Faculty of Veterinary Medicine, Beni-Suef University, Beni-Suef, Egypt

Mahmoud M. Kamel
College of Medicine, Taif University, Al-Taif, Saudi-Arabia
Department,of Clinical Pathology, National Cancer Institute, Cairo University, Cairo, Egypt

Mater I. R. Al-Malky
Pediatric Hospital, Al-Taif, Saudi Arabia

María G. Cárdenas-Mondragón, Ricardo Carreón-Talavera, Margarita Camorlinga-Ponce, Alejandro Gomez-Delgado, Javier Torres and Ezequiel M. Fuentes-Panana
Unidad de Investigación Médica en Enfermedades Infecciosas y Parasitarias (UIMEIP), Hospital de Pediatría, CMN Siglo-XXI, Instituto Mexicano del Seguro Social (IMSS), Mexico City, Mexico

Romain Banchereau and Alejandro Jordan-Villegas
UT Southwestern Medical Center, Dallas, Texas, United States of America

Nicole Baldwin, Hui Xu, Jose Rossello-Urgell, Phuong Nguyen, Derek Blankenship and Virginia Pascual
Baylor Institute for Immunology Research, Dallas, Texas, United States of America

Jacques Banchereau
Baylor Institute for Immunology Research, Dallas, Texas, United States of America
Hoffmann-Laroche, Nutley, New Jersey, United States of America

Damien Chaussabel
Baylor Institute for Immunology Research, Dallas, Texas, United States of America
Benaroya Research Institute, Seattle, Washington, United States of America

Monica Ardura, Asuncion Mejias and Octavio Ramilo
Nationwide Children's Hospital, Columbus, Ohio, United States of America

Elizabeth Saye and Clarence B. Creech
Vanderbilt University School of Medicine, Nashville, Tennessee, United States of America

Lin Wei, Qingyun Zhou, Shengping Hou, Lin Bai, Yunjia Liu, Jian Qi, Qin Xiang, Yan Zhou and Peizeng Yang
The First Affiliated Hospital of Chongqing Medical University, Chongqing Key Laboratory of Ophthalmology and Chongqing Eye Institute, Chongqing, P. R. China

Aize Kijlstra
University Eye Clinic Maastricht, Maastricht, The Netherlands

Jenifer Mason, Miren Iturriza-Gomara, Sarah J. O'Brien, Winifred Dove and Nigel A. Cunliffe
Institute of Infection and Global Health, University of Liverpool, Liverpool, United Kingdom

Bagrey M. Ngwira
Department of Community Health, College of Medicine, University of Malawi, Blantyre, Malawi

Martin C. J. Maiden
Department of Zoology, University of Oxford, Oxford, United Kingdom

Emmanuelle Ecochard-Dugelay
Inserm, CESP Centre for research in Epidemiology and Population Health, U1018, Reproduction and Child Development Team, Le Kremlin Bicêtre, France

Jean Bouyer
Inserm, CESP Centre for research in Epidemiology and Population Health, U1018, Reproduction and Child Development Team, Le Kremlin Bicêtre, France, Université Paris Sud 11, Kremlin Bicêtre, France

Vincent Gajdos
Inserm, CESP Centre for research in Epidemiology and Population Health, U1018, Reproduction and Child Development Team, Le Kremlin Bicêtre, France, APHP, Paediatric Department, Hopital Antoine Béclère, Clamart, France
Université Paris Sud 11, Kremlin Bicêtre, France

Muriel Beliah, Caroline Boisson and Francis Perreaux
APHP, Paediatric Department, Hopital Antoine Béclère, Clamart, France

Philippe Labrune
APHP, Paediatric Department, Hopital Antoine Béclère, Clamart, France
Université Paris Sud 11, Kremlin Bicêtre, France

Jocelyne de Laveaucoupet
APHP, Radiology Department, Hopital Antoine Béclère, Clamart, France

Ralph Epaud
APHP, Paediatric Department, Centre Hospitalier Intercommunal, Créteil, France
Université Paris Est, Créteil, Val de Marne, France

Hubert Ducou-Lepointe
APHP, Paediatric Radiology Department, Hôpital Trousseau, Paris, France
Université Paris, Paris, France

Rahul Pradhan, Umesh Shrestha, Samir C. Gautam, Stephen Thorson, Kabindra Shrestha and Neelam Adhikari
Pediatric Research Unit, Pediatric Department, Patan Academy of Health Sciences, Lalitpur, Nepal

Bharat K. Yadav
General Practice and Emergency Medicine, Patan Academy of Health Sciences, Lalitpur, Nepal

Dominic F. Kelly and Andrew J. Pollard
Oxford Vaccine Group, Department of Pediatrics, University of Oxford; and the NIHR Oxford Biomedical Research Centre, Oxford, United Kingdom

David R. Murdoch
Department of Pathology, University of Otago, Christchurch, New Zealand; and Microbiology Unit, Canterbury Health Laboratories, Christchurch, New Zealand

Gwo-Hwa Wan and Ju-Ping Huang
Department of Respiratory Therapy, College of Medicine, Chang Gung University, Tao-Yuan, Taiwan

Su-Li Yang
Department of Laboratory Medicine, Chang Gung Memorial Hospital, Tao-Yuan, Taiwan

Chung-Guei Huang and Kuo-Chien Tsao
Department of Laboratory Medicine, Chang Gung Memorial Hospital, Tao-Yuan, Taiwan
Department of Biotechnology and Laboratory Science, Research Center for Emerging Viral Infections, Chang Gung University, Tao-Yuan, Taiwan

Yhu-Chering Huang and Tzou- Yien Lin
Division of Pediatric Infectious Diseases, Chang Gung Memorial Hospital, Tao-Yuan, Taiwan
College of Medicine, Chang Gung University, Tao-Yuan, Taiwan

Robert C. Holman, Christine M. Hughes, Jason M. Mehal, Arianne M. Folkema, Inger K. Damon and Mary G. Reynolds
Division of High-Consequence Pathogens and Pathology, National Center for Emerging and Zoonotic Infectious Diseases, Centers for Disease Control and Prevention, Atlanta, Georgia, United States of America

Andrea M. McCollum
Division of High-Consequence Pathogens and Pathology, National Center for Emerging and Zoonotic Infectious Diseases, Centers for Disease Control and Prevention, Atlanta, Georgia, United States of America
Epidemic Intelligence Service, Scientific Education and Professional Development Program Office, US Centers for Disease Control and Prevention, Atlanta, Georgia, United States of America

John T. Redd and James E. Cheek
Division of Epidemiology and Disease Prevention, Office of Public Health Support, Indian Health Service, Albuquerque, New Mexico, United States of America

Elena Critselis, Maria N. Tsolia and Vassiliki Papaevangelou
Second University Department of Pediatrics, ''P. & A. Kyriakou'' Children's Hospital, National and Kapodistrian University of Athens School of Medicine, Athens, Greece

Panagiotis T. Nastos
Laboratory of Climatology and Atmospheric Environment, Department of Geology and Geoenvironment, National and Kapodistrian University of Athens, Athens, Greece

Kalliopi Theodoridou and Maria Theodoridou
First University Department of Pediatrics, ''Aghia Sophia'' Children's Hospital, National and Kapodistrian University of Athens School of Medicine, Athens, Greece

Christos Hadjichristodoulou
Department of Hygiene and Epidemiology, University of Thessaly School of Medicine, Thessaly, Greece

Lina Qurei, Zaidoun Salah and Maysa Azzeh
Virology Research Laboratory, Medical Research Center, Al-Quds University, East Jerusalem-Abu Dies, Palestine

Donald Seto
School of Systems Biology, George Mason University, Manassas, Virginia, United States of America

Index

www.ingramcontent.com/pod-product-compliance
Lightning Source LLC
LaVergne TN
LVHW060600210926
848485LV00005B/1347